READER'S DIGEST
SOUTH AFRICAN FAMILY GUIDE TO

Natural Medicine

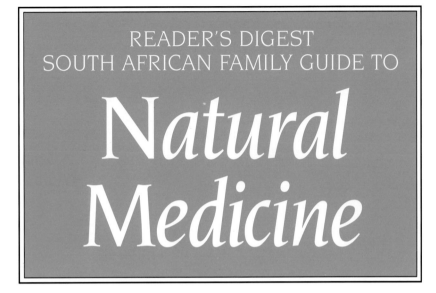

READER'S DIGEST
SOUTH AFRICAN FAMILY GUIDE TO

Natural Medicine

PUBLISHED BY
THE READER'S DIGEST ASSOCIATION SOUTH AFRICA (PTY) LIMITED
CAPE TOWN

READER'S DIGEST SOUTH AFRICAN FAMILY GUIDE TO NATURAL MEDICINE
was edited and designed by
The Reader's Digest Association
Cape Town

First South African edition © 1992

The Reader's Digest Association
South Africa (Pty) Ltd
130 Strand Street, Cape Town 8001

Project editor: Tim O'Hagan
Project co-ordinator: Carol Adams
Indexer: Ros Lavine

ISBN 0-947-008-87-X

Contributors

The publishers wish to express their thanks to the
following who, as contributors and consultants,
assisted in preparing this book:

Consultant editor
Dr Nick Lee MB BS MRCS LRCP Dip Av Med
Editor, South African Medical Journal

Principal contributor
Jeremy Lawrence

Contributors and consultants
Anthony Attenborough
Dr Daniel J Benor, MD
John Blackwood, MA
Paul T Brown, PhD, DipPsych, FBPsS
Simon Brown
Brian H Butler, BA
Dr Derek Chase, MRCGP
Jean Coleman, BSc, MScPsychol, MScPsycoth
Dr James Cox, MB, BS, MRCGP, DObstRCOG
Keir Davidson
Arnold Desser, BA, CAc (Nanjing), MRTCM
Dr David Dowson, MB, ChB
Dr James A Dyson, MRCS, LRCP
Dr Sarah Eagger, MB, BS, MRCPsych
Mark Evans, MNIMH
Simon Fielding, DO, MRO
Theophilus Gimbel, DCE, MIACT, NFSH, MLHRC
Edelweiss Gouws, MSc, Dip Hosp Dietetics
Dr Waguih R Guirguis, DPM, MRCPsych
Nicola M Hall, FBRA
Fiona Harrold
Gabriella Hatfield
Leslie Hawkins, BSc, PhD, MIBiol, CBiol
Eileen Herzberg
Sara Holden, BA, MInstGA
Ian M Hutchinson, DC
Dr Julian N Kenyon, MD, MB, ChB
Dr Kai Kermani, BSc, DRCOG, MRCGP, MBFATT
Dr George T Lewith, MA, MRCP, MRCGP
Glynn Macdonald, BA, MSTAT
Dr Isaac M Marks, MD, FRCPsych
Dr Sheena Meredith, MB, BS
Beverley Milne
Robin Monro, MA, PhD

Dr Susan Morrison, MB, BS, MRCGP
Dr Roger Neighbour, MA, FRCGP
Paul Newham, BA
John Newman
Prof Tim Noakes, MB, ChB, MD, FACSM
Dr Patrick C Pietroni, FRCGP, MRCP, DCH
Miriam Polunin
Shirley Price, DipEd, MBABTAC, MISPA, MIFAT, MIFA
Melanie Reinhart, BA, DFAstrolS
Stanley Richardson, FSSCh, FMAA, MSF, MSAAc
Ray Ridolfi, MRSS
Dr Alan J Riley, MSc, MB, BS, MRCS, DObstRCOG, MFPM
Dr Brian Roet, MB, BS, DA, FFARACS
Gaston Saint-Pierre, BA
Dr Farida Sharan, MD, MH, ND, FBRI
Franklyn Sills, MA, RPT
Dr Peter Smith, MB, ChB
Michael Turner, PhD, FIFST, FRSH, FIBiol
Roger Newman Turner, BAc, ND, DO, MRO, MRN
Dr Paul Wallace, MSc, MRCGP
Diane Waller, MA, DipPsych, ATC, DPhil
Auriel Warwick, RMTh
Clive Wood, MSc, DPhil
Dr David Zigmond, MB, ChB, MRCGP, DPM

Artists
Andrew Aloof
Richard Bonson
Baird Harris Limited
Biz Hull
Rosalyn Kennedy
Tim Pearce
Malcolm Porter
David Thorpe

Photographers
Roger Bell
Chapman/Collins & Partners
Diana Miller
Vernon Morgan
Andra Nelki

Introduction

Your guide to natural medicine

Medicine can be regarded as existing in two main streams: the scientifically based discipline of modern medicine, which has led to amazing advances in diagnosis and treatment, and alternative, *natural* or *complementary* medicine, which has developed over centuries through observation and practice.

What is complementary medicine?

Natural or complementary medicine is a broad term which encompasses a variety of practices, some of which are widely accepted, whereas others are regarded as being more *on the fringe*. These fall into four different categories: complete healing systems, diagnostic techniques, complementary therapies and self-help measures.

Complete healing systems offer theories about what causes disease, and how it can be diagnosed, investigated and treated. These systems include naturopathy, homoeopathy, chiropractic, acupuncture, herbal medicine and ayurvedic medicine. Most of these systems have well-established training schemes, and a code of ethical guidelines which governs practitioners in the same way that the South African Medical and Dental Council regulates the activities of conventional doctors.

Diagnostic techniques include hair analysis for nutritional deficiencies, pendulum diagnosis for a wide variety of diseases, iridology which examines the eyes for a clue to diagnosis, and kinesiology, which tests muscle strength to detect allergies. Although all aspects of a patient's being are important when trying to arrive at a diagnosis, most conventional doctors would have some difficulty using these techniques without being able to see a convincing connection between what is being observed and the disease process.

Complementary techniques are not concerned with the diagnosis of a patient's condition or establishing the exact cause of the disease. They simply claim that they work. Examples are massage, reflexology, aromatherapy, spiritual healing and hydrotherapy – and most of them are used in addition to orthodox treatment.

Self-help measures are those aimed at improving the general level of health without attempting to treat specific conditions. They include breathing exercises, relaxation techniques, yoga, meditation and special diets. Many conventional doctors find most of these measures acceptable.

Complementary medicine in South Africa

Complementary medicine in this country is much more widespread than orthodox medicine – particularly if the large number of traditional healers, herbalists and spiritual healers of the indigenous African populations is taken into account.

Even in the medical profession there is a growing interest in the practice of complementary medicine as evidenced by the formation recently of the South African Complementary Medicine Association (SACMA), and the fact that the Science and Education Committee of the Medical Association of South Africa (MASA) is examining the role that complementary medicine plays in health care today.

A recent issue of the MASA's continuing medical education journal for doctors was devoted entirely to complementary medicine.

Using this book

As the cost of conventional medical care rises, more and more people are taking responsibility for their own health, and are turning to complementary medicine. This book attempts to give a comprehensive overview of the field as well as the point of view of orthodox practitioners. However, a word of warning is necessary: As we have already said, complementary medicine encompasses a field which includes a whole host of approaches to healing, some of which may help and some of which may be positively harmful.

It is therefore important to state that it could be a mistake to rely on a therapist who has had no recognised courses of training or professional regulation.

Similarly it would be inadvisable to rely on complementary therapies for the treatment of life-threatening conditions such as cancer, without consulting an orthodox medical practitioner. For the above reasons, Reader's Digest cannot take responsibility for any unforeseen results attendant on consulting this book.

Taking responsibility for your own health means careful study of the available options and maintenance of your critical faculties at a high level of awareness. We hope this book will help you to do so.

Dr Nick Lee *Editor, South African Medical Journal*

Special Features

The Reader's Digest South African Family Guide to Natural Medicine includes the following special features on vital, health-related topics that affect most people at some time or other. The special features complement existing entries in the book, providing the reader with a more comprehensive, in-depth view of the topic covered.

ABSENT HEALING

Projecting healing powers over a distance

As its name suggests, absent or distant healing is performed in a patient's absence. The healers, including those who practise SPIRITUAL HEALING, use prayer, MEDITATION or VISUALISATION THERAPY to link themselves to divine or mystical healing forces which are then channelled to patients, activating their power to heal themselves. The patients may not even know that they are being healed, although most healers will send healing only when requested by a patient.

Healers usually discover this ability by accident, and see it as a gift which they must use in the service of others. Most regard themselves as channels for powers which come from beyond them, and not as being personally able to heal. Often, training or religious belief helps them to develop their gifts, and many belong to church or spiritual groups. They work alone or in groups, and regular meetings are held at which people who are in need of help are prayed for or meditated upon.

Who it can help Any mental, physical or spiritual distress can be treated. The patient need take no active part, and may still benefit, although it is thought that a relaxed patient is likely to be more receptive to healing energies liberated within him.

Because the patients do not have to participate actively in the healing process, exponents of absent healing believe it is particularly suitable for babies, young children and animals, for very ill or unconscious patients, or for the mentally disordered.

Chronically ill people whose vitality and self-healing powers have been exhausted by lengthy illness may gain special benefit.

Absent healing is also particularly suitable for those who are too ill to travel.

Finding a healer Some therapists offer healing among a variety of treatments, others work as healers only. For advice, and to find a healer in your area, write to the Southern Africa Federation of Spiritual Healers (which is affiliated to Britain's National Federation of Spiritual Healers): Cape Province – 10 Corvette Avenue, Sun Valley, Fish Hoek 7975; Natal – 18 Ebony Drive, Glen Anil, Durban 4051; Transvaal – 6 Roos Street, Monument, Krugersdorp 1739.

The Southern Africa Federation of Spiritual Healers is not registered with the South African Medical and Dental Council or similar statutory organisations. Its members do not ask a fee for their services, although voluntary donations may be accepted to cover incidental costs incurred.

Healing forms part of the ministry of most religions, and an approach can often be made through a minister or other religious worker, or through a spiritualist society. Healing meetings are also sometimes advertised in local newspapers and church notices.

Healers who publicly make claims for themselves (some healers tend to attract considerable media coverage) may not necessarily be charlatans – their claims may simply reflect an absolute faith in the powers they work with.

Consulting a healer Healers should not attempt to examine or diagnose patients, and should advise you to see a doctor if you have not already done so. Healing is usually a gradual process of helping patients to heal themselves. Instant cures cannot and should not be expected, especially where illness is the result of long-term factors such as unhealthy diet or ongoing STRESS in a family or work situation.

In such cases, healing may help, but it is not offered as a replacement for more direct, orthodox therapies.

Often, healing is sought as a last resort, when the body's defences are already depleted and, although it has proved successful in some cases regarded by orthodox medicine as incurable, patients should not expect healing to succeed immediately where all else has failed. Progress is often slow – sometimes even preceded by worsening symptoms as the body seeks to regain its ability to fight the illness.

Spiritual healers never accept that a case may be incurable, and this alone encourages many seriously ill patients. Healing of any type is likely to have positive psychological effects, and even where a condition cannot be reversed or improved, a patient may be relieved of distress and brought to accept his or her condition.

Many people even experience a sense of inner harmony through this kind of therapy, and this tends to have a positive effect on others around them.

The only danger arises when conventional treatment, which may help, is neglected in favour of absent healing, which may not.

An orthodox view

In spite of numerous claims to the contrary, most medical authorities remain sceptical of the benefits of absent healing.

Many good results are ascribed by doctors to temporary psychological effects; the patient is helped by what he or she believes will help – at least in the short term. In recent years, some orthodox doctors have co-operated with healers.

Whatever their attitude, however, practitioners of all kinds generally agree that absent healing can do no harm at all, provided

it does not take the place of other treatment and provided the patient's hopes are not raised unrealistically.

ACID STOMACH

A variety of symptoms is covered by this emotive term. Usually, it refers to regurgitation of acid or partly digested food from the stomach into the oesophagus (food pipe) or mouth. Other symptoms may include heartburn (a burning sensation behind the breastbone), belching and a feeling that food is becoming stuck after swallowing.

The causes include overeating or drinking, being overweight, wearing constrictive clothes, or bending, lying down or physical exertion too soon after eating. Regular attacks accompanied by a feeling of burning or constriction in the throat may be caused by a loose muscle at the base of the oesophagus, allowing acid to flow back from the stomach. Occasionally the symptoms indicate a more serious disorder, such as a stomach ULCER or hiatus hernia – if they persist, consult a doctor.

What the therapists recommend

NATUROPATHY

Self help Eat small, regular meals based on wholefoods such as fruit, vegetables, wholegrain cereals and moderate amounts of proteins such as lean meat, fish, eggs, cheese and nuts. Cut out fatty foods and those that contain possible irritants such as chemical FOOD ADDITIVES or hot spices. Avoid drinking immediately before meals, and drink sparingly during meals.

Hot compresses (see p. 193) over the stomach are said to improve the blood supply in the area and relax the muscles.

Consultation You will be given individual advice about improving your diet, and reducing the level of STRESS in your life – factors considered most important for regulating the digestive system.

HERBAL MEDICINE

Consultation In addition to advice about diet and way of living, practitioners may recommend comfrey root, marsh-mallow root and slippery elm to reduce irritation and inflammation of digestive organs. Despite rumours, comfrey has not been shown to cause liver damage, but it is advisable to use the remedy only on a short-term basis – for up to three weeks. For persistent problems see a qualified medical herbalist.

Comfrey and marsh-mallow would be taken as infusions or decoctions (p. 184); slippery elm can be taken either in tablet

Wilde als (a species of wormwood) is used to treat acid stomach and a number of other conditions – from bronchitis to gout. It is one of the oldest medicinal shrubs.

form or a teaspoon of powder dissolved in a cup of hot water.

To tone and heal the whole digestive system, the bitter herbs wormwood ('wilde als'), rue, gentian and golden seal may be suggested, but should not be taken for long periods or in large doses because of potentially poisonous effects.

This is particularly true during pregnancy, because these herbs tend to stimulate the uterine muscles or can cause vomiting.

Yarrow and sweet flag are said to have the same action, but with a milder effect. Yarrow can be taken as an infusion. Camomile tea and infusions of fennel may also help.

Do's and don'ts for acid stomach

Do take time to relax, allowing about 20 minutes of leisure before and after eating. Eat slowly, chew well, and make meals enjoyable occasions.

Don't smoke – it will irritate the stomach lining.

Do make sure you get enough sleep.

Don't take aspirin or other pain-killers in large quantities – they can cause gastrointestinal bleeding.

Do make sure that your clothing is always loose and comfortable – especially over the stomach – and avoid tight belts and girdles.

Do reduce the amount of coffee and tea you drink, and avoid them entirely during an attack.

Other alternative treatments

Acupuncture This is said to relieve many digestive disorders, including excess acidity and inflammation of the stomach lining.

Homoeopathy *Nux vomica* is used to relieve discomfort due to overeating or to relieve a HANGOVER. Take one tablet every hour for three hours, then one every two hours, if required.

Use the 6 or 30 centesimal potency.

An orthodox view

Doctors agree that diet is important in treating acid stomach. They recommend a bland diet of small, regular meals which include foods such as rice, milk, fish, chicken and cereals to reduce acidity. Fried and fatty foods are excluded, as are heavy meals, large amounts of alcohol, coffee, tea, and hot, spicy or very acid foods.

If the symptoms persist, the doctor may also prescribe an antacid preparation – an alkaline substance such as aluminium hydroxide or magnesium trisilicate that neutralises acidity in the stomach. Alternatively, if one of the more serious disorders mentioned earlier is diagnosed, some other form of treatment may be advised.

ACNE

The facial spots and scars of acne usually tend to appear at puberty, the time when young people are most concerned about their looks (see PUBERTY AND ADOLESCENCE). The chest, shoulders and back can also be affected. The cause of acne is not fully understood, but heredity, hormonal fluctuations, hygiene and diet may all play a part.

An oily substance called sebum, produced by the skin's sebaceous glands, acts as a natural lubricant for the skin, but when too much is produced the glands can become blocked and inflamed, causing blackheads and pimples. Sometimes the blocked glands become infected – pus and sebum build up under the skin, forming larger pimples or cysts which can leave scars and pitting.

The fluctuating hormone levels of puberty are known to have an important role in the onset of acne. In particular, the male hormones, produced in large quantities during puberty, appear to affect the total amount of sebum released.

The severity of an attack can vary from week to week as hormone levels change, and women often find that the condition gets worse just before a period. The problem usually clears up as the sufferer reaches the early twenties.

What the therapists recommend
NATUROPATHY

Self help Keep the skin scrupulously clean, washing frequently – up to five times daily – but taking care that it does not become too dry. Use gentle cleansers made from natural ingredients or herbs, rather than harsher chemical preparations.

If you prefer soap, make sure that you use a mild, unscented brand. To remove as much oil as possible, first wash the skin, then apply a hot facecloth for two minutes, splash with cold water and wipe gently with a ball of cotton wool soaked in witch hazel. Repeat as necessary and always use a clean facecloth, towel and cotton wool to prevent the spread of infection.

Women should avoid heavy make-up, but light, non-greasy products will do no harm and may boost self-confidence. Remove make-up thoroughly every evening with a natural cleanser followed by toner and moisturiser if the skin feels taut or dry. Most health food shops stock natural cosmetics and skincare products, and some can easily be made at home. For example, you can make a cheap, effective toner by mixing equal parts of rose water and witch hazel.

Other natural skin remedies include GARLIC, which acts as a natural antibiotic when rubbed onto spots. An ointment made with propolis (a resin substance extracted from flowers by bees) can be dabbed on several times a day. For the chest, shoulders and back, vigorous body rubbing with a loofah or dry towel stimulates circulation to the skin, and regular outdoor exercise is also an important factor.

Consultation Practitioners regard acne as a sign of some underlying disorder or imbalance in the body. Skin eruptions are seen as the body's attempt to rid itself of poisons from a system too overburdened with impurities for normal methods of elimination. Treatment is long term and the body must first be helped to cleanse itself and eliminate waste products.

Other herbal remedies

To make an antiseptic lotion for spots that have been picked or squeezed Squeezing pimples is never advisable, but if you are tempted to do so, you can prevent infection spreading by gently bathing the whole face with a lotion made from a teaspoon of calendula tincture (which is usually available from many chemists and health shops) in a glass of cold water.

To bring pustules to a head Make a paste from a teaspoon of powdered marsh-mallow root or slippery elm mixed with hot water. Spread it onto the acne and leave for about 20 minutes. Wash the mixture off with comfrey infusion.

To heal damaged skin An infusion of comfrey leaves also makes an excellent facial wash, and comfrey in any form will promote healing and the growth of new tissue.

To improve circulation and disinfect the area Paint lemon juice onto spots.

To cleanse the skin from within Take the following herbs as infusions, tablets or medicinal extracts: blue flag, echinacea, nettle, dandelion root.

Correct skin care is important. The therapist will advise on natural methods and may also recommend purifying treatments.

The therapist may recommend a diet to fortify the body against infection and as an aid in regulating hormone levels. The diet will be rich in natural wholefoods – wholegrain cereals, fresh fruit salads and vegetables – and free from oily, refined products such as cheese, fatty meat, cakes, white bread and sweets (see EATING FOR HEALTH).

Vegetables are eaten raw or lightly cooked, as high temperatures destroy many vitamins and enzymes (see RAW FOOD DIET). Food is grilled, steamed or baked, rather than roasted or fried. Chocolate should be avoided, and skimmed milk replaces full-cream milk. Supplements of vitamin A and zinc may also be advised.

HERBAL MEDICINE
Self help For an anti-inflammatory and antibacterial skin wash there is a choice of three homemade preparations:

Calendula Mix a teaspoon of tincture of calendula (available from health food shops

or made following instructions on p. 184) in a glass of water.

Camomile Simmer a teaspoon of dried flowers or a camomile tea bag for ten minutes in a cup of water, covered.

Yarrow, elder or lavender Pour a cup of boiling water over a handful of fresh or dried flowers, cover, and steep for ten minutes.

To use the preparations, strain as necessary and then bathe the affected areas with the solution, dabbing on gently with cotton wool. Alternatively, use the solution to make a compress (see p. 184).

Some therapists recommend a facial steam bath to reduce inflammation and infection by pouring a jug of boiling water into a bowl containing a handful of camomile flowers. Use lime flowers or sage leaves instead to detoxify; or lavender, to promote healing. Place the bowl on a table, sit with your face a comfortable distance above it, and cover your head and the bowl with a towel. Steam your face for as long as is comfortable, but never longer than 15 minutes. Take great care not to knock over the bowl or to scald the skin, and always stop if in doubt. Afterwards apply a toner to close the skin pores.

Consultation To remove toxins from the system a herbalist may make up an individual prescription for each patient, using herbs such as burdock leaves, artichoke leaves, greater celandine leaves, sage flowers and marsh-mallow roots and flowers.

For women, certain herbs such as chasteberry and false unicorn root may be recommended with the aim of regulating the hormonal system. However, these must be used only under the therapist's direct supervision.

Other alternative treatments

Biochemic Tissue Salts For outbreaks of acne during adolescence, *Calcarea sulph.* is prescribed. Take four tablets an hour for the first two days, then four times a day until the skin improves – usually within about two to four weeks.

Aromatherapy Bathe the affected skin with distilled water containing six drops of essential oil (two each of lavender, juniper and cajuput). Stir well, as essential oils do not dissolve easily in water. Afterwards apply a vegetable oil or non-greasy lotion containing any or all of these oils – use a total of 20 drops in 60 ml of water. Tea-tree oil applied directly onto spots with a cotton bud is claimed to stop infection.

Bach Remedies These may help to cope with the emotional problems that often accompany acne. Try Wild oat and Walnut for adolescent emotional problems, Crab apple for shame and embarrassment, Gorse for feelings of hopelessness.

Homoeopathy Practitioners recommend *Kali bichromicum* for chronic acne, and *Sulphur* for inflamed or infected pustules that are worse when washed. *Psorinum* is advised for severe and itchy infections.

An orthodox view

Some doctors will, like alternative practitioners, advise a change of diet – again avoiding fatty or oily foods. Others believe that diet has little or nothing to do with acne. This view is supported by scientific research which has so far found no evidence that acne can be aggravated by eating certain foods.

Chemists sell many anti-acne preparations. However, a doctor can quite easily recommend an appropriate product for your skin, and may prescribe antibiotic creams such as Actinax or NeoMedrone. Serious cases of acne will be treated with a six-month course of antibiotic pills or capsules in low doses.

Do not use a sun lamp and make sure you do not sunbathe too much without a doctor's advice, as ultraviolet light can damage the skin (see SUNBURN).

ACUPRESSURE
An ancient massage skill

We all use this instinctive form of healing when we press our hands against our foreheads to soothe a headache. Massage is an inborn skill, but traditional oriental medicine, practised over 3 000 years ago in China and Japan, developed this skill into a healing art with a system of special massage points. Acupressure is a mixture of MASSAGE and ACUPUNCTURE, and is thought to be the forerunner of acupuncture. It is still widely used at home by Japanese families.

Instead of inserting needles into the skin, practitioners use firm thumb or fingertip massage on pain-relieving 'pressure points'. These points are the same as those that are used in acupuncture.

Acupressure is said to improve the body's own healing powers, increase vitality and prevent illness. Like acupuncture, it is used to balance a flow of energy called Qi, which is believed to run through invisible channels known as meridians.

Who it can help Acupressure can only relieve symptoms and must be used in conjunction with other treatments. Practitioners claim success in relieving many ailments, including ALLERGY, ARTHRITIS, ASTHMA, BACK PAIN, CIRCULATION PROBLEMS, DEPRESSION, DIGESTIVE PROBLEMS, INSOMNIA, MIGRAINE and TENSION.

But always remember that some painful symptoms are warnings of serious illness, so always consult your doctor before using acupressure for any but everyday ailments you would normally treat at home.

Finding a therapist South Africa has no association of acupressure therapists, but this technique of healing massage is related to both acupuncture and shiatsu, and therapists in either of these two methods may be able to help you. Consult the 'Finding a therapist' sections under ACUPUNCTURE and SHIATSU in this book.

Consulting a therapist There are several forms of acupressure, including Shin Tao, Jin Shin Do and Shiatsu. The difference lies mainly in the combination of pressure points and the amount of pressure used. However, all practitioners start by compiling your case history. You are then questioned about your diet and way of life, and your pulses are taken, as in acupuncture.

For treatment, you are asked to sit or lie on a firm table or a mattress on the floor. No equipment or oils are used and you do not undress, but you are advised to wear loose-fitting clothes that will not obstruct the therapist's touch.

Each therapist has his own way of working and applies pressure in a variety of ways to tone or sedate the energy channels. He may use his thumbs, fingers, palms, knees, elbows – even feet.

The points may be tender and you may feel some discomfort such as a deep chill or pain. However, this massage is believed to produce swift results, so that the tenderness soon decreases.

Sessions last between 30 and 60 minutes, and the number of sessions varies according to your condition and response to therapy. Weekly treatments are advised for specific disorders, or you can go whenever you feel in need of a 'tune-up'.

Pain relief for sudden conditions may be rapid, but long-standing problems may take longer. Dietary changes, EXERCISE and a self-healing technique such as VISUALISATION THERAPY may also be prescribed.

Some acupressure treatments are not recommended for women during PREGNANCY. Your therapist will advise you.

Self help Acupressure is safe to use at home for common ailments such as HEAD-ACHES and nausea (see right) but may occasionally induce minor aggravations – such as a short-term worsening of symptoms – if pressure points are overstimulated. Although you can use acupressure on yourself, it is a better proposition to get a friend or relative to massage you. A course with a qualified practitioner is the best way to learn. If common ailments persist, you should see your doctor.

How to do acupressure massage Make sure that anyone you are treating is calm and relaxed, that the room is comfortably warm and that his clothing is not too tight. Ask him to sit or lie down on a firm mattress or soft rug, preferably on the floor. If seated, the spine should be straight.

Find the pressure points you need to work on by pressing deeply over the body and noting those areas which are tender – if an organ is not functioning properly, its corresponding point on the body may be tender to the touch.

Start deep, firm massage on the tender points, using your thumbs or fingertips. Exert

Treating some common ailments

These recommendations are only general guidelines, as there are several points that can be used for each condition.

For headache, toothache, menstrual cramps and constipation: Squeeze the point 'Large Intestine 4' firmly for about five minutes between thumb and forefinger of either hand. This point is located in the web of flesh between the thumb and index finger. The pressure should be towards the index finger. Most facial aches and pains may be relieved at this pressure point.

a downward pressure of about 4,5 kg, and appreciably less for small children and babies. (You can practise this by pushing down on your bathroom scales.) Massage must be in the direction of the meridian's energy flow. Your pressure should cause some discomfort, but not pain. The tenderness will soon pass. Be sure to avoid any painful pressure on the face, abdomen or directly over joints.

Use rapid movements, about 50-100 times a minute and do not use oils or creams – they are not necessary. Take your time: adults need about 5-15 minutes of massage at each pressure point; small children about five minutes;

For nausea from any cause, such as travel sickness, pregnancy or anxiety: Press with your thumb on the point 'Pericardium 6' as shown, about 50 mm from the wrist, for five to ten minutes.

To stimulate energy and to soothe babies' colic and babies' and adults' digestive problems: The point 'Stomach 36' is used for these disorders and to tone-up the system generally. This point is about 75 mm below the knee joint on the outer side of the leg. It is often slightly

tender to touch, so it is usually easy to find. The point is considered to be one of the great Qi or energy 'balancers' in traditional Chinese medicine and is used often in both acupuncture and acupuncture. Press gently with your thumb for five to ten minutes.

and babies half a minute using only gentle pressure.

With self-help acupressure you can repeat the massage as often as necessary. Two or three treatments every hour are usually enough for sudden, painful conditions. Up to 20 treatments may be necessary for long-standing painful conditions, given two or three times a week, with a longer interval between as the condition improves.

Do not try to learn complicated routines or treat specific illnesses such as arthritis – know your limitations. For best results, visit a trained therapist first.

An orthodox view

There has been little direct research into how acupressure works, but the use of acupressure bands ('sea bands') on the wrists to combat Motion Sickness and other forms of nausea (see NAUSEA and VOMITING) has been scientifically studied. Research at the Department of Anaesthetics at Belfast University has shown clearly that acupressure or an acupressure band worn on a point called the 'Pericardium 6' (see p. 13) does relieve nausea caused by general anaesthesia, pregnancy, travel sickness and some drugs.

ACUPUNCTURE

Using needles to treat diseases and ailments

In this ancient Chinese therapy, patients are treated by inserting needles into their skin at particular points. These acupuncture points lie along invisible energy channels called 'meridians', which are believed to be linked to internal organs. The needles are said to unblock, increase or decrease a flow of energy (called Qi) through the meridians.

Traditional Chinese medicine views the body as a balance between two opposing yet complementary natural forces called 'yin' – the female force – and 'yang' – the male.

Yin force is passive and tranquil, and represents darkness, coldness, moisture and swelling. Yang force is aggressive and stimulating, and represents light, heat, dryness and contraction.

An imbalance of yin and yang is believed to cause diseases and ailments. For example, too much yang may cause sudden PAIN, inflammation, spasms, HEADACHES and high BLOOD PRESSURE; too much yin may cause dull aches and pains, chilliness, fluid retention, discharges and TIREDNESS.

In acupuncture, diagnosis and therapy are aimed at identifying any imbalance and correcting it by inserting needles at appropriate

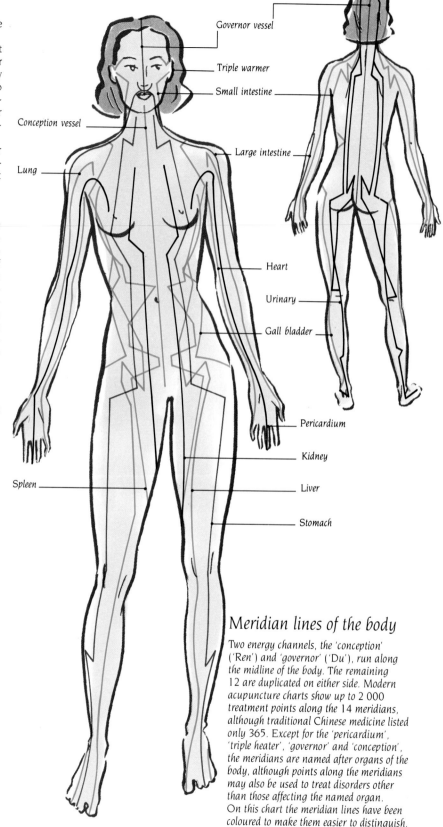

Labels: Governor vessel · Triple warmer · Small intestine · Conception vessel · Large intestine · Lung · Heart · Urinary · Gall bladder · Spleen · Pericardium · Kidney · Liver · Stomach

Meridian lines of the body

Two energy channels, the 'conception' ('Ren') and 'governor' ('Du'), run along the midline of the body. The remaining 12 are duplicated on either side. Modern acupuncture charts show up to 2 000 treatment points along the 14 meridians, although traditional Chinese medicine listed only 365. Except for the 'pericardium', 'triple heater', 'governor' and 'conception', the meridians are named after organs of the body, although points along the meridians may also be used to treat disorders other than those affecting the named organ.
On this chart the meridian lines have been coloured to make them easier to distinguish.

points. There are by tradition 365 points, but many more have been discovered over the centuries and there are up to 2 000 on modern charts (see illustration).

Most of the important points are on the 14 meridians, each named after an organ which it represents – the heart, small intestine, bladder, kidney, gall bladder, liver, lungs, colon, stomach and spleen, plus two organs not recognised in Western medicine – the pericardium, which controls circulation and is important in sexual activity, and the 'triple heater' (or 'warmer') which controls endocrine (glands) activity and acts effectively as the body's thermostat. Two extra meridians called the 'Ren' (or 'conception') and the 'Du' (or 'governor') run vertically up the midline of the body.

Various physical, emotional and environmental disorders are said by practitioners to alter the flow of Qi (also called Ch'i or Shi) making it either too fast or too slow; or it may even be blocked or diverted to the wrong organ. An acupuncturist aims to return the flow to its normal rate.

Who it can help In the West acupuncture is used mostly to treat a variety of painful conditions such as ARTHRITIS, BACK PAIN and RHEUMATISM, but it has also been found to help people suffering from ALLERGY, ANGINA, ANXIETY, ASTHMA, BRONCHITIS, COLITIS, DIGESTIVE PROBLEMS, gall-bladder problems, INSOMNIA, STRESS, tiredness and ULCERS. Success has been claimed in relieving withdrawal symptoms after giving up SMOKING and other types of ADDICTION.

Finding an acupuncturist As the law at present stands, anyone may use the title 'acupuncturist' whether or not he or she has been properly trained. Qualifications are not easy to obtain within South Africa, although a five-year course available at the Natal Technikon's Department of Homoeopathy in Durban includes acupuncture among a range of other therapies taught. Many acupuncturists in South Africa have acquired their qualifications elsewhere, including the Far East.

For information on where to find a qualified acupuncturist in your area, you should write to the South African Medical Acupuncture Society, P O Box 2229, Dennesig 7601; the South African Physiotherapists Acupuncture Society, c/o The Physio School, King Edward VIII Hospital, Private Bag, Congella 4013. Alternatively, write to the South African Homoeopathic Association, 20 Botanic Grove, Berea, Durban 4001.

Consulting an acupuncturist A traditional acupuncturist uses Chinese diagnosis and follows an ancient set of rules to select the points. He will inspect your tongue, skin texture and colouring, hair texture, posture and movement, and listen to your breathing and the sound of your voice.

He will ask about your way of life, diet, exercise, quality of sleep, phobias and reactions to stress. He will also feel the 12 pulses of traditional acupuncture, six in each wrist, each pulse representing one of the 12 main organs and functions in acupuncture. This process is called 'palpating' and is the means used by acupuncturists to diagnose disturbance in the flow of Qi and any disease of the internal organs.

Fine, stainless-steel needles are then inserted – usually a quick, painless and bloodless procedure – and rotated between his finger and thumb, to 'draw or disperse energy' from a point.

You will feel a slight numbness or tingling sensation over each point. Most lay acupuncturists insert the needles so that they just penetrate the skin, or go in about one or two centimetres. The Chinese use even deeper insertion into the muscle tissue – up to eight or nine centimetres.

The number of needles used varies from one to as many as 15, but in general the more experienced the acupuncturist, the fewer needles he uses. They may be left in for just a few minutes or up to half an hour (depending on the particular patient, reaction to previous treatment, and the condition being treated), during which time there may be a heaviness of the limbs and a pleasant, pervasive feeling of relaxation.

A good acupuncturist now uses disposable acupuncture needles from sealed, sterilised packs, or he will sterilise them in a machine called an autoclave. Boiling water is not adequate, as acupuncture needles can transmit blood-borne diseases such as hepatitis and the HIV virus responsible for AIDS.

Instead of rotating the needles with finger and thumb, some acupuncturists prefer to use an electrical stimulator or laser device to achieve the same effect.

Consultations may last up to an hour, particularly if a detailed history and 'palpation' is necessary.

Patients usually start feeling better within the first four to six visits – especially if the condition is long-standing, with clear and persistent symptoms. However, a complex problem such as asthma may need more sessions before there is a clear improvement.

Sometimes the patient may even feel worse after initial treatment – but this usually means that the acupuncturist has overstimulated the body's energies, and will use fewer needles for a shorter time in the next session. In general, acupuncture works in

The acupuncturist places needles in the neck and shoulder of a patient sent to her by an osteopath, to relieve pain and muscle tension caused by thinning discs in the neck vertebrae.

How acupuncture developed

The word 'acupuncture' is a European term meaning 'to prick with a needle'. It was coined by a Dutch physician called Willem Ten Rhyne who introduced the practice to Europe following a two-year stay in Nagasaki, Japan, in 1683.

Acupuncture has been practised in China for some 3 500 years, but the exact date of its origin is unknown. A legend says that this complex healing system developed when it was noticed that soldiers who survived arrow wounds in battle sometimes also recovered from other long-standing ailments.

The first medical textbook on acupuncture was the Nei Ching Su Wen (the 'Yellow Emperor's Classic of Internal Medicine'), which dates from about 400 BC. The first therapeutic success with acupuncture appears in records of around the same time, when a physician named Pein Chueh used it to revive a dying patient in a coma.

The practice was gradually developed and refined until the Ching dynasty (AD 1644-1911), when Western medicine became more popular. Since the Communist revolution, however, acupuncture has been revitalised and is now widely used throughout China.

Acupuncture was used extensively by British doctors in the early 19th century for

This Chinese amulet shows the yin (black) and yang (red) symbol.

the relief of pain and also for the treatment of FEVER. In 1823 the first edition of The Lancet, the famous medical journal, carried a detailed report of the successful use of acupuncture in treating RHEUMATISM.

Acupuncture points can also be stimulated by a low-frequency electrical current applied with a probe (electro-acupuncture), or with finely tuned laser beams. Electro-acupuncture may also be used to detect acupuncture points (which pass an electric current more easily than other areas of skin), and to give a greater stimulation effect to acupuncture needles.

See also ACUPRESSURE; AURICULAR THERAPY; MOXIBUSTION; REFLEXOLOGY.

Moxibustion, related to acupuncture, as shown in a 700-year-old Chinese picture.

---

stages and improvement should build up in successive sessions. However, if there is no improvement after six to eight sessions, acupuncture is unlikely to work.

Many traditional acupuncturists recommend three or four visits a year at changes of season for a general body 'tune up' to balance the pulses and maintain health.

An orthodox view

The Chinese have published volumes of research into the use of acupuncture to treat many conditions, claiming a high success rate, but their methods of conducting clinical trials do not meet Western standards, and their conclusions are interpreted with caution. However, orthodox research based on a number of experiments involving animals, and the use of drugs on humans, has now discovered that it is possible to stop a 'pain signal' reaching the brain by 'closing a gate' on the nerve along which the signal travels from the source of pain.

This stops you feeling pain, and it is thought that acupuncture may work in a similar way. But doctors point to a danger that acupuncture may mask certain symptoms –

including some associated with CANCER – which are warnings that call for orthodox treatment.

A further discovery has revealed that the body produces opiates called endorphins and enkephalins, which dull the senses and are part of its pain-relieving system. Worldwide studies have shown that acupuncture releases these opiates into the body's central nervous system, and that the amount of pain relief felt after acupuncture relates directly to the amount of opiates that are released.

This may explain the successful use of acupuncture to relieve pain during dentistry, childbirth and surgery. It is used widely in China as a replacement for chemical anaesthetics, where it is held to be 90 per cent effective for suitable patients. A small number of Western teaching hospitals and pain clinics also use acupuncture to relieve pain after operations, if they have doctors trained in the skill.

There is considerable evidence to suggest that acupuncture points are important medically. Western doctors recognise that treating areas of skin made tender by disease with injections, massage and heat can give pain re-

lief. These areas, called 'trigger points', are often some distance from the diseased organ, and recent research has shown that over 70 per cent of them are also Chinese acupuncture points.

Research also shows that acupuncture points can be detected with electronic instruments because they have a lower electrical resistance than the surrounding skin. There is, however, no evidence as yet to prove the physical existence of 'meridians'.

ADDICTION

Vicious cycle of dependence

To most people the word 'addiction' conjures up pictures of heroin addicts injecting themselves with dirty injection needles, or Mafia gangs, pushers and street fights. But hard drug addiction is only one aspect of a growing problem – and is not even the most common or the most important. For addiction has become a part of everyday life.

In South Africa, SMOKING is responsible for at least 12 000 premature deaths each year, a figure that is rising out of proportion to the population increase. Some 104 000 people are known to be confirmed alcoholics. Thousands of men and women are addicted to tranquillisers and sedatives – and a large proportion of the population needs its 'fix' of coffee several times a day.

Addicts can be people of all ages from all kinds of backgrounds. The underlying cause is often a problem or situation in life which they cannot face or escape from, social pressure to conform, or simply a wish to experiment, out of curiosity.

As the body gets accustomed to the stimulation induced by the mood-changing substance, more and more of it is needed to get the same effect.

Addiction is a dependence on a substance which alters the body chemistry and so changes the user's moods. Illegal drugs such as cannabis, cocaine, crack (a form of cocaine that is smoked), acid (LSD) and heroin all do this. However, medically prescribed tranquillisers and sleeping pills, the nicotine in cigarettes and the caffeine in coffee also have a similar effect.

This is known as acquiring a 'tolerance' for it. For example, the heavy drinker starts to need an extra scotch or two, the caffeine addict makes his coffee ever stronger and the smoker gets through more cigarettes each day. This process eventually levels out, but by then the next stage has set in – withdrawal symptoms if the addicts cannot get the substance to which they are addicted.

These symptoms may include stomach pain, ANXIETY, loss of appetite, HEADACHES, INSOMNIA , muscle cramps, NAUSEA and VOMITING, PALPITATIONS, panic attacks, shaking, sweating and tearfulness. In severe cases there will be CONVULSIONS and hallucinations – usually seeing frightening things that are not really there.

At this stage addicts have to continue taking whatever fix they are hooked on just to feel normal, and a cycle of dependence is established. Curing dependence means giving up all illegal drugs, and doctors avoiding the over-prescription of potentially addictive medical drugs (see DRUGS AND THEIR DANGERS); it means stopping smoking and reducing alcohol intake to moderate levels (see ALCOHOLISM); it means cutting down on stimulants such as tea and coffee – using decaffeinated coffee to reduce caffeine intake, for example.

What the therapists recommend

ACUPUNCTURE

Practitioners believe this to be an effective treatment for breaking addiction habits, because it deals with the problem at every level

Signs and symptoms of drug abuse

The earlier an addiction is discovered, the better chance the addict has of recovery. General symptoms are:
Behaving out of character when there is no obvious explanation.
Mood swings, anxiety, depression, fear, lethargy and tiredness.
Unusual laziness; poor performance at school or work.
Neglecting food and appearance.
Constant sniffing, dry cough and skin peeling around the lips.
Specific symptoms include
Pinpoint-size eye pupils – a sign of heroin and morphine addicts.
Unsteadiness, trembling of the limbs and confusion, sometimes resembling drunkenness, are indicators of tranquilliser dependence.
Red eyes, over-relaxed and drowsy are the signs of a cannabis user.
Disorientated or giggly: telltale behaviour of an LSD user (and terror during a 'bad trip').
Signs to look for include Unusual smells or substances around the house – tubes of glue, tablets, capsules and powder, greenish-brown 'tobacco', homemade cigarette stubs and hypodermic needles.
Uncharacteristic dishonesty – stealing, perhaps to buy drugs.
Changes in the person's circle of friends, attitudes and interests.
Needle injection marks and/or bruises on the inside of the elbow.

– investigating the underlying cause of addiction, alleviating withdrawal symptoms, breaking the habit and rekindling enthusiasm for life. Diet (see EATING for HEALTH) and EXERCISE will be recommended, and the therapist may advise professional counselling or PSYCHOTHERAPY such as group therapy. The therapist will probably treat points in the arms and legs, corresponding to the small and large intestines, heart and lungs and also points in the ear, corresponding to the brain. Recent research by conventional doctors in the USA has confirmed that acupuncture works well against alcoholism.

BACH REMEDIES

Agrimony is prescribed for those who maintain a cheerful façade and drink to conceal tension and inner pain; Larch for addiction

masking a lack of confidence; Star of Bethlehem where addiction follows a shock or sudden loss; Clematis for desire to escape reality; Wild oat for difficulty finding one's way in the world; Gorse for hopelessness; Willow for resentment, feeling victimised by life; Rescue Remedy for withdrawal symptoms. See also DEPRESSION.

HOMOEOPATHY

Consultation A homoeopath will deal with each patient's individual needs. Treatment is said to help reduce withdrawal symptoms; increase the addict's ability to succeed in breaking his habit; and help him come to terms with the underlying cause.

On a self-help basis, advice may be offered that Nux vomica is recommended for tranquilliser addicts and alcoholics when the underlying cause is TENSION, pressure or irritability. For a sudden, acute attack take a dose of 200th potency half-hourly – three or four doses should suffice. For an ongoing, chronic problem, take 3rd or 6th potency three times daily for a month.

NATUROPATHY

Consultation Whatever the addiction, a balanced diet is advised to build stamina and help the body to heal itself. Fasting may be recommended to clear poisons from the system, as well as exercise and relaxation routines such as MEDITATION. Naturopathy treatment can be combined with ACUPUNCTURE, psychotherapy and HYPNOTHERAPY.

Cravings for stimulants like tobacco have sometimes been found to be associated with low blood sugar, which could induce tiredness. The therapist will advise cutting out sugar, honey and sweet foods.

To overcome mild tranquilliser addictions a high-potency vitamin B-complex (100 mg taken twice a day with food) and vitamin C (500 iu twice a day) may be recommended; smokers are said to need extra vitamin B_1, B_6, B_{12} and C to make up for the loss of various B vitamins in the body, which are destroyed by the presence of nicotine.

An orthodox view

There are several approaches to treatment, but one thing is essential to them all – addicts have to realise that they have a problem, and be convinced that they want to change. Although many people are reluctant to talk to their doctor about these problems, most doctors are only too happy to offer help and advice.

For most forms of addiction it is best to start with self help. Read about how to tackle the problem – a doctor can advise on pamphlets and publications. Addicts should seek proper counselling and support from self-help organisations such as the South African

National Council on Alcoholism (SANCA), and Alcoholics Anonymous. Both organisations offer help at various centres throughout South Africa, and anonymity is guaranteed. AA not only assists people with a drinking problem, but also holds closed meetings for families and friends.

If the doctor feels that the addict is really motivated, he may arrange to see him regularly during a withdrawal period. And if specialist help is required (which may include going into hospital) he can usually arrange it. Alcoholics may need detoxification and psychotherapy. Group psychotherapy may also be used to help the families of alcoholics and drug addicts.

Prescribed-drug addicts will have to work with their doctor, coming off the drug gradually, perhaps aided by psychotherapy or hypnotism. Illegal drug users may be given less-harmful substitute drugs in limited amounts, and be sent to special detoxification clinics and rehabilitation centres.

ADENOIDS

The body, like an exclusive club, has a team of 'bouncers', whose job it is to keep out undesirables. One of the most effective of these is the pharyngeal tonsil, a small pad of tissue at the back of the nose. Just as a bouncer can get the worst of a tussle, so the tonsil can suffer in its battle against infections or ALLERGY. It can become enlarged or inflamed – rather like the palatine tonsils in an attack of TONSILLITIS. When an infection persists, or the pharyngeal tonsil has to deal with repeated infections, it can become chronically enlarged, causing breathing problems. This is commonly called 'adenoids'.

Babies are born with a small pharyngeal tonsil, which grows from the age of three until about five years later, after which it shrinks. Most cases of adenoids are in children aged between five and seven. They seldom occur after puberty.

The child breathes through the mouth and snores as the flow of air from the nose to the throat is blocked by swollen tissue. Sometimes he will also have a blocked nose or nasal speech, or the Eustachian tube connecting the middle ear to the throat may become blocked, causing deafness. Usually the pharyngeal tonsil returns to normal size, but see a doctor if the symptoms last more than a month, or there is earache or deafness.

What the therapists recommend
NATUROPATHY
Self help If a child has frequent infections and adenoid problems, his general health

should be improved. Strengthen general resistance to infection by introducing a wholefood diet (see EATING FOR HEALTH) rich in vitamin C and including foods such as citrus fruit, berries, leafy green vegetables, potatoes, sweet potatoes, tomatoes, onions, garlic and leeks.

Consultation The naturopath will examine the child thoroughly before beginning treatment. He will then give advice about improving the child's health in a variety of ways, including diet, relaxation and EXERCISE.

Food supplements such as VITAMINS and MINERALS may be suggested, depending on the child's individual needs. Dairy products (milk, butter and cheese) may also be cut from the diet for a short time, and replaced with soya milk and other calcium-rich foods.

HERBAL MEDICINE
Self help Herbal infusions (see p. 184) made from red sage, horehound, marsh-mallow and fenugreek may all help to relieve discomfort. A useful mixture can also be made from horehound, mullein, eucalyptus, coltsfoot leaves and wild-cherry bark. Use a teaspoon of each to a cup of boiling water.

Extracts of the following herbs are used to counteract infections: echinacea as tablets or drops, myrrh and wild indigo. Garlic – the fresh herb or in capsule form – can also be effective against infections.

A herb said to be useful for any inflammation connected with the lymphatic system is cleavers (also known as goosegrass or clivers). Make an infusion by pouring a cup of boiling water onto 2-3 teaspoons of the dried herb and leave it to infuse for 10-15 minutes. Make and drink the infusion three times a day, or take 2-4 ml of the tincture (see p. 184) three times a day.

Other alternative treatments
Ionisation An ioniser placed in a bedroom at night can help if there is nasal congestion.
Hydrotherapy Adding mustard to a hot bath may be useful in all cases of infection.

An orthodox view
Doctors feel that vitamin and mineral food supplements may act simply as a PLACEBO, there being no good evidence to suggest that such preparations offer any specific help against adenoids.

Most cases of adenoids will be left untreated. When the child's body overcomes the infection, the swollen tissue shrinks and the symptoms disappear.

Severe infections are treated with antibiotics. Very occasionally surgery may be decided on to remove the pharyngeal tonsil, sometimes together with the palatine tonsils. However, this is now done far less frequently than it was 30 years ago.

AEROBICS

Any exercise that increases the body's need for oxygen is a form of aerobics. This includes activities such as walking, as well as sports such as rowing, JOGGING, swimming, and the popular 'aerobics' fitness exercises.

Aerobic exercise is a vital part of body fitness, since it strengthens the heart and lungs and builds up stamina, or the ability to keep going without running out of breath. Everybody needs regular aerobic exercise, but it is vitally important to start slowly and follow a sensible plan (see EXERCISE).

AGORAPHOBIA
When going out is a nightmare

People with an irrational fear of open spaces are suffering from agoraphobia. The term also applies to the state of acute ANXIETY suffered by those who dread finding themselves in public places of any kind. Faced with such situations, they become agitated, break into a sweat and their pulse rate soars. Their fear is very real to them, even though they admit it is unreasonable. Often, agoraphobics will go to any length to avoid public places, making it impossible for them and their families to lead normal lives.

What causes agoraphobia is not really understood, but the condition is thought to be strongly connected with other psychological states of anxiety.

Sometimes it develops in people who suffer from panic attacks, as a response to a general fear of panicking in public. Or it can be an unconscious mental device used to evade responsibilities in the outside world.

What the therapists recommend
NATUROPATHY
Self help A wholefood diet (see EATING FOR HEALTH), with an emphasis on raw foods and juices, is said to be beneficial. For example, a mixture of lettuce juice and carrot juice – 150 ml of each – might be taken, twice during the day and once at bedtime. This should have a gentle, calming effect on the nervous system. Dietary supplements may also include a high-potency vitamin B stress complex (vitamins B_1, B_6 and pantothenic acid are held to be particularly important). In addition, you can take vitamins C, E, and zinc, calcium and magnesium in chelated form – in which the minerals are easier for the body to absorb.

These supplements are all thought to help regulate the nervous system's functioning

and, in particular, its ability to cope with STRESS. The amino acid tryptophan is also said to have calming and relaxing effects.
Consultation The practitioner will pay attention to the patient's way of life as well as his symptoms. The practitioner will ask about diet, how any stressful experiences are dealt with, and how much time is devoted to EXERCISE and relaxation.

On the basis of this information, the patient is then told which aspects of his life may be causing or building anxiety, and ways of changing them will be suggested.

The patient will also be shown RELAXATION AND BREATHING exercises to help at times of stress, and will be told how to relax generally. The practitioner will probably work in conjunction with other therapists (see HYPNOTHERAPY, REFLEXOLOGY).

HERBAL MEDICINE
Self help To allay fear or anxiety, try a tea made from three or four sprigs of lemon balm – fresh leaves taste best – infused in a cup of boiling water. This is said to be relaxing and can be drunk as often as the sufferer feels it necessary.

AROMATHERAPY
Self help Several oils are recommended, including marjoram, basil and Roman camomile. Put a few drops of any of these, or mix a drop of two of them, or all three, on a ball of cotton wool or paper tissue and put it into your blouse or shirt, or sprinkle a few drops on your clothing. Use only pure essential oils obtainable at health shops, and not those which are in a vegetable carrier oil.

Other alternative treatments

Homoeopathy Usually, most remedies are chosen to suit individual patients, but some general ones which are believed to help agoraphobics are: *Aconitum* for sudden panic attacks, fears and confusion; *Arsenicum album* for chronic anxiety with occasional panic attacks, especially in overtidy or obsessive types of people.
Bach Remedies Try Mimulus if the fear is well-defined; Aspen if there is apprehension or a secret dread, and Rock rose if it escalates into panic. If there is a fear of losing control or of doing something dreadful, try Cherry plum. Larch should ease the loss of confidence caused by fear, and Pine a tendency towards self-reproach.
Biochemic Tissue Salts *Kali phos.* is recommended for anxiety: take four tablets every two or three hours.
Acupuncture and Reflexology Both these therapies are claimed to relieve anxiety and to restore tranquillity.
Psychological Therapies Various practitioners offer many different kinds of psycho-

logical therapy. There is no register of these therapists in South Africa – so choose one with whom you are in sympathy and feel you can trust.

Some use techniques that are also part of orthodox therapies, such as psychoanalysis and BEHAVIOURAL THERAPY. More often, treatments use methods based on HUMANISTIC PSYCHOLOGY or transpersonal psychology that are not generally accepted by conventional psychology.

For more about these approaches, see ROGERIAN THERAPY, ENCOUNTER GROUPS, GESTALT THERAPY, PSYCHODRAMA, TRANSACTIONAL ANALYSIS, CO-COUNSELLING, BIOENERGETICS, POLARITY THERAPY, METAMORPHIC TECHNIQUE, REBIRTHING, PSYCHOSYNTHESIS.

An orthodox view

Some doctors use methods similar to those of alternative therapists – such as listening to a patient's problems and discussing them sympathetically.

But when necessary, a GP will also prescribe tranquillisers such as Valium (diazepam), Librium (chlordiazepoxide), Ativan (lorazepam) or Inderal (propranolol) to help the patient cope with anxiety. If these do not work, the patient may then be referred to a qualified psychiatrist or psychotherapist (see PSYCHOTHERAPY).

Psychiatrists are medically qualified physicians who specialise in the wide range of psychological disorders that exist. They treat these disorders with drugs. Psychotherapists, however, treat disorders through behavioural therapy or psychoanalysis.

For agoraphobia, behavioural therapy is often successful. Psychiatry, however, has a poor track record for treatment of agoraphobia and, as the drugs and other therapies are often drastic or involve side effects such as sleepiness or memory loss, many general practitioners avoid it.

AIDS

The human body has no defence against Acquired Immune Deficiency Syndrome (AIDS) because the complex, everchanging virus that causes this widespread disease attacks the very cells that should be helping the body to fight off infection.

This Human Immunodeficiency Virus (HIV) is usually – though not always – passed on through casual sexual intercourse, or by injecting drugs with a needle which has already been used by someone who carries the virus. Before tests for infected blood were developed, a number of people caught the HIV from blood transfusions.

The catastrophic damage that the HIV can cause to the IMMUNE SYSTEM can leave the body prey to infections of the lungs, skin, nervous and digestive systems, and a variety of cancers. This is AIDS, which eventually develops in practically all people who catch the HIV. Even though HIV-infected people have no visible symptoms in the early stages, they are still carriers of the virus and can pass it on to others.

There is no known cure, and the fear of AIDS that has spread worldwide since 1981, when cases were first diagnosed in the USA, has led to serious misconceptions about the disease, with distressing social consequences for sufferers.

It cannot, as many think, be passed on simply by touching a sufferer, or by drinking from the same glass or using the same cutlery – or even by kissing, as long as there are no cuts or sores on the mouth. The virus dies in the air and is also destroyed outside the body by soap and detergent. The disease is not, as many think, confined to homosexual men – it can be spread by unprotected sexual contact with any infected person.

As a protection against sexually transmitted AIDS, the health authorities recommend using the condom, designed originally as a contraceptive. This works because the virus can be passed on through prolonged contact of body fluids – and the condom prevents contact with fluids such as the partner's semen or vaginal secretions during intercourse. For drug addicts, who can get the virus from a used syringe contaminated by the infected blood of an HIV carrier, official advice is to use a new disposable syringe for each injection.

People with haemophilia have also caught the HIV after being given transfusions of HIV-infected blood or blood products. However, blood is now screened for infection. Also at risk are babies whose mothers carry the HIV.

Symptoms of AIDS infection include weight loss, EXHAUSTION, DIARRHOEA, FEVER, coughing, breathlessness and swollen glands in the groin, armpits and neck. Some sufferers develop Kaposi's sarcoma, a rare skin cancer. Others suffer less serious complaints such as THRUSH, COLD SORES, milder SKIN DISORDERS or BOWEL DISORDERS.

Nobody knows why the few HIV carriers who do not develop AIDS remain well. However, there is a general feeling among both conventional and alternative practitioners that healthy living, a positive mental attitude and learning to cope with STRESS can help.

AIDS is prevalent worldwide. It is endemic in some places, such as parts of central and southern Africa, where those people affected are mostly heterosexuals.
Alternative treatments Because AIDS is a relatively new disease, and because those in-

fected can get a wide range of complaints, alternative therapists have been unable to lay down hard-and-fast overall methods of treatment. Generally, however, practitioners tend to concentrate on a holistic approach, trying to treat simultaneously the sufferer's body, mind, emotions and spirit.

To achieve this, collaboration between the various different specialist therapies would be advisable. These might include the following therapies: ACUPUNCTURE, AUTOGENIC TRAINING, HERBAL MEDICINE, HOMOEOPATHY, MASSAGE, NATUROPATHY, REFLEXOLOGY and SPIRITUAL HEALING.

What the therapists recommend

NATUROPATHY

Self help A preparation of natural fats known as AL721 has been patented in the United States and reportedly used with beneficial effects there and in Israel. (AL stands for 'active lipids', which are fatty substances; 7:2:1 is the ratio of the ingredients used.) The mixture is designed to protect mucous membranes and blood cells which fight viruses.

HERBAL MEDICINE

Self help For secondary infections, particularly thrush, two tablets of dried golden seal root are recommended twice a day; one to three GARLIC capsules a day are also very effective. For bowel disorders, about 20 drops of golden seal in liquid form should be taken three times a day between meals. Acidophilus is also believed to help against thrush and bowel infections: take ¼ teaspoon of Superdophilus twice a day between meals.
Consultation To ensure protection against viruses, a herbalist might recommend the powerful herb echinacea. Dosage would be 500 mg of dried root powder. Up to three garlic capsules a day might also be prescribed.

BACH REMEDIES

Self help If you or your partner is found to be HIV positive, you might benefit from learning about the Bach Remedies in some depth, to support you through the crisis. They include: Mimulus for fear of getting ill; Mimulus and Aspen for apprehensiveness and fear of death; Holly and Willow for anger, resentment and desire for revenge; Gorse for feelings of hopelessness; Sweet chestnut for extreme despair; Walnut to assist the transition in lifestyle and values; Pine for guilt and self-blame; Wild rose for apathy, resignation or collapse; Honeysuckle for regrets over the past. See also GRIEF and TERMINAL ILLNESS.

An orthodox view

The only conventional drug which has been shown to be effective on a limited scale in some cases is Retrovir (Zidovudine). But one of its side effects can be to inhibit bone-marrow production, which in turn necessitates continual blood transfusions for a few patients.

A doctor will recommend EXERCISE, which will be dependent on the victim's ability to take it. A simple, nutritious diet, with plenty of FIBRE, fresh fruit and vegetables may also be advised. If thrush is present, mushrooms, sugar and yeast should be avoided.

In addition, to improve the state of the immune system, supplements such as amino acids, vitamins and trace elements may be prescribed. The most important vitamins include A (preferably in the form of beta-carotene, 12 500 iu up to three times a day), B group, C (up to 6 g a day, depending on tolerance and side effects), and E (100 iu daily). The recommended trace elements include selenium (100-300 micrograms daily) and zinc (15-300 mg, depending on the basic salt that is taken).

ALCOHOLISM

One of the most common forms of ADDICTION is alcoholism. It develops when the drinkers' bodies become so used to absorbing large amounts of alcohol that they can no longer function normally when they do not drink. The symptoms are a continual craving for alcohol, an inability to drink moderately and, as the illness develops, a need to drink more to get the same effect.

Mostly, alcoholism develops slowly over years of steadily increasing consumption. The victim may start by drinking to be 'one of the crowd', or to give himself a lift, or to help him to forget his worries. Later his system becomes dependent on alcohol and, if he cannot get it, he suffers withdrawal symptoms such as feverishness, sleeplessness and tremors, accompanied by hallucinations – *delirium tremens* (DTs).

Alcoholism should always be treated by a doctor, since continual heavy drinking can cause serious LIVER DISORDERS, brain damage, mouth, throat and pancreatic CANCER, OBESITY, ANAEMIA, SEXUAL PROBLEMS and disorders of the stomach, nervous system and heart. There may be high BLOOD PRESSURE, and vitamin deficiencies if meals are neglected. Social and psychological problems are also common.
Self help Prevention is the best method of dealing with alcoholism. Control social drinking by counting and measuring all drinks – even at home. Set a daily limit and stick to it; and eat something while drinking, to slow down the absorption of alcohol into the blood. If you meet friends in a pub, buy your own drinks rather than taking part in rounds. Drink slowly – no more than one unit in half an hour – and make every second drink non-alcoholic. Do not drink at all if you are going to drive, and ask your doctor first if you are taking medicine.

What the therapists recommend

Naturopathy The practitioner will advise about diet, EXERCISE, avoiding drink, and coping with STRESS and other emotional problems. Naturopathic remedies are believed to be particularly effective used in conjunction with PSYCHOTHERAPY, ACUPUNCTURE and HYPNOTHERAPY.
Herbal Medicine Evening-primrose oil is said to be helpful, since it is rich in GLA (gamma-linolenic acid) which the body of an alcoholic is often unable to manufacture for itself. It is believed to help in preventing recurrent mood swings and various degrees of liver damage.

Milk thistle, which is gentle in its action, is believed to help liver cells to regenerate.

Facts about alcohol abuse

Each year in South Africa alcohol abuse costs more than R1-billion in damage to health, in accidents, crime, family breakdown and loss of production at work. Loss of production alone accounts for nearly R1-million of this total sum.

More than 25 000 motorists annually are arrested for being under the influence of alcohol, while one in four hospital admissions is directly or indirectly related to alcohol abuse. Though fewer females are heavy drinkers than men, suicide attempts by alcohol-addicted persons are more common among women than men.

Apart from the many harmful physical effects of alcoholism, there are also severe psychological effects, with widespread social repercussions.

Alcoholism is not restricted to adults, married or otherwise. The increase in alcoholism among teenagers and schoolchildren, which is inferred from the general rise in convictions for drunkenness and consumption of alcohol, is one of the most alarming social trends of the past two decades.

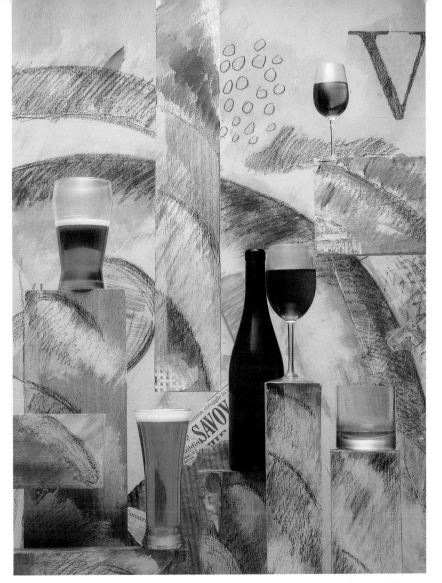

About 21 units of alcohol a week for men but only 14 for women is the recommended 'safe' intake. One unit is any one of the drinks which are illustrated above: about 166 ml of strong beer or ale, about 250 ml of ordinary beer or lager, a glass of wine, a small glass of sherry, or a single measure of spirits or aperitif. Pregnant women should preferably avoid all forms of alcohol. If they do drink, they should never drink more than four units in a week.

Herbal remedies are also said to help in overcoming any withdrawal symptoms.

Infusions of skullcap, pasque flower (use carefully in low doses), motherwort, oats and lavender are recommended.

Bach Remedies These remedies are said to help people to deal with the reasons for their drinking problems: Agrimony is used where cheerfulness hides deep anxiety; Larch where there are feelings of failure; and Crab apple where the drinkers feel ashamed of themselves. White chestnut is recommended to overcome obsessive thoughts.

Hypnotherapy Treatment under hypnosis involves trying to strengthen the willpower and the determination which is needed to stop drinking altogether, and planting subconscious 'drinking is bad' thoughts deeply in the patient's mind.

An orthodox view

A doctor may recommend AVERSION THERAPY, using a drug such as Antabuse, which makes you violently ill if you drink anything alcoholic. BEHAVIOURAL THERAPY and group therapy are also used.

Where to seek help

For help with drinking problems contact your local branch of Alcoholics Anonymous (AA), a worldwide organisation that, as its name implies, operates in strictest confidence. Look the organisation up in your telephone directory, or contact the AA's General Service Office, P O Box 23005, Joubert Park 2044 (telephone 011-3337219).

Al-Anon helps the families of problem drinkers and holds regular group meetings.

Is someone in danger?

Few people find it easy to admit to a drinking problem, but if someone you know seems in danger, these tests may show whether he should seek help:

Does the drinking follow one or more of these patterns?

Drinking to forget a personal or emotional problem.

Drinking bouts with periods of abstinence in between, which gradually diminish.

Drinking small amounts throughout the day, so that although the drinker is never really drunk, he does not stop drinking for more than short periods of time.

Only the last two patterns are definitive signs of a physical addiction to alcohol, but all are considered dangerous and show that help is needed.

Ask the drinker to answer the following questions honestly YES or NO.

Do you:

1 Look forward to drinking and plan other activities around it?

2 Drink as happily alone as when you are in company?

3 Get a special 'lift' from your drinking?

4 Use alcohol to help you relax, sleep or cope with emotional problems?

5 Set aside both time and money for your drinking?

6 Often end up drinking more than you meant to?

7 Drink more than other people can?

8 Sometimes forget things that happen when you are drinking?

Four YES answers may indicate addiction to alcohol – the drinker should see a doctor or contact one of the organisations below.

You can find the address and telephone number of an Al-Anon Information Service centre in your local telephone directory, or contact the Al-Anon General Service Office at P O Box 2077, Johannesburg 2000 (telephone 011-296696).

SANCA – the South African National Council on Alcoholism and Drug Dependence – has out-patient and in-patient facilities for alcoholics, as well as highly efficient after-care hostels. The headquarters of SANCA are at 318 Happiness House, cnr Wolmarans and Loveday streets, Johannesburg 2001 (telephone 011-7255810).

ALEXANDER TECHNIQUE

Improving your health through better posture

By using the Alexander Technique you can learn to improve your posture so that your body is able to work in a more natural, relaxed and efficient manner. It is said to be entirely safe, to promote a harmonious state of both mind and body, and to help a number of medical conditions, ranging from BACK PAIN to HEADACHES.

The method was developed by an Australian actor, Frederick Matthias Alexander (see box), who found himself losing his voice on stage and discovered that he could cure the condition by improving his posture. His discovery became the basis for a whole technique for retraining the body's movements and positions. Today there are Alexander training schools and teachers in many parts of the world. People are taught individually and teachers refer to them as 'pupils' rather than patients.

Anyone feeling that they could benefit from the technique can test themselves by observing their posture in front of a mirror and performing some of the simple procedures illustrated.

Who it can help Teachers claim that the Alexander Technique has helped people of all ages and from all walks of life, by improving their health, emotional well-being, mental alertness and resistance to STRESS. The British writer Aldous Huxley said that the technique not only improved his physical and mental health, but caused a 'general heightening of consciousness on all levels'.

The Dutch zoologist and ethologist Professor Nikolaas Tinbergen, awarded the Nobel Prize for Physiology and Medicine in 1973, said in his acceptance speech that the Alexander Technique had brought 'striking improvements in such diverse things as high blood pressure, breathing, depth of sleep, overall cheerfulness and mental alertness… and also in such a refined skill as playing a stringed musical instrument'. He had become a pupil of the technique while working at Cambridge.

As a result of improved posture, those who have benefited from the training actually become taller because they stand more upright. The training has also been used to improve the performances of athletes, dancers and public speakers. Success has been claimed in treating EXHAUSTION, DEPRESSION, ANXIETY, tension HEADACHES, high BLOOD PRESSURE, various RESPIRATORY DISORDERS, peptic ULCERS, IRRITABLE BOWEL SYNDROME,

COLITIS, RHEUMATOID ARTHRITIS, OSTEOARTHRITIS, lower back pain, SCIATICA and ASTHMA.

Finding a teacher All reputable teachers of the technique have completed a three-year course, either in South Africa or abroad, at a training school recognised by the South African Society of Teachers of the Alexander Technique (SASTAT). To find a teacher near you, contact SASTAT at 35 Thornhill Road, Rondebosch 7700 (telephone 021-6868454).

Seeing a teacher The teacher begins by watching how you use your body. Even simple activities such as walking or reading a book involve the use of many muscles, and a certain amount of muscular tension and 'spring' is needed just to react against the pull of gravity. Children move naturally, but usually acquire bad habits as they grow. In addition, stress can result in misplaced muscular effort, seen in such simple actions as holding a pen too tightly, opening a jam jar or driving a car.

Some people suffer from chronic muscular tension, which throws the head, neck and back out of alignment, causing rounded shoulders, a bowed head and arched back. If this is not corrected the spine develops a curve, and a hump may appear at the base

Even the way you stand can cause problems . . .

For much of the time people do not adopt the right posture, even when simply standing up. This may lead to aches and pains. They may stand in a slouched, round-shouldered way that looks and can feel uncomfortable (*right*). And in trying to correct themselves, they may stand too stiff and upright (*centre*) which can be equally harmful. A teacher can show you how to 'stand tall' in an aligned and balanced way (*far right*).
This is one of the many means by which the technique aims to rehabilitate – or redeploy – the body's entire muscular system. The goal is to return to the natural stance and movements of childhood which need the minimum of muscular effort.

Slouched   *Over-correct*   *Aim for*

Teachers use gentle manipulation to set pupils on the right path. A teacher may help a pupil to relax, then carefully pull her neck, stretching her body (*below*). Others employ gentle pushing techniques, of the hips, stomach and back, for example.

F M Alexander 1869-1955

An answer in the mirror

The originator of the Alexander Technique, Australian actor Frederick Matthias Alexander, found his career faltering when he began to lose his voice on stage. Medical treatment did not help, but he noted that his condition improved with rest and wondered whether something he was doing while on stage might be causing the problem. Acting out his stage role before a mirror, he saw that when the moment came for him to speak a startling physical change occurred: he shrank in height and had difficulty breathing.

He decided that the combined effort of having to remember his lines and project them for an audience was causing him to lower or duck his head, a natural reflex action to stress. He could feel that this put pressure on his vocal cords and tightened his throat, interfering to some extent with his breathing and creating tension throughout his body. Further, he found that even the thought of projecting his voice triggered off these reactions, leading him to believe that mind and body must be very closely related.

By observing and correcting himself, Alexander began to change the way he thought about his task and to overcome what he called his 'startle reflex pattern'. He recovered his stage voice and came to use his body in a more natural way.

Alexander began to teach his technique. In 1904 he came to London where he was soon much in demand by the acting profession, which quickly saw the benefits of his method. And so did many public figures, including Aldous Huxley (1894-1963), the British author.

Alexander moved to America, and the technique rapidly gained international recognition. He suffered a stroke when he was 78, but astonished his doctors by using his method to regain the entire use of his body and faculties.

of the neck. This causes back pain and strains the heart, lungs and digestive system.

The teacher shows you how to change these harmful postures and regain the habit of using muscles with minimum effort and maximum efficiency.

While you stand, sit or lie down, the teacher gently manipulates your body into a more natural position. Meanwhile, you should concentrate on the teacher's instructions about posture. You are encouraged to think of the technique as a way of working not just on your body, but on your total awareness.

Gradually, by constantly practising and thinking about good posture, you should learn to release tension and use your body correctly. The teacher uses no force and there is no wrenching or clicking of joints – just a subtle adjustment as you learn to walk, sit,

How to help yourself

Bad habits, such as a bad posture, are often so ingrained that they feel natural, and it may be difficult to rehabilitate your muscles to get rid of them. The technique is learnt from a qualified teacher, but you can help yourself: like Alexander watch yourself in a mirror, while standing, walking or sitting, for example, and aim for a relaxed stance and movements, with minimum muscular effort.

Walking
Avoid *Slouched posture, with head down, shoulders stooped and tense (above).*
Aim for *Keeping the balance of the head on top of the spine, freely poised and shoulders relaxed. Feel yourself transferring your weight onto alternate feet as you walk (right).*

Sitting

Aim for Holding your head freely poised, shoulders relaxed, knees a little apart (crossed legs twist the pelvis and spine) and feet firmly on the floor (right).

Avoid Sitting with your head down, shoulders rounded and stomach compressed, resulting in restricted breathing (above). Or trying to sit so straight that your back is unnaturally curved.

Getting in and out of a chair

Aim for Keeping your spine and neck in alignment and simply bending at the hip, knees and ankles. When getting into a chair imagine you are squatting down. Adopt the same posture when rising.

Getting into a chair
Avoid Collapsing into a chair by throwing your head back, sticking your bottom out and arching your lower back.

Rising from a chair
Avoid Jutting your head forwards, folding your body and then straightening up.

Working at a desk
Avoid Slouching over the desk, stomach tight, breathing restricted and arms tense (above).
Aim for Sitting correctly (see top) and simply bending forwards at the hip joint, keeping your bottom firmly in the seat (left). Do not grip a pen too tightly, or tense your arms when typing, writing or working at a word processor or computer. Make sure your chair is chosen or adjusted to be a comfortable height in relation to the desk top.

stand and move all over again, in a free, released way.

Lessons last about 30 or 45 minutes, and a course of 30 is usual, after which you should have learnt enough about the technique to be able to continue on your own.

An orthodox view

Recent scientific research has confirmed Alexander's views about natural posture and the connection between anxiety and physical tension. The technique does not conflict with orthodox opinion and although doctors may not always suggest this therapy, they do not oppose it.

ALLERGY

Streaming eyes, sneezing and skin rashes are just three of the many symptoms resulting from the body's allergic reactions to substances to which it is abnormally sensitive, such as pollen, house dust, various pets and certain types of food. Hundreds of thousands of people throughout the world are victims of one form or allergy or another, enduring short- or long-term irritation and discomfort as a result. See A BATTLE GOING ON IN YOUR BODY, p. 26.

ALLOPATHIC MEDICINE

Treating illness with the cure of opposites

When the 18th-century German physician Samuel Hahnemann developed a new system of medicine, he needed to distinguish it from the conventional medicine of the day. He described the conventional system as 'allopathic' – from the Greek words *allos* meaning 'different' and *pathos* meaning 'suffering' – because it treated illness by prescribing drugs that had effects opposite from the symptoms. He called his new system HOMOEO-PATHY – from the Greek words for 'the same' and 'suffering' – and it was based on the principle that 'like cures like'.

In allopathic medicine, a patient who develops a high temperature as a result of infection is treated with a drug such as aspirin to lower the temperature. A homoeopath prescribes (in minute amounts) a remedy that *causes* a high temperature in a healthy person, so using 'like to cure like'.

Allopathic medicine views symptoms of illness as something wrong with the body

that treatment will put right. Homoeopathy treats symptoms as signs of the body's *resistance* to disease, and works with them rather than against them. Allopathy is sometimes wrongly used to refer to all conventional medicine. In fact, orthodox medicine today makes use of many different techniques, some of which rely on principles closer to those of homoeopathy.

ALZHEIMER'S DISEASE

The dilemma of growing old at an early age

This early onset of 'old age' is also known as pre-senile dementia. Symptoms are similar to those of senile dementia, or senility, but strike in middle age or even earlier. The patients' intellect, personality and physical condition all deteriorate in a way similar to the normal process of ageing. They become confused and forgetful, unable to think clearly and incapable of carrying on a conversation. They tend to lose track of time – often wandering about at night – and movements become stiff and unco-ordinated. Eventually they become bedridden and incontinent.

The cause is a loss of nerve cells in the brain, which shrinks, but how this comes about is not fully understood. However, research has found that both types of dementia – and particularly Alzheimer's disease – may be linked to levels of aluminium in the body. A shortage of the B-complex vitamin choline may also be involved.

A doctor should be consulted if any of the symptoms start interfering with normal activities or cause social problems.

What the therapists recommend

ACUPUNCTURE

A practitioner may advise treatment to alleviate symptoms and to improve general health, depending on the patient's condition.

HERBAL MEDICINE

Rosemary, which is believed to stimulate circulation and have a tonic effect on the nervous system, would be advised, but results are likely to be limited to reducing symptoms and slowing the rate of decline.

An orthodox view

There is as yet no cure, conventional or alternative, but a doctor may use drugs to alleviate symptoms and treat any attendant disease, and arrange for care in a nursing home or hospital if necessary.

AMNESIA

Loss of memory is seldom caused by the fiction-writer's favourite device of a knock on the head, though such an injury can be a cause. More usually it is brought on by severe emotional SHOCK, HYSTERIA, drink, or drug ADDICTION. A number of diseases can also cause amnesia, including meningitis, syphilis, brain tumour and EPILEPSY.

There are several forms of memory loss, and sufferers are said to have 'retrograde' amnesia if they cannot recall events before losing memory, or 'anterograde' amnesia if they cannot recall events afterwards. If an emotional disturbance is the cause, sufferers may also lose their identity.

In many cases, memory returns when the underlying condition clears up. However, if the cause is concussion, memories prior to a head injury may be lost forever.

What the therapists recommend

HYPNOTHERAPY

Consultation The technique known as hypnoanalysis can be used as a drug-free alternative to narco-analysis (see below), but because it is impossible for an unwilling patient to be hypnotised, not everyone is susceptible to this treatment. In a state of hypnosis, the conscious mind is bypassed so that the hypnotist can communicate directly with the subconscious mind (which monitors mental and physical functions, and is believed to remember most – if not all – of our life experiences).

In this state it may be possible for someone with amnesia to recall repressed painful memories.

BACH REMEDIES

Self help Clematis for lapses in consciousness, disorientation, mental numbness and vagueness; Star of Bethlehem if the cause was shock or grief; and Rescue Remedy if the cause is an accident or trauma.

An orthodox view

When the cause is an underlying mental illness, a doctor may give anaesthetic drugs to make the patient feel drowsy, yet talkative, and able to speak about his or her emotional problems in a way that would not have been possible normally. This type of therapy, narco-analysis, may be given in hospital or to outpatients.

It may also be used with exploratory PSY-CHOTHERAPY, in which a counsellor (usually a psychiatrist or psychiatric social worker) explores and assesses the patient's personality and situation by asking a series of intimate questions, the aim of which is to enable him to cope with problems.

A battle going on in your body

A number of seemingly unrelated ailments such as ASTHMA, HAY FEVER and ECZEMA all have something in common – they are caused by allergies. They erupt when your body reacts to something it is abnormally sensitive to – pollen, house dust, animal fur, foods such as shellfish, eggs and chocolate, to name but a few of these 'allergens', as they are called. If you are allergic, eating, breathing in or simply touching even tiny amounts of an allergen will cause your body to defend itself by releasing substances which are known as 'antibodies' – proteins designed to neutralise allergens and other antigens (see IMMUNE SYSTEM).

The ensuing battle between antibodies and allergens triggers the release of histamine and other chemicals from surrounding cells, which causes the allergic symptoms. Doctors use drugs called 'antihistamines' to control symptoms produced by allergies.

Some medical authorities believe that one person in every six has some kind of allergy; others argue that this figure is far too high. One reason for their disagreement is the difficulty in telling the difference between a true allergy, sensitivity and intolerance.

Unlike a true allergy, a sensitivity depends on how much of the substance you come into contact with. For example, almost everyone is sensitive to chlorine, but while some people have painful eyes after just a few minutes in a chlorine-treated swimming pool, others can tolerate it for much longer without ill effects. If you are among those quickly affected, you are more sensitive to chlorine than most, but probably not allergic to it.

An intolerance is different again – an adverse reaction, which may have psychological overtones, and which is particular to you. For example, a certain cheese may

make you ill, but other cheeses may not affect you. In this case, you are probably not allergic to the offending cheese, more likely just intolerant of it.

The controversy deepens when such conditions as DEPRESSION, INSOMNIA, HYPERACTIVITY and inability to concentrate are attributed to allergy. There is no doubt that this is sometimes the case, but to suggest that it is always so (as some 'fringe' allergy clinics may do) would be misleading. Because orthodox medicine has, until now, not been very successful in detecting and treating allergies, a host of these clinics has opened to fill the gap. Many employ unqualified staff, and their techniques are dubious. However, other alternative treatments do help.

Causes of allergies

Environment Grass pollen, dust mites, animal hair, feathers, certain plants, and chemical and industrial pollutants can all provoke uncomfortable and irritating allergic responses such as runny, itchy eyes; HEADACHE; rashes and skin irritation; COUGHS and SNEEZING; WHEEZING, asthma, hay fever and eczema.

Diet Almost any food can bring on an allergic response, such as NAUSEA and VOMITING and DIARRHOEA. The commonest allergens in order of frequency are: milk and other dairy products such as cheese; eggs; nuts; fish and shellfish; wheat and flour; chocolate, and artificial colorants. Some young babies suffer WIND, CONSTIPATION and diarrhoea because they are allergic to milk protein, and they may in time go on to develop asthma and eczema.

COELIAC DISEASE is due to a sensitivity to wheat protein (gluten). MIGRAINES seem sometimes to be brought on by certain foods, particularly chocolate, cheese and red wine. And it is now widely accepted that some children are affected by FOOD ADDITIVES, especially tartrazine and benzoate, leading to hyperactivity and behaviour problems.

Other factors It is possible to be allergic to just about anything. Certain soaps, perfumes, detergents, printers' ink, insect bites, stings, nickel in jewellery, antibiotics, cosmetics – all of these can be culprits.

Coping with an allergy

Like any problem, such as a cold or flu, that affects the immune system, the severity of an allergic attack depends as much upon your general health as on the allergen. Eating sensibly, relaxing and taking care of yourself will help you to cope with, and minimise, an allergic response. In addition to maintaining your health, there are three steps to be taken when dealing with an allergy. Firstly do all you can to identify the

---

Do's and don'ts for allergy

Do try to trace a pattern in your symptoms. Sneezing when doing housework might mean that you have an allergy to house dust, while an allergic reaction to perfume could show as a rash on the neck.

Do breastfeed a new baby for the first six months if possible. It will strengthen the baby's immune system and avoid the allergens in cow's milk. This is important if the mother suffers from asthma or eczema or other allergic symptoms, as the baby may also be allergic.

Do take steps to deal with STRESS, ANXIETY and TENSION as these can increase the frequency and severity of allergic reactions.

Do try to improve your health as much as possible. Good nutrition from a balanced diet (see EATING FOR HEALTH), and adequate rest and relaxation will all be beneficial.

Don't assume without first consulting your doctor that your symptoms are caused by an allergy – they could also indicate another kind of illness. For example, a rash that may develop if you are treated with penicillin could be due to your illness rather than an allergy to the antibiotic itself.

cause, or allergen; secondly, avoid it; and thirdly, if avoidance is impossible, treat the symptoms.

Food and chemical-induced allergies can be extremely difficult to track down. Your doctor may decide to use skin testing to identify the cause, or suggest that you scrupulously follow a course of elimination dieting (completely cutting suspected foods out of your diet one at a time and observing the effect).

Warning Many fringe clinics' techniques are not always reliable, and their suggested treatments, especially full-scale elimination dieting undertaken without medical supervision, can be dangerous. Always check with your doctor first.

Self help Tracking down an allergen calls for good record-keeping.

Keep a diary Note everything you do and eat. It may establish an unsuspected, yet decisive, link between your allergic reaction and a particular food, or something like scent that you wear or cat's fur.

Elimination dieting On a small scale, elimination dieting may be helpful. If you suspect that a certain food – eggs or chocolate, for example – is at the root of your problem, you should cut it completely out of your diet for a week or two and see what happens. (In cases of eczema, you may have to eliminate a food for up to three weeks or longer to be sure of its effect.) Otherwise, you should follow your normal daily diet. Under no circumstances should you drop more than one food item from your diet at a time; it not only makes the eventual identification of the allergen more difficult, but it can also lead to an unbalanced and non-nutritious diet.

Warning While it is possible to suffer from multiple allergies, or that the particular allergen affecting you is present in a wide variety of foods, do not attempt an ambitious elimination programme without medical supervision. Without proper controls, the results of medical tests will be virtually impossible to interpret correctly.

Alternative identification methods Despite the reputation of some dubious allergy clinics, alternative practitioners can be very successful in identifying allergens. Avoid using anyone who claims to be able to make a diagnosis by post, get your doctor's advice before going on an elimination diet, and you should come to no harm.

Clinical ecology The study of how the physical environment affects health focuses mainly on food allergies and chemical sensitivities. Many practitioners are trained doctors, and combine

Avoiding an allergen

Avoidance is the most effective way to deal with an allergy, but it is not always easy. However, there are precautions:

Check food labels Choose fresh, unprocessed foods; if you suspect food additives, read labels carefully and avoid those additives as far as you can.

Choose household products with care When using detergents, particularly biological detergents, take extra care. Rinse your washing thoroughly. Wear rubber gloves when using any household cleaners or chemicals. Keep notes of what you use, and a process of elimination may help.

Vacuum frequently To get rid of dust mites and prevent a build-up of animal hairs, vacuum daily.

Change your garden Few people are driven to such desperate lengths, but if your hay fever is really troublesome you could try paving over the lawn and growing non-flowering foliage plants. This will not, of course, prevent pollen drifting from your neighbours' gardens, but some hay fever sufferers say that their weekends have been made bearable by such action.

If your efforts to avoid or eliminate the allergen have failed or are impracticable, the solution is to treat the symptoms. Remember that most allergens are, in themselves, harmless. It is your body's response, not the allergen, that does the damage, so coming into contact with the offending substance will not hurt you as long as you can control your reaction to it.

orthodox techniques with others such as cytotoxic testing (which uses white blood cells), muscle testing and electrical testing. If you suspect that you are suffering from an allergy, consulting a clinical ecologist could prove helpful. See CLINICAL ECOLOGY.

Kinesiology This is a more controversial technique. Practitioners believe that a person's muscle power is affected by allergy, and measure your muscular response to suspected substances to identify an allergen. Evidence in support is limited, but kinesiology can do you no harm.

Other alternative treatments

Homoeopathy You may have to take far more personal responsibility for your cure than if you had consulted a conventional doctor. You may also have to change your diet and lifestyle as well as taking prescribed remedies.

Ionisation An ionising machine artificially produces negatively charged particles of air (ions) which are found naturally by running water, at the seaside and in pure mountain air. Ionisation may help symptoms such as asthma and hay fever.

Bach Remedies Clematis is prescribed for general oversensitivity; Mimulus for fear of getting an allergic reaction; Impatiens if there is irritation of the skin or mucous membranes. Beech is claimed to be able to help various food intolerances and other allergies.

Biofeedback Practitioners train you to recognise your body's response to an allergen by electrically measuring such functions as skin resistance and brain waves. When you have learned to identify the onset of an allergic reaction you can take steps to control it.

Hypnotherapy Just how HYPNOTHERAPY works to counter allergies is hard to define, but sufferers have successfully used stress reduction and desensitisation techniques to alleviate, or even entirely remove, allergic conditions such as asthma and eczema.

An orthodox view

A doctor may prescribe antihistamines, cortisone sprays and creams, nose drops or bronchodilators to treat various allergic reactions. All of these may provide effective relief, but some of the drugs used cause side effects, such as drowsiness, and others, particularly nose drops containing isoprenaline, can be habit-forming (see ADDICTION). Desensitising injections – under careful medical supervision – can be effective.

AMOEBIASIS

Amoebiasis is an infectious disease most prevalent in tropical and subtropical areas, where standards of public hygiene are poor. The infection is caused by a tiny, single-celled animal parasite, *Entamoeba histolytica*, which scavenges for food in the large intestine, where it multiplies. The disease is spread by food and water contaminated by flies carrying the germ from human faeces.

In its advanced state amoebiasis develops into full-blown amoebic DYSENTERY. But the diarrhoea characteristic of the disease may be mild and intermittent.

Another symptom of amoebiasis is abdominal cramps, while if the infection spreads to the liver an abscess will develop. The liver then becomes painfully enlarged, and the victim is a prey to fever, chills and weight loss.

What the therapists recommend

Acupuncture A consultation with the patient will enable the acupuncturist to decide on the appropriate point to be stimulated.
Homoeopathy Homoeopathic treatment is possible to alleviate amoebiasis; the form it takes depends on the homoeopath's assessment of the patient.
Naturopathy Complete rest for the bowel and warmth for the abdomen are regarded as essential. The patient will be taken off drugs and injections, and may be advised to fast for a few days.

An orthodox view

Severe attacks of amoebic dysentery can be fatal, so early diagnosis and specific therapy are essential. After checking the patient's stools for the parasite amoebae or their cysts, the doctor will prescribe an antiamoebic drug such as metronidazole or iodoquinol. A liver abscess may have to be drained.

ANAEMIA

The name anaemia is given to a range of illnesses that involve a lack of the oxygen-carrying substance haemoglobin in the blood. Anaemia can be caused by loss of blood, an inability to produce enough red blood cells, or an inherited abnormality.

Symptoms include DIZZINESS, TIREDNESS, HEADACHES, INSOMNIA, shortness of breath, paleness, disturbances of vision, swollen ankles, loss of appetite, PALPITATIONS and, in older people, chest pains. The four main types of anaemia are iron deficiency, pernicious, megaloblastic and sickle cell.

Iron deficiency anaemia, the commonest form, results from a shortage of iron, an essential constituent of haemoglobin. This shortage takes place through poor diet, blood loss, illness or infection. Women of childbearing age tend to have low stores of iron as a result of their menstrual blood losses. Therefore they tend to become anaemic more quickly if iron losses exceed iron intake. Pregnant women are particularly at risk because, although they no longer have menstrual losses, the growing baby exerts an even greater drain on their iron stores.

Pernicious anaemia develops when a lack of a stomach enzyme called 'the intrinsic factor' prevents the body from absorbing enough vitamin B_{12} to make an adequate supply of blood. It is usually treated with regular injections of Vitamin B_{12}.

Megaloblastic anaemia is caused by a deficiency of B_{12} or another vitamin, folic acid (one of the many B vitamins), which is found in liver and fresh vegetables. Either of these deficiencies interferes with the production of red blood cells in the bone marrow. Pregnant women and elderly people are most affected.

Sickle cell anaemia is an inherited blood disorder which is found among some people of African and Middle Eastern descent. Symptoms appear in childhood and include yellowing of the skin and the whites of the eyes (JAUNDICE, FEVER), and a feeling of weakness or fatigue after physical exertion.

Always consult a doctor if you suspect anaemia, as medical diagnosis is necessary before beginning any type of treatment.

What the therapists recommend

NATUROPATHY

Self help Plenty of iron-rich foods such as dark green leafy vegetables, walnuts, raisins, brewer's yeast, wheat germ, strawberries, parsley, nettles, apricots and pumpkin seeds are prescribed, and meats such as liver and kidneys. In moderation, full-bodied red wines may also help.

For pernicious anaemia caused by inadequate diet, a naturopath will suggest that you eat foods which are rich in vitamin B_{12}, such as dairy products, eggs, liver and kidneys.

All forms of anaemia may benefit from raw juices such as spinach, carrot, nettle and horseradish. Molasses is held to be good for building strong red blood cells, and high potencies of pollen may also help.

Consultation The cause will be investigated before treatment. You will be referred to a doctor or, if the naturopath is a doctor, given orthodox treatment if the symptoms are severe, if another illness is causing the anaemia, or if you are losing blood regularly or in large quantities.

The naturopath will then give detailed individual advice about STRESS, diet and lifestyle. Dietary supplements may be prescribed – for example, iron gluconate (a naturally occurring form of iron) taken together with 500 mg to 1 g of vitamin C at each meal, plus zinc, since extra iron can interfere with zinc absorption.

HOMOEOPATHY

Self help Therapists may prescribe *China* to strengthen red blood cells and give energy, particularly after a severe illness with loss of fluids. *Ferrum metallicum* can help replace iron in the blood. Pernicious anaemia is said to respond to *Arsenicum*; and pale, sensitive people who overexert themselves and become weak and breathless may be helped by *Phosphorus*, which is said also to be good for children who outgrow their strength.

AROMATHERAPY

Self help The essential oils of Roman camomile and lemon are recommended. Add ten drops of each to about 3 tablespoons (50 ml) of vegetable oil or bland white lotion (see p. 36), and apply daily to the whole body after a bath or shower. A tea made with two drops of lemon and one of Roman camomile oil may also help.

HERBAL MEDICINE

Self help Popular remedies include infusions (see p. 184) of angelica, wild chicory leaves, horsetail, nettle, rosemary flowers or leaves, strawberry and thyme, and decoctions (see p. 184) of wild chicory root, dock root, plantain and walnut. Take about three cups a day. Carrot as a juice or vegetable is also said to significantly increase red blood cell production in the body.

You may find herbal remedies in the form of tonic wines more palatable. They can be made easily at home, but always use a good quality wine and sterilise all containers, which must be non-metallic, with boiling water before you start. Two tonics recommended for anaemia are:

Dock wine Soak together for 24-48 hours in 2 litres of red wine in a covered container: 180 g yellow dock root, 8 g liquorice root, 4 g juniper berries, 120 g brown sugar. Then boil the mixture gently in a double boiler until reduced by a third, strain and bottle. Drink half a wine-glassful every morning before eating.
Consultation The underlying cause of the anaemia must always be properly diagnosed by a doctor beforehand. Pernicious anaemia may be treated with vitamin B_{12}, and dock root – especially yellow dock – is used for iron deficiency. Herbs containing iron, vitamins B and C – such as parsley, nettle and turnip tops – may be given, while the bitter herb gentian is said by some to tone the digestive system and increase the absorption of nutrients such as iron.

An orthodox view

Doctors agree that taking supplements such as iron, vitamin B$_{12}$ or folic acid and eating foods rich in these nutrients will help many people with anaemia, provided that treatment is based on an accurate diagnosis.

Deficiencies are made up with iron or vitamin tablets or injections, and, if another disorder is causing the anaemia, this will also be treated.

Sickle cell anaemia cannot be cured, but blood transfusions can keep it under control.

ANAL PROBLEMS

An itching bottom is a common – sometimes embarrassing – irritation, often aggravated by persistent scratching, which inflames the skin. Sweat, poor hygiene in hot, sticky weather, rough or tight clothing, WORMS, THRUSH, rashes, PILES, various irritating soaps or lotions and sitting down for lengthy periods of time – all of these may be contributory causes.

Anal bleeding or pain can also have a number of causes, including piles, BOWEL DISORDERS, ULCERS or anal fissures – splits in the skin lining the anal passage made by passing hard motions.

Occasional anal pains that disappear after a few hours and do not recur are probably due to muscular spasms. You should not hesitate to consult a doctor if you find that itching, irritation or pain persists, or when there is bleeding.

What the therapists recommend
NATUROPATHY
Self help Wear loose cotton underwear to allow air to circulate. Avoid using harsh soaps or detergents on skin and clothes. Chronic itching may be helped by scrupulous hygiene: wash the anal area several times a day with warm water, dry with a soft, clean towel and apply wheat-germ oil. Vitamin E cream may also be applied.

Occasional itches may be soothed considerably by applying a paste made from baking soda or oatmeal and water; calamine lotion; lemon juice; witch-hazel lotion; or wintergreen alcohol.

You can also try wetting the area and rubbing in a little salt, if you are sure it will not irritate your skin.
Consultation If signs indicate that the problem is a symptom of a bowel disorder or other illness, you will be given tests to investigate the cause. Treatment will depend on diagnosis, but is likely to include advice on diet and exercise.

For a simple fissure you will probably be advised to increase the amount of FIBRE in your diet, which should soften motions and so prevent constipation.

HERBAL MEDICINE
Self help Fissures may be eased by making a decoction (see p. 184) of a handful of calendula flowers in a litre of milk, and adding this to a hip bath. If the fissures are caused by constipation, try infusions (see p. 184) of laxative herbs such as linseed and psyllium seed to soften the motions and reduce straining.

A decoction of dandelion root can also be used for a gentle laxative effect.

AROMATHERAPY
Self help For itching, most therapists would recommend that you take a warm bath containing three drops of Roman camomile and three drops of tea-tree essence. You must stay in the bath for at least ten minutes.

Alternatively, mix three drops of sandalwood oil, three drops of lavender oil, two drops of camomile oil and one drop of peppermint oil in about 3 tablespoons (50 ml) of vegetable oil, and apply to the affected area as required.

An orthodox view

Doctors approach anal problems in similar ways to those of alternative therapists. Small fissures usually heal themselves and pain can be eased by a hot bath; holding a hot, wet sponge to the anus; using a painkilling ointment such as Anusol or Anacal; or eating plenty of laxative foods – fruit and bran, with ample fluid – to soften the motions.

In all cases of anal itching, avoid scratching and keep the area clean and dry. If you use talcum powder, choose a mild type and stop using it if irritation returns.

ANGINA

The symptoms of angina are vice-like spasms in the upper chest, which usually occur when the victim is involved in some activity or exertion. These spasms can be extremely frightening, and it is advisable to seek immediate medical help to make sure that the pain is not due to a heart attack.

The chest spasms last a few minutes and may spread to one or both arms – particularly the left – and the neck, throat, jaw or back. The spasms are most often accompanied by feelings of exhaustion, choking, suffocation, nausea or impending death. The pains vary from mild to severe and may crush, burn, ache or numb the chest – but they are not sharp or throbbing.

The cause of angina – medically referred to as *angina pectoris* – is an inadequate supply of blood to the heart. In moments of extra exertion, such as climbing stairs, running for a bus – even losing your temper – the body needs extra oxygen. To meet this need, the heart beats faster, and BLOOD PRESSURE rises to speed the circulation of the blood and so take more oxygen to the body tissues.

Sometimes, however, the heart cannot function properly because the arteries carrying the blood are too narrow for an adequate flow (see ARTERIES [HARDENING]). This is when angina pains are felt – a warning sign that the heart cannot work any harder, and that you should stop and rest immediately.

Angina itself does not cause permanent damage. Except during an attack, the narrowed coronary arteries of an angina patient are able to supply the heart muscle with sufficient blood for normal activities – the supply is never completely cut off and there is no death of heart tissue.

But if, in the course of time, the arteries continue to narrow, the risk of a heart attack increases (see HEART DISORDERS).
Warning No alternative practitioner should treat chest pains without first finding out the cause. The advice given below is for *diagnosed* cases of angina.

What the therapists recommend
NATUROPATHY
Consultation Practitioners advise that diet is important as a way of stopping cholesterol from clogging the arteries and reducing any strain on the heart. In general the diet should be based on raw or lightly cooked vegetables, fresh fruit and a variety of salads, whole grain cereals, pulses such as beans and lentils, fish, and lean meat and chicken. Equally important is giving up smoking, which is a major risk factor.

Oatmeal porridge and oat bran are believed to reduce the level of blood cholesterol and should be eaten regularly, along with grilled, oily fish such as mackerel and maasbanker. You will be asked to replace animal and dairy fats with unsaturated margarine, vegetable oil and low-fat products, and avoid large amounts of sugar, salt and alcohol to reduce blood pressure, although a glass or two – no more – of wine daily may help.

Avoid coffee and other caffeine-containing drinks such as tea, cola drinks and cocoa, as they increase blood pressure and pulse rate. Drink herbal teas and coffee substitutes made from figs, chicory and cereals instead.

Treatment will then focus on relieving STRESS. You may be advised to change your attitude to work or even change your job.

RELAXATION AND BREATHING techniques will be recommended as may regular, gentle EXERCISE such as walking, swimming and cycling – depending on your general state of health. The therapist will give you individual advice about how much exercise is safe, but good general advice is never to do more than allows you to stop and hold a conversation at any time. Patients taking conventional drugs prescribed by a doctor, such as glyceryl trinitrate and beta blockers, will, however, be told to avoid vigorous exercise.

Dietary supplements may be suggested, including calcium and magnesium, which are believed to promote a healthy heart and nervous system. Vitamin B-complex is recommended for anyone suffering from stress or TIREDNESS, and vitamin C to counteract cholesterol in the blood.

If you eat a lot of margarine and vegetable oils, you may be told to take extra vitamin E, which is said also to help the coronary arteries to function normally. You will start with low doses of 100-200 iu a day – especially if your blood pressure is high – and gradually increase to 400-600 iu if there is no increase in blood pressure.

Some naturopaths may recommend raw juice, FASTING or a raw fruit and vegetable diet – to be taken under supervision – as a means of lowering blood pressure and improving circulation to the heart and lungs.

HERBAL MEDICINE
Self help A popular herbal remedy that may be prescribed for angina is an infusion (see p. 184) of hawthorn berries, mixed with yarrow, for high blood pressure, or an infusion of lime blossom for arteriosclerosis.

Garlic, added to food, or in capsule form, is said to bring down the level of cholesterol

When to get help

If it is your first attack (see symptoms, main text).
If the attacks become more frequent or occur for reasons other than those which usually cause them.
If the pain is worse than it usually is, follows a different pattern or simply feels 'different'.
If the attack includes a cold sweat.
If you have pain at night, keeping you from sleep, or if it wakes you.
If angina recurs after treatment for a heart attack.
If your usual methods of dealing with an attack have no effect.
If the pain lasts longer than usual – if it lasts more than ten minutes call a doctor immediately.

in the blood and to reduce the risk of blood clots blocking already narrowed arteries. Oats, usually taken as porridge, are another effective way of reducing cholesterol.

Other alternative treatments

Acupuncture Angina patients are likely to be considered too *yang* – or active and assertive – by an acupuncturist, who will give treatment to restore the correct balance of *yin* and *yang* to body and mind. Acupuncture can also relieve the pain of angina and help the patient to relax.

Osteopathy and Chiropractic Many angina sufferers also experience tension in the neck, shoulders and back, which aggravates their chest pains. Osteopathy and chiropractic can relieve muscular tension.

Bach Remedies Try Elm if overwhelmed by responsibility; Hornbeam for mental exhaustion; Impatiens for impatience or tension; Olive for overwork; White chestnut for insomnia; Rescue Remedy for shock and fear.

Other useful relaxing and healing therapies recommended for angina sufferers include: ALEXANDER TECHNIQUE, AUTOGENIC TRAINING, MASSAGE and REFLEXOLOGY.

An orthodox view

Doctors, like alternative practitioners, believe that there is more than one cause of angina. Most significant is a blockage of the coronary arteries – atherosclerosis. Smoking, STRESS, TENSION and various emotional upsets can also cause or contribute to angina. If you are in a competitive job, or are constantly experiencing tensions or domestic conflicts, reactions within your nervous system mount up and increase your chances of developing angina.

The doctor will carry out tests, and if you do have angina, further tests will determine the causes. Once they are found, drugs such as glyceryl trinitrate or beta blockers may be prescribed. The doctor will also advise you to avoid stress and prescribe a low-fat diet.

Coronary bypass operations are often performed when the patient's arteries are badly blocked. A piece of healthy vein or artery is taken from another part of the body, and grafted so that blood can flow around the blockage. The blockage can also be opened by inserting an inflatable catheter into the blocked coronary artery.

ANOREXIA

Teenage dieting, or sudden weight loss due to illness or STRESS, often trigger off this so-called 'slimmer's disease'. The victims become addicted to being thin, seeing it as

some sort of solution to their problems: pressures at home and at school, feelings of insecurity and low self-esteem, and the traumas of growing up.

Adolescent girls in particular may feel that they are generally losing control of their bodies as they start to menstruate and develop a womanly shape.

They see starvation as a way of turning back the clock and regaining control; the body reverts to its pre-adolescent shape, periods stop and the worry and attention that their emaciated state arouses in others makes them feel special.

Some doctors and practitioners also see a connection between anorexia and media tendencies to promote a trim figure as a recipe for health, success and happiness. Even women in their twenties are vulnerable, and statistics reveal that men – especially young, ambitious professionals – are also increasingly susceptible to the illness.

Whatever influences are at work on the victim, anorexia is a food phobia which is thought to be caused by an underlying mental disturbance of some kind.

Anorexics do have an appetite, but choose to ignore their hunger, occasionally overeating, then getting rid of the food by self-induced vomiting, or taking laxatives and diuretics (see BULIMIA), or by fasting and taking too much exercise.

Paradoxically, anorexics are often obsessed with food, and feel a need to cook, or to study recipes and menus.

As a sufferer's condition deteriorates, a number of serious side effects occur – and are endured – in order to stay slim. These include DEPRESSION, ANXIETY, INSOMNIA, ANAEMIA, INFERTILITY, loss of sexual drive, impaired thinking, CONSTIPATION, perspiration, slow pulse rate, low BLOOD PRESSURE, reduced body temperature, changes in colour and texture of hair, nails and skin, and excessive hair growth on the body.

Eventually chronic illness sets in and if the condition is not treated effectively, the sufferer may die from malnutrition, HYPOTHERMIA or dehydration.

Since the weight loss is apparent to everyone but the sufferer (who imagines that his or her body is larger than it really is), family pressure to eat properly can make matters worse. A doctor must be consulted and he will stress that a proper understanding of the problem by the family is crucial.

What the therapists recommend

Home treatment is not advisable. Most alternative practitioners agree that help in hospital is essential in the early stages of recovery. All alternative therapies should be used in conjunction with orthodox treatment or COUNSELLING. Some which may help are:

ACUPUNCTURE

Practitioners believe that this can help to relieve stress, balance the body's energy and promote well-being.

ART THERAPY

The therapy gives patients a creative outlet for pent-up feelings, and a discussion of the work they produce can, in return, give the therapist and patient pointers to emotional states and the progress being made. For example, patients may at first paint 'pretty' pictures which they assume will please the therapist. Later, however, they may paint pictures that reflect their inner turmoil.

DANCE THERAPY

This is a good outlet for pent-up feelings and has proved especially useful in treating adolescents who are withdrawn and suffer with neurotic illnesses. It may encourage them to feel a sense of purpose and identity.

Despite their weight loss, anorexia victims imagine they are heavier than they really are. The priority in treatment is persuading them to accept medical advice and help.

HYPNOTHERAPY

The therapist will discuss a patient's problems and try to establish a rapport, so that the sufferer is receptive to hypnosis. Ideally the patient is then susceptible to any suggestions the hypnotist may make about changes in behaviour, and will be given posthypnotic suggestions, among which will be a positive feeling towards eating, instead of a revulsion to food. In addition, the patient should try to maintain an 'ideal' weight.

NATUROPATHY

Supplements containing multivitamins, minerals and high doses of zinc are given to build up strength until the appetite returns. A wholefood diet (see EATING FOR HEALTH) is gradually introduced, with plenty of freshly squeezed fruit and vegetable juices.

BACH REMEDIES

Heather is recommended if the patient's refusal of food is seen as a plea for attention; Beech is suitable for an emotional inability to accept food (or love). If the patient collapses, Wild rose is suggested. In the case of adolescents, Wild oat and Walnut could be offered.

An orthodox view

Because, as most therapists would admit, alternative treatments are on the whole supplementary, the first vital step in treating anorexia is to persuade the patient to accept orthodox medical help.

As sufferers tend to make themselves vomit after eating, in many cases the best course is close supervision in hospital by experienced nurses, who will encourage the patient to reach a target weight.

Once discharged, the patient needs supportive counselling and the help of a psychiatrist or psychotherapist to prevent the condition recurring. Underlying problems, general health and lifestyle are explored, and patients are encouraged to adopt a more positive outlook.

Doctors have found that some anorexics recover spontaneously if their personal problems resolve themselves.

See also PUBERTY AND ADOLESCENCE.

ANTHROPOSOPHICAL MEDICINE

Illness and the path to spiritual growth

In the early 1920s a group of doctors working on the Continent began practising a new system of holistic medicine. They were followers of the ideas of Rudolf Steiner (1861-1925), an Austrian philosopher and founder of anthroposophy – from the Greek words meaning 'man' and 'wisdom' – which was the basis of the new system.

Steiner believed that the structure and functioning of a living organism could not be explained in purely physical or chemical terms. Instead, he maintained that as well as a physical body, all living things possessed an 'etheric' body which distinguished them from the dead mineral world.

In addition, Rudolf Steiner taught that animals and man had 'astral' bodies which represented their emotions; and that man alone had an individual spiritual core, which he called the ego.

Steiner was not a qualified doctor and only assumed an advisory role in medical matters. He collaborated with the Dutch physician Dr Ita Wegman (1867-1943), leading to the foundation of the first anthroposophical clinic in Arlesheim, Switzerland, and their joint authorship of *Fundamentals of Therapy*. In anthroposophical medicine, Steiner's four aspects of man – the physical, etheric and astral bodies, and the ego – are held to correspond to the four ancient Greek elements: earth, water, air and fire. They are connected to each other by means of three interpenetrating bodily systems. These are called the digestive/metabolic system, the nerve/sense system and the rhythmic system.

The digestive/metabolic system is governed mainly by the physical and etheric bodies, and includes processes such as excretion and the functioning of the glandular system, as well as all the restoring and rebuilding processes that take place in the body without our knowledge.

The nerve/sense system, by contrast, is dominated by the ego and the astral body, which control conscious processes such as thought, perception and self-awareness. It controls the body during the day, but gives way at night, when the digestive/metabolic system takes over. This allows the physical and etheric bodies to replenish themselves every night, and repair the wear and damage caused during the day by the activities of the astral body and the ego.

The rhythmic system is formed by the alternation of the other two systems, and controls processes such as circulation and breathing. Steiner believed that tension between the two types of activity was an inevitable part of life, and went on until the moment of death. Good health was a sign that a temporary balance between the two states had been achieved, but this could not continue for any length of time, or the individual would stop developing. Instead, anthroposophical doctors believe that by becoming more aware of these two opposing processes, each individual can start to take responsibility for his own development and the course of his life. Illness can in some cases be the key which starts off this process. As anthroposophy is also founded on a belief in reincarnation, practitioners consider that all illness has a deeper meaning either in terms of a previous life or as preparation for a future life, and never view it as a simply

Anthroposophical remedies

A whole range of special medicines is used by anthroposophical doctors. Some of them date from the early days of anthroposophy and Steiner's own instructions, others were developed by his followers, and new ones are continually being investigated.

The remedies are composed of mineral, plant and animal substances which are thought to counterbalance specific ailments.

Steiner believed that many natural substances were related to aspects of physical health – for example, seven metals (lead, tin, iron, gold, copper, mercury and silver) corresponded to bodily organs. So an anthroposophical doctor may prescribe a homoeopathic remedy or ointment made from tin for a patient with liver trouble, or one with copper to regulate the kidneys.

The essential oils of plants are also used to improve circulation, or cause a temperature rise in patients with degenerative diseases such as CANCER.

physical problem. A wide variety of different treatments is used to help patients, including special anthroposophical medicines (see box); herbal remedies (see HERBAL MEDICINE); homoeopathic remedies (see HOMOEOPATHY); and a type of movement called EURHYTHMY, developed by Rudolf Steiner; and also conventional drugs and surgery when they are necessary.

Who it can help All anthroposophical doctors are fully medically qualified, so they can be consulted for any sort of physical or mental illness. People who want to use drugs or surgery as little as possible, while still being safely treated, may find anthroposophical medicine a good alternative, since the broad range of therapies used by practitioners often allows them to prescribe conventional treatment more sparingly than orthodox doctors.

Finding a therapist All anthroposophical practitioners are qualified medical doctors who have usually completed a post-graduate course recognised by the Anthroposophical Medical Association. In addition to their medical studies, most anthroposophical doctors have also undertaken a general study of anthroposophy, and many also follow an anthroposophical path of inner development, such as MEDITATION.

Some anthroposophical doctors work as general practitioners in Rudolf Steiner (Waldorf) schools and homes for children in need of special care. There are a number of such communities (Camphill communities) in South Africa, staffed by a dedicated, hard-working group of people.

Further information can be obtained from the Anthroposophical Society, P O Box 65119, Benmore 2010 (telephone 011-726-8272), or Bonair, Price Drive, Constantia 7800 (telephone 021-7946445).

Consulting a therapist Consultations are much like visits to a family doctor, but in ad-

The scientist and philosopher Rudolf Steiner (1861-1925; left) founded the Anthroposophical Society to explore new approaches in education, science, religion – and medicine. It has its headquarters in the Steiner-designed Goetheanum (above) in Switzerland. An earlier version of the building was destroyed by fire in 1923.

The anthroposophical view of illness

'According to anthroposophical medicine, illnesses are divided into two main groups – inflammatory, or feverish, conditions, which are more common during childhood; and degenerative, or hardening, conditions, which tend to affect older people.

Inflammatory diseases are thought to arise when the individual's digestive/metabolic system becomes too strong, producing a heating, dissolving effect on the body. Such diseases include all fevers, and childhood diseases such as CHICKENPOX and MEASLES, which are believed to strengthen the child's IMMUNE SYSTEM and prevent the ageing process from setting in too soon. For this reason, anthroposophical doctors do not necessarily always try to reduce a fever.

Degenerative diseases, by contrast, are said to arise from the hardening, contracting influence of the astral body and ego on the nerve/sense system. They include conditions such as CANCER, hardening of the arteries and diseases in which the immune system is deficient, and are often accompanied by symptoms such as INSOMNIA, ANXIETY and a low temperature. Anthroposophical doctors believe that these conditions often develop as a result of events much earlier in the patient's life.

Anthroposophical practitioners say that the pattern of illness has changed considerably during the 20th century, with inflammatory diseases becoming less common, but degenerative conditions alarmingly on the increase.

They attribute this to the growing intellectual and materialistic emphasis in education and society, which is held to be reinforcing the astral and ego forces, while at the same time depleting healing physical and etheric ones in man and the earth as a whole. Consequently, they consider humanity to be fast approaching a critical point in evolution when a new approach to illness and health could be crucial for our long-term survival.

dition to describing your symptoms you will probably be asked about other aspects of your life and daily routine, such as how well you sleep, what foods you eat, and whether you often feel anxious or tense. A diagnosis is made in the normal way, and appropriate treatment given which could be anthroposophical, homoeopathic, herbal or conventional, depending on the condition.

While they aim first of all to relieve suffering, anthroposophical doctors often also try to treat the underlying imbalance that they think is causing an illness. They may suggest eurhythmy, ART THERAPY or MUSIC THERAPY, and send the patient to a specialist in one of these. Some Steiner doctors also work with therapists qualified in a special type of rhythmic massage designed to harmonise the breathing and circulatory systems, and stimulate general vitality. The relationship between doctor and patient is considered an important part of the therapy, and many practitioners will also refer patients in need to qualified counsellors.

Although anthroposophical doctors believe that illness is connected with the patient's personal destiny, they do not claim to have any special insight into his past or future lives. Nevertheless, some do feel that their philosophy helps them to work with difficult or incurable conditions, and that active therapy will benefit patients in a future life, even when a physical cure is not possible during the present one.

An orthodox view

Most doctors are not aware of the underlying principles of anthroposophical medicine, but those who are tend to agree that its treatment may be beneficial.

ANXIETY

Everyone needs to feel anxious at some time or another – anxiety causes a reaction which pumps the hormone stimulant adrenaline into the system. It spurs people to do challenging and uncongenial tasks and prepares them to cope adequately with difficult situations. What is not desirable is for anxiety to become a problem – for normal, temporary feelings of uncertainty, worry or fear to eventually become a persistent or uncontrollable state of mind.

Normal anxiety almost always has a cause of which you are aware – for example, an important interview or a test of some kind may be looming up. But anxiety can become a problem when worry or apprehension is experienced for no apparent reason, or is much worse than the situation warrants.

Although anxiety is an emotional state, it can induce physical symptoms that are not 'all in the mind' – PAIN (particularly in the head, chest, abdomen and back), INSOMNIA, muscular TENSION and DIZZINESS. Often there is NAUSEA and VOMITING, DIARRHOEA or frequent urinating. The sufferer may show signs of panic such as SWEATING, PALPITATIONS and abnormally deep breathing, or feel tired, weak and listless. Generally, the symptoms disappear when there is no longer a reason to be anxious. Yet some people suffer from recurrent attacks over a period of years – an illness known as 'chronic anxiety'.

What the therapists recommend

NATUROPATHY
Self help A wholefood diet is advisable, with plenty of raw fruit, vegetables and salads, and extra protein if required. Avoid red meat, alcohol and smoking. Raw carrot juice and lettuce juice are believed to strengthen the nervous system and have a calming effect. Try two cups of either during the day and a third before going to bed. Cups of camomile tea may be used instead.

Consultation You will be given advice about coping with STRESS, taking EXERCISE, and RELAXATION and BREATHING techniques. KINESIOLOGY can test for ALLERGY.

Dietary supplements may be recommended, including vitamin B-complex and vitamin C to help in coping with stress; vitamin E, said to improve the functioning of the central nervous system; and minerals such as calcium, magnesium and zinc.

HERBAL MEDICINE
Self help As sedatives and to treat insomnia, you can try infusions (see p. 184) of camomile, valerian root and lime flowers. Other remedies recommended for anxiety include infusions of hawthorn flowers, rosemary, betony (not more than two small cups a day, or it may cause vomiting), hops (but avoid if you are depressed), passion flower, and hyssop (avoid if pregnant).

HOMOEOPATHY
Self help If the anxiety is in anticipation of some sort of test or unpleasant event, and you feel fearful, go weak at the knees, or tremble all over, try *Gelsemium*.

If you suffer from fear and apprehension – such as stage fright – or panic in a crowd or closed space, or are compelled to do things in a hurry, *Argentum nitricum* may help. In such cases, a dose of 30th or 200th potency taken the night before, and hourly for two or three hours beforehand on the day itself, should be adequate. Remember that such symptoms are worse in hot weather.

For panic, shock, fear or feelings of being restlessly troubled, try *Aconite. Arsenicum albi-*

cum is recommended by most practitioners for persistent bouts of anxiety with occasional panic attacks.

Other alternative treatments

Biofeedback Stress-related complaints, especially anxiety, were among the first areas to be tackled using biofeedback. A method called respiration biofeedback, in which the patient listens to his own amplified breathing and tries to regulate it accordingly, is said to be successful in treating anxiety.
Biochemic Tissue Salts To combat general anxiety three doses of *Kali phos.* should be taken daily for a month. An adult dose is four tablets and a child's is two tablets. A dose taken every half-hour on the day of a test or event – such as going for a daunting job interview – can be helpful.
Aromatherapy If struck by panic, deeply inhale a few drops each of essential oils of basil, clary sage, lavender and sandalwood on a tissue. If your anxiety is accompanied by a headache, or is causing muscular tension, add drops of marjoram and camomile

oils to the others already recommended. In order to relax, try some drops of frankincense and patchouli. Ylang-ylang is believed to combat insomnia, and melissa is said to help to raise your spirits.

Hydrotherapy Try a tepid bath, cold friction or hot-and-cold compresses.

Bach Remedies An acute attack of anxiety may be helped by Rescue Remedy. White chestnut is recommended for anxious thoughts that go round and round in your mind, possibly preventing sleep. For anxiety accompanied by indecision, take Scleranthus. Agrimony helps to present a bright and cheerful front, although you may be troubled and anxious underneath.

Acupuncture Treatment depends on the cause of the anxiety – such as disturbed sleep or exhaustion – but can be very successful. A practitioner will advise you.

Other therapies that can help anxiety victims – mainly by teaching relaxation – include AUTOGENIC TRAINING, DANCE THERAPY, HYPNOTHERAPY, MEDITATION, OSTEOPATHY, REFLEXOLOGY and YOGA.

An orthodox view

Like alternative therapists, a doctor will be concerned to uncover the root cause of a patient's anxiety, but will also check whether any physical symptoms are being caused by some other illness.

You will be asked to discuss aspects of your life that may be causing anxiety – such as marriage problems, money worries and difficulties at work. Most doctors are skilled, sympathetic listeners who can offer support and advice, but if this is not sufficient, tranquillisers or sedatives may be prescribed. They are not a long-term cure, however; they are simply a way of helping you to cope with some of the symptoms of anxiety and they can be addictive if used for long periods.

If your anxiety is so severe that it interferes with your work or relationships, you may be referred to a psychiatrist, who will probably prescribe stronger tranquillisers and may also offer PSYCHOTHERAPY.

APHRODISIACS

Do they really stimulate sexual desire?

Over the centuries, many foods, drugs and herbs have been held to stimulate or enhance sexual desire, from such folklore favourites as oysters and nasturtium leaves to exotic concoctions made from crushed, dried beetles (in a toxic drug called 'Spanish Fly') and powdered rhinoceros horn. Most of the controversial aphrodisiacs have been discredited after scientific scrutiny, but other stimulants are used in alternative medicine.

What the therapists recommend

AROMATHERAPY

Aromatherapists list several essential plant oils which they believe to be aphrodisiacs: jasmine, patchouli and ylang-ylang.

Jasmine is considered a sensual stimulant and antidepressant, and it is said also to ease pain in the female reproductive system. Patchouli is thought to be an antidepressant and stimulant for the nerves and mind, and ylang-ylang's exotic scent is held to stimulate the senses and induce feelings of well-being. Use the oils for MASSAGE, inhale them (see p. 36), or add five to ten drops to a full bath, relax and breathe deeply.

HERBAL MEDICINE

In South Africa and abroad, the herbal therapists' most favoured stimulant is GINSENG. It is generally available in the form of tablets, tonics or teas from your health food shop. Alternatively, you can make an infusion by adding half a teaspoon of the powdered root to a cup of boiling water and simmering it gently for ten minutes.

Drink the infusion three times a day. Therapists say that ginseng must be taken for several months before any proper results can be expected. However, you should exercise care if you are using it over a prolonged period as it can slightly raise the blood pressure.

A stimulating infusion which is believed to strengthen the reproductive system can be made from a mixture by weight of the following herbs: ginseng root, 3 parts; saw palmetto berries, 2 parts; false unicorn root, crushed, 6 parts; Irish moss, whole or flakes, 2 parts; and motherwort leaves, 3 parts.

To make the infusion put a teaspoon of the mixture in a cup of water and simmer for five minutes. To test its effectiveness, drink two or three cupfuls a day for a month.

NATUROPATHY

Practitioners might suggest 1-5 g of pollen or one or two generous teaspoons of royal jelly (the food of queen bees) every day to aid male or female potency by increasing stamina and combating fatigue.

An orthodox view

Conventional doctors recognise the complexity of the factors that influence sexual desire, but do not accept that it can be aroused by simply taking any particular substance. However, many doctors do accept some of the claims made for ginseng as an overall tonic and stimulant. Research indicates that the herb may help the body to cope with STRESS, overcome fatigue, boost energy and enhance its powers of recovery. Aromatherapy, too, has gained some acceptance, since research has shown that scents can affect the mind.

A doctor will treat IMPOTENCE and FRIGIDITY by dealing with any underlying physical problems and referring the patient to a counsellor or psychotherapist.

APPENDICITIS

This fairly common complaint occurs when the appendix – a small, blind tube attached to the beginning of the large intestine – becomes inflamed or infected.

A mild inflammation of the appendix can cause occasional discomfort in the lower right quarter of the abdomen – the so-called chronic or 'grumbling' appendicitis. Some doctors do not believe in such a condition and suggest that other causes should be looked for.

Symptoms of a serious inflammation – known as acute appendicitis – take from four to 48 hours to develop, and begin with a dull pain near the navel, nausea and sometimes vomiting. However, not all cases present in the same way. The sufferer usually refuses food and drink, and is often constipated. After a few hours the pain increases and moves to the lower right section of the abdomen. The temperature may rise slightly and the breath smell unpleasant. Sometimes the pain disappears after a few hours, but this does not necessarily mean that the illness has passed.

Call a doctor as soon as possible for symptoms of acute appendicitis. If you delay, the appendix may burst, causing an inflammation of the lining of the abdominal cavity – known as peritonitis – which can cause death. Even if the inflammation is confined to a

---

Do's and don'ts if you suspect appendicitis

Do lie down, keep warm and use a hot-water bottle to ease the pain.
Don't eat or drink. Rinse your mouth out with a little water if necessary.
Don't take laxatives, painkillers or any other types of medicine.
Do call a doctor if the pain gets worse, or it becomes constant or it has not gone after four hours.

small area, the result will be an abscess on the appendix, which will have to be drained. If the appendix is not removed, acute attacks will probably recur.

Warning Always consult a doctor before seeking any alternative treatment for chronic appendicitis. There is no safe alternative treatment for acute appendicitis. In China the condition is sometimes treated by acupuncture, but in the Western world it would be considered too dangerous to delay surgery while trying this method.

What the therapists recommend

HERBAL MEDICINE
Self help For chronic symptoms, an infusion (see p. 184) of agrimony, which is used as an anti-inflammatory herb, is suggested. Take one cupful three times a day.

ACUPUNCTURE
Consultation Treatment would probably begin with acupuncture in the neck, followed by acupuncture and/or MOXIBUSTION at points in the abdomen or leg.

AROMATHERAPY

The healing power of plant essences

Enhancing health with highly concentrated oils extracted from plants is known as aromatherapy. These highly scented extracts – called essences or essential oils – contain the substances that give plants their smell. Aromatherapists believe that many also have therapeutic properties.

Essential oils are produced by tiny glands in the petals, leaves, fruit, seeds, nuts, roots, stems, bark and wood of many plants and trees. In nature they are released slowly, but when heated or crushed the oil glands burst, releasing the plant's aroma more strongly. To extract pure essential oil a distillation process is used, which involves vaporising the plant essence in steam which is then cooled down and separated into water and essential oil. If the oil is dissolved in alcohol, or some other solvent, the product is called a resin or absolute. Though less pure than essential oil, since traces of the solvent remain, even after purification, many resins and absolutes also have valuable therapeutic properties.

Essential oils are used in a variety of ways, but mostly for MASSAGE treatments. They can also be inhaled, added to baths or used for compresses (see p. 36). Oils of guaranteed purity are sometimes swallowed. Inhaling is believed to work quickest, because smell has been shown to have an immediate effect on the brain. Scientists have shown that the oils can also penetrate the skin – possibly through sweat pores and hair follicles – and are absorbed into the body fluids and bloodstream, to work internally.

Warning Essential oils must be used with care as they are highly concentrated and could cause ALLERGY or skin irritation. Oils must be ingested only when prescribed by a medically qualified practitioner.

Who it can help Practitioners believe that the correct use of essential oils is safe and suitable for people of all ages, even babies. As a whole body therapy it is held to be a

Revival of an ancient art

Nobody really knows exactly where and when the ancient healing art of aromatherapy began. The medicinal use of plant oils is recorded in some of the earliest Chinese writings. The ancient Persians, too, valued flower waters distilled from roses and orange blossom, and used them both as cosmetics and as remedies for sickness. In the 11th century the well-known Persian philosopher and physician Avicenna refined the distillation process and produced much purer essential oils.

Chinese knowledge of medicinal oils is thought to have reached the west by way of the Greeks and Romans, but the first recorded use of plant oils in Britain was in the 13th century. From then on, manufacture increased and the oils became widely used as perfumes, antiseptics and medicines, until the 19th century. Cheaper, chemical copies of the oils were then made; they did not have the same medicinal properties, but they almost ended the therapeutic use of natural oils.

The early 20th century saw a revival of interest in natural treatments, and with it an increasing demand for natural plant oils. The pioneer of their use in modern medicine was a French chemist, Professor René Gattefossé, who accidentally discovered the healing power of lavender essence when he plunged his hand into it after receiving a bad burn. In a short time the burn had healed without forming a blister or leaving a scar.

Gattefossé went on to treat soldiers wounded in the First World War, and discovered many other healing oils. Later, his work was built on by a French physician, Dr Jean Valnet, and Marguerite Maury, a French biochemist and beautician. Valnet used essential oils to treat CANCER, tuberculosis, DIABETES and other serious illnesses, and claimed many successful cures. Marguerite Maury developed techniques such as massage and various beauty and skin-care treatments using essential oils.

The pressing of flowers to make medicines is shown in this Egyptian relief of about 600 BC.

preventive treatment that improves one's resistance to stress and disease.

Aromatherapists can help to relieve the symptoms of many illnesses and often see improvement in nervous problems such as DEPRESSION, anger, STRESS and symptoms such as HEADACHES and INSOMNIA.

Almost all the oils have proven antiseptic qualities and many, such as lavender, tea tree and geranium, are said to be effective against various infections.

Apart from treating illnesses, the oils are valued for their gently stimulating or calming effects on the mind and their ability to impart a sense of well-being. They are also said by practitioners to be able to prevent illness.

Finding a therapist Aromatherapists have an above-average knowledge of anatomy and physiology equivalent to that which is required in first-year nursing, and they have completed a six-week training course in the therapy. Often therapists will have training in SHIATSU, REFLEXOLOGY and TOUCH FOR HEALTH techniques, as well as aromatherapy itself. To find a qualified therapist in your area, you should contact the Association of Aromatherapists (Southern Africa), P O Box 23924, Claremont 7735.

Consulting a therapist The visit begins with a discussion of your general health, and any problems you may have had in the past, and your way of life, including diet, exercise,

posture, appearance and sleeping habits. The therapist does not diagnose at this stage. He may test your foot reflexes to help him build up a picture of your overall health.

The therapist then selects the oils that are considered right for you as a whole person and, depending on the nature of the problem, gives an aromatherapy massage treatment if applicable, and may mix oils for you to use at home.

The treatment lasts for up to two hours. Therapists believe that massage treatments often lead to a permanent improvement, which can be maintained by using the oils at home. In other cases, repeated treatments may be considered necessary.

Aromatherapy at home

Here are methods by which you can treat yourself at home, using the oils recommended for your condition:

Bath Disperse six to eight drops of essence in a warm bath, lie back and breathe deeply. Stay in the bath for 10-15 minutes. Bath treatments with appropriate oils are recommended for INSOMNIA, TENSION, sore muscles, poor circulation, PERIOD PROBLEMS, COUGHS, COLDS, HEADACHES and fluid retention.

Inhalation Put two or three drops of the appropriate essential oil onto a paper towel or handkerchief and inhale. Placing the paper towel or hankie on your pillow at night should ease breathing if you have a blocked nose. Steam inhalations can be made by placing four to six drops of the appropriate essence and half a cup of hot water into a bowl on a table. Sit with your head a com-

fortable distance above the bowl and cover head and bowl with a towel to keep the vapour in. Breathe deeply through your nose until the smell has almost gone, and repeat three times a day. Avoid steam treatments if you have ASTHMA or sensitive skin.

Foot and hand baths Add eight to ten drops of suitable essential oil to a large bowl of hand-hot water. Soak the hands

A leg is massaged to relieve a circulation problem (above). Oils such as sage and lemon are used, and strokes must be applied from foot to knee. Tense shoulder and neck muscles caused by stress are massaged with, circular finger movements for about three minutes (left). Juniper, lavender, sweet marjoram, camomile, neroli or rose otto oil can be used.

or feet in it for 10-15 minutes, swirling them around occasionally, and adding additional warm water if the bath gets cold. Complete the treatment by wrapping your hands or feet in a dry towel for another 15 minutes and then rubbing in aromatherapy massage oil (see below).

Compresses Add eight to ten drops of essential oil to 500 ml water. In it soak a small towel or old sheeting, folded into four thicknesses and large enough to cover the area being treated. Wring it out, place it over the affected area and cover with cling film.
Make sure that you leave it in place until it reaches body temperature, and repeat the process as you find necessary. Use hot water for old injuries, muscular pain, toothache, menstrual cramps, cystitis, boils and abscesses. Use iced water for recent injuries such as sprains, bruises, swelling, inflammation and headaches.
Some oils can be used undiluted on local areas, for example, lavender on burns and stings, lemon on warts, bergamot on cold sores, tea tree for nail-bed infections, and camomile for bruising.

Massage Normal massage techniques can be used to apply essential oils in a plant oil base to the skin. To mix an aromatherapy massage oil, combine in a 50 ml dark glass bottle about 25 drops of essential oils, and top up with almond oil. A teaspoon is enough to treat the whole back, and less is needed for smaller areas. Massage the oil well into the skin to relieve stress, muscular aches and pains, breathing problems, arthritis and skin disorders.

Self help Some workshops and short courses are available which teach the principles of aromatherapy for home use. See box, *Aromatherapy at home*, left, for an introduction to self help with aromatherapy.

An orthodox view

Doctors and nurses are becoming increasingly aware of the benefits of aromatherapy, and many hospitals in Britain now offer it as an additional treatment.

Scientists have proved the medicinal properties of many plants, and accept that these properties are present in many aromatherapy oils. Research has shown that the scent of the oils affects the cells in the nose which send messages to the brain, and that the oils can, indeed, penetrate the skin.

Research is in progress into the therapeutic properties of essential oils at a number of universities and hospitals in many parts of the world.

Do's and don'ts for aromatherapy

Practitioners say that aromatherapy is safe and suitable for home use, provided that you follow the following guidelines:

Do buy only high quality oils, from a specialist aromatherapy supplier. The label should say that the contents are pure, undiluted essential oil, or an essential oil diluted with vegetable oil or alcohol. If the label says that the oil can be applied directly to the skin, it has probably been diluted, since pure oils are too strong for this.

Don't use essential oils when pregnant except under the guidance of a qualified therapist.

Don't apply pure, undiluted oils directly to the skin except in emergencies such as insect bites and stings, or if using lavender on its own.

Don't swallow any oils unless they are supplied by an aromatherapist and used under his supervision.

Oils for mind and body

Hundreds of plants around the world have been used for the production of essential oils, but aromatherapists generally rely on a repertoire of about 50 to treat most conditions. The list (right) is a useful guide to some of the better-known oils.

Aromatherapy oils

OIL	EFFECTS	USES
Benzoin (resin, not essential oil)	Warming, relaxing	Tension, cystitis, chest complaints arthritis
Bergamot	Uplifting, refreshing, relaxing	Herpes, ulcers, sore throat
Black pepper	Stimulating	Digestive problems, food poisoning, catarrh
Camphor	Cooling, stimulating	Constipation, insomnia, acne, rheumatism
Cedarwood	Sedative	Anxiety, bronchitis, coughs
Clary sage	Warming, relaxing	High blood pressure, period problems
Cypress	Toning, refreshing	Varicose veins, diarrhoea, cellulite
Eucalyptus	Clears head	Headaches, coughs and colds, muscular pain
Fennel	Eases wind, stomach pains	Digestive problems, kidney stones, menstrual problems
Frankincense	Relaxing, rejuvenating	Cystitis, stress, skin problems, cough
Geranium	Refreshing, relaxing	Urinary disorders, viral infections
Jasmine (absolute, not pure oil)	Relaxing, warming	Apathy, catarrh, dry skin, depression
Juniper	Refreshing, relaxing, detoxifying	General poor health, rheumatoid arthritis
Lavender	Refreshing, relaxing, sedative	Good for children, depression, digestive problems, burns, headaches
Lemon	Refreshing, stimulating	Poor circulation, high blood pressure, acne
Lemon grass	Toning, refreshing	Indigestion, oily skin, colitis
Marjoram	Warming, strengthening	Migraine, bruises, cramp
Myrrh	Cooling, drying	Mouth ulcers, thrush, catarrh, infections
Orange blossom (neroli)	Deeply relaxing	Panic, stress, insomnia, depression, shock, grief
Patchouli	Relaxing	Depression, dry skin, wounds
Peppermint	Cooling, refreshing	Motion sickness, headaches, indigestion
Pine needle	Refreshing, antiseptic	Asthma, cystitis, influenza
Roman camomile	Refreshing, relaxing	Good for children, depression, headaches
Rose (rose otto)	Relaxing, soothing	Good for children, depression, headaches
Rosemary	Invigorating, refreshing	Poor memory, mental fatigue, bronchitis
Sage	Improves circulation	Poor circulation, viral infections, rheumatism
Sandalwood	Relaxing, soothing	Cystitis, dry skin
Tangerine	Sedative, soothing	Babies, pregnancy
Tea tree	Antiseptic, cleansing	Thrush, colds, sore throats

ARTERIES (HARDENING)

Hardening of the arteries is a natural process that occurs as you grow older and your arteries lose some of their original elasticity and flexibility. In itself, normal hardening of the arteries – also known as arteriosclerosis – does not cause illness. However, STRESS, SMOKING, an unhealthy, fatty diet or high BLOOD PRESSURE, can cause atherosclerosis, a condition with which arteriosclerosis is often confused, and which is due to cholesterol plaques clogging the arteries.

Depending on which arteries are affected, symptoms of severe atherosclerosis can include chest pains (see ANGINA), leg pains, and temporary disturbances of sight, speech, balance and use of the limbs. A common cause of artery damage is when atherosclerosis is associated with high levels of cholesterol and other fatty substances in the blood. They form deposits on the artery walls, where they harden, prevent blood from flowing freely, increase the risk of blood clots, and sometimes cause a complete blockage. Drinking too much (see ALCOHOLISM) and being overweight can also cause problems.

Atherosclerosis tends to run in families and affects men more than women. It is also more common in the West, where a fatty diet often accompanies a sedentary lifestyle.

Warning See your GP if you have symptoms indicating hardening of the arteries.

What the therapists recommend

NATUROPATHY
Self help Stop smoking! Adopt a wholefood diet based on fresh fruit, vegetables and salads, wholegrain cereals, fish and lean meat. Reduce your intake of saturated animal and dairy product fat, salt, sugar and alcohol (see EATING FOR HEALTH) as much as possible. Eat plenty of oatmeal porridge, oat bran, lentils and beans for FIBRE to help lower your cholesterol level.

Consultation You will be advised about diet, the adverse effects of stress and smoking, and the advantages of EXERCISE and relaxation. Supplements may be prescribed, for example vitamin B-complex, said to relieve stress, or vitamin C, believed to reduce cholesterol and prevent blocked arteries. Eating more unsaturated fats is also thought to increase the body's need for vitamin E – you will be advised to start with small daily doses of 100-200 iu if you have high blood pressure, and increase this amount slowly to 400-600 iu if your blood pressure does not rise. A teaspoon of lecithin taken with meals, and vitamin A, may also be prescribed in order to counteract cholesterol.

Eating to help your arteries

Here are some healthy alternatives to foods that can damage your arteries:

FOOD	HEALTHY ALTERNATIVES
Butter, animal fats such as suet and lard	Margarine (read the label and look for a polyunsaturated kind), vegetable oils
Milk, cream	Skimmed or low-fat milk, soya milk, yoghurt
Meat	Fish, chicken, lean cuts of meat, venison, vegetable protein such as beans, tofu and soya dishes
Hard and high-fat cheeses	Cottage cheese, low-fat cheese, tofu for cooking
Fried foods such as chips	Boiled, grilled, steamed or baked foods such as baked or boiled potatoes
White bread and white flour, potatoes, products such as pasta	Wholegrain bread, oats, brown rice
White sugar	Brown sugar, fructose, honey, in moderation. Eat fresh or dried fruit if you want something sweet
Salt	Low-sodium salt, vegetable salt
Alcohol	One or two glasses of wine a day will do no harm, and may even help. Drink beer and spirits only occasionally; try low/non-alcoholic beers and wines, or fruit and vegetable juices and spring water

HERBAL MEDICINE
Self help Garlic, onions and ginger, raw or cooked, are believed to reduce cholesterol in the system. Yarrow infusions are said to help in preventing blood clots, lime flowers to improve circulation generally, and lemon to lower blood pressure.

An orthodox view

Doctors agree that not smoking, switching to LOW-FAT DIETS, taking moderate exercise and adopting a less stressful lifestyle will help many people with arteriosclerosis. In addition, conventional medicine can offer drugs to reduce high blood pressure, and surgery to replace blocked sections of artery with pieces taken from healthy veins or arteries, and techniques to open up the blockage using a balloon catheter.

ARTHRITIS

There are more than 100 different types of arthritis, all involving some disorder or inflammation of the joints. Two of the most common forms are osteoarthritis and rheumatoid arthritis, which affect millions of people worldwide; a third common form is GOUT, caused by crystals of a body waste, uric acid, collecting in the sufferer's joints.

Osteoarthritis causes swelling, pain and stiffness and sometimes deforms the joints.

The parts most affected are the hips, knees, spine and hands. Shock-absorbing cartilage between the bones of the joints becomes rough and worn, allowing the bones to rub together and wear when the joints are flexed. Muscles and ligaments are also weakened. Women are more at risk than men.

Rheumatoid arthritis also affects more women than men. During an attack the tissue, tendons and ligaments of the joint become inflamed. Feet and fingers are usually the first parts to be affected; then the wrists, knees, shoulders, ankles and elbows. Symptoms include swelling, stiffness and pain in the joints; red, shiny skin over the joints; and a general feeling of stiffness and restricted movement. Sometimes there is numbness in the hands (see CARPAL TUNNEL SYNDROME), loss of weight or appetite, FEVER, or a general sense of being unwell.

The causes of arthritis are largely unknown, but various factors such as heredity, injury and stress on the joints may play a part. Many therapists believe that certain forms may be associated with a breakdown of the IMMUNE SYSTEM – possibly triggered off by an ALLERGY or by VIRUS INFECTIONS.

Always see your doctor if you suspect that you may have arthritis.

What the therapists recommend
NATUROPATHY
Self help A wholefood, largely vegetarian diet (see EATING FOR HEALTH), with plenty of salads and lightly cooked vegetables is rec-

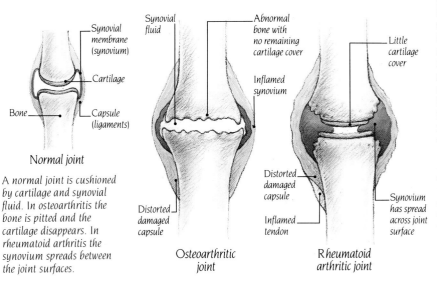

Normal joint

A normal joint is cushioned by cartilage and synovial fluid. In osteoarthritis the bone is pitted and the cartilage disappears. In rheumatoid arthritis the synovium spreads between the joint surfaces.

Synovial membrane (synovium)
Cartilage
Bone
Capsule (ligaments)
Synovial fluid
Distorted damaged capsule

Osteoarthritic joint

Abnormal bone with no remaining cartilage cover
Inflamed synovium
Distorted damaged capsule
Inflamed tendon

Rheumatoid arthritic joint

Little cartilage cover
Synovium has spread across joint surface

ommended. Cut out foods, such as dairy products, that can cause allergies. However, modest amounts such as one or two eggs a week and a little fish or chicken every second day may do no harm.

Avoid red meat and white flour products. Use goat's milk and the cheese and yoghurt made from it, instead of cow's milk and its products. Avoid also acid fruits such as lemons, oranges, grapefruit and strawberries, rhubarb, spinach, tomatoes, salt and sugar (use honey), tea, coffee, alcohol and products containing FOOD ADDITIVES. Drinking raw fruit and vegetable juices may also help. For cases of acute inflammation, two to four cups of celery juice and one cup each of carrot, cucumber and beetroot juice daily are generally recommended.

Consultation Before prescribing a course of treatment, the naturopath will examine you thoroughly, and ask general questions about your health, and what your eating habits are. The naturopath will then probably do some tests – for example, to find out if you have any specific allergies.

Correct diet is thought by many naturopaths and their patients to be effective in controlling the symptoms of arthritis, so the therapist will then advise about the best diet for your individual needs. He may suggest a RAW FOOD DIET one day a week, or recommend sulphur-rich foods (see MINERALS) such as garlic and live yoghurt. If necessary you will be urged to lose weight (see SLIMMING THE NATURAL WAY).

Arthritis sufferers with vitamin or mineral deficiencies may be recommended to take vitamins A, B-complex, especially B_{12}, C and E, and minerals such as zinc and calcium. Other supplements used include evening primrose oil, pollen tablets, kelp or seaweed.

You will probably be advised to keep active and use your joints with specific exercises, except in severe stages of rheumatoid arthritis, when it is better to rest.

TRADITIONAL MEDICINE
Self help Remedies include a warming lotion made from glycerine and cayenne pepper (not if the skin is broken), and hot poultices and compresses (see p. 184) of pounded fresh ginger, powdered sulphur or green clay (available at health food shops or from chemists, to special order). Another lotion may be made by mixing one part cayenne to four parts olive oil and eight parts spirit of camphor.

Cider vinegar, honey and cod-liver oil are traditional cures – try 2 teaspoons of cider vinegar in a glass of water with a little honey, first thing in the morning and again at every meal; or take 2 teaspoons of cod-liver oil for five days before going to bed. Some sufferers also claim to have been helped by copper bracelets (see COPPER THERAPY).

HYDROTHERAPY
Self help Swimming and bathing take the weight off joints, and warm water relaxes muscles and relieves pain. Sea water is believed to be particularly beneficial (see THALASSOTHERAPY), as are seaweed baths. You can buy dried seaweed for this purpose at health food shops or herbalists. An Epsom salts bath may also help – simply add 3-4 tablespoonfuls to a hot bath.

HOMOEOPATHY
Self help Two generally used homoeopathic remedies are *Ruta* and *Rhus tox*. The second is also claimed to be a specific remedy for pains that become worse after resting and

in damp weather, and are relieved somewhat by continuous activity. For very painful joints that hurt if moved, try *Bryonia*, and after an injury, *Arnica*. If pain is eased by pressure and cold, and increased by heat and movement, *Bryonia* may help. *Pulsatilla* is used when pains seem to move from joint to joint, neck and shoulders 'crack' on movement, legs feel heavy in daytime and ache at night. Symptoms tend to worsen in a hot and stuffy atmosphere. Gentle movement and pressure can give relief.

MOXIBUSTION
Consultation Arthritis is seen as due to a blockage of Qi, or energy. The therapist will diagnose the organs affected and base his treatment on the diagnosis. The general treatment for all forms of arthritis is moxibustion at points in the back, abdomen, arms and legs. Acupuncture may be given also at points in the neck, back, abdomen and legs. Additional local treatment will also be given at the affected joints.

HERBAL MEDICINE
Self help Devil's claw is claimed to have given good results – research by drug companies has confirmed that the herb contains several glycosides that are powerful anti-inflammatory agents. For this reason, however, it is best not used during pregnancy. Alfalfa (lucerne) – as tablets or infusion (see p. 184, do not boil) – is used as a nutritional supplement, as is celery. Infusions of parsley and ginger root are said to clear poisons from the system, and extracts or infusions of willow, primula, aloe vera and feverfew are all believed to reduce inflammation. Wild yam and lignum vitae ('thuja') may be helpful for attacks of rheumatoid arthritis.

ACUPRESSURE
Self help For the best results you should carry out self treatment daily, morning and evening until the symptoms are relieved. In each case press the points indicated firmly for one to two minutes – and massage in a clockwise direction if required.

Hands: Press the point at the end of the crease between forefinger and thumb towards the finger bone. *Hips:* Press strongly inwards at the hollow at the sides of the hips at the joint between pelvis and leg. *Knees:* Press in and under the kneecap in the outer depression. Or – and this is said to be particularly effective – press inwards at the point three thumbs' width down from the kneecap in the hollow on the outer edge of the shin.

Other alternative treatments

Acupuncture Practitioners treat more patients with arthritis than those with any other complaint. Both osteoarthritis and rheumatoid arthritis are said to respond well to acupuncture techniques. In addition, good results have been achieved in other similar diseases such as BURSITIS and fibrositis, or 'muscular rheumatism'. All are best treated before they become chronic and cause degenerative changes that lead to restricted movement and severe pain.

Bach Remedies Oak for those who are dutiful, stoic and long-suffering; Beech for rigidity and intolerance; Pine for those with autocratic, domineering personalities. When there is resentment and bitterness, Willow. Rock water for the self-critical, with punishingly high standards, and Vervain if the arthritis is thought to be a response to over-extension of one's resources, or if the sufferer has fixed, fanatical ideas.

Aromatherapy Try rubbing camomile onto painful joints. Ten drops each of rosemary, marigold and lavender oil in 3 tablespoons of almond oil make another massage oil. Pine, lavender or juniper oil can be added to a hot bath.

Osteopathy, Chiropractic, Massage, Alexander Technique and other manipulative therapies These can be effective, especially if begun in the early stages. However, they need to be practised with great care or harm

may result. Always ask your doctor's advice before adopting any of these therapies and do not use them if there is inflammation – for example, in the acute phase of rheumatoid arthritis.

Reflexology Massage to the reflex areas relating to the joints affected may help relieve pain and inflammation. So, too, may direct massage to zone-related areas (shoulder for hip, elbow for knee, wrist for ankle, hand for foot and vice versa). Massage to the reflex areas for the pituitary, adrenals and parathyroid glands, the kidneys and the solar plexus may also be helpful. A good general treatment to all the reflex areas is also recommended. See chart, p. 295.

Yoga, Tai-chi Ch'uan, Eurhythmy and Dance Movement Therapy Gentle exercises such as these can help to prevent stiffness and keep the joints supple. They may also relieve STRESS and help you to relax. Exercises are not recommended for severe cases of rheumatoid arthritis, for which rest is advised. The improvement of breathing is also important and may assist severe cases of rheumatoid arthritis and osteoarthritis.

Psychotherapy, Autogenics and Hypnotherapy These may help to overcome anxiety and depression, and encourage a

more positive attitude to life. Some practitioners believe that unexpressed negative emotions such as fear, anger and grief may be a cause of rheumatoid arthritis and must be dealt with before a cure can take place.

An orthodox view

Doctors have made comparison tests of acupuncture and orthodox treatments for arthritic pain in joints such as the knee, back and shoulder, and have found it to be as effective as claimed. In general, however, little is known about the root causes of arthritis, and doctors can only treat the symptoms. Drugs are prescribed to relieve pain and swelling, and physiotherapy is often recommended by doctors to keep the joints flexible and strengthen weak muscles.

In severe cases, arthritic joints can often be replaced with artificial ones; hip replacements are particularly successful. Where this is impossible, a wide range of aids and appliances is available to help arthritis sufferers remain independent.

Self-help yoga exercises

Foot rotation (right): *Sit down and put one ankle across the other thigh. Rotate the foot using your hand. Rotate it in the opposite direction. Then exercise the other foot.*

Shoulder rotation (below): *Sit down with your arm on the chair arm. Rotate the shoulder on that side using the other hand. Rotate the other way. Repeat for the other shoulder.*

ART THERAPY

Healing through self-expression

People with emotional problems can be helped to express their deepest thoughts and feelings visually through art therapy. Instead of being given drugs to suppress their symptoms, patients are encouraged to communicate their feelings to others by way of drawing and painting.

Often fears and needs are expressed that are so deeply buried that the person is not normally even aware of them. Giving these a visual form in paint, clay or some other art medium may be the first stage in the healing process of helping the patient to recognise and eventually overcome his problems.

This relatively new form of therapy was first practised in England during the 1940s, mainly as a result of the work of the artist Adrian Hill and psychotherapist Irene Champernowne (see box, p. 42), and has grown steadily since then. Today art therapy is practised in many parts of the world.

Who it can help All those with emotional or psychological problems, or who want to find out more about themselves, may benefit, especially if they find it hard to express themselves in words. Group art therapy is particularly recommended for those people who experience difficulty relating to others, or who suffer from such ailments as ALCOHOLISM, drug ADDICTION, ANOREXIA, BULIMIA, or physical or mental handicaps which interfere with communication.

Symbolic portraits

One way in which group members are encouraged to express their feelings about one another is by drawing 'symbolic portraits'. Each member draws the others not as they really appear, but in terms of the shapes, colours and images he associates with them.

Symbolic portraits of a group member (above and right) were done by two other members of the group.

The young woman they were drawing seemed small and meek, but was drawn as a cat-like creature with sharp claws, ready to pounce. She was taken aback by this, but as she thought about it she came to realise that she was using her meek appearance to suppress her natural aggressiveness, and that this made her feel tense and knotted up inside. The realisation should help her to release her aggressiveness and channel it in a creative and positive way.

This clay mask (above) was made collectively by a small group of patients who had been drug addicts. At first, one member of the group, Aldo, dominated the others and insisted that they should use the clay to make a model prison. At first they agreed but soon became dissatisfied and lost interest, and began to bicker among themselves. The therapist urged them to find a way to resolve the problem and would not let them leave the room — even for a cigarette.

Eventually, the group smashed up the prison and began discussing what they should make instead. They hit enthusiastically on the idea of masks and each made one. They then joined in creating a group mask, which was made with great care, loving attention, and lavishly applied colouring.

They ended satisfied with their achievement, pleased at finding a creative solution to their problem by working together. Even Aldo felt relieved that he had been able to co-operate with the others, instead of having to dominate them.

Another man drew the woman therapist as a conductor in charge of the group (above). She looks quite fierce, and the patient explained that he had been afraid when he found out that the therapist would be a woman, since he feared women in authority.

One patient in the group was drawn as a closed box, tied up with string (left). He agreed that he felt cut off from others and unable to be open with them, and decided that he wanted to change.

Two early pioneers of art therapy

The first experiment with art as a form of therapy took place by chance early in the Second World War when the artist Adrian Hill was recovering from tuberculosis in a Sussex sanatorium.

Bored with the tedium of his convalescence, he turned to his art as a way of passing the time creatively, and began introducing other patients to painting and drawing to take their minds off their illnesses and traumatic wartime experiences.

To his surprise, Hill found that not only were they enthusiastic, but that they used their pictures to express fears and anxieties that had been suppressed in their personalities for years. They also started using pictures to portray frightening scenes they had witnessed in the war. Unintentionally, Adrian Hill had become Britain's first art therapist.

Another pioneer was Irene Champernowne, who studied psychotherapy under the Swiss psychoanalyst Carl Gustav Jung.

Champernowne was very impressed by Jung's use of painting and modelling to help patients with emotional problems express their unconscious feelings, and she herself was similarly helped through an emotional crisis.

In 1942, Irene and her husband Gilbert set up a centre for 'psychotherapy through the arts' at their country house, Withymead, near Exeter, where they employed artists, musicians and dancers as well as medical experts.

Although they worked in very different ways – Hill as an enlightened art teacher and Irene Champernowne as a psychotherapist – they laid some of the foundations for the profession of art therapy.

Long-term hospital patients can be helped to return to the community by learning to communicate better with others, and people with a low opinion of themselves can gain self-confidence and a sense of achievement.

Finding a therapist Art therapists in South Africa, like drama therapists and music therapists, fall under the category of 'single-medium' therapists. No formal training is available, nor are there any registered art therapists, but if you wish to consult one, contact the Professional Board for Occupational Therapy, c/o The South African Medical and Dental Council, P O Box 205, Pretoria 0001 (telephone 012-286680 or 3241626). Patients treated by doctors trained in ANTHROPOSOPHICAL MEDICINE may be given art therapy as part of their overall treatment.

Consulting a therapist Most patients are referred to an art therapist only when their emotional difficulties become so severe that they are admitted to hospital, either as outpatients or in-patients.

Often these people find it extremely hard to talk about their personal problems because deep or frightening feelings are involved, or they do not understand why they are troubled or unhappy.

Art therapists are specially trained to be sensitive – and, when the time comes, to be good listeners – who not only recognise a patient's need to share his problems, but also understand how difficult it can be to express innermost feelings, especially when distressed and confused.

Patients who are worried about not being able to draw or paint very well are reassured from the beginning. They are told that they do not need to be 'good at art', because making images, marks and symbols is a natural human activity which all children do spontaneously at play, but tend to give up as they grow older. Patients are helped to rediscover the ability to play creatively, and by doing so express and understand themselves and their problems better.

The patient is offered various art materials such as easy-to-use paints, crayons, charcoal, coloured and plain paper, clay, Plasticine, and old magazines and newspapers with which to make collages. 'Junk' material such as scrap wood, boxes and plastic containers which can be used to make three-dimensional constructions may also be provided. The patient is free to use the materials in any way he wishes, with the therapist offering help only if he seems stuck.

At first some people may find it hard to work spontaneously with unfamiliar materials and in front of a stranger. But most patients, once they begin to use paint, clay or whatever, become so involved in their creation that they forget fears and inhibitions, and express themselves freely.

Often the images created are unexpected, frightening or disturbing, and even the patient may be surprised or shocked at his work. Sometimes first attempts are just nervous doodles or splodges of colour, but the therapist will always be responsive, encouraging the patient to talk about himself through his work, though never offering an over-simplistic judgment or interpretation. Art therapy is often used with groups of about eight to ten patients, each member working on individual pieces but also being encouraged to help others and co-operate on group projects.

As the different members get to know one another, they become a sort of 'family' – and start to behave as they would with their own families. Then, as old conflicts, fears and needs emerge in their work and personal relationships with one another, the therapist helps the patients to work through their feelings and resolve their problems.

Self help After receiving art therapy from a qualified practitioner, patients are encouraged to continue to paint and draw on their own, as a way of understanding and developing themselves.

An orthodox view

Art therapy is considered to be 'alternative' because it combines visual arts such as painting and collage with psychotherapy in a way that is still new and unusual in medicine. However, art therapy is accepted by doctors as an effective form of treatment, and many patients have been helped by it, even when more conventional psychiatry or psychotherapy has failed.

ASTHMA

How to deal with breathing problems

Attacks of asthma occur when inflammation or muscular spasm causes the bronchial passages of the lungs to contract, making breathing difficult and causing a WHEEZING sound, as the breath is exhaled. Other symptoms may include coughing, a fast pulse – up to 90 beats a minute – and, in serious attacks, going blue in the face. Often the victim feels restless and panicky, and may turn pale, rather than blue. While most attacks last just a few minutes, serious bouts may go on for hours and must always be treated by a doctor or there is a risk of collapse or death from lack of oxygen, strain or exhaustion.

Asthma is usually due to several interacting inherited or environmental factors such as ALLERGY (especially to pollen, house dust, animal hair, feathers, or mould and fungi spores), climate and temperature, or to infection, STRESS, ANXIETY, or any kind of physical exertion.

Asthma that runs in families tends to start in childhood or adolescence, and is sometimes associated with ECZEMA or HAY FEVER. Often it disappears after a year or two. Among adults, asthma sometimes develops after recurrent chest infections or as a result of HEART DISORDERS.

What the therapists recommend

NATUROPATHY

Self help Adhere to a wholefood diet (see EATING FOR HEALTH) and avoid eating anything containing FOOD ADDITIVES such as the colouring agent tartrazine – which can trigger allergic reactions. Also avoid refined products such as white flour and sugar, and reduce your intake of dairy products.

Include plenty of fresh fruit and vegetables – especially garlic and onions, said to counteract the production of mucus – and raw juices such as carrot, celery, spinach and grapefruit. Some therapists may recommend one or two teaspoons of cider vinegar with a little honey to be taken in a glass of water three times a day.

Osteopathy may be recommended to keep the rib cage moving freely to help with normal breathing.

Consultation You will be advised about a suitable diet, and also about RELAXATION AND BREATHING techniques and reducing stress. The therapist will usually test for allergies – possibly by using KINESIOLOGY – and tell you to cut out any otherwise harmless foods to which you may be allergic – dairy products and wheat, for example.

If you also have THRUSH or are taking antibiotics, you will be advised to eat plenty of live yoghurt or take acidophillus tablets, which are believed to restore friendly bacteria to your digestive tract. Vitamins A, C and E, propolis tablets and honey may all be prescribed against coughing and inflamed bronchial passages.

BIOCHEMIC TISSUE SALTS

Self help *Kali phos.* is recommended for nervous asthma or a tight chest and difficulty in breathing; and *Kali mur.* alternated with *Kali phos.* for thick, white phlegm that is hard to cough up.

If asthma is caused by muscular spasms in the bronchial tubes, alternate *Magnesia phos.* with *Kali phos. Calcarea phos.* is a general remedy believed to be suitable for all types of asthma.

HERBAL MEDICINE

Self help Generally, asthma is best treated by a practitioner, but infusions (see p. 184) of euphorbia and thyme are recommended to relax muscular spasms and loosen phlegm; and passion flower and pasque flower (always the dried herb, not the fresh plant) to relieve TENSION.

Elecampane is held to be good for the lungs and to loosen mucus when used in an infusion made from elecampane root that has been soaked for eight to ten hours in water. Add 30 g to 600 ml of water, bring to boiling point and make sure you allow to cool before drinking. Camomile is said to have an anti-inflammatory action, and may be helpful if stress is a problem.

HOMOEOPATHY

Self help *Arsenicum album* is used to treat difficult breathing; also when the sufferer needs to bend forward to breathe, or feels exhausted and finds the symptoms worse between midnight and 2 am. If attacks peak between 3 and 5 am, *Kali carbonicum* is recommended, and *Aconite* if they occur after exposure to cold or a dry wind. *Ipecacuanha* can help acute breathlessness and may assist if there is a cough or loose mucus in the chest.

Other alternative treatments

Massage To allow mucus to drain out during massage, the patient should lie face down with head lower than chest. Massage the back with long, gliding strokes, and knead the shoulders. Then use cupping movements on the middle and upper back, paying special attention to the lung points between the shoulders. See MASSAGE.

Ionisation This has made difficult breathing easier for a number of asthma sufferers. Keep an ioniser switched on whenever possible – at home or at work.

Osteopathy, Alexander Technique and Chiropractic These therapies can help by teaching asthma sufferers to breathe properly. By correcting the posture and breathing of asthmatic children, therapists aim to reduce the risk of spinal and chest deformities which could possibly result from years of difficult breathing.

Reflexology Massage to the reflex areas relating to the lungs and bronchi, plus areas relating to the solar plexus, diaphragm, adrenal glands, heart, digestive system, spine (cervical and thoracic regions) and pituitary gland is recommended. See chart on p. 295.

Biofeedback and Yoga These are thought to help, especially attacks brought on by tensions or stress. Yoga postures to open the chest include corpse posture, shoulder stand, mountain, fish, pelvic lift, back roll and cobra. Attention is usually given to deeper breathing and prolonging breathing out.

Hydrotherapy Hot and cold compresses (see p. 193) applied to the back and chest are believed to help the lungs work better, by stimulating circulation and muscular activity.

Aromatherapy A few drops of oils such as eucalyptus, juniper and wintergreen can be added to a teaspoon of carrier lotion and applied to the chest nightly. The same oils, plus peppermint or rosemary, can be inhaled from a tissue when breathing is difficult.

Acupuncture Some sufferers have found that treatment reduces the number of attacks they experience. The acupuncture is often applied to the ear.

Bach Remedies Mimulus is recommended if the sufferer is generally fearful and oversensitive; Rescue Remedy for a sudden attack, plus Olive for exhaustion afterwards. If attacks are brought on by anger, try Holly. Try Aspen for apprehension, or Rock water for self-restricting attitudes.

An orthodox view

Doctors recognise that allergies can play a part in causing asthma, and a doctor may offer allergy tests. Asthma itself is controlled mainly by cortisone and other drugs – often in the form of aerosol inhalers – that reduce inflammation in the bronchial tubes and open up the air passages. Antibiotics are used if the cause is a chest infection. Asthma should invariably be managed under a doctor's supervision.

ASTIGMATISM

This is a common eyesight defect causing distortion and blurred vision, and sometimes headaches and aching eyes, and is due to irregularities in the shape of the eye's lens. It may be hereditary, or caused by problems in the lens or in the transparent cornea of the eye, through which light passes. See EYESIGHT PROBLEMS; BATES METHOD.

ATHLETE'S FOOT

Dealing with inflamed and itchy feet

Keen runners and swimmers are among the typical victims of this common foot infection. It is a type of RINGWORM caused by the fungus *Tinea pedis*, which is often picked up in public places such as changing-rooms and swimming pools, and once contracted it can be hard to get rid of. It is commonly found among adolescents and young men.

The skin on and between the toes becomes inflamed and itchy, and may crack or flake off, exposing red, tender skin underneath. Sometimes small blisters and rashes appear. In time, the nails may also be affected and may start to crumble or separate from the nail beds.

What the therapists recommend

NATUROPATHY

Self help Apply propolis ointment or vitamin C powder to affected areas, or bind cotton wool containing honey or cider vinegar into place over the area and leave it on overnight. Go barefoot whenever you possibly can – except in public places where reinfection could occur – and wear socks made from natural fibres such as wool or cotton, which allow the skin to breathe. Make sure when you remove your socks that you put them back on the same feet to avoid spreading the infection to the other foot. A skin tonic can also be made from the juice of fresh strawberries mixed with pulped fresh dates – drink about two cups a day.

HERBAL MEDICINE

Self help Daily herbal footbaths may be recommended for fungal infections – either a strong infusion (see p. 184) of golden seal root or a mixture of 30 g each of red clover, sage, calendula and agrimony, with 2 teaspoons of cider vinegar added to the water. Bathe the feet for half an hour, then be sure to dry well and powder with arrowroot or powdered golden-seal root.

Calendula cream is said also to soothe irritated skin and effectively combat infection. In addition, essential oil of tea tree applied neat to the affected area may help reduce the irritation.

Other alternative treatments

Aromatherapy Add two drops each of lavender, tea tree and tagetes oil to a bowl of warm water. Soak the feet for ten minutes each night. Alternatively, make a small compress with the same oils. Place it on the affected area and keep in place with a cotton bandage or a sock.

Each morning, add a tablespoon of calendula oil to the same essential oils and apply to the affected area.

Reflexology Although reflexology treatment cannot be given to the areas of the foot affected by athlete's foot, sometimes the general effect of the treatment in stimulating the body's healing forces may encourage the condition to clear. This is particularly so if other alternative treatment is being given at the same time.

An orthodox view

The antifungal properties of certain herbs have been extensively demonstrated by herbal practitioners in experiments. However, doctors prefer to rely on more powerful chemical preparations, whose effectiveness has been proven.

Most pharmacies keep a selection of these proprietary foot powders and creams, which can be bought over the counter without a prescription.

In cases of minor infection, doctors will generally prescribe a cream containing antifungal preparations and, if this does not work or if the infection recurs, tablets of more powerful antifungal preparations can be taken orally.

The aura around the hand of an aura therapist is shown on this Kirlian photograph. The photograph is thought to show the extra level of electromagnetic energy that is emitted during the act of healing.

AURA THERAPY

Using visible magnetism to fight disease

Practitioners who use this therapy describe the aura as a magnetic field around the body that interacts continually with other auras in the environment. These individual auras are said to be in contact with a universal field of spiritual energy, from which they draw their power. Many practitioners – particularly spiritual healers – say that they can see auras as areas of light around their patients, and use them to aid treatment.

Artists and mystics have claimed from ancient times to have seen and portrayed this effect – for example, works of art as diverse as ancient Indian sculptures, aboriginal rock paintings in Australia, and American Indian totem poles all show figures surrounded by areas of light or lines emanating from their bodies. The halo in Western religious art is also believed to derive from a golden aura seen glowing around the subject's head.

Aura therapists say that although we are not usually aware of it, the aura determines our first responses to people and situations, and is a quicker and more sensitive gauge than many more rational faculties. They believe the unease you may feel in some people's company results from an aura that vibrates out of harmony with your own; that a sense of peace in a place may mean you are surrounded by harmonious auras there.

The auras of plants, animals and minerals are said to communicate and interact continually with one another as part of a single living system. Each person's aura is thought to be made up of all the radiations from the cells and chemicals in his body, and their interactions.

The visible aura is said to be an oval extending from a few centimetres to a few metres around the body, and sometimes more at the head. The light is composed of seven different coloured rays, each associated with particular organs of the body as well as higher functions; and the shapes, colours and strengths of the rays are said to vary from person to person, reflecting each individual's unique make-up.

Who it can help Aura therapists say that anyone may be helped, particularly those interested in developing themselves spiritually and those whom conventional medicine cannot help. Like other spiritual healers, aura therapists do not accept that anyone's condition is incurable.

Finding a therapist There are no formal qualifications in aura therapy, but people who practise it are usually healers or qualified alternative therapists who have a particular interest in spiritual awareness. Generally their ability to see and use auras therapeutically has been developed over many years of dedicated practical experience with their patients, as well as with much work on their own spiritual development.

Finding an appropriate aura therapist of established credibility can be difficult, as

Learning to see auras

While some people believe that only specially gifted psychics can see auras, others think that we can all develop the ability to some degree. We could therefore start by training ourselves to be perceptive to subtle effects that we do not normally notice.

Begin by setting aside all doubts about auras and try to believe sincerely that they are there and that you can see them. Try to react to people and situations with as much empathy as possible. People who see auras speak of the ability as a subtle process of 'tuning in' to life forces.

Learn to look at people carefully. Watch their movements: are they tense and jerky or smooth and flowing? Are their clothes comfortable on them, and do the colours suit the person and his personality?

Try to understand the sort of messages people are sending out about themselves, and what they may be holding back. Try to imagine yourself in another person's position – how would you feel in similar circumstances and what would your reactions be?

there is no national association in South Africa. If you are consulting an alternative practitioner such as a naturopath, homoeopath or healer, he or she may be able to refer you to someone who practises aura therapy.

Look too at the advertisements in alternative health and healing publications, where aura therapists may also style themselves 'clairvoyant', 'psychic consultant' or some other term.

Consulting a therapist A therapist starts by observing – or, more rarely, actually touching – a patient's aura to interpret his state of health. A dull aura, for example, could show poor health or a need for change, which is exhausting the patient, while dark patches over certain organs are said to indicate the presence of disease.

Therapists believe that personality and emotions can also be interpreted from auras. For example, an aura with soft, fringed edges may be seen as a sign that the person is too susceptible to the influence of others; firm but fluid boundaries mean openness but not vulnerability, and a hard, distinct outline may indicate a defensive attitude and a tendency to view the world as hostile, owing to a

deeper insecurity. Colours, too, are held to be important: lots of red in an aura is believed to indicate anger, and blue, idealism.

Once the therapist has achieved a clear view of the patient's aura, and feels he understands the problem, he can offer treatment in a number of ways. Sometimes this could involve 'feeding' extra colour into a dull or depleted aura, or introducing a complementary colour to help balance one that is too strong. Therapists say that they do this not by using the energy of their own auras, but by making themselves into channels through which universal spiritual energy can flow into the auras of others. This can be done by touching the patient's aura or using visualisation to transmit the energy.

Self help Practitioners who use auras therapeutically tend to emphasise the need for patients to take an active part in the healing process. Part of the therapy usually involves helping the patient to become more self-aware and more in touch with his own spiritual nature. This can involve learning to see and strengthen your own aura by means of visualisation, COLOUR THERAPY, SOUND THERAPY or even by drawing, writing or keeping a journal. However, they emphasise that support and guidance from an experienced therapist are usually also needed.

Colours of the aura Colours emanating from an individual are believed to reveal his or her nature and physical and emotional state. Here are some basic guidelines, though a proper interpretation of someone's aura can be complex since the colours have to be interpreted in relation to one another:

Red The colour of life and physical vigour, red represents strength, energy and passions, and is associated with the co-ordination of the individual as a whole. Tension or nervousness may show as light red; anger or sensuality as dark red. An excessive amount of red in an aura is said to indicate selfishness, wilfulness or an overvaluing of material things. Therapeutically, red is associated with the nerve endings, excretory functions and the sex glands.

Orange This is associated with energy and health and indicates a strong personality which is also considerate of others. But too much orange shows an overemphasis on selfish goals or ambitions. Orange is also the colour of the adrenal glands, sexual functioning and the spleen; it can also indicate fear, illusion or disillusionment.

Yellow Intellect and optimism are indicated or, in some cases, frustration or worry. If the yellow happens to be very pale there may be weakness or indecisiveness, but golden-yellow is a sign of spiritual development and insight. Yellow is also associated with the pancreas, digestive system and reproduction and childbirth.

Green The colour of nature, regeneration and healing, green shows a lively, adaptable personality and a versatile mind. It is associated with the thymus gland, the heart and circulatory system.

Blue Idealism, integrity and inspiration are associated with blue. Pale blue indicates a potential for learning and scholarship. Physically, blue is the colour of the thyroid gland, and is associated with the ears, nose and throat, and with breathing and speech.

Indigo This indicates a tendency to act on intuition and a search for spiritual truth. It indicates moral values and transcendence of the physical world. A predominance of indigo in an aura signifies calmness and benevolence or, if it is not well balanced, irritability. It is also associated with the pituitary gland and the lymphatic system.

Violet The colour of spiritual enlightenment, insight and love. It represents the pineal body, the nervous system and the integration of the whole body.

Black and grey These colours show that the aura has been damaged by negative thoughts or emotions, STRESS or illness, or by undergoing anaesthesia.

White Perfection, the ideal and truth are represented by white. It has a balancing effect on black or grey in the aura.

An orthodox view

Although there is no scientific evidence for the existence of auras, some doctors believe that they exist – in the form of emissions of energy, from both living and dead tissue. The degree of emissions varies, but may indicate the presence of disease. However, orthodox practitioners do not feel that auras can always be detected, or that they can be 'interpreted' accurately.

AURICULAR THERAPY

Curing it by ear

By treating only one part of a patient's body – the ear – auricular therapists claim that they can cure sickness in other parts of his system. For instance, a painful right shoulder is usually treated by means of the right ear; but treatment given to the left ear is often just as effective.

The therapists' method is similar to ACUPUNCTURE, and they claim that the ear has more than 200 acupuncture points which are physically related to specific areas of the body. By stimulating nerve endings at appropriate points, a 'healing wave' is sent along the nerve to the part that is ailing. Therapists also contend that any problem or diseased part of the body has an effect on its corresponding point in the ear. This may show itself in the form of nodules, white marks, scars or ECZEMA.

While admitting that they do not fully understand how their art works, practitioners point out that it is being practised in many parts of the world as a significant therapy.

Who it can help The therapy is said to be very useful in controlling and alleviating various types of ADDICTION – including alcohol, drugs, food and tobacco. It can also help people suffering from ARTHRITIS, ASTHMA, INDIGESTION and MIGRAINE, and those with NERVOUS DISORDERS and URINARY PROBLEMS.

It is said also to be highly effective in controlling pain and is widely used as an anaesthetic in countries such as China and Sri Lanka – especially in childbirth, dentistry, and major surgical operations, during which the patients remain awake, relaxed and apparently free from pain.

Finding a therapist Although auricular therapy is on the increase in South Africa, there are as yet no officially listed clinics in the country. However, the therapy is closely related to ACUPUNCTURE, and a specialist in this branch of complementary medicine should be able to direct you to an auricular therapist, or in some instances treat you himself. For information on where to find a qualified acupuncturist in your area write to the South African Medical Acupuncture Society, P O Box 2229, Dennesig 7601, or the South African Homoeopathic Association, 20 Botanic Grove, Berea, Durban 4001. Practitioners of other alternative therapies (such as naturopathy and homoeopathy) may also be able to help you find one.

Consulting a therapist The therapist will compile a complete case history. As well as general health details – and those of parents and, possibly, grandparents – the patient will be asked about his family life, work relationships, SMOKING, drinking, what he eats and how much, and also his hobbies and spare-time interests.

The patient's ear is then examined thoroughly for any unusual marks or deformities. The therapist will also inspect skin texture, by which he claims to learn a lot about a patient's state of health. For example, dry and flaky skin over the lung acupuncture point can indicate asthma or a lung infection.

Therapists will usually want to see patients once a week. However, in the early stages of an acute illness, this may well be increased to a daily visit for the first two or three days.

Diagnosing acupuncture points The therapist usually does this with a small, blunt-ended probe. He passes the probe over the skin of the ear until the patient feels discomfort. This indicates the point, or points, which should be treated.

Another method employs an electrical point detector. The patient holds a metal bar electrode which is wired to a meter. The therapist holds another electrode which looks like a ballpoint pen with a blunt end. He passes this over the patient's ear points, and any abnormality is duly recorded on the meter.

Types of treatment Many therapists use acupuncture needles placed in the chosen acupuncture points and manipulated.

The therapist may pass a tiny electric pulse down the needles. No pain is felt and patients usually find the treatment relaxing. Electrical stimulation may also be given without needles. The patient holds a metal rod which is attached by wire to an electrical stimulator. Another wire leads from the stimulator to a pen-shaped electrode held by the therapist. He places the tip of the 'pen' on the chosen area and a mild, stimulating current is passed into the relevant point.

Rediscovering an ancient art

In the 1950s Dr Paul Nogier of Lyons, France, noticed that many of his patients had strange cauterisation marks on their ears. They had been made by a local lay practitioner and were a 'certain cure' for sciatica.

Dr Nogier began seeking clinical proof of this, and he gradually discovered that each one of the acupuncture points on the ear could act as a reflex, or health mirror, of a particular part of the body.

His researches also showed him that joining the various points formed the outline of an unborn baby lying upside-down in its mother's womb. From this he concluded that the ear is a reflection in miniature of the entire human body. He has published books and developed a sophisticated system of treatment at his clinic in Lyons.

The art of 'needling' a patient's ear was a standard treatment in Mediterranean countries four centuries before Christ. There is also proof of it being practised in ancient India, China, Greece and Egypt, though it had largely been abandoned until Dr Nogier revived it.

A third method – for very young children and people who are afraid of needles – is the use of a laser. Stimulation is carried out by the electrical frequency of the light source, and patients experience no sensations at all.

Self help Patients who cannot get to their practitioner regularly can treat themselves by using press needles, or semi-permanent needles as they are also called. These are mainly used to treat conditions such as ANOREXIA and heavy smoking. Press needles are very fine pins with heads like drawing pins. Or else they may resemble small, pointed studs.

The needles are fitted by the practitioner and left in place for several days at a time, covered by a small piece of plaster to keep them clean. To stimulate the pressure points, the patient simply presses the heads of the needles gently. In cases of addiction the needles should be pressed every hour and whenever the craving comes on. Otherwise, they should be pressed once every hour, especially in cases of painful joints and certain forms of arthritis.

An orthodox view

Although auricular therapy has long been used in China with reportedly good results, it still has to prove itself in South Africa. Approach it, therefore, with caution.

AUTISM

An autistic child lives in a world of its own, unable to communicate and relate to other people – including its parents, to whom this can cause great distress. Autism is a rare mental illness that appears without known cause during the first three years of a child's life. It affects more boys than girls and may be related to SCHIZOPHRENIA in adult life.

Cut off from normal, everyday life, autistic children often give the impression of being deaf or mute. However, they are not physically handicapped – though they are usually mentally retarded and therefore notoriously slow developers.

Temper tantrums are often their only sign of emotion, and they may react violently to any change in their daily routine or environment – for example, if a meal is late or if furniture in the home is rearranged.

Normal play is also impossible for the autistic child, who prefers simple, repetitive games, toys and mechanical objects to playing with other children. A few autistic children display exceptional ability at tasks such as computing numbers, working out dates, recognising addresses, or memorising pieces of music at first hearing.

What the therapists recommend

Dance Therapy Some autistic children are able to express themselves through dance, and by analysing their 'movement content' the therapist can then help them adjust to the condition.

Faith Healing A process called 'psychic-visualisation' is used. The healer 'visualises' both the child's illness and the energies that he believes can help to cure it. For example, the healer may choose to imagine the child's mind as a vast, dark city, that is gradually lighting up.

Hair Diagnosis As autism is difficult to diagnose, hair diagnosis is claimed to be useful as part of nutritional diagnosis.

Bach Remedies Water violet is recommended if the patient is withdrawn, aloof and does not seem to want contact; Mimulus if there is actual fear of contact; Aspen if there is apprehension; Crab apple if the patient performs obsessive rituals. Beech is advised if the individual seems impervious to others' love, and Pine if there is periodic violent behaviour, which tyrannises others.

Music Therapy The appeal of music has been found to arouse an emotional response in autistic children. The therapist uses the music to hold a 'conversation' with the child by playing an instrument and singing, usually improvising, while the child is encouraged to respond with its voice, a percussion instrument, or both. As the child's mood changes during the session, the therapist meets each change with a suitable style of music. The child's responses give it a means of expressing feelings and relating to something outside its closed world. Music therapy can also be used in conjunction with drama, ART THERAPY and DANCE MOVEMENT THERAPY and has helped some autistic children to improve.

Naturopathy Consultation is necessary, and usually a wholefood diet is recommended (see EATING FOR HEALTH), perhaps with vitamin and mineral supplements.

An orthodox view

Doctors did not recognise autism until the early 1940s; before that autistic children were often thought by some people as 'backward' or 'difficult'. Even today diagnosis remains lengthy and difficult, calling for close co-operation between parents, family doctor and a paediatrician.

Autistic children need specialist care and special schooling. There is no known cure for autism, although some children may benefit from PSYCHOTHERAPY treatment, occasionally in the form of child psychoanalysis, or various calming drugs. Doctors also consider using alternative therapies – particularly those involving music and art – to be helpful in many cases.

AUTOGENIC TRAINING

Exercising your mind towards health

The basis of this relaxation therapy is a series of six simple mental exercises (see box, p. 48) which are aimed at relieving STRESS and helping the body to cure itself. Autogenic comes from the Greek word for 'self-producing', or 'coming from within', and the training has links with AUTOSUGGESTION, MEDITATION and YOGA.

Training requires no special clothing, or the adoption of difficult and awkward postures, and has been compared by some of its

Three main autogenic positions

Using these positions, training exercises can be carried out in various places and situations – such as at work, on a train, or while taking it easy in the park. Each position is taken up with your eyes shut, thinking about something peaceful and pleasant.

The reclining position *This enables the patient to achieve a more beneficial level of sleep.*

The armchair position *This is particularly useful for practising the therapy in cars, trains and buses – and while relaxing at home and possibly at work.*

The simple sitting position *This allows the patient to experience deeper levels of relaxation in the neck and shoulders – one of the body's main tension areas.*

practitioners to learning to drive a car: first make yourself comfortable behind the wheel; then start off properly (calmly and without jolts); next change gear (alter your physical and mental states); and finally come to a smooth, safe halt.

Before starting the therapy you will be given a brief checkup to make sure the training is suitable for you. You will also be asked to fill in a form giving your full medical and mental history. Some patients will only be treated under appropriate medical supervision – for example, those suffering from glaucoma or serious heart conditions. Modified treatment is given to asthmatics, diabetics, epileptics, expectant mothers, and people with emotional problems.

Who it can help Therapists claim that autogenic training has proved itself in treating a variety of ailments – including AIDS, ANXIETY, BRONCHITIS, COLITIS, DEPRESSION, ECZEMA, INSOMNIA, IRRITABLE BOWEL SYN-DROME, high BLOOD PRESSURE, INDIGESTION, MIGRAINE and ULCERS. Its calming effect helps the body to cure itself they say. It is also said to be particularly helpful to people who want to avoid or cut down on drugs such as sleeping pills and tranquillisers.

Athletes and sportsmen who want to relax mentally and emotionally are said to benefit;

their bodies make more efficient use of oxygen, so improving their performances – and they also recover faster from injuries and exertions.

Businessmen also use the therapy to help them relax; airline crews and passengers have had tuition to counter the effects of JET LAG. Apart from children under six, the train-ing is held to be suitable for people of any age. Children over six – an age when they are held to be capable of understanding the

training – are said to behave better and do better at school after a course, with improved concentration and behaviour.

Finding a therapist   Although there are pri-vate clinics which specialise in autogenic training abroad, this type of therapy is not yet well established in South Africa. However, you can look at alternative health and healing publications, which may list telephone num-bers or addresses of autogenic training ther-apists. Alternatively, a homoeopath or

Six ways of willing good health

Therapists claim that by silently repeating a set of six phrases – such as 'My right arm is heavy' – patients can induce various physical sensations. In turn, these are said to lead to states of deep relaxation, promoting good health and preventing and curing illness. The exercises can be practised in all or any of the three main positions (see illustrations p. 47).

Heaviness exercise focuses thoughts on heaviness in arms, legs, neck, shoulders.

Warmth exercise concentrates on awareness of warmth in the limbs.

Heartbeat exercise involves concentrating on the heartbeat.

Breathing exercise cultivates an awareness of breathing.

Stomach exercise focuses on a feeling of warmth in the abdomen.

Forehead exercise concerns itself with coolness of the forehead.

Increased energy

More than 3 000 scientific papers have been published throughout the world recounting the success of autogenic training as a medical aid to thousands of people, but nobody knows exactly how it works.

Medical research strongly suggests that accumulated stress – which is brought to bear on the immune system by a wide variety of factors – can contribute to making people ill in various ways. In addition, muscular tension caused by stress can lead to CRAMP, strained muscles and BACK PAIN. This can affect the proper co-ordination of body and mind, making people accident prone.

Practitioners claim that there is a link between repressed emotions such as grief and anger and the onset of several ailments, and that autogenic training can be effective for such conditions.

A characteristic feature of the training is experience of so-called 'autogenic discharges' – fleeting impressions of touch, taste, smell and so on, related to past memories. These discharges are often intense and dramatic, and may be followed by feelings of increased energy.

naturopath may be able to put you in touch with a therapist.

Consulting a therapist A therapist's technique varies according to the patient's individual needs, but it usually follows a general pattern. Once satisfied that the patient can be helped by the training, the therapist shows him the three main autogenic positions (see p. 47) in which the basic exercises are done.

Autogenic training is usually taught in groups of six to eight patients. The sessions last for about 1½ hours and are usually held once a week for eight to ten weeks.

During the first two to four sessions the therapist focuses on *The heaviness exercise*, the

The road to relaxation

Autogenic training was developed in Berlin in the late 1920s by a German neurologist, Dr Johannes Schultz, who treated his patients by means of hypnotism. He noted how they benefited from states of hypnotic relaxation, and wondered if he could get equally good results without hypnotism.

He devised a set of relaxation exercises based on his clinical observations. By the silent repetition of certain phrases, patients brought on feelings of heaviness, warmth, slowed heartbeat, regular breathing and a warm abdomen. To these he added a sixth sensation – that of a cool forehead – after observing how psychologically disturbed patients benefited even more from therapeutic warm baths when ice packs were put on their foreheads.

first of six basic exercises (see p. 48) in which the patients silently repeat phrases aimed to gradually produce feelings of deep relaxation and tranquillity.

To begin with, they are performed in clean, quiet, comfortable rooms with subdued lighting. Later on, the exercises can be done almost anywhere.

Each weekly session begins with patients comparing notes on how they spent the previous six days, and how they got on with their exercises at home.

The patients are encouraged to keep a comprehensive diary as an aid to memory and a guide to the therapist. At this stage any special problems are carefully sorted out by adjusting the therapy to meet the individual's specific needs.

As the sessions progress, the patients in the group may also perform a series of 'intentional exercises'. These exercises are intended to throw off hitherto repressed feelings of sadness, bitterness, anger and fear, which otherwise may lead to physical discomfort.

Self help Although autogenic training is usually taught in group sessions, the therapist will ask you to practise the basic exercises at home or anywhere that is convenient. To begin with, the exercises need last for only a minute or two, three times a day. Towards the end of the course they will gradually be extended to about 15-20 minutes three times a day.

An orthodox view

Autogenic training is a well-accepted approach to relaxation and has been extensively researched. It is particularly helpful in conditions where the sympathetic nervous system (which unconsciously stimulates certain bodily functions) is overactive, and in PSYCHOSOMATIC ILLNESS.

AUTOSUGGESTION

Healing yourself by hypnosis

People can use this form of simple HYPNOTHERAPY on themselves. It is believed to work by releasing the unconscious healing powers of body and mind. Autosuggestion is also known as Couéism after Emile Coué (1857-1926), a French apothecary who developed the technique towards the end of the 19th century.

Coué's method is based on a form of meditation which aims to empty the mind of conscious thoughts by the repetition of words or phrases such as the maxim for which he later became famous: 'Every day, in every way, I am getting better and better.'

He believed that if this phrase was repeated regularly while in a relaxed state of mind, it would become implanted in the imagination, and would then direct the unconscious processes of the body and mind in a positive way.

Who it can help People who practise autosuggestion generally do so to enhance their overall well-being, health and happiness. It can also speed recovery and help to alleviate PAIN and suffering caused by physical and mental illnesses. TENSION, ANXIETY, PHOBIAS and ADDICTIONS (for example to food, alcohol or SMOKING) are said to respond well to autosuggestion. ASTHMA, ALLERGY and PSYCHOSOMATIC ILLNESSES may be helped, but take longer.

Autosuggestion can also be effective in controlling pain and FEAR – for example during childbirth (see NATURAL CHILDBIRTH) or among the terminally ill.

Finding a therapist This is a self-help technique, but if necessary a medically qualified hypnotherapist may be able to give you advice and instruction. In South Africa there is no registered association of clinical hypnotherapists, but a group called the South African National Association of Hypnotherapists has recently been formed. Its address is 22 Ladbrook Street, Kenwyn 7764 (telephone 021-7614829). Consult your general practitioner or, if you seek autosuggestion therapy for dental work, you should speak to your dentist.

Self help Learning autosuggestion is simply a matter of practising regularly on your own while relaxing. Find a suitable time and place to do so every morning and evening – Coué suggested in bed just before falling asleep and just after waking up.

Meditate if you know how to (see MEDITATION) or empty your mind of all distractions, and concentrate on Coué's formula, repeating it continuously at any speed, either aloud or silently. Do not, however, think about its

How autosuggestion developed

From what Coué saw in his practice as an apothecary, he became interested in the role of the mind in healing illness. He observed the work of doctors who used hypnosis to help their patients and performed some experiments himself. From the results he drew two conclusions:

1 That the healing effects of hypnotism were not due to the hypnotist's skill, but rather to powers within the subject's unconscious mind – so that all hypnosis was, in a sense, autosuggestion.

2 That doctors paid too much attention to the will and ignored the patient's imagination, which Coué thought was more powerful.

Coué believed that having the will to live or get better was of no use if a patient had an imaginary fear that he could not recover. As an example of the effect of imagination on the body, Coué pointed to the process of salivating, which cannot be willed to happen but which is easily brought on by imagining tempting food.

Coué believed also that if the will did not interfere, the imagination could be influenced by autosuggestion, to help in healing physical and emotional problems of all types. He devoted the rest of his life to developing and teaching techniques of autosuggestion that people could practise on their own.

During the 1920s, Coué's methods became world famous and autosuggestion is now an integral part of many other therapies – particularly AUTOGENIC TRAINING and VISUALISATION THERAPY.

Emile Coué thought that 'education of the imagination' by autosuggestion led to cures.

meaning or imagine that it is a command to yourself – just repeat it as an incantation. About 20 repetitions are all that is necessary on each occasion, but it is important to practise regularly every morning and evening, otherwise the suggestive effects will tend to be weakened.

Coué believed that his formula was suitable for any circumstances, but followers have since developed other suggestions – for example, it is claimed that pain or tension may be relieved by repeating 'It is passing off', while passing your hand rapidly over the affected part.

For relaxation and tranquillity, a phrase such as 'I am completely at peace' is recommended.

You can also experiment with your own suggestions, keeping in mind that some therapists believe suggestions should always be phrased positively.

For example, a suggestion such as 'I am not depressed' may not work as well as the more positive statement 'I am happy'. To stop smoking, eating or drinking too much you could try saying, 'Smoking is not good for my body', 'Overeating is not good for my stomach', or 'Drinking is harming my liver'.

Warning Some therapists warn that hypnotic states are not suitable for everyone, and you should always talk over any proposed treatment with your practitioner. Where the conscious mind is opposed to the idea of hypnotism or suggestion, it is better not to try – in this state of mind you are not likely to be suggestible in any case.

There may also be a danger that some people with psychotic mental disorders or deeply repressed emotions could lose touch with reality – as a result of which their conditions could worsen. If in doubt, consult a qualified psychotherapist or hypnotherapist (see PSYCHOTHERAPY).

An orthodox view

The medical profession of the time was extremely hostile to Coué's theory. Though some doctors were prepared to admit that a patient's will might influence his health, they were more sceptical about the role played by the imagination.

Nowadays many doctors and psychologists are more sympathetic to this and other aspects of the therapy, and autosuggestion has been shown to influence both the mind and the body (see COGNITIVE THERAPY).

Autosuggestion is considered to be safe and can be used in conjunction with any other therapies. However, it should never take the place of orthodox treatment for serious disorders – particularly those which are life-threatening.

AVERSION THERAPY

This is a technique used in BEHAVIOURAL THERAPY. It is a type of learning by punishment in which the patient is taught to associate an undesirable habit or behaviour with an unpleasant experience. For example, alcoholics are sometimes given the drug Antabuse (disulfiram) which makes them violently sick when they drink – and heavy smokers are occasionally given similar treatment so that the very smell of tobacco makes them feel quite sick.

According to the therapists, the behaviour and the unpleasant experience that follows become so connected in the subject's mind that the habit of addiction is broken and his behaviour changes for the better.

However, much depends upon the patient's WILLPOWER and the determination he has to break his addiction, whatever it is. If he develops the right attitude of mind then aversion therapy stands a far better chance of working. With positive effort on the patient's part the technique is said to be successful in about one out of five cases.

AWARENESS THROUGH MOVEMENT

Group lessons in the FELDENKRAIS METHOD are known as 'awareness through movement'. During the lessons a teacher instructs the participants in a series of slow, simple movements which are performed while sitting or kneeling on the floor. The purpose is to improve the students' postures and bodily awareness. As a result, their self-image and emotional well-being are also frequently enhanced.

AYURVEDIC MEDICINE

The all-healing 'science of life'

Every aspect of people's physical, mental and spiritual health is dealt with in this all-embracing traditional Indian system of medicine. The name 'Ayurveda' comes from two Sanskrit words: *ayur* meaning 'life', and *veda* meaning 'knowledge'. It is the main form of medicine in India, where orthodox doctors and Ayurvedic physicians work alongside each other. Ayurveda is also growing in popularity in the West, where more and more patients are seeking advice from its practitioners.

Its doctrine of prevention means that people are often treated *before* showing signs of illness. This involves their keeping in constant, close touch with a therapist, who will monitor his patient's entire way of life – diet, hobbies, sex life, choice of spouse, conditions at home and work, religious beliefs, personal habits, and so on – and advise changes as necessary.

If illness does occur a wide variety of remedies and techniques is used – from conventional surgery to plant-based drugs and mineral supplements specially prepared for the needs of each individual. Altogether there are some 8 000 different medicines designed to heal patients – and to keep them healthy and well adjusted.

Who it can help Practitioners claim that all can benefit from Ayurvedic treatments, which they believe are particularly successful in relieving STRESS and TENSION.

A host of illnesses including ARTHRITIS, ASTHMA, DIABETES, ECZEMA, INDIGESTION, tuberculosis and ULCERS, have reportedly been treated with particular success.

Finding a practitioner The South African Association of the Age of Enlightenment in Johannesburg has a list of practitioners in South Africa. You can write to them at P O Box 87483, Houghton 2041 (telephone 011-6157127).

In India, there are three methods of training: by learning directly from a fully qualified teacher; by qualifying in orthodox medicine and then taking a course in Ayurvedic medicine; or by attending one of a hundred or so officially accredited colleges. A five-year college course leads to the degree of Bachelor of Ayurvedic Surgery and Medicine.

Consulting a practitioner The practitioner will start by finding out all he can about your personal and professional life, and details of your medical history and eating habits. He then helps you to relax by means of breathing exercises and takes your pulse, by which he aims to learn a great deal about your physical and mental condition.

Further diagnosis may involve examining your urine, stools, sputum, eyes, skin, nails and tongue. The practitioner will also listen carefully to your voice. By all these means he can assess your condition and choose an appropriate treatment.

As Ayurveda is a holistic system, no disease is ever treated in isolation. However, all conditions are divided up into four principal categories:

Accidental These arise from any kind of blow, cut, sting, bite or physical accident. Treatment for such cases is usually by first aid or surgery.

Physical Internal ailments such as tissue degeneration, tumours, inflammations and blockages come into this category. These are treated by a carefully balanced combination of medicines, diets and practices.

Mental These largely take the form of anger, fear, hatred, laziness, misery and pride. They are treated by a variety of means such as MEDITATION and COUNSELLING.

Ayurvedic medicine does not regard SCHIZOPHRENIA and manic-depression as purely mental diseases – but rather as a mixture of physical and mental states.

Natural The problems of birth, GROWING OLD and dying are included in this category and are treated by taking part in various religious ceremonies and rites. The natural consequences of hunger, thirst and tiredness have their own natural remedies.

Treatments These fall into three main sections: medicinal, dietary and practical.

Medicinal remedies The drugs used are made from natural substances such as herbs, vegetables and minerals. Getting the right balance of ingredients for each individual patient can take several weeks or even months of painstaking preparation.

In general, herbal and vegetable drugs are believed to start to lose potency if kept, and should be taken when fresh; on the other hand, mineral drugs are held to gain strength the longer they are kept. In addition, various homoeopathic and orthodox medicines and treatments are sometimes prescribed by Ayurvedic practitioners.

Dietary regimes Food is prepared in accordance with the season, weather, time of day, and – most importantly – the needs of the individual patient.

For instance, to increase your energy you may be advised by the practitioner to introduce spices and meat into your diet; in order to lower your energy dairy products may be prescribed.

Food should be eaten slowly, well chewed, swallowed in a happy state of mind; patients are told to concentrate on savouring and enjoying their meals. In some cases, FASTING is recommended.

Practical aids These involve various practices including MASSAGE, emetics, enemas, oil treatments, steam baths, breathing exercises, meditation and YOGA.

An orthodox view

Many doctors agree that Ayurvedic medicine, with its emphasis on health as much as illness, is probably the most complete health system so far developed. Its underlying principles – such as the prevention of disease – are more important than its actual remedies and healing techniques.

However, any serious and potentially life-threatening illnesses – such as acute APPENDICITIS and heart attacks – should always be conventionally treated.

Ayurveda's three basic forces

According to Ayurvedic teaching, everyone and everything in the universe consists of three basic forces or elements. In Sanskrit they are called *Vata*, *Pitta* and *Kapha* (often pronounced Vat, Pit and Kaph). They are thought to control all physical and mental processes.

Vata is likened to the wind, which is constantly on the move, and controls the central nervous system.

Pitta is like the sun, a source of energy. It controls the digestive system and all biochemical processes.

Kapha governs the balance of tissue fluid, controlling cell growth and the firmness of the body.

Good health is believed to result from the three forces being in harmony. Bad health is said to occur when they are out of balance. Their relative strength in a person is determined at the time of his conception, and continues throughout life.

The practitioner's task is to discover the patient's inborn disposition and to pinpoint any imbalance that is causing him physical or mental distress.

Vata imbalance for example, can be caused by irregular meals, too little sleep, leading a promiscuous sex life, outbursts of anger and jealousy, and any form of overexertion – physical, mental or vocal.

Pitta imbalance is often triggered by INDIGESTION, acidity, alcohol abuse, and feelings of grief or fear.

Kapha imbalance can result from lack of exercise, sleeping during the day, and the effects of the seasons. Using the concepts of *Vata*, *Pitta* and *Kapha*, Ayurvedic physicians try to understand their patients' basic dispositions, taking into account their age and stage of development – childhood, maturity and middle age, and old age.

BACH REMEDIES

Flower treatments for all disorders

This series of 38 preparations made from wild flowers and plants is called after its originator, an English physician named Dr Edward Bach (1880-1936). He began his career as a medical doctor and bacteriologist in London in 1915. In addition to orthodox medicine he also practised homoeopathy, and he firmly believed that a wide spectrum of natural cures exists for every ailment.

After a severe illness of his own in 1917, Bach found he could intuitively judge the healing properties of different plants, and the illnesses they can cure. In 1930, he gave up his busy Harley Street practice and settled in Wales, where he continued to search for healing plants.

Bach believed that the dew on flowers was somehow 'impregnated' with their medicinal properties, and he collected it to give to his patients. Soon he found he could not collect enough for all who asked for treatment, so he experimented and decided that floating freshly picked flowers on clear spring water in sunlight could produce the same result as dew. This enabled him to bottle and sell his remedies, and the same production method is used today.

The remedies are designed to treat the whole person, not just symptoms of illness. The principle behind their use is that every kind of disorder arises because of an inner imbalance for which nature has provided a cure in the form of healing plants, sunlight, spring water and fresh air.

Who it can help Users of the Bach remedies say that anyone may benefit from them. Although they are chosen according to psychological and emotional symptoms, they may also help physical ailments, and are safe provided that orthodox treatment is given if necessary.

Self help Dr Bach intended his remedies to be simple enough for anyone to use without consulting a professional therapist. When choosing a Bach remedy, try to examine as honestly as possible your mental and emotional state, and your habits, attitudes and typical ways of behaving, and then select the remedy or remedies most suited to you (see box). Use no more than five at one time; generally, the fewer the better. Dr Bach believed that there is a 'type remedy' corresponding to each individual's nature and personality, and that this may need to be taken for a lengthy period, while other remedies can be used for temporary problems. Finding the right remedies can be a difficult task, but most therapists advise users

Bach stock remedies need to be diluted. Almost fill a 20 ml dropper bottle with pure, uncarbonated spring water; then add two drops of each chosen stock remedy.

simply to select those that appeal to them and experiment.

Bach remedies can be bought from most health food and natural medicine shops. They come in a concentrated form known as *stock remedy* – an infusion of flowers in water, preserved with alcohol. This must be diluted with spring water before use.

Take four drops of the dilute remedy four times a day, including first thing in the morning and last thing at night. The drops can either be taken in water or dropped straight onto the tongue, provided that your tongue does not touch the dropper, as this may transfer bacteria to the solution and cause it to spoil. Dr Bach advised that as you take each dose you should imagine it as a healing light penetrating your whole being.

Bach remedies are said to be safe for babies and children, and even for animals. A 20 ml solution of the remedies will be enough for about ten days, after which you may want to try a different combination. Stop taking the remedies whenever you feel that you no longer need them, and resume doses if the problem comes back. If symptoms persist, see a doctor or psychotherapist, and never delay seeking such advice because you are taking a Bach preparation.

Although stock remedies last indefinitely if kept in a cool, dark place, dilute remedies last for only about three weeks: to prolong their life, add about one-third as much alcohol – brandy is traditionally used. In hot weather, keep dilute remedies in a fridge and add a little brandy or cider vinegar to prevent spoiling. Discard any solutions that develop a sediment or musty smell.

Finding a therapist Bach remedies are used in conjunction with other forms of treatment by many therapists who practise HERBAL MEDICINE, HOMOEOPATHY or NATUROPATHY. However, there is no register of these practitioners, and no Bach courses or qualifications are offered.

Consulting a therapist The therapist will encourage you to talk about yourself and your work, relationships, health and feelings,

before choosing the most suitable remedies. He will explain what each one is for, how it should be taken and what effects it should have. You may be asked to keep a record of any changes in your general condition.

An orthodox view

Many case studies and personal accounts have testified to the effectiveness of the remedies. Scientists cannot explain these claims, for chemical analysis of the remedies shows only spring water and alcohol.

Some practitioners defend the remedies by saying that scientific research may not yet be sophisticated enough to measure their healing properties, and point out that some RADIONICS techniques claim to show a distinctive energy field around the remedies. Many psychotherapists also believe the remedies to be beneficial since, when chosen with care, they encourage people to think about their behaviour, attitudes and lifestyles, and this self-awareness can help the healing process.

BACK PAIN

At some time in their lives, most people in this country are affected by back pain. It is usually caused by damaged discs in the spine, or strained muscles resulting from bad habits of lifting and carrying heavy loads. See DEALING WITH BACK PAIN, p. 54.

BAD BREATH

Causes and treatment of an embarrassing problem

This common symptom can have a number of causes. Eating spicy food, onions or garlic can leave an unpleasant smell on your breath for hours after a meal. Persistent bad breath, however, is usually caused by TOOTH AND GUM DISORDERS, or an infection such as THRUSH.

What the therapists recommend

Herbal Medicine Try chewing parsley, drinking infusions (see p. 184) of peppermint or fenugreek, or taking chlorophyll tablets.

Homoeopathy *Kali phos.* is recommended to remove any bitter taste in the mouth on waking. For a metallic taste, try *Merc. sol.*, in the 6X potency, twice a day for ten days.

An orthodox view

As with alternative therapies, bad breath is treated conventionally according to its underlying cause. Occasional symptoms can

The 38 Bach remedies

The Bach Centre in England gives these guidelines for using the remedies:

Agrimony Those who hide worries behind a cheerful face.

Aspen Apprehensive for no known reason.

Beech Critical and intolerant of others.

Centaury Weak willed; easily exploited or imposed upon.

Cerato Those who doubt their own judgment, seek confirmation from others.

Cherry plum Tension, fear, uncontrolled or irrational thoughts.

Chestnut bud Refuses to learn by experience – continually repeats same mistakes.

Chicory Possessive (self-centred), clinging, overprotective, especially to loved ones.

Clematis Inattentive, dreamy, absent-minded, escapist.

Crab apple The 'cleanser'; for self disgust, prudishness, or shame at ailments.

Elm Feelings of inadequacy, overwhelming responsibility.

Gentian Despondency.

Gorse Feelings of hopelessness, pessimism, defeatism.

Heather Talkative (obsessed with own troubles and experiences).

Holly Hatred, envy, jealousy, suspicion.

Honeysuckle Living in the past, nostalgia, homesickness.

Hornbeam 'Monday morning' feeling, mental fatigue, procrastination.

Impatiens Impatience, irritability.

Larch Lack of self-confidence, feelings of inferiority, fear of failure.

Mimulus Fear of known things. Shyness, timidity.

Mustard 'Dark cloud' that descends, feeling sad and low for no known reason.

Oak Naturally strong/courageous, but no longer able to struggle bravely against illness or adversity.

Olive Exhaustion, feeling drained of energy by long-standing problems.

Pine Guilt, blaming oneself even for the mistakes of others. Always apologising.

Red chestnut Obsessed by care and concern for others.

Rock rose Suddenly alarmed, scared, panicky.

Rock water Rigid-minded, self-denying.

Scleranthus For those with uncertainty/indecision/vacillation; fluctuating moods.

Star of Bethlehem For all the effects of serious news, or fright following an accident, shock and grief.

Sweet chestnut Utter dejection, bleak outlook, despair.

Vervain For those with over-enthusiasm, fanatical beliefs.

Vine Dominating, inflexible, tyrannical, autocratic, arrogant. Usually good leaders.

Walnut Assists in adjustment to transition or change – eg, puberty, menopause, divorce, new surroundings.

Water violet Proud, reserved, aloof; enjoys being alone.

White chestnut Persistent unwanted thoughts. Preoccupation with some worry or episode. Mental conflict.

Wild oat Unsure of direction in life.

Wild rose Resignation, apathy.

Willow For those who are resentful, embittered, always thinking 'poor old me!'

Dr Bach also combined five of the remedies – Cherry plum, Clematis, Impatiens, Rock rose and Star of Bethlehem – into an all-purpose treatment he called **Rescue Remedy**.

This treatment can be used for any kind of SHOCK, illness, injury or trauma, and is said by practitioners to help restore calmness after accidents or bad experiences. Rescue Remedy is available as a stock remedy or a cream – for use on cuts, grazes, burns and bites, as well as skin conditions such as ECZEMA. It is not intended for long-term use and does not replace medical treatment.

---

be alleviated by using proprietary breath fresheners and mouthwashes containing perborate. These are available from chemists and some other stores.

If you find that bad breath persists for more than a week or two, you should see a dentist or doctor for thorough investigation and treatment. As well as treating your teeth and gums, a dentist will be able to teach you the correct way to brush your teeth, and how to keep them in good shape permanently. In addition, he may refer you to a dental hygienist for a proper clean-up.

BALDNESS

The problem begins when new hair does not grow fast enough to replace the normal daily loss caused by the body's fluctuating rhythms and hormone levels. As the thinning process continues, new growth stops altogether in certain parts of the scalp.

Most permanent baldness is due to a common hereditary condition – sometimes combined with other factors such as STRESS, poor diet or poor circulation – that affects men more than women. Thinning usually begins at the temples and crown, and can start as early as the teens, although it is generally most noticeable in middle age. Hair loss is often slow and all the hair is seldom lost. Women are rarely as severely affected, and usually not until after the MENOPAUSE.

Temporary baldness or loss of hair (see HAIR PROBLEMS) can be caused by ANAEMIA, a deficiency of the thyroid hormone, scalp infection, illness, pregnancy, or drugs such as the contraceptive pill, steroids or various antibiotics.

What the therapists recommend

NATUROPATHY

Self help To improve your general health, try embarking on a wholefood diet (see EATING FOR HEALTH) rich in protein foods such as pulses, fish, lean meat, eggs, cheese and nuts – and a cup of fresh lettuce juice every day may also help.

Consultation The naturopath will give advice about diet, coping with stress and learning to relax. He will tell you about HAIR CARE and recommend the best products for you. Supplements may be prescribed – brewer's yeast, vitamin B-complex, multiminerals or kelp, for example. To improve your circulation, you will be advised to take regular outdoor exercise and not smoke.

Other alternative treatments

Traditional Medicine Rural people use an infusion of the leaves of the Cape willow (*Salix mucronata*) to stimulate hair growth. A recipe, used for the same purpose, consists of an oil brewed from these leaves, maidenhair fern leaves, cloves, nutmeg, brandy and maize or sunflower oil. You can also try massaging your scalp with warm almond oil. Leave for an hour, then wash out.

Aromatherapy Mix five drops each of sage and cedarwood essential oils in 30 ml of surgical spirit and massage a sprinkling firmly into the scalp every day. Keep the fingers in the same place and rub so that you feel the skin moving over the bone beneath.

Homoeopathy *Lycopodium* is said to help premature baldness and greying – take the 6X potency twice a day for a month. Hair loss caused by hormones after childbirth or at the menopause, and accompanied by feelings of indifference to loved ones, may be helped by *Sepia* 6X twice a day for a week.

An orthodox view

Doctors support the use of vitamin supplements and tonics for patients who seem run down, but appear to have no other reason for their hair loss. A drug called minoxidil can also be applied to stimulate hair growth. If your appearance worries you a great deal a hair transplant or a wig may help.

Dealing with back pain

At some time in their lives, most people will be stricken with back pain of some sort or other. In all, millions of working days are lost each year in South Africa because of it. Back pain makes more people, including many doctors, seek alternative treatment than any other ailment. Fortunately, however, back pain seldom lasts for more than a few days or weeks, and often goes away on its own. If the pain persists, you should see a doctor in case there is a serious underlying cause. But in most cases back pain is caused by sprains, strains and bad posture. Alternative practitioners believe that, in time, back trouble can be effectively reduced by at least 70 per cent by adopting some simple exercises or therapies.

Most back pain has a simple physical cause – such as inflamed or strained muscles, restricted joints, or pressure on nerves. It can keep recurring, and may not be helped by the routine conventional treatment of painkillers such as aspirin and paracetamol, muscle relaxants and anti-inflammatory drugs.

Conversely, simple expedients such as applying heat and cold can help. A hot-water bottle placed on the painful area can bring temporary relief – as can a pack of crushed ice cubes.

Hold the ice against the area after injury to prevent tissue swelling. After a few days, alternating hot and cold applications can be most effective.

ACUPUNCTURE and MASSAGE, postural training as taught in the ALEXANDER TECHNIQUE, and the manipulative work of osteopaths and chiropractors often prove effective. They also give the victim a chance to take an active part in treating the problem himself.

Nevertheless, you should always be sure to consult a general practitioner before undertaking any alternative treatment – if the back pain does not have a simple physical cause, but is a symptom of something more serious, inappropriate treatment could be potentially dangerous.

If conventional treatment fails to rectify the problem, discuss the matter further with your doctor before you seek alternative treatment.

Finally, although back pain is such a physical ailment, psychological elements should not be overlooked. STRESS and ANXIETY can contribute significantly to back problems, and you are more likely to damage or weaken your back if you, and your back muscles, are tense (see TENSION).

You and your spine

Think of your spine as the central pole that holds up a tent (your body) and the ligaments and muscles supporting it as the guy ropes. If they are tense or distorted they tilt the 'tent', making your back ache.

The spine consists of 24 small bones called vertebrae. There are seven in the neck (cervical); 12 in the upper back (thoracic); and five in the lower back (lumbar). In addition, five fused bones form the continuation of the spine called the sacrum; and four more small bones form the 'tail bone', or coccyx.

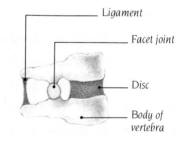

— Ligament

— Facet joint

— Disc

— Body of vertebra

The spinal cord runs through a hole in each of the vertebrae. The body's nerve roots are attached to the cord, linking them to the brain. Pressure on the cord can cause anything from pins and needles to acute pain and even paralysis.

Spinal joints are held together by a network of ligaments, or tough bands of fibre, and a series of facet joints. Together they restrict the movement of the spine in any given direction. The vertebrae are protected by fibre disc 'shock absorbers'.

Spinal muscles Each joint is surrounded by tough, fibrous muscles that receive messages from the brain, making the muscles contract. In turn, this causes the various joints to move as required, usually in pairs, with one contracting while the other one relaxes.

It strikes in many forms...

The pain is most often in the lower back, but it can lead to conditions such as SCIATICA in the leg when the spinal root of the sciatic nerve is irritated, or has been damaged by dislocation of the hip joint.

Sudden (acute) back pain is usually associated with an injury or with a SLIPPED DISC, pulled muscle or torn ligament. It can strike when you are playing games – particularly games that involve sudden, erratic movements – lifting heavy objects, twisting around sharply or simply moving awkwardly. Joint displacement,

or a straining of muscles and ligaments, can also lead to severe pain of the lower back known as LUMBAGO.

Continuous or recurring (chronic) back pain is frequently caused by a longstanding habit of poor posture – for example, if you are inclined to sit slumped in an armchair, stand with your back and shoulders hunched, or walk with a slight stoop. By placing extra strain on the muscles, those who are overweight are particularly likely to develop bad posture.

Sleeping in the wrong position or on the wrong sort of bed often adds to the problem of back pain (see BEDS AND BEDDING). These faults, at least, can quite easily be remedied.

Self-help exercises – designed to bring relief

The following exercises have been specially designed to relieve acute back pain. Start them as soon as you can move without too much discomfort – probably within a day or two of the start of the attack.
Repeat the exercises every few hours daily, until the pain goes. Once you have recovered, Exercise 4 will help to stop further pain.

If you cannot straighten up fully, or if the pain is appreciably worse when you are standing or walking, do not attempt the exercises. Go to bed, rest, and get medical advice as soon as possible.
If the exercises make the pain worse or it spreads to other parts of the body, stop immediately and see a doctor.

Exercise 1
Lie face down with your arms beside your body and head to one side. Take a few deep breaths and relax for four or five minutes.

Exercise 2
Remain lying face down. Place your elbows under your shoulders and lean on your forearms. Take a few deep breaths, then allow your lower back to relax completely, and remain in this position for five minutes.

Exercise 3
Place your hands on the floor beneath your shoulders, straighten your elbows and push up the top half of your body, allowing your back to sag. Hold the position for a few seconds then repeat up to ten times, letting your spine arch upwards a little more with each repetition.

Exercise 4
Stand upright, feet slightly apart, and hands in the small of your back. Bend your trunk backwards as far as you can, keeping the knees straight. Hold for a second or two, then straighten up. Repeat up to ten times, each time trying to bend back as far as you can without losing your balance. Use this exercise also to prevent further back pain, doing it once in a while when working in a forward bent position.

Taking avoiding action

Since his beginnings several million years ago, man has been coping with the discomfort and inconvenience of back pain. Evolution has not completely adapted his spine, which was originally intended for four-legged movement and stance, to functioning on two legs. The spine is involved in every muscular effort, no matter how small, which is why many people cannot attribute their back pain to a specific cause. In some cases it disappears as mysteriously as it appeared. But some everyday activities – such as rising from a chair, getting out of bed and getting dressed – must be done correctly in order to avoid pain.

Getting in and out of an armchair

1 Bring your feet as close as you can to the front of the chair, if possible under the edge. Keep your knees at least a shoulder width apart to provide a good balance.

2 Keep your spine straight, and place your hands on the arms of the chair.

3 Slowly straighten your legs and at the same time bring your buttocks vertically above your feet. Then push yourself out of the chair with your arms.

4 To sit down in a chair, stand with your back to the chair and your feet a shoulder width apart, close to the front of the chair. Keep your back straight, and lower yourself slowly. Place your hands on the arms of the chair as soon as you can.

Getting dressed

Whatever the cause of your back pain, these tips will help you to start the day without straining your back. Avoid sitting down and bending over to put your clothes on – it will strain your back needlessly.

1 Roll your clothes up so that you can put your arms or legs through quickly and easily.

2 If you have difficulty pulling on tights or trousers, try dressing while lying on your back on the bed. Pull your knees up to your chest to get the clothes over your feet, then straighten your legs as you pull the clothes up. Do not arch your back to pull the clothes over your hips.

Alternative treatments

Many victims of back pain despair of ever finding a cure. Alternative treatment can help in many such cases, often providing immediate relief and avoiding prolonged bed rest and time off work. Among the treatments offered are:

Chiropractic A qualified chiropractor will determine if the cause is mechanical – or if another medical condition is to blame. If mechanical, he will apply precise and gentle manipulation to restore normal movement to the joints of the back, allowing them to function properly.

The manipulation may involve gentle twisting, pressing and pulling. Only one session may be needed to correct a ricked back, but a course of treatment to eradicate a bigger problem such as a SLIPPED DISC may call for six or more sessions.

If the chiropractor cannot help you, or suspects that an underlying illness may be causing the back pain, he may refer you to a physician.

Massage Techniques These are gentler than those of chiropractic – and may provide lasting help in dealing with occupational stress and strain, postural tension and muscle fatigue. The aim of massage techniques is to relax the muscles and so relieve and prevent recurrence of pain.

Although occasionally massage does not solve certain structural back problems, it works well against such painful conditions as LUMBAGO and chronic muscle tension. The basic techniques are fairly easily learned and can be practised in the comfort and privacy of your home (see p. 225).

Acupuncture As well as providing relief, this has been found useful when the back pain is too severe for other treatments to take place. For example, muscle spasms and tension can be eased enough to allow massage to be used. For more information on ACUPUNCTURE see p. 14.

Alexander Technique You can be taught during a course of lessons to use your body in a more natural way – and so prevent or alleviate back pain.

See also ACUPRESSURE; HYDROTHERAPY; REFLEXOLOGY; ROLFING; T'AI-CHI CH'UAN.

Getting out of bed
1 Bring your knees up to about hip level and roll over onto your side.

2 Lower your feet to the floor and use your arms to push yourself up into a sitting position. Reverse this procedure to get back into bed.

What the therapists can do

Most forms of back pain can be treated by any one of several alternative therapies – including acupuncture, the Alexander Technique, chiropractic and other massage techniques. Most back pain occurs in the lower back, where strained ligaments are often the cause, and this can be relieved – if not cured – by therapists. However, if there is a more fundamental reason for the pain – such as a kidney complaint (lower back pain) or pleurisy (upper back pain) – then it should be treated by conventional means.

Alexander Technique

Teachers claim that nearly everyone has some kind of postural defect which can be rectified by studying how they move, stand and sit. Sitting problems can be helped by the teacher placing the pupil in the right posture, so that his middle and lower back and neck have the correct amount of curvature.

Chiropractic

A physical examination will be carried out in order to reach a diagnosis. In the treatment of back pain, the patient may be manipulated while sitting upright or lying on one side so that it is easier for the therapist to work on the affected joint. A rapid thrust, without much force, is used to open up the joint and allow it to move.

Acupuncture

At the first consultation, the acupuncturist will ask the patient for a full history of his back pain symptoms, as well as details about his personal life. He will lie the patient on a couch and insert sterilised needles into the appropriate points in the back and legs. The depth of penetration of each needle is said to help to restore body balance and treat the pain.

Massage Techniques

The most common form of massage treatment is Swedish massage which, when applied to the back, includes – stroking; kneading, rolling and squeezing; rubbing in small circular movements against the bone; and flicking and clapping to tone and strengthen the muscles. One of its therapeutic benefits is the feeling of ease and well-being it induces.

Caring for your back

*Many people who suffer from back pain for short or long periods do so
because they do not know how to take care of their backs. Any kind of
physical activity – from running to catch a bus, to sneezing – can affect
the back. In addition, heavy work such as digging in the garden and
carrying loaded shopping bags can result in severe and sometimes
long-lasting pain. In most cases this is cleared up by rest and basic
treatment such as the application of heat to the affected area. However, it is
better to try to avoid pain altogether by taking the following precautions.*

Carrying heavy loads

Wrong *If you have a heavy load when out shopping do not put
all your purchases into one large shopping bag to be carried in one
hand (below right). If you do this, it makes you lopsided and puts
undue strain on the spine.*

Right *Carry two evenly loaded shopping bags, one in each hand,
so that you are well balanced (below). Do not overtire yourself and
rest if necessary, putting the shopping bags down on the ground.*

People who are prone to back pain

There are several 'high risk' occupations associated with a
painful back. If you fall into any of them, take extra care.

Manual workers About 22 per cent of miners, furniture
removers, construction workers, dockers and other manual
workers are regular sufferers.

Nurses About 17 per cent of nurses – who regularly have to
lift bedridden patients, and carry and bend in their work – are
stricken each year.

Office workers Typists and computer operators are prone,
because they often use badly designed chairs that do not give
enough support to the small of the back, and so encourage
the operatives to slouch.

Drivers Long-distance truck drivers, tractor drivers and those
who spend a lot of time behind the wheel are liable to get
lower back pain due to poor posture and the vibration they
experience in their vehicles.

Housewives and mothers Bending to make beds, cleaning,
lifting and carrying babies and small children frequently cause
back problems. Many women start getting back pain during
pregnancy (see *Relieving back pain in pregnancy*).

Athletes Any sport that involves vigorous activity (for
example, football, tennis or squash), or one that makes great
use of a particular set of muscles (for example, weightlifting
or golf), can put undue strain on the back.

The elderly The older you are, the less supple your joints
and muscles are likely to be. Back pain and stiffness may result
– and there is a risk of OSTEOPOROSIS developing.

Previous sufferers If your back has already pained you, it is
liable to 'go' again. Exercise and good posture (see illustrations) help to strengthen the spine and prevent recurring
trouble.

Sitting and driving

Wrong *Do not slouch or slump when
seated (above right), and do not hunch
when driving or reading. Slouching may
feel more comfortable, but it puts great
strain on the back.*

Right *Choose chairs which support the
small of your back – and avoid those
that are too soft or bucket-shaped.
Adopt an upright position and, when
reading, hold the book up and away
from your knees (right).*

Working in the garden
Wrong Do not bend from the hips with straight legs to pick out weeds (above left). This action, and not the digging itself, is the commonest cause of backache in the garden.
Right Go down on one – or both – knees as close to the weeds as possible to save stretching (above right). This applies to picking up any object, not just pulling weeds in the garden.

Lifting an awkward object
Wrong Never stoop when lifting an object such as a tea chest or packing case (below left). Lifting and handling in the wrong way are common causes of back pain.
Right Squat by the object to be lifted (below right). Keep your feet about 30 cm apart. Keep close to the load and pull it into your body while carrying. Wear loose clothes.

Relieving back pain in pregnancy
Many women suffer from low back pain during pregnancy – particularly in the last three months. This is caused mainly by poor posture as the baby gains weight. The mother leans backwards to counterbalance the change in weight distribution – and this often makes the ligaments supporting the spinal joints overstretched and slack. In addition, the ligaments naturally become more elastic so that the pelvis can expand at the moment of birth. The following exercises should help to relieve back pain. If they prove too uncomfortable or difficult, try sitting crosslegged for short periods; or sit on the floor with your legs slightly apart and straight out in front of you; or get on your hands and knees and arch your lower back a few times.

Standing extension (right)
1 Stand up straight with your feet pointing directly forwards, about a shoulder width apart. Place your hands on the small of your back and breathe in deeply.
2 Breathe out slowly. As you do so, bend backwards, supporting your back with your hands, so that your lower back is arched. Repeat ten times.

Pelvic tilt (below)
1 Lie on the floor with your arms at your sides, your feet flat on the floor and your legs bent.
2 Gently press the back of your waist against the floor and tilt your pelvis forwards by tightening your abdominal and buttock muscles. Hold for six seconds, relax slowly, and repeat up to ten times.

Postnatal leg rolls
Practise this toning-up exercise daily from about a week after the birth until your check-up at six weeks. Lie on the bed with arms outstretched, knees bent and feet together. Roll your legs from side to side, and each time you reach the midway position, press your back against the bed. Make sure you feel no discomfort and slowly repeat several times.

BATES METHOD

Can you improve your eyesight without glasses?

Most people who have failing eyesight regard it as part of GROWING OLD, and become resigned to wearing stronger spectacles. Followers of the Bates Method, however, assert that some simple eyesight exercises can help to keep your eyes strong and healthy and prevent them from being misused. The exercises were created by Dr William H Bates, a New York eye specialist.

To achieve and maintain healthy eyesight, most Bates practitioners also recommend a well-balanced diet – not necessarily vegetarian – along with nutritional supplements (see EATING FOR HEALTH) and the use of HOMOEOPATHY. This should be done under the appropriate professional guidance.

The exercises have an educational and not a medical basis. Therefore they are not intended to cure eye diseases such as CATARACTS and glaucoma. In such cases expert medical help should always be sought.

Who it can help Anyone, no matter how good or poor their sight may be, may benefit.
Finding a teacher The Bates method does not form part of ophthalmic or optometric training in South Africa, but there are Bates

The doctor who healed himself

At the end of a particularly tiring day in 1900, Dr William H Bates (1860-1931), a New York ophthalmologist and specialist in children's eye complaints, noted how much his own eyes ached. It reminded him of how often his patients complained of eyestrain and headaches – even after they had responded well to medical treatment.

In the quiet of his darkened office, he rested his elbows on his desk and cupped his palms over his eyes. After ten minutes his eyes stopped aching and he felt mentally refreshed.

Uncupping his hands, he found that objects in his room seemed much clearer and brighter. His observations led him to evolve his 'method of eyesight training', which is described in his best-selling book of 1919, *Better Eyesight Without Glasses*. By the time Bates died his method had gained disciples and practitioners on both sides of the Atlantic.

Seven Bates eye exercises

The seven basic exercises described here were first devised by Dr Bates between 1900 and 1931. The first three are not illustrated, and 'Remembering' is done while you are doing the fourth – 'Palming' (right).

Remembering (not illustrated)
While palming your eyes, try without straining to recall an object or experience in great detail and bright colours. According to Dr Bates, at least one patient found his eyesight was improved by visualising a beautiful yellow buttercup. Remembering things in the mind's eye helps people to see them more clearly in reality, said Dr Bates.

Shifting (not illustrated)
Do not stare fixedly at an object (as spectacle wearers tend to). Instead, move your gaze constantly from one point of interest to another. As your eyes become more relaxed, so the movement becomes smaller, helping your sight to become clearer.

Blinking (not illustrated)
Get into the habit of blinking regularly, once or twice every ten seconds, to clean and lubricate the eyes – especially if you wear glasses or contact lenses.

Palming
Sit comfortably and relaxed at a desk or table. Close your eyes, rest your elbows on a cushion on the table, keeping your back and neck straight and your head level. Then cover your eyes – without touching them – with your cupped palms. Think of something pleasant, such as a favourite holiday spot, or listen to a radio talk, show or play. Do this exercise for about ten minutes, at the very least twice each day – or whenever your eyes feel tired or ache.

Near and far focusing
Hold two pencils, or your index fingers, in front of your face – one about 75 mm away, the other at arm's length. Focus on one with both eyes, then blink and focus on the other. Repeat several times whenever an opportunity arises.

Splashing
First thing every morning, splash your closed eyes 20 times with warm water and then 20 times with cold water to stimulate circulation. Reverse the process last thing at night.

Swinging
Stand with feet apart and sway gently from side to side, letting your eyes swing along with your body's movement. Be aware of the visual movement as this relaxes your eyes and helps them to become more flexible. Repeat whenever an opportunity arises. It often helps to play music while doing this exercise.

The case of Aldous Huxley

In 1939, when the writer Aldous Huxley was 45 years old, he was rapidly losing his eyesight, and needed thick magnifying spectacles to read. Then he heard of the Bates Method, and within two months of starting lessons reported that he was able to read without spectacles, and was doing so without strain or fatigue.

Later he reported that the opacity in his corneas, which had not changed for 25 years, was beginning to clear up. 'My own case is in no way unique,' Huxley continued. 'Thousands of other sufferers from defects of vision have benefited by following the simple rules of that Art of Seeing which we owe to Bates and his followers.'

teachers practising in England. These teachers have no medical qualifications, but have been trained by other teachers. Information locally may be found by consulting books in the public library.
Consulting a teacher Practitioners base their treatment on Dr Bates' principles outlined on the previous page.
Self help Once the basic exercises have been learned, they can easily be practised at home or at work. The simplest ones – such as blinking every few seconds to lubricate the eyes – can be done at any time.

An orthodox view

Eye exercises have proved their value time and again in treating several eye conditions. The Bates Method is, however, a very systematic approach and may be difficult to follow, but anecdotal evidence presented from numerous sources does suggest that it can be a helpful therapy.

Do's and don'ts about your eyes

Bates teachers recommend the following do's and don'ts for those who want to take up the exercises:
Do practise regularly – success is said to depend on persistence.
Do your best to relax when doing the exercises: a stiff neck or tensed shoulder muscles will not help your eyes to relax.
Do read in a good light, and look up briefly at the end of every page.
Do rest your eyes – preferably by palming – when using visual display units (VDUs), for one minute in every twelve.
Don't do the exercises while wearing spectacles or contact lenses.
Don't overwork or strain your eyes while doing the Bates exercises – the aim is to ease tension and relax them, not to force them.
Don't do anything – such as watching a lot of television with the lights off – that blurs vision.

BATHING

Invigorating cures for body and mind

Bathing of many different types has long been practised for its reputed relaxing and health-giving effects. The best known form is probably HYDROTHERAPY, which uses steam or water baths of various types to treat illness, improve circulation and aid the elimination of many impurities from the body. Sunbathing is also very popular and can help some skin conditions such as ACNE. However, great care is needed to avoid SUNBURN.

Herbal baths – particularly hand and foot baths – are an important part of HERBAL MEDICINE and combine the curative powers of herbs with those of water. Many SPAS are famous for their mineral-rich waters, and sea water is used therapeutically – see THALASSOTHERAPY. Mud baths and MUD THERAPY with specially rich soils are also used to treat a variety of complaints including SKIN DISORDERS, ULCERS, ARTHRITIS and RHEUMATISM.

BEDS AND BEDDING

Getting a good night's rest

Most people spend about a third of their lives asleep but pay relatively little attention to their choice of a bed. In fact, everyone has different needs and finding just the right bed for each member of the family is most important. Your bed affects how deeply you sleep and how rested you feel when you wake up. If chosen carefully it will protect your health and speed recovery from illness. A badly chosen bed, however, or one that provides little support, can cause chronic BACK PAIN or muscular TENSION, and may leave you feeling tired after a restless night.

Hard or soft?

It is not always true that the harder the bed you sleep on the better it must be for your back – choosing the right firmness is, more often than not, a matter of compromise. Too soft a bed will not provide the right amount of support and you will sink into the mattress, twisting your spine and suffering varying degrees of discomfort.

However, if a bed is too hard, your muscles will not be able to relax fully and your sleep will be disturbed and restless as you try to get comfortable. You may also suffer from pins and needles or numbness on pressure points such as the hips, shoulders, base of the spine or heels, where the blood flow can become restricted.

Choosing a bed

Base Whatever type of mattress you use, it is advisable to put it on some kind of a base and not just on the floor. Every night your body loses quite a lot of moisture in brea-

thing and sweating, and much of this is absorbed by your mattress. Placing a mattress on the floor prevents air from circulating through it and traps moisture, encouraging the growth of bacteria which may eventually cause rot or mould.

Three main types of base are available:

Solid-topped bases These are hollow, wooden bases which are usually perforated to allow air to circulate. They are covered with a single layer of padding to provide very firm support.

Slatted bases The wooden slats allow air to circulate through the mattress. Some slatted bases are more flexible than others, but generally they provide good support.

Sprung bases These are less firm than the other types, but will support you well if they are combined with the right kind of mattress. They also help the mattress to last longer, as they absorb some of the nightly wear and tear. Avoid sprung bases with firm edges, for although they are cheaper they reduce the sleeping area of the bed and when the springs in the middle start to wear, the edges will remain firm, creating a central hollow.

Mattress In the past, mattresses were just fabric covers filled with whatever materials that were available – straw, horsehair or fea-

thers. Today, a variety of different types is made to cater for our different needs. The mattress is undoubtedly the most important part of any bed and it is essential to take time and care over your choice.

Pocket spring mattresses About a thousand small springs positioned in individual calico pockets support each part of your body independently. These mattresses come in a range of different firmnesses which combine comfort with support, but they need to be used on a spring base. You might find them expensive.

Open-coil spring mattresses These come in a variety of different firmnesses and designs, and are by far the most popular mattresses available in South Africa. They are cheaper than the pocket spring sort, and contain from about 300 larger springs. They do not mould quite as well to the body, but many are still excellent. Special advantages are lightness and good ventilation.

Foam mattresses Many different varieties of these mattresses are available and you need to choose carefully. The best are made from layers of rubber latex or polyurethane which mould to the shape of your body while also providing good support. They are available in different firmnesses and are good in-

Night-time comfort

The perfect mattress combines an underlying firm support with sufficient softness to give where your body presses hardest. In this way you can relax without sagging (right), and can turn over easily. Elderly and heavy people, children and bedridden invalids should have a firm mattress; thin people need more softness. Put the mattress on the correct type of base, which absorbs a proportion of the stress and also enables the mattress to breathe, and it should last the 10-15 years you can expect from a good-quality product.

Too hard

Too soft

Correct

Too hard a mattress may cause numbness on shoulder and hip when you lie on your side, or on the base of the spine and heels when you lie on your back. Too soft a mattress will cause discomfort by letting your spine sag.

Pocket spring mattress *There is maximum independent movement for the springs in this construction, which makes for greatest comfort, particularly for couples of differing weights.*

Open-coil spring mattress *Fewer and larger springs are linked to hold them in place – which reduces individual adjustment to your body contours and weight.*

Foam mattress *A sandwich construction of soft and firm foams is best for combining comfort with support. Foam is dust-free but the base must allow thorough airing.*

sulators, although latex allows more air to circulate and is cooler.

These mattresses will help if you suffer from ALLERGY or ASTHMA as they do not collect dust. However, if you are extremely sensitive to dust it may be better to consider one of the special sterile non-allergenic foam mattresses that are available. Whatever your needs, however, you should avoid the very cheapest type, which distort permanently after only a short time.

Natural-fibre mattresses Wool, horsehair, cotton flocking and coir fibre from coconuts are still used in the manufacture of some mattresses. Many people find natural fibres more comfortable and better ventilated than other types, but these mattresses do tend to be expensive.

Orthopaedic mattresses Very firm mattresses of all designs are sold locally as 'orthopaedic'. In fact, they cannot cure an orthopaedic condition, but do, nevertheless, provide excellent support and can sometimes relieve or prevent back pain.

Futons These Japanese mattresses are becoming increasingly popular in the West, and particularly so in South Africa. Futons are not sprung, but simply consist of layers of cotton or wool felt, sometimes mixed with synthetic fibres. They need a slatted base to allow air movement, and come in different thicknesses. Three layers is the best thickness for a futon, but to get firm, comfortable support you will need to stack two of them, one on top of the other.

It is very important to see that futons are aired and rolled up every day, and a regular shaking out helps to keep the layers even and separate. On the right sort of base they can also be used to sit on and are very useful if you are short of space. They are claimed to help relieve backache and improve health generally, although fragile and elderly people may find them too heavy to handle easily.

Waterbeds These can be effective in providing firm support evenly to all parts of the body, and are used in some hospitals for patients with burns or bedsores.

Double beds Choosing a double bed can be difficult as the needs of both partners – which invariably differ – must be taken into account. If the springs on a double bed are weak or there is a weight difference of more than about 30 kg then the heavier partner is likely to end up sleeping in the middle of the bed and the lighter to be pushed to one side. Even with a smaller weight difference the heavier partner may create a dip in the mattress into which the lighter one rolls. In such cases you may need to buy a good pocket spring mattress or – if there is a big weight difference – separate single units which can be zipped together to form a double bed suited to each partner.

In constant use, a good bed should last about ten years, a cheap one less, and a really expensive one a bit more. After that, it is unlikely to be giving you the comfort and support you need.

Pillows

The choice of pillow is very important. The purpose of a pillow is to support the neck more than the head, and you should, therefore, make sure that you never sleep with only your head on the pillow, or you may strain your neck and upper back muscles. Choose a feather pillow for air circulation, foam if you suffer from allergies, or a contoured one for extra neck support. Herb pillows may help defeat INSOMNIA.

Bed coverings

Duvets are lighter and warmer than blankets, and allow more air to circulate while you are sleeping.

When buying a duvet, choose the filling that suits you best. Down is warmest and lightest but also the most expensive, a feather and down combination is adequate for most needs and allows good ventilation, but if you are allergic to house dust or feathers look for a synthetic filling.

Care for your duvet by shaking it out regularly to keep the filling evenly spaced, or it will collect in the edges and corners and you may feel cold.

Do's and don'ts for buying a bed

Do make sure the bed is at least 15 cm longer than you are – or than the taller partner if you are buying a double bed.

Don't buy a bed or a mattress without lying down on it to see that it supports you well and is comfortable. Couples should try out beds together.

Do buy the best and largest bed you can afford and that will fit into your bedroom. Space is essential, as we move about constantly during sleep and a comfortable bed is necessary for good health.

Do remember that someone who sleeps on his side actually takes up more space – not less – than someone who sleeps on his front or back.

Don't economise on your bed or you may pay the price in terms of health and discomfort. Buy the best you can afford.

BEDWETTING

There are two sorts of bedwetters – children who are never dry, and those who are sometimes dry but then start wetting the bed again. The medical terms for their conditions are primary and secondary enuresis. Both alternative and conventional practitioners stress the importance of not making the child feel shame, and of avoiding all forms of punishment or forceful methods of trying to make the child overcome the problem. Indeed, bedwetting should not even be considered a problem before the child is three or four years old, as children develop bladder control at differing times.

By the age of two and a half, two out of every three children are usually dry in the daytime, and half of them are dry through the night. Six months later, 85 per cent are dry by day and night, barring an occasional accident. At the age of five, only 9 per cent of children are bedwetters; by the time they are 15, only 2 per cent are.

However, though relatively few children have the problem, it can cause much misery and disrupt family relationships. It has been around for as long as clothes have been worn, and some bizarre and painful remedies have been suggested in the past – placing burning leaves between the child's legs; making the child eat the crop from a cock; sprinkling dried sow's bladder over its head.

Only in recent times has a more enlightened and understanding approach been followed. Most primary enuresis is caused by a slow development of bladder control – much as some children are slower than others in learning to read. The usual cause of secondary enuresis is some ANXIETY or psychological upset, such as parental rows or a new baby arriving. Parents can also foster anxiety by starting pot training too soon, or being too fussy or insistent about it.

Other causes of bedwetting are urinary infections (see BLADDER PROBLEMS) or a congenital bladder abnormality. Occasionally there may be complex causes – certainly if the child has been punished or abused the problem may not only get worse, but his distress and psychological disorder may deepen. Finally, bedwetting can also be used by the child as an attention-seeking ploy. Until the problem is overcome, fit the bed with a waterproof sheet or mattress.

What the therapists recommend
BEHAVIOURAL THERAPY
Self help Gentle conditioning, in which the child is encouraged to become involved, has proved very successful. A special pad is placed under the sheet in the bed. Any water (urine) penetrating to the pad activates a

buzzer, which wakes the child who can then switch it off. Three out of every four bedwetters given a buzzer become dry. See also An *orthodox view*, below.

COUNSELLING

Consultation Both parents and the child are involved, and the child is given a positive role – for example, keeping a calendar or diary in which stars are awarded for 'dry nights', with perhaps a small prize or reward for stars accumulated, and praise and encouragement offered for each dry night.

HERBAL MEDICINE

Consultation If there are psychological factors, such as anxiety, a herbalist would probably concentrate on trying to relieve them. St John's wort may be prescribed as a gentle relaxant and antidepressant. Horsetail tea may be suggested to help empty the bladder and gently tone the muscles.

An orthodox view

A doctor may well recommend the counselling or 'buzzer' conditioning treatments outlined above, and can advise on where to obtain a pad. But he will first encourage both parents and child to keep in mind that the problem is most likely to disappear of its own accord, and to accept bedwetting as part of the child's natural development. This may give the child enough confidence to talk about his worries or fears (of darkness, perhaps), and he should be urged to do so.

On a practical level, the child may be told not to drink just before going to bed, and to visit the lavatory last thing. Those who fail to respond to the buzzer (some sleep so soundly they never even hear it) may be given an antidepressant drug to reduce wetting – though whether this works by relieving some subconscious depression or by a direct effect upon the bladder is not known. In difficult cases, perhaps involving a physical abnormality, the doctor may call for a specialist opinion.

BEE STINGS

When a bee stings it leaves both its sting and a poison bag in the skin. The poison is not dangerous unless it causes an allergic reaction (see ALLERGY), but pain is immediate and lasts from three to six hours. Swelling, inflammation and itching follow – usually clearing up after a few days.

If the sting becomes infected, the victim may become feverish and have painful joints for two or three days. An allergic reaction will cause severe swelling, which can spread over the body. In rare cases, where the victim is extremely sensitive, there may be anaphylactic SHOCK, with difficulty in breathing, unconsciousness and sometimes even death. See a doctor as soon as possible if symptoms indicate an allergic reaction.

Self help Remove the sting by easing it out with a fingernail in the opposite direction to the line of entry, taking care not to burst the poison bag.

What the therapists recommend

Traditional Medicine Dabbed onto the sting, an infusion of the leaves of either the wild dagga (*Leonotis leonurus*) or klipdagga (*Leonotis leonitis*) plant can provide relief. You can also apply crumbled leaves of plantain – the common, broad-leaved weed – to the wound. Alternatively, heat crumbled or broken plantain leaves gently over a match flame until they wilt (do not burn), then squeeze them and apply the juice.

Homoeopathy *Ledum* is believed to be most effective, helping to relieve redness, swelling, stinging and pricking pains. Take a dose every one to three hours until the discomfort stops.

Apis mellifica is recommended if *Ledum* has not reduced the pain and swelling after four hours, or if the site of the sting is painful, swollen, red and feels hot. Take one pill every four hours. For very severe reactions, use the remedies in the 200X potency, taken every half hour for two or three doses. Otherwise, use the 30X potency.

Naturopathy Plunge the affected area immediately into a bowl of water, with a teaspoon of bicarbonate of soda and ice cubes – cold slows the circulation and helps to stop the poison spreading. Swift relief may also be obtained by holding or taping a freshly cut slice of raw onion over the affected area, or by smearing the site gently with wheat-germ oil, placing an ice bag on top, then applying soothing calendula cream.

An orthodox view

Except in serious cases, the only treatment needed after removing the sting is to clean the area with an antiseptic or smooth on an antihistamine cream, available from chemists, to prevent infection.

If there is a severe reaction to the sting, a doctor will prescribe steroids, antibiotics, antihistamine tablets or painkilling drugs to combat inflammation or infection.

Some people are highly allergic to bee stings and may need rapid emergency treatment. Such people should wear a Medic-alert bracelet or necklace, and a doctor should be consulted immediately. An antihistamine injection will be given for acute allergy and the victim taken into hospital and treated for anaphylactic shock.

Insect repellents available from chemists may help to prevent bee stings. See also MOSQUITO BITES, WASP STINGS.

BEHAVIOURAL THERAPY

Learning to overcome problems

When you laugh at a friend's joke, raise your voice in anger, punish a naughty child or reward a good one, you are practising a subtle sort of behavioural therapy. In dozens of everyday situations like these we all encourage other people to behave in the way we would like them to. We want our friends to be amusing, our enemies to feel intimidated and our children to get on with others and to do well.

In the same way, behavioural therapists use rewards – and sometimes punishments – to help people to overcome harmful or antisocial behaviour such as SMOKING, drinking too much, personal violence or giving in to unreasonable FEAR.

The therapy is based on the idea that bad behaviour is often something that has been learned – from whatever source or example – and can be 'unlearned' by training, to be replaced by something better. Accordingly, children may actually be taught to behave badly by parents or teachers, who reward disruptive behaviour with extra attention; or young people may learn to drink heavily to conform and win acceptance among their drinking friends.

Many disaster victims have found that their experiences leave long-lasting behaviour problems, such as a fear of enclosed spaces (see CLAUSTROPHOBIA). Therapists aim to overcome these difficulties by teaching victims to respond to them in different and more constructive ways.

Finding a therapist Behavioural therapy is covered in most clinical training courses. Clinical psychologists are listed in the Yellow Pages of all telephone directories but for details of specific therapies practised contact the Psychological Association of South Africa, P O Box 2729, Pretoria 0001 (telephone 012-3261981).

Consulting a therapist The therapist will talk over your problem in detail, asking when it began, exactly what happens on each occasion, and in what manner you and others close to you cope with it. He will then choose an appropriate treatment and begin a course of behavioural retraining, usually involving one visit a week. A typical course might last for three months.

How the principles of modern behavioural therapy developed

In the late 19th century, a Russian scientist named Ivan Pavlov (1849-1936) became internationally renowned for experiments in which he trained dogs to salivate at the sound of a bell, which they immediately associated with the arrival of food. He called this process *conditioning* and used it to study how some human behaviour was learned.

In America J B Watson developed similar ideas in the early decades of the 20th century, and they became known as Behaviourism. The underlying principles that the two dedicated psychologists established still form the basis of modern behavioural therapy.

After the Second World War, another American psychologist, Burrhus Skinner, got animals and people to play an active part in the learning process – unlike Pavlov, whose dogs were passive participants.

Skinner developed the theory of *reinforcement* – a kind of reward or pleasant experience that makes it more likely that the behaviour required will be repeated.

For example, AGORAPHOBIA, an irrational, overpowering fear of open spaces, may become more entrenched by the relief a person experiences when staying indoors.

This relief encourages him to remain indoors longer and longer until he cannot go out at all.

Skinner's solution to this sort of problem was to get the person to associate his unwillingness to go outside with bad experiences, while associating ventures outdoors with some sort of reward. Today, these methods are still used to help people overcome their difficulties.

However, Skinner took Behaviourism to extremes by suggesting that it could be used to control *all* human behaviour and so create a perfect society run by psychologists.

Fortunately, most behavioural psychologists were not impressed with these extreme ideas and did not take them very seriously, but universally behavioural techniques are still used on a purely personal level, with the patient's full knowledge and consent.

PHOBIAS and fears can often be overcome using a technique known as *systematic desensitisation*. The patient practises relaxation exercises while imagining increasingly disturbing or frightening situations. When he is able to stay completely calm, the therapist gradually allows him to experience the real situations, while still helping him to relax. Eventually the relaxed response becomes so well learned that it comes naturally, and the fear or phobia is overcome.

A quicker 'shock' method of dealing with some fears is called *flooding* or *forced exposure*. The patient is confronted with the situation he most fears.

At first he is terrified, but as time passes, the fear begins to exhaust itself and rational control gradually starts to take over again. Many patients, to their delight, have learned to tolerate insects, heights, confined spaces and snakes in this way.

ALCOHOLISM is sometimes treated by AVERSION THERAPY, a method which involves taking a drug such as disulfiram (Antabuse) that causes a feeling of nausea when a person drinks alcohol.

Eventually the mind starts to associate drinking and nausea so closely that all desire for alcohol is lost.

A less drastic form known as *imaginal aversion* uses imaginary unpleasant associations to break bad habits – for example, it may be easier to stop smoking if you imagine each cigarette smeared with something repulsive before putting it to your lips.

Who it can help Therapists claim most success in treating specific problems such as smoking, excessive drinking, OBSESSIVE-COMPULSIVE BEHAVIOUR, phobias and fears, and children's problems such as BEDWETTING and school phobias.

Some special techniques, such as desensitisation, tend to work best for children and adults who do not think much about their motives and why they behave as they do; other kinds of techniques, such as *imaginal aversion*, are used for motivated and imaginative patients.

Like most forms of PSYCHOTHERAPY, the training is most effective when you have a feeling of empathy towards the therapist and feel that he is genuinely helpful, kind and interested in your problem. It is also more successful when the undesirable behaviour is not pleasurable – it is easier to overcome a fear of snakes than to give up smoking or heavy drinking.

An orthodox view

Behavioural therapy is based on scientific research into how people learn, and doctors accept that it can often help patients to overcome problems which conventional medicine cannot treat.

BILHARZIASIS

How humans serve as hosts to a persistent parasite

A parasitic worm, the schistosome, is responsible for the spread of bilharziasis (or bilharzia), a disease named only in the mid-19th century but known to have existed in antiquity. Water is essential to the complex life-cycle of the parasite, and it is the medium by which a person may become infected, when larvae in the water penetrate the skin.

Having travelled to the liver the larvae develop into adult worms that mate, then travel to other parts of the body. Here the eggs are laid; and when these are excreted in the urine and faeces they survive only if they enter fresh water. Essential at this stage, too, is the presence in the water of particular species of snail, which act as hosts to the bilharzia hatchlings. It is from these snails that the bilharzia larvae are in due course emitted.

A few days after a person has come in contact with infected water a skin rash will develop. An allergic reaction follows later, with the development of influenza-like symptoms including fever, chills and muscular pains. Severe symptoms occur after about three months: diarrhoea, abdominal pain, blood in the urine or faeces, and a burning sensation during urination.

What the therapists recommend

Homoeopathy The nature of the treatment will depend not only on the immediate symptoms but on the homoeopath's wider assessment of the patient's health and character.

An orthodox view

A course of drugs is prescribed to eliminate the parasite. A single dosage of the drug praziquantel may be sufficient to achieve this. No vaccine against bilharziasis is available.

BILIOUS ATTACK

Bile, also called gall, looks like motor oil and is a bitter, yellow-brown or yellow-green fluid produced by the liver, and stored in the gall bladder. About half a litre or more is produced daily, and its job is to break down food passing through the duodenum (the first part of the intestine), allowing it to be digested and absorbed. Bile also helps the liver to detoxify poisonous substances. During a true bilious attack, bile is brought up from the duodenum into the mouth, but this is rare. The term is often used loosely by lay people for any episode of NAUSEA AND VOMITING, particularly one from an ACID STOMACH.

BIOCHEMIC TISSUE SALTS

Mineral remedies for everyday ailments

A correct balance of the natural mineral salts found in the body is essential for health, and biochemic tissue salts can help to maintain or restore that balance, say practitioners who prescribe them.

They believe that an imbalance or lack of these salts can cause a range of illnesses, while replacing them in small, easily absorbed doses restores balance and allows the body to heal itself.

Biochemics was developed in the 1870s by a German homoeopathic physician, Dr Wilhelm Schuessler, who coined both the terms 'biochemics' and 'tissue salts'. He named 12 tissue salts as being vital for good health, and he described exactly what each of them did in the human body. Dr Schuessler also listed the ailments which he claimed could be cured by patients using tissue salts as medicines in tablet form.

The 12 tissue salts (see box) are also listed in the homoeopathic range of medicines, and are prepared in the same way – but the two therapies are quite different. While biochemics makes good the mineral deficiency believed to be causing the disease, the homoeopathic philosophy of 'like cures like' prescribes remedies to induce the symptoms of the disease in a healthy person, and is also concerned with the patient's mental and emotional levels.

Who it can help Biochemics claims to help alleviate many everyday aches and pains, and the tissue salts should be used to treat only simple, easily recognised symptoms that are usually self-healing, such as those associated with INDIGESTION, COLDS, HAY FEVER, TENSION, muscular PAIN, minor SKIN DISORDERS, cuts and burns. It may be possible to use tissue salts alongside medications prescribed by a doctor.

Consulting a therapist Naturopaths, herbalists and homoeopaths often prescribe tissue salts when they believe that the body is not producing enough mineral salts for good health, but biochemics is principally a self-help treatment. However, if you are already being treated by a doctor or an alternative practitioner, you should consult him or her before using any of the biochemic remedies.

Self-help Tissue salts are available from health stores and some chemists. They are prepared in highly diluted doses – their usual potency being 6X, which means one part of the active ingredient is mixed with nine parts

The tissue salts and their uses

Here is a list of Schuessler's 12 tissue salts with their numbers, names, chemical names, what they are claimed to do and the conditions for which they are believed to be useful.

1 *Calc. fluor.* Calcium fluoride
Helps promote elasticity of tissues. Used for PILES, ruptures, strained tendons, VARICOSE VEINS, muscle weakness, stretch marks, CIRCULATION PROBLEMS, COLD SORES at the corners of the mouth, cracked tongue and lips.

2 *Calc. phos.* Calcium phosphate
Helps build new blood cells, strengthens bones and teeth, aids digestion. Used for poor circulation, CHILBLAINS, indigestion, lowered vitality, iron-deficiency ANAEMIA, and during convalescence. Also for decaying teeth and teething problems.

3 *Calc. sulph.* Calcium sulphate
Blood constituent and purifier. Used for spots during adolescence, sore lips, slow-healing skin and wounds.

4 *Ferr. phos.* Iron phosphate
Constituent of red blood corpuscles which helps to distribute oxygen in the body. Used for inflammation of the skin, feverishness, chestiness, sore throat, coughs, colds, chills and muscular RHEUMATISM.

5 *Kali mur.* Potassium chloride
Used for respiratory disorders such as ASTHMA and BRONCHITIS; also for CATARRH, colds, WHEEZING, sore throat, TONSILLITIS, sluggish digestion.

6 *Kali phos.* Potassium phosphate
A nerve soother and nutrient. Used for tension, HEADACHES, indigestion, DEPRESSION, loss of sleep and irritability due to worry or excitement.

7 *Kali sulph.* Potassium sulphate
Promotes and maintains healthy skin. Used for minor skin eruptions with scaling, sticky or yellowish discharge, discharge of the nose or throat, catarrh, and poor condition of nails, hair and scalp.

8 *Mag. phos.* Magnesium phosphate
Nerve and muscle fibre nutrient. Used to relieve darting pains, CRAMP and menstrual pains, acute spasms, HICCUPS, COLIC and WIND.

9 *Nat. mur.* Sodium chloride
Controls distribution of water in the body. Used for watery colds with flow of tears and runny nose; loss of smell or taste.

10 *Nat. phos.* Sodium phosphate
Acid-alkaline regulator of the cells. Used for acidity, HEARTBURN, gastric indigestion and rheumatic pains.

11 *Nat. sulph.* Sodium sulphate
Balances body water. Used for queasiness, MORNING SICKNESS, DIGESTIVE PROBLEMS, BILIOUS ATTACK, colic, INFLUENZA symptoms and headaches.

12 *Silica* Silicon dioxide
Conditioner and cleanser, eliminates waste. Used for toxic accumulations, PIMPLES AND SPOTS, BOILS, STYES.

The combination biochemic tissue salts
The following are combination remedies – in which salts have been chosen for their effects on different aspects of a problem – and their uses.
Combination A, for NEURALGIA, neuritis, SCIATICA.
Combination B, for nervous exhaustion, edginess, general debility and during convalescence.
Combination C, for acidity, heartburn.
Combination D, for minor skin ailments.
Combination E, for flatulence, indigestion and colic.
Combination F, for nervous and MIGRAINE headaches.
Combination G, for backache, LUMBAGO and piles.
Combination H, for hay fever.
Combination I, for fibrositis, muscular pain.
Combination J, for COUGHS, colds and chestiness.
Combination K, for brittle nails, hair loss.
Combination L, for VARICOSE VEINS.
Combination M, for rheumatic conditions.
Combination N, for menstrual pain.
Combination P, for aching feet and legs, and also chilblains.
Combination Q, for catarrh, sinus disorders.
Combination R, for infants' teething pains.
Combination S, for biliousness and stomach upsets.

lactose (milk sugar) and the process repeated a further six times, as in HOMOEOPATHY. The patient notes his symptoms and takes the salt or combination of salts recommended for him – though time and patience may be needed to find exactly which salts work best for individual cases.

Each salt is known by a certain number and an abbreviated name, and combination remedies are known by a letter. Homoeopa-

Dr W Schuessler (1821-98), who developed the tissue salts, was a physician in Oldenburg, near Hamburg in Germany.

Bioenergetic exercises

Some typical exercises performed in bioenergetic classes include:

Grounding   The way you stand and 'ground' your feet is seen as a sign of your emotional security. Bioenergetics regards the legs and feet as the primary way we maintain contact with the reality of our lives. Exercises in grounding include getting group members to explore different ways of using their feet – such as tip-toeing or stamping – and then discussing how each person responded to them.

Animal game   Each member of the group chooses an animal with which he identifies, and then imitates its stance and behaviour. For example, a person may find that he readily identifies with a leopard, which is 'always on the hunt', and this may help him to learn more about his personal relationships.

Breathing   This plays an important part in bioenergetics, and the ability to breathe freely and fully is held to reflect emotional well-being.

Nervousness, fear, anger and depression can all cause unnatural breathing patterns. The subject will be encouraged to correct these by practising regular diaphragmatic breathing.

thic chemists can supply them as required. The small, moulded, lactose-based tablets are dissolved in the mouth.

The frequency and regularity of doses taken is considered to be most important – every half hour if the symptoms are sudden and short-lived; every two hours if they are long-lasting.

The tablets are absorbed quickly into the bloodstream, and give prompt relief in sudden, short-term conditions such as colds and flu. Response to long-standing ailments can be slow, taking six months or more.

It is claimed that the tissue salts will not mask any symptoms they cannot treat; instead the symptoms will persist – an indication that the patient should seek orthodox medical advice.

Warning   Because the tablets are lactose-based, anyone with a milk-sugar intolerance (see ALLERGY) should buy them in another form in case of side effects. Diarrhoea, a bloated stomach and FLATULENCE occurring after drinking milk can be indications of lactose intolerance.

An orthodox view

Research has now shown that there are at least 12 tissue salts in the body. Doctors do not agree that all diseases treated by biochemics are due to tissue salt imbalance, however, and there is currently no scientific evidence that biochemic remedies have any therapeutic effect.

But it is generally agreed that the salts are gentle, non-toxic and non-habit-forming and that Dr Schuessler's dozen are basic to the maintenance of good health.

There are no side effects unless a person is allergic to lactose. If there is a danger, it is that someone with a serious condition may continue self-treatment when he is in need of medical attention.

BIOENERGETICS

A healthy integration of body and mind

Those who practise bioenergetics believe that a form of energy creates an interaction between our body and mind, governing both our physical and our mental states. Although nobody has yet been able to find or measure this energy force – known variously as Qi (chi), prana, life force, vitalism, and so on – it is said to affect everyone.

Bioenergetics counsellors or therapists cite as one example of its effect the common experience of 'up' days, when we feel bright and full of energy, and 'down' days, when we feel dull and lethargic.

The concept of a body-mind energy forms the basis of Eastern therapies or philosophies such as YOGA, T'AI-CHI CH'UAN and ACU-PUNCTURE, which collectively have a massive following worldwide. Sigmund Freud, the founder of psychoanalysis, made use of a similar idea – which he called 'libido' or psychic energy.

This concept of Freud's was taken further by one of his followers, Wilhelm Reich, who renamed it 'orgone' and identified it with sexual energy (see REICHIAN THERAPY and OR-GONE THERAPY).

Although Reich's theories eventually fell into disrepute, one of his American pupils, Dr Alexander Lowen, used aspects of Reich's work as a basis for the theory of bioenergetics. He first developed these ideas during the 1960s, and bioenergetics is now recognised as a legitimate form of therapy by many psychotherapists.

Our everyday language is full of expressions that acknowledge how our emotions affect our bodies. We speak of being 'flushed with pride', 'overburdened with grief', of being 'tickled pink'. And sometimes even talk of having 'butterflies in the stomach' – an allusion to nervousness.

Bioenergetic therapists believe that personal psychological problems, STRESS, negative attitudes and emotions such as anger and FEAR all affect the way we sit, stand, move and breathe. For example, therapists observe that an obstinate, defensive type of person tends to adopt a characteristic body posture which involves almost literally 'digging his heels in'.

The purpose of bioenergetic therapy is primarily to help people to become aware of their habitual postures and body movements – known as 'character armouring' – and the emotions that are associated with them. By doing certain exercises they are then taught ways of 'unlocking' this armouring, so that the body regains its ability to function freely and naturally.

Through the 'unlocking' process, the original emotional problem is effectively 'released' and COUNSELLING can then help.

Who it can help   As with many newer therapies, bioenergetics offers a range of different benefits to different people. Because of its focus on personal growth rather than the treatment of illness, many people use bioenergetics simply to learn more about themselves.

Other people, however, have reported that it has helped them with a variety of complaints ranging from severe MIGRAINE and AS-THMA to IRRITABLE BOWEL SYNDROME and peptic ULCERS.

Some people also practise bioenergetics as a Western form of yoga, using it to keep fit and increase their general bodily awareness. It claims to help those who suffer from a poor self-image – those who may feel too fat or too thin, or are otherwise unhappy with their looks – to develop a more positive attitude to their bodies.

Nearly all participants – whatever their reasons for joining a group in the first place – report having 'more energy' or feeling 'more alive' after a bioenergetics class.

Finding a therapist Although bioenergetics is very popular in some European countries, and in parts of the United States of America, there are few practising therapists as yet in South Africa, and classes can be difficult to find.

Seeing a therapist The first consultation is usually an individual one, but for later sessions the subject normally joins a group of about eight or ten people for either a two-day workshop or a series of weekly meetings. There is no set procedure for the way that groups are conducted, but classes usually combine a series of exercises (see box on previous page) with a period of discussion.

An orthodox view

Since no way has yet been found to measure bioenergy objectively, scientists and doctors have not been able to confirm or repudiate the claims made for bioenergetic therapy. The only evidence that exists is the accounts of participants, and these are considered too subjective to constitute scientific proof.

BIOFEEDBACK

Machines to measure body and mind

The lie detector used by police and courts in the United States is just one of many biofeedback machines and instruments developed to monitor changes in people's physical and mental states.

Therapists in biofeedback use the machines to let patients actually observe these changes – for example, in their body temperature and brain wave patterns. The patient is then taught to carefully control these bodily functions by techniques such as VISUALISATION THERAPY, RELAXATION AND BREATHING, and MEDITATION. This is called biofeedback training.

The instruments themselves do not affect the workings of the body in any way, but simply provide information. As the patient becomes increasingly expert at recognising and altering his responses, he is able to avoid conditions such as ANXIETY or raised BLOOD PRESSURE.

How biofeedback training techniques work is not fully understood, but it is clear that they can affect the part of the nervous system that determines how active or relaxed our bodies are. This is known as the autonomic nervous system, and governs responses such as blood pressure, skin temperature, digestion and muscular TENSION, which until quite recently were thought to be entirely involuntary. Biofeedback has shown that this is not so, and that most people can learn a certain amount of control.

Who it can help Proper biofeedback training can be used to teach people relaxation and meditation techniques or to help a number of illnesses. For example, MIGRAINE attacks and tension HEADACHES – which are associated with cold hands – have been prevented by teaching patients to raise the temperature of their hands. Many people have used it to reduce their blood pressure without taking drugs.

HYPERVENTILATION – a symptom of panic or anxiety – may be controlled by learning breathing techniques with the aid of biofeedback. Therapists also claim that many illnesses and stress-related conditions can be avoided by using biofeedback techniques to learn how to relax at times during the day.

Finding a therapist Biofeedback is not widely used in South Africa, where it is still in its infancy. It is usually combined with other therapies, and the equipment for it is imported. To find a therapist, consult the psychology department of your local university or hospital.

Consulting a therapist Patients are usually seeking help in learning to relax, or to overcome specific physical or psychological problems. The therapist selects the most suitable equipment – an electrical skin resistance gauge for anxiety, or hand-held thermometer for headaches, for example – and explains how it works. The patient is then attached to the equipment so that he can see or hear a continuous signal measuring his responses.

However, before training actually starts, the therapist may demonstrate that the act of willing alone is not sufficient to bring about changes in the physical states being measured. Depending on which responses are being tested, the patient will be asked to try to cause a change – for example, to raise the temperature of his hand or to lower the tension in his facial muscles. Most people find that the harder they try, the more they tense up.

To overcome this problem, the therapist can use a number of special techniques that work at a deeper, less conscious level. These include diaphragmatic breathing (see p. 299), progressive muscular relaxation (see p. 301), autohypnotic suggestion, visualisation and meditation.

Most of these techniques involve the subject suspending the conscious will and trying to change the physical state indirectly or by using imagination – a process which is called 'passive volition'.

When the patient does this successfully, the signal from the biofeedback equipment changes, indicating that his physical state has been influenced.

This makes it easier to learn the passive volition techniques, for the patient knows when he is making progress and can adjust his behaviour accordingly.

For treatment to be effective, the patient must also practise the new techniques at home without the aid of biofeedback equipment. Training sessions – usually six, one a week – continue until physical responses can be controlled at will. After that, continued good health depends on regular practice.

Instruments used in biofeedback include the hand-held thermometer (above), which can measure anxiety levels because the hands grow colder as anxiety rises. The electric skin resistance (ESR) gauge (left) is similar to a lie detector. Anxiety and fear cause the hands to sweat, reducing the skin's resistance to a small electric current.

Sample biorhythm chart

The purple, green and red waves show respectively the subject's fluctuating intellectual, emotional and physical cycles for a particular 33 day period. When a wave is above the caution line, it is in an active, high-energy phase; when below the caution line, in a passive phase storing energy for the next peak; and when crossing the line a 'caution' day occurs and accidents or mistakes may happen. The most difficult days are when two curves cross the caution line – June 2 on the chart, for example.

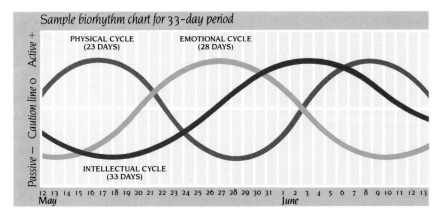

Self help Biofeedback equipment for use in the home is usually imported. Enquire at the psychology department of your nearest university or hospital.

An orthodox view

Biofeedback training is one of the few alternative therapies that is based on scientific principles. Most of the instruments were originally designed for use in scientific and medical research, and the effects they measure are accepted by doctors as accurate indications of bodily processes. Even though doctors do not know how activities such as meditation and breathing can influence these processes, they accept that measurable changes do often occur.

One scientific study in the mid-1970s found that after biofeedback training, about a third of patients taking drugs for high blood pressure were able to bring their pressure ratings down to normal without drugs. Another clinical experiment found that biofeedback helped four out of five migraine patients to relieve their symptoms.

BIORHYTHMS

Explaining life's ups and downs

We all have our 'up' days, when everything runs smoothly, and 'down' days, when however hard we try, nothing goes right, we lack concentration and feel accident prone. These physical, emotional and intellectual ups and downs are thought to be controlled by three internal body clocks or 'cycles', called 'biorhythms'. The physical and emotional cycles were charted quite independently by two doctors, Wilhelm Fliess and Herman Swoboda, around 1900, and the third was discovered by an engineer, Professor Alfred Teltscher, 20 years later.

The physical cycle lasts 23 days, and is said to govern vitality, strength, endurance, confidence, sex drive, and immunity to and recovery from illness. The 28 day emotional (sensitivity) cycle is held to govern moods, nervous reactions and creative ability, and the 33 day intellectual cycle decision-making, memory and learning ability.

An individual's cycles can be shown on a graph as waves moving above and below a horizontal line called a 'caution' line. The graph gives an at-a-glance picture of the kind of ups, downs and caution (or 'critical') days the person may expect in the weeks ahead.
Who they can help It is believed that everyone can benefit from understanding the relationship between their pattern of biorhythms and their pattern of behaviour. A chart cannot predict whether someone is going to have an accident or catch a cold, but it may help them to avoid one.

It is believed that the date of a surgical operation, if chosen with care using a chart, can enhance the patient's chances of making a good recovery, although this has not received any orthodox approval, or been proved scientifically.
Finding out about biorhythms Individual biorhythmic forecasts calculated by computer for six to 12 months ahead are available from various agencies which advertise in alternative and health magazines, and in the personal columns of some newspapers.

Alternatively, if you prefer, you can work out your own chart with the aid of books which contain charts to make this process easier. There are calculators that will work out your cycles accurately when you key in your birthdate.

An orthodox view

Biorhythms offer a scientifically acceptable theory for human mood swings. However, while many scientists accept the concept of biorhythms, most do not consider it a sufficiently accurate basis on which to predict or treat patients.

BLACKOUT

This momentary loss of consciousness happens when the brain does not get enough oxygen. There are a number of causes, a very common one being a drop in BLOOD PRESSURE – for example, when you stand up suddenly or have to stand for long periods. If you suffer from blackouts, see a doctor for diagnosis and treatment. See also DIZZINESS and FAINTING.

BLACKWATER FEVER

When red blood cells in the body are under siege

This potentially life-threatening illness develops as a complication of malignant tertian MALARIA (the most dangerous form of the disease), and it may also result when BILHARZIA cases are neglected. There is a 20-30 per cent chance of death.

Red blood cells in the body are destroyed at a great rate, and when the products of these cells find their way to the kidneys the urine is dyed black or very dark – hence the name blackwater fever. Various other body tissues are discoloured yellow (jaundice); the patient is subject to chills, vomiting and kidney failure.

What the therapists say

Naturopathy Blackwater fever is a medical emergency, to be dealt with in hospital. Post-hospital naturopathic treatment would be similar to that for other fevers. The patient is secreting a much-diminished supply of digestive juices and cannot cope with normal meals, so should be discouraged from eating for some days.

An orthodox view

A doctor should be consulted immediately, and the patient should be hospitalised as soon as possible. In hospital the patient will be given renal support.

He or she will be encouraged to drink plenty of alkaline fluids, and may also be given an intravenous drip of glucose and bicarbonate of soda. A blood transfusion may be needed.

The quinine taken by malaria patients may be a factor contributing to blackwater fever, and this drug should therefore be stopped.

BLADDER PROBLEMS

Embarrassing symptoms such as INCONTINENCE make sufferers reluctant to talk about bladder problems, so they are much more common than is generally realised. Over the age of 65, one woman in every 12 and one man in every 70 is bladder incontinent – making it by far the most common problem. It takes several forms:

Stress incontinence Women are the main sufferers – the condition is usually the result of childbirth or a surgical operation weakening the pelvic muscles. The first symptom may only be a few drops of urine leaking whenever you cough or strain; eventually any slight physical effort such as bending can cause a leakage.

Urge incontinence Both sexes are vulnerable. Sufferers usually cannot reach the lavatory in time when the need arises. This can happen unexpectedly several times an hour and be exhausting.

Dribbling incontinence This is more common among men – a leakage of urine can occur at any time without the man even being aware of it. PROSTATE PROBLEMS are the usual cause: the bladder is never properly emptied, so urine continues to dribble out.

Incontinence can also result from a bladder infection (see CYSTITIS), or a stroke or spinal injury, so it is important to see your general practitioner immediately if you develop the condition. Many of the measures that help to combat incontinence can also help to prevent it.

Problems other than those of incontinence include bladder CANCER and bladder stones – both relatively rare. Bladder cancer can result from working near certain dyeing chemicals, and SMOKING can also increase the risk of contracting it. Symptoms may not appear until the cancer has grown quite large, and include blood or mucus in the urine.

What the therapists recommend

Naturopathy A practitioner will generally recommend a diet which is high in FIBRE, and the avoidance of CONSTIPATION, which aggravates bladder problems. The diet will also be low in kilojoules (see EATING FOR HEALTH), as being overweight puts extra, unwanted pressure on the bladder. Regular EXERCISE, especially any designed to strengthen the abdominal and pelvic muscles, will also be recommended.

Herbal Medicine Many South African indigenous plants, infused in water, are still used in rural areas to alleviate bladder ailments; the best known is buchu (Agathosma betulina), while others include the cancer bush, the wild rose geranium, the water lily (root and stem) and the wild olive (root). A tea made from the root of the bitter apple (Kei apple) clears a bladder infection. A herbalist may advise a naturopathic diet and exercise, and may also prescribe arbutus (ground laurel).

An orthodox view

Many doctors in this country and abroad feel that with most common bladder problems prevention is much more effective than cure, and will recommend the same sort of general good health guidelines on diet and exercise as a naturopath.

If a doctor suspects a bladder infection, the urine will be tested and if necessary an antibiotic prescribed.

If prostate problems are diagnosed, an operation may be required. In the case of bladder stones, large ones can be removed surgically; sometimes they can be disintegrated by powerful sound waves.

BLISTERS

These small swellings are formed by pockets of watery fluid collecting underneath the skin. They can be caused by friction (for example, by wearing badly fitting shoes), burns, SUNBURN, insect STINGS AND BITES, or by coming into contact with irritating substances. Some infections, such as COLDSORES, CHICKENPOX, SHINGLES and IMPETIGO, may also cause blisters.

What the therapists recommend

Traditional Medicine Applying the leaves of the spekboom, the water lily or traveller's joy (old man's beard) are among traditional South African means of relieving blisters. Blisters can also be soothed by the fruit and leaf of the bitter apple (Kei apple), or the juice of the bulbinella.

Biochemic Tissue Salts For immediate relief adults should try taking four tablets of Nat. mur. half-hourly until the pain has gone. For children two tablets should be taken half-hourly.

Aromatherapy Dab the blister carefully with lavender essential oil.

An orthodox view

If there is an infection antibiotics may be prescribed. Tests may also be made to determine the cause of infection.

BLOOD PRESSURE

By taking your blood pressure it is possible to establish exactly how hard your heart has to work to pump blood through your body. Depending on what you are doing, blood pressure changes throughout the day, although the brain needs a constant supply of about 900 ml of blood every single minute.

Abnormally high blood pressure is known as hypertension; low blood pressure is called hypotension.

Regular medical check-ups on your blood pressure levels (see box, opposite above) are advisable, as both conditions may require treatment – though hypertension is usually regarded as the more dangerous.

Blood pressure varies constantly, so a diagnosis of high blood pressure should never be made without taking several readings on different occasions.

The condition is more common among middle-aged people – about one in every ten

Do's and don'ts for high blood pressure

Don't smoke.
Don't take the contraceptive pill; try other methods of contraception instead.
Do increase the amount of FIBRE in your diet.
Do lose weight if you need to (see SLIMMING THE NATURAL WAY).
Do restrict alcohol consumption to two to four glasses of wine a week.
Do take regular aerobic EXERCISE of a non-competitive kind such as walking, swimming or cycling. Begin gently if you are not fit and never push yourself beyond what feels comfortable. Ask your doctor if you are uncertain.

Measuring blood pressure

This is done by placing an inflatable cuff around the upper arm. The cuff is pumped up until it exerts enough pressure to stop the flow of blood in the arm's main artery. As the cuff is slowly deflated and the blood begins to flow again readings are taken on a gauge at two points in the heart's pumping cycle. One reading, called the systolic pressure, is taken at the moment when the pulse actually beats and measures the peak pressure; the other, called the diastolic pressure, is measured between heart beats and shows your lowest level of blood pressure.

The two readings are combined as a fraction – systolic pressure over diastolic pressure – to give your blood pressure measurement. Normal for an adult is a systolic pressure of about 120 and a diastolic pressure of about 80 – or a blood pressure reading of 120/80 ('120 over 80'). Systolic pressures of 100-140 and diastolic ones of 60-90, slightly less in children, are usually considered within normal bounds.

is affected – and among men. Often they do not know that they have a problem, as there are usually no obvious symptoms – although some report headaches, dizziness and ringing in the ears.

Most cases of hypertension are the result of a number of interacting factors, such as drinking too much, eating too much salt, being overweight and taking too little exercise. A general narrowing or hardening of the arteries (see ARTERIES [HARDENING]), taking the contraceptive pill, SMOKING, or an inherited tendency to hypertension are other factors.

If tests show that you have high blood pressure it is important to take immediate steps to bring it down, otherwise it may contribute to serious conditions such as ANGINA, heart attack, stroke, haemorrhage or KIDNEY COMPLAINTS.

What the therapists recommend
NATUROPATHY

Self help Naturopaths suggest you should adopt a wholefood diet based on fruit, vegetables, wholegrain cereals – brown rice is particularly recommended – beans, fish and chicken (see EATING FOR HEALTH). Onions, GARLIC and strawberries are believed to lower

blood pressure, and HONEY may also help by calming the nerves.

Include plenty of fibre in your diet and reduce salt, sugar, animal fat and red meat to a minimum. Replace tea, coffee and cold drinks with herb tea, fruit juice, coffee substitutes or mineral water. See also LOW-FAT DIETS; SALT-FREE DIETS.

Consultation You will be given individual advice about diet, and supplements such as vitamin E, lecithin, garlic, pollen and magnesium or green buckwheat (rutin) may be recommended. Sometimes rutin tea or raw juices are recommended – about two to four cups a day of celery, grapefruit, orange, cucumber, pear or pineapple juice, separately or in combination.

The therapist will also advise you on reducing STRESS – by changing your daily routine, for example, to allow more time to relax or exercise; by adopting a co-operative rather than competitive attitude to others; or by practising various RELAXATION AND BREATHING techniques.

The practitioner will monitor your blood pressure, but may at times insist that you

take medication from your doctor to aid in the safe control of the problem.

AROMATHERAPY

Self help Add a few drops of lavender, lemon and/or ylang-ylang essential oil to your bath water, or to a base oil (see p. 37) for MASSAGE. Clary sage, melissa and marjoram can also be used. Or you can try three or four drops of essential oil taken in tea (see p. 52) two or three times a day.

HOMOEOPATHY

Self help *Arg. nit.* may help if you suffer from nervous tension, worry or overwork, but consulting a homoeopath who could get to the root of the problem is advised.

Consultation Homoeopathic remedies are designed to treat the whole person, not just an illness, so your overall physical and emotional state will be assessed, and medicines prescribed for your circumstances.

ACUPUNCTURE

Consultation Acupuncture has been used successfully to help lower blood pressure,

Low blood pressure (hypotension)

This is not generally as serious as high blood pressure, and is usually temporary, caused by getting up suddenly after sitting or lying down. It affects mostly elderly people, and the symptoms are momentary giddiness or FAINTING on standing up, due to slower than normal response to changes in position. Persistent low blood pressure may be due to an underactive adrenal gland.

The symptoms can sometimes be alleviated by standing up more slowly, but a number of alternative therapies may help to treat the underlying causes.

What the therapists recommend

Acupuncture For a systolic pressure lower than 100, accompanied by symptoms such as tiredness, lack of energy, headaches, dizziness, palpitations or cold hands and feet, points in the abdomen, back, neck, upper arm and lower leg would probably be treated. Further specific treatment would depend on individual symptoms.

Naturopathy Adopting a wholefood diet (see EATING FOR HEALTH) may help. It is also important to see that you get plenty of rest and take regular gentle exercise. Avoid artificial stimulants such as tea, coffee, alcohol and tobacco. A naturopath would give advice on

a healthier diet and lifestyle. Supplements such as vitamin E and MINERALS may be suggested.

Herbal Medicine A herbalist may recommend infusions (see p. 184) prepared from herbs such as broom, which is said to increase blood pressure. Other herbs may be used to tone and stimulate the whole system – kola, oats, gentian, wormwood (wilde als) and crataegus (hawthorn) are a few.

Aromatherapy You are advised to add hyssop, rosemary, sage or thyme essence to a massage oil or to your bath, or take them in a tea (see p. 37).

Bach Remedies Olive is prescribed for general exhaustion and depletion; Wild rose for resignation and apathy; Star of Bethlehem for uncompleted mourning, chronic sadness; Willow for resentment and self-pity; Clematis for loss of interest in life and mental confusion; Honeysuckle for nostalgia or regrets about the past.

An orthodox view

Hypotension for reasons other than those given above is not regarded as a dangerous condition. Recommendations by alternative therapists – although not harmful – would not be seen as affecting this condition.

although it is not known whether it does so by adjusting the overall functioning of the body, or simply by promoting relaxation – usually it does both. Treatment is combined with advice about diet and lifestyle, and varies according to how serious the condition is. Generally points in the abdomen, lower trunk, back, foot and head are stimulated, sometimes giving immediate relief.

BACH REMEDIES

Self help Oak and Elm for those feeling overwhelmed by responsibilities; Impatiens for irritability and impatience; Agrimony for the 'life and soul of the party', who hides his anxieties; Vervain for over-enthusiasm and strain; Vine for those who are ruthless and driven by ambition; Rock water for those with impossibly high standards; Beech if advice from others is refused. The last three are also for those who find relaxation difficult. If the condition is rooted in repressed emotion: Holly for anger, hatred and desire for revenge; Mimulus for fear of poverty; Star of Bethlehem for shock and grief.

Other alternative treatments

Hydrotherapy Try hot and cold foot baths twice a day.

Reflexology As high blood pressure is often caused by stress, the general relaxing effect of a full treatment is often beneficial. The most important areas requiring massage will be those relating to the heart, kidneys, adrenal glands, solar plexus, head, eyes, lungs, neck and spine. See chart on p. 295.

Yoga The corpse pose and YOGA meditation are likely to help. Practising yoga regularly can also relieve stress (avoid inverted postures). See also BIOFEEDBACK, MASSAGE, ACUPRESSURE.

An orthodox view

Doctors agree that diet is important and that cutting down on salt intake, and reducing excess weight should help.

   They make careful tests to find the cause of the hypertension and determine if it has had any effects on the body that need treating. You will be advised to cut your alcohol intake and stop smoking.

   If these measures do not help, drugs such as beta blockers (which lower the heart rate), diuretics (which increase production and excretion of urine) or vasodilators (which enlarge the blood vessels) may be prescribed. However, all of these drugs treat only the symptoms and not the underlying cause, so they have to be taken until the condition is effectively cured by some other means. Your doctor will probably tell you of any serious side effects, such as IMPOTENCE and TIREDNESS, that are attributable to the drugs you are taking.

BOILS
Dealing with a common infectious disorder

These inflamed, pus-filled areas of infection on the skin often start in a hair follicle – the minute hollow in the skin where a hair grows. The follicle and surrounding cells in the skin are killed by bacteria – usually staphylococci – and form thick yellow pus. As the pocket of pus gets bigger, the boil gradually comes to a head and, usually within a week or two of starting, the pus bursts out and disperses.

   In some cases several follicles become infected, giving rise to a cluster of boils, called a *carbuncle*. Both boils and carbuncles are a form of *abscess*, and generally erupt in hairy areas such as the neck, nostrils, armpits and wrists. They may also erupt where there is friction, such as between the legs and buttocks. The most common place for abscesses to form is in the gums, where they are commonly called gumboils (see TOOTH AND GUM DISORDERS).

   Boils are most likely to appear when you feel run down, are extremely tired, weakened by poor nutrition, or suffering from DIABETES.

   Although boils are a common minor disorder, they should not be ignored. If untreated, the infection can spread, eventually causing fever and general debility, particularly if pus enters the bloodstream. And it is for this reason that boils should never be squeezed.

   Medical treatment should be sought for carbuncles or a series of boils; if the boils are particularly painful; if the inflammation spreads without coming to a head; or if no pus is discharged even though a head has formed on the boil.

Warning Bacteria from boils can also find their way into warm food, where they rapidly multiply and can cause food poisoning. Sufferers should wash their hands thoroughly before dealing with food – and should not use anyone else's towel, as discharging boils are highly infectious.

What the therapists recommend

Traditional Medicine Apply a kaolin or magnesium sulphate poultice – available from chemists – to bring the boil to a head. Draw out the pus with a magnesium poultice. Or apply a bread poultice every three to four hours. Crumble a slice of bread into boiled milk or water, wrap it in gauze, drain and apply hot.

Naturopathy Practitioners regard a wholefood diet as the key to treating boils – or avoiding them altogether (see EATING FOR HEALTH). A cleansing diet of raw vegetables and fruit is recommended for the first two to

seven days. Naturopaths also recommend that close attention should be paid to personal hygiene and skin care (see NATURAL AIDS TO BEAUTY).

   A poultice can be made from crushed fenugreek seeds. Wrap a teaspoonful in foil and simmer for about ten minutes in a cup of water. Strain and then apply the seeds on a piece of lint, lightly held in place. Alternatively, apply a hot, softly baked onion to bring boils to a head – or bandage a slice of lemon on the area.

Homoeopathy *Hepar sulph.* is used to help a boil to come to a head, and *Silica* to speed the discharge of pus once it has burst.

Biochemic Tissue Salts Among those frequently recommended by practitioners are *Ferr. phos.* and *Kali mur.* Given alternatively in the early stage they are said to prevent swelling and pus. In cases where the boil bursts but the discharge continues and the wound is slow to heal, practitioners recommend taking *Calc. sulph.*

Herbal Medicine Herbalists traditionally believe that boils are the manifestation of internal impurities – and that the blood can be purified by drinking strong teas made from herbs such as barberry, burdock, cayenne, echinacea, golden seal and yellow dock. Use a teaspoonful of the chosen herb to a cup of boiling water and, when the tea is cool enough, drink a tablespoonful every two to three hours.

   Poultices made by mixing a paste of slippery elm and hot water and applied warm for several days are said to help clear up boils and heal the wounds.

An orthodox view

If a boil refuses to burst, a doctor may lance it so that the pus drains away. He may also prescribe an antibiotic such as penicillin to kill the bacteria and prevent the infection spreading any further. If he thinks that diabetes is the underlying cause, he may test your urine.

BONESETTING

The art of bonesetting – the treating of broken bones and dislocated limbs by manipulation – dates back to the Stone Age. The bonesetters' skills reached a peak in the 18th and 19th centuries, when their relatively gentle use of hands for correcting bone and muscle problems was preferred to the more vigorous methods of conventional physicians and surgeons.

   Today traditional bonesetters have mostly been replaced by practitioners of osteopathy and CHIROPRACTIC – whose methods are partly based on those of their predecessors.

BOWEL DISORDERS

There are a number of bowel disorders, all of which have pronounced symptoms. The two most common of these are CONSTIPATION and DIARRHOEA. In some cases there may be bleeding, with blood in the faeces or discharged from the anus. Both can indicate the presence of PILES or, more seriously, CANCER. Any such symptoms – or any marked changes in otherwise well-established bowel habits – should be reported to your doctor as soon as possible.

See also COLIC, COLITIS, DYSENTERY, INCONTINENCE, IRRITABLE BOWEL SYNDROME, WIND and WORMS.

BREAST PROBLEMS

Most women will have a breast problem at some time in their lives. Fluctuations in hormone levels – associated with the menstrual cycle or with the rise and decline of fertility over the years – generally cause the problems. These frequently right themselves as the hormone levels stabilise.

The breasts consist of glandular tissue and fat, which fibrous bands called ligaments support on the chest wall. Hormones in the female bloodstream make the breast tissue develop during puberty, produce milk after childbirth, and dwindle after the menopause.

Men have little breast tissue and rarely suffer breast problems. A man who has any pain or swelling in the breast area should get professional advice.

The most common disorders are mastalgia (painful breasts) and fibrocystic disease (lumpy breasts). The most serious is breast CANCER. Some women who are breastfeeding experience discomfort or difficulties that will respond to simple treatment (see below and box).

Many women have painful breasts before a period. Some pregnant women have pain early in pregnancy. The raised level of oestrogen and of sodium in their blood causes water to be held in the fatty tissue of the body. Since there is a large amount of fat in the breasts, so much water is retained that the breasts feel overfull, tight and sore.

In about half the women aged 30-55 increases of fibrous (*fibro-*) and glandular (*-cystic*) tissue occur in the breasts, which may then feel tender and lumpy, especially before a period. A soft, sore lump (an adenoma) may develop in a breast. Because the lump seems to slip away when you try to grasp it, it is often

Remedies to ease breastfeeding

	LACK OF MILK	CRACKED NIPPLES	BLOCKED MILK DUCT (pain in one segment)	ENGORGEMENT (over-full breast; poor flow)
Self help	Take extra drinks and rest. Eat pears and strawberries. Have your back massaged.	Make sure the whole areola is in the baby's mouth and the nipple well back in the mouth. Use a softening cream.	Soak breasts in a warm bath. Stroke breasts towards nipples to express milk. Empty breasts after feed.	Apply hot compresses before and during feeds, cold compresses after feeds. Let baby feed at affected breast.
Acupressure	Use a matchstick to stimulate the outer side of both little fingers just below the nail.	As for lack of milk.	Stimulate inside the wrist in central hollow, on breastbone, halfway along the shoulder towards the back, on chest wall beneath each breast.	As for blocked duct.
Aromatherapy	Massage with oil of aniseed, caraway, fennel, verbena.	Massage with oil of camomile.	Massage with oil of geranium or mint.	Massage with oil of garlic.
Herbal medicine	Take infusions of milkwort, fenugreek, holy thistle, fennel.	Rub in calendula cream.	As for cracked nipples.	Massage with calendula cream, honey, almond oil.
Homoeopathy	Take Causticum, Urtica urens.	Take *Caster equii*.	Take *Silica*.	Take *Phytolacca*.

called a 'breast mouse'. Sometimes an olive-sized cyst develops, mostly in the upper and outer part of the breast towards the armpit.

Avoiding and relieving problems

Women can reduce the risk of some breast problems by examining their breasts regularly (see illustrations, p. 74) for early warning of troubles, and by following a healthy lifestyle with a few extra measures added specifically to aid breast care.

Diet Cut down on salt and salty foods. This will help to curb the retention of water in the fatty tissue, which is one cause of mastalgia. Eat plenty of fresh fruit and vegetables to make sure you get enough VITAMINS. Vitamin B_6 eases WATER RETENTION by acting as a diuretic (making you pass more urine) and it may restore your oestrogen balance. Cut down on coffee, tea, chocolate and cola.

Give up smoking and regular drinking of alcohol, which seem to increase the risk of contracting cancer. Cut down on animal fats – many researchers believe that as the body breaks down these fats, by-products are

formed that can encourage breast cancer. Eat soya bean products, which are thought to counteract the harmful by-products of fat.

Exercise Fat will be burned off instead of stored in the body if you take regular exercise. Swimming, especially breaststroke, and skipping are good general muscle toners and are particularly good for firming the chest muscles behind the breasts. Strong muscles and a well-fitting bra help to prevent sagging.

An effective exercise for the muscles round the breasts is to put your hands together as hard as you can while you count to five. Relax, then repeat four or five times.

Do not let your chest muscles sag. Maintain a good posture with a straight back whether you are standing or sitting. Breathe properly to help to open up your chest.

YOGA can help to relieve tension and exercise chest muscles.

Breastfeeding You need plenty of rest and a nourishing diet while breastfeeding, with ample vitamins, calcium and iron (see EATING FOR HEALTH). As well as your usual fluids, drink a glass of water after each feed.

Examining your breasts

Set aside 10-15 minutes each month to check your breasts. Immediately after a period is the right time to do it. In the week before and during a period, your breasts may feel swollen and sore but this is not abnormal. After the menopause, carry out the examination at a fixed time each month – perhaps on the first day of the month. Once you have done a few monthly checks, you will know what is the normal appearance and structure of your breasts and notice immediately anything unusual. Some women are made too anxious by carrying out their own examination and prefer to have a six-monthly checkup by a health worker.

1 Strip to the waist and face a mirror in a good light. Look for any changes in the shape of either breast, for any puckering or dimpling of the skin, and for changes in the condition of either nipple.

3 Raise and lower your arms and see if both nipples move by the same amount.

4 Squeeze each nipple gently to make sure there is no discharge. Look for any rash or flaky skin on the nipples.

5 Lie flat with a small cushion or a folded towel under your left shoulder blade and with your left hand behind your head. Keeping your right fingers flat, use them to work round and round your left breast in tiny circles, pressing firmly as you go and gradually spiralling from the outermost part towards the nipple. Make sure you cover every part.

2 Put your hands behind your head and look again. Turn sideways for another look and then lean forward and check again.

6 Again working the flat of your fingers in tiny circles, test from your armpit down towards your breast. Then use your left fingers to check your right breast.

If you find anything unusual, see your doctor within a few days. Do not keep feeling any lump while you wait to see the doctor and remember that the great majority of breast lumps are harmless.

While feeding, sit up straight in a high-backed chair and support the baby on a pillow on your lap to lift it well up to the breast without straining your back and arms. Make sure you are relaxed with plenty of time and no distractions so that the milk will flow. A warm bath and your favourite peaceful music may help you if tension is making feeding difficult.

You can ease many discomforts yourself, as shown in the chart, but if you are feverish with hard, painful breasts and greenish milk, you may have MASTITIS and should get professional help. If you have the same symptoms and a localised swelling, you may have an abscess and should again seek help.

What the therapists recommend

NATUROPATHY

Self help Maintain a healthy weight and eat plenty of watercress, turnips, cabbage and all other plants of the cabbage family. Make up a vegetable juice from half turnip and half watercress and then add an equal quantity of carrot juice. Have some of the juice each day. Splash or spray your breasts with cold water every day.

Consultation A diet will be worked out to rid your body of waste that has accumulated. A course of BIOCHEMIC TISSUE SALTS may be suggested and vitamin supplements prescribed as required for your individual diet – perhaps A, B$_1$, B$_6$, C and E. Capsules of calcium, arginine, kelp, oil of evening primrose or flaxseed oil are claimed to relieve the discomforts of fibrocystic disease.

Other alternative treatments

Aromatherapy Make up a cream of one part essence of geranium, five parts white wax, 12 parts water, 20 parts sweet almond oil. Massage the cream into your breasts at bedtime to ease soreness. Alternatively, bathe them with a bowl of water, boiled then cooled to a pleasant warmth and three to four drops of essence of geranium added.

Homoeopathy *Calc. ostrearum* and *Calc. phos.* are generally recommended to ease painful breasts and *Conium flaculatum* for pregnant women whose breasts hurt.

Reflexology Massage is applied from the second to the fifth zone on top of the feet to treat fibrocystic disease.

An orthodox view

For mastalgia, a doctor is likely to prescribe a diuretic drug to relieve the water retention. Alternatively he may prescribe a synthetic hormone to balance out the patient's excess oestrogen level.

For cysts that cause pain in fibrocystic disease, your doctor may send you to a hospital to have fluid drawn off from the cyst by a syringe, or to have the cyst removed. Occasion-ally a biopsy may be recommended to confirm that any breast lumps are not malignant.

A small sample of the suspect tissue is removed under a local or a general anaesthetic so that cells can be carefully examined under a microscope. Even if the lump is not malignant, and is fibrous tissue, you may still be advised to have it removed.

Some women run a greater risk of developing cancer than others, particularly those with a family history of cancer. Any woman who feels she may be at risk of developing cancer should examine herself regularly, and also be screened by her doctor at regular intervals. Screening can be by mammogram, an X-ray taken with the breasts held firmly between two photographic plates, or by an ultrasound scan, in which a small, high-frequency sound instrument is passed over each breast. If a cancerous lump is found, you will be referred to a specialist unit for surgery, radiotherapy, chemotherapy or a combination of these treatments.

BRONCHITIS

When the large air passages (bronchi) which carry air from the windpipe to the lungs become inflamed the result is bronchitis. It can be brought on by a variety of viruses and bacteria.

Symptoms include persistent COUGHS, WHEEZING, breathlessness, chest pains, FEVER, HEADACHES and loss of appetite. The condition may come on suddenly (acute bronchitis), or develop in a more serious form, as a prolonged disorder (chronic bronchitis) that gets progressively worse: In its serious form, the lining of the bronchi narrows and the lungs' air sacs are gradually destroyed, cutting down the supply of oxygen to the blood. This form occurs in occupations where air pollution is common, such as coal mining and in the building trade.

Warning Anyone developing symptoms of bronchitis should see a doctor before seeking alternative treatments. Both conventional and alternative practitioners will recommend smokers to stop SMOKING – the most common cause of the disease.

What the therapists recommend

NATUROPATHY

Self help Avoiding dairy products and eating only wholefoods (see EATING FOR HEALTH) is believed to help in reducing mucus. Also avoid dry, overheated rooms.

Consultation Naturopaths believe that bronchitis is generally caused by poor living habits, which poison the system and can lead to the build-up of poisonous waste in the bronchi. Lowered resistance caused by overwork, EXHAUSTION, a sudden CHILL, or exposure to coldness, is thought to trigger the symptoms.

Many practitioners do not agree with the prescription of conventional drugs or medicines for bronchitis except in severe cases, but may suggest such supplements as GARLIC capsules and vitamins B and C.

For prolonged cases, an all-fruit diet for three to five days is recommended (under constant supervision), followed by ten to 14 days on a diet of raw salads, vegetables and sweet fruit – all to be eaten according to appetite. After this, a more varied, normal diet of fish or poultry and fresh vegetables may be resumed, but still with no dairy products and with two or three days each month on the all-fruit diet.

For a sudden onset of bronchitis, an initial fast until the fever and other symptoms have eased is recommended. This can be followed by two or three days on an all-fruit diet.

Naturopaths also recommend measures such as dry friction baths – self-massage with a brush or sponge – Epsom salt baths (see HYDROTHERAPY), RELAXATION AND BREATHING exercises, and outdoor exercise.

HERBAL MEDICINE

Consultation Practitioners may prescribe one or more plant-based remedies including gum plant, coltsfoot, squill, liquorice, comfrey, boneset, white horehound, heartsease, wild thyme, ginger and elder flower. The exact prescription will depend much on the individual patient. Echinacea may be added, to build up the immune system.

These herbal prescriptions may be supplemented from time to time with vitamin C, plus iron to help form haemoglobin, the blood's oxygen carrier.

Once the patient is well enough, the practitioner will recommend a combination of rest and gentle exercise, such as walking, gradually going on to more vigorous activities such as swimming.

Prescriptions are reviewed regularly during consultations, with emphasis on healing the damaged bronchial tissues, restoring the body's resistance and building up the nervous system.

Other alternative treatments

Aromatherapy Essential oils of eucalyptus, hyssop and sandalwood are generally recommended as effective inhalants. Eucalyptus is considered to be very good for clearing your head when it feels all clogged up; hyssop is recommended as a decongestant and sandalwood as a relaxant. Use them as drops on a paper towel or in a bowl of hot water in the following proportions: six eucalyptus, two hyssop, two sandalwood.

The same oils can be applied during massage, in a ratio of 15:10:5. Many less expensive oils may also help, including pine, cajuput and niaouli.

Biochemic Tissue Salts In the first stages of bronchitis, *Ferr. phos.* 6X potency is recommended. If the condition worsens, *Kali mur.* 6X potency should also be taken, along with *Nat. mur.* 6X potency.

Homoeopathy For sudden attacks, when the patient finds movement difficult and wants long, cool drinks, try *Bryonia.* Chronic sufferers should consult a homoeopath personally. Other aids recommended include *Aconite,* at the onset of feverishness; *Kali bich.* if the mucus is stringy, tough and thick, and difficult to cough up; and *Pulsatilla* if the cough is dry, or the mucus is loose and green and the patient does not feel thirsty.

Acupuncture Points on the lung, bladder, stomach and spleen meridians are treated.

Reflexology Massage to the reflex areas relating to the bronchi, lungs and throat, together with the solar plexus, adrenal and pituitary glands, lymphatic system and spine is recommended. See chart on p. 295.

An orthodox view

While many alternative therapists disagree about using drugs to treat bronchitis, a doctor may prescribe medicine to ease the cough, a balsam inhalant to aid breathing, and antibiotics to fight the infection. However, some doctors reject cough-suppressing drugs, because coughing and spitting prevent infected matter being inhaled.

The patient will be advised to get plenty of rest in a warm room, to avoid moving from a hot to a cold atmosphere, and to avoid dusty places. Smokers with progressive bronchitis will be advised to give up, otherwise their health will continue to deteriorate, leading to complications such as EMPHYSEMA, PNEUMONIA and HEART DISORDERS.

A conventional doctor would be concerned if someone with a cough were treated by an alternative practitioner without an accurate diagnosis being made. All patients should consult a doctor if a cough persists, as it may be a symptom of a serious disorder.

BRUISING

Most bruises are the result of a fall or blow which causes bleeding in the tissues under the skin. This can be slowed down – reducing discomfort and the extent of the bruising – if you apply an ice pack or a cold, damp cloth over the bruise with moderate pressure for about ten minutes. Aspirin or paracetamol will relieve the pain. Do the same for a 'black

eye' – despite popular belief, putting raw steak on it is a waste of time.

A badly bruised limb should be rested for 24-48 hours. In the case of a leg, lie down and raise it on pillows to reduce blood flow.

Unless bruising appears for no apparent reason, or does not clear up within a fortnight, there is usually no need to see a doctor.

What the therapists recommend

Naturopathy Many naturopaths believe that people who bruise easily may lack vitamin K, a vital blood-clotting protein. Eating 150 g of yoghurt daily is thought to stimulate the micro-organisms that produce the vitamin. Fresh green vegetables are recommended, with fresh pineapple or its juice, which contain enzymes that are said to speed the disappearance of bruising.

As an immediate measure, spray the area with cold water to stimulate local circulation.

Herbal Medicine A cold compress soaked in comfrey infusion (p. 184) or oil of lavender, or comfrey ointment is recommended.

Homoeopathy Rub *Arnica* oil or ointment gently into the bruised area.

BULIMIA

The consequences of compulsive eating

Strict dieting or a desire to be thin can bring on bulimia – which, like ANOREXIA, is an eating disorder with a psychological basis. The victim has sudden uncontrollable cravings for food, which lead to periodic bouts of overeating, called 'bingeing', which are followed by the taking of laxatives or self-induced vomiting to get rid of the food.

Strangely, victims are usually of normal weight for their age and height, and seldom appear to be ill. But beneath the surface they conceal a constant fear of food and of their inability to stop eating.

Bulimia has become a more common eating disorder than the much better known anorexia, and can affect both men and women of any age – although most of its victims are women in their twenties. It has been estimated that about 45 per cent of those suffering from anorexia will later develop bulimia.

It is a dangerous condition that can cause a variety of physical and mental symptoms such as low BLOOD PRESSURE, PERIOD PROBLEMS, TENSION, ANXIETY and DEPRESSION. Regular use of laxatives and vomiting can cause KIDNEY COMPLAINTS, URINARY PROBLEMS, dehydration and poor circulation. In extreme cases, overeating itself may eventually lead to death.

Do's and don'ts for overcoming bulimia

Do try to eat full, regular meals, and make mealtimes happy and relaxed occasions. Take your meals with other people whenever possible – this makes it impossible to binge.

Do plan your day so that you stay busy. Boredom and loneliness spark off more binges than hunger.

Do try to express your feelings to others. Pent-up anger or frustration is responsible for much overeating.

Do give yourself a treat now and again. An occasional chocolate or packet of crisps does little harm and may stop you becoming obsessive about 'forbidden foods'.

Don't keep large supplies of high-calorie snack foods such as biscuits, sweets, nuts or ice cream.

Don't take laxatives or make yourself vomit if you do overeat occasionally. Rare indulgences won't make any difference to your weight, but laxatives can be habit-forming and may damage your health.

Don't eat between meals – this could turn into a full-blown binge.

Warning Anyone who thinks he may be suffering from bulimia – or is trying to help a family member with the disorder – should consult his doctor before any of the alternative treatments are embarked upon.

What the therapists recommend

NATUROPATHY

Self help See SLIMMING THE NATURAL WAY for advice about how to stay slim while also taking in all the nourishment your body needs. Include plenty of raw foods (see RAW FOOD DIET) and freshly squeezed raw fruit and vegetable juices in your diet.

Consultation The naturopath will help you to work out an individual diet plan. It will be supplemented with extra vitamins and minerals where necessary.

The practitioner will also advise you how to cope with STRESS and take EXERCISE, especially outdoor exercise. The naturopath may work alongside a psychotherapist.

Other alternative treatments

Bach Remedies Complex emotions may underlie this condition. Crab apple is recommended for self disgust and anxiety about weight and appearance; Heather for being self-obsessed and craving love; Scleranthus for instability and mood swings; Beech for difficulty in receiving food and love in appropriate measure; Pine for guilt about the condition; Aspen for fear of being found out; and Holly for negative feelings such as jealousy, hatred and the desire for revenge.

Psychotherapy Patients are often started on BEHAVIOURAL THERAPY, followed by COGNITIVE THERAPY to deal with underlying causes such as a poor self-image, fear of failure, and social or personal problems.

Among other therapies, DANCE THERAPY, YOGA, EURHYTHMY, T'AI-CHI CH'UAN and BIO-ENERGETICS may help bulimia victims feel more positive about their bodies.

An orthodox view

Doctors agree that bingeing, taking laxatives and vomiting can do serious damage. Your general practitioner can help you to work out a safe diet if you want to lose weight or avoid putting it on. If deep psychological problems are an underlying cause, you will be referred to a psychologist or psychotherapist.

BUNIONS

Bunions are often caused by ill-fitting shoes which put pressure on the big toe. The joint swells, the skin over it becomes hard, red and sore – and the toe is forced inwards. Middle-aged women who have always worn narrow shoes, children, teenagers and young adults are particularly prone to bunions. Unless treated, an operation may eventually be needed to cure them.

What the therapists recommend

Naturopathy Bathe the feet for 20 minutes daily in a bowl of hot water in which a tablespoon of Epsom salts is dissolved. Alternating footbaths of hot and cold water may also

Avoiding bunions

Make sure socks are not tight, and that shoes are wide enough for comfort, with plenty of room for the toes.
Remove shoes whenever possible and do toe-flexing exercises.
Wiggle and massage your toes when you are in the bath.
Loop a strong rubber band around both big toes and move the feet outwards to try to make a 'V'. Do it as often as is practicable.

help, and gentle, circular massage helps to keep movement at the joints.

Herbal Medicine Bio-Strath Willow formula – a modern preparation made from extract of willow and primula – is said to relieve inflammation. It can be taken long-term in liquid form – available from health shops – and is said to have no side effects. Celery seeds are also thought to help. Make an infusion (p. 184) with 1 teaspoon of seeds. Take 1 tablespoonful three times daily, cold (but *not* during pregnancy). Celery helps you to lose more uric acid, so it is also appropriate for GOUT and related conditions.

Aromatherapy Massage the feet every night with oils of patchouli (if the skin is dry) and lavender. Camomile and geranium are also helpful.

Acupuncture Therapists say that pain can be relieved – but only if the source of pressure on the big toes, such as tight shoes, is avoided.

An orthodox view

A doctor may recommend the wearing of felt pads to ease the inflammation – as long as they are not so bulky that they put unwanted pressure on the affected area. The patient would then probably be sent to a chiropodist. If the foot is seriously deformed, the doctor may prescribe painkillers, or an operation may be advised.

BURSITIS

Housemaid's knee and TENNIS ELBOW are two common forms of bursitis. This is the name given to any inflammation of the small liquid-filled sacs – or bursas – which lubricate the joints, helping skin, muscles and tendons to move smoothly over the bones.

In bursitis, excess liquid collects in the sac, and this prevents the free movement of the joint, causing heat, swelling and pain. The condition is usually caused by repeated bumping or overuse of the joint, ARTHRITIS, GOUT or infection.

What the therapists recommend

NATUROPATHY

Self help Rest the joint as much as you possibly can, and stop any activities that may be causing pressure or bumps at the joint. If the elbow is affected, it may help if you put the arm in a sling. Use a crepe bandage or tubular bandage as a support for the joint, and apply cold (not ice) compresses (see p. 193) for five to ten minutes three times daily.

When the pain and swelling begin to decrease – usually after about seven to ten days – start using the joint again. Go carefully at

first, increasing the range of movements until you are using the joint normally again.

A nourishing, complete wholefood diet supplemented with vitamins A and C is also recommended (see EATING FOR HEALTH and VITAMINS). If symptoms persist for ten days or more, see your doctor.

HYDROTHERAPY

Self help Apply cold compresses (see p. 193) to the joint during the first few days, when swelling and pain are worst. Leave them on overnight and for several periods of about 20 minutes during the day, renewing them whenever they no longer feel cold. Alternate or replace with hot compresses once improvement begins.

For acute inflammation, a bag of frozen peas can be applied as an ice pack (it will conform to the contours of the affected part). First smear the skin with olive or cooking oil to prevent frostbite. Apply three times daily, on for five minutes, off for five minutes, then on for ten minutes.

HERBAL MEDICINE

Self help After the first few days, hot herbal poultices (see p. 184) may be helpful. Comfrey, linseed, marsh-mallow and slippery elm are recommended, either individually or in combination. If you find that heat is helpful, gently boil a tablespoon of cayenne pepper in 600 ml of cider vinegar for ten minutes. When it is cool, soak a clean hand towel in the mixture, wring it out slightly and wrap it around the joint. If the skin begins to burn, protect it by applying a thin layer of oil or diluting the mixture with water.

Drinking herbal infusions (see p. 184) may also help. Camomile is recommended.

Other alternative treatments

Aromatherapy Mix five drops each of lavender, juniper, eucalyptus and rosemary essential oils in almond or peanut oil and massage into the affected area every day.

Homoeopathy For swelling, redness and pain, *Apis* 6X potency every two hours is recommended. If attacks recur, try *Rhus tox.* 6X potency twice a day for two weeks.

An orthodox view

Doctors support the naturopathic advice to rest the joint at first and avoid banging or applying pressure to it to prevent further attacks.

Generally-accepted orthodox treatment involves anaesthetising the area and draining excess fluid from the bursa with a fine needle. Sometimes cortisone is injected to reduce the risk of another attack, and antibiotics are given if there is an infection. If the bursitis does not clear, the bursa may be removed under local anaesthetic.

When the body's cells go out of control

Cancers can develop when the body's own policing system fails to destroy cells with the wrong genetic code and allows them to multiply unchecked. Orthodox medicine recognises that environmental factors seem to stimulate faulty cell division and that prolonged grief or depression makes the policing system less efficient. But it is still far from unravelling the complexities of this multi-form illness. It can see also that factors outside hospital clinics and operating theatres play a vital part in the outcome of orthodox treatment. Alternative therapies generally tend to concentrate on this aspect – fostering positive control by patients over their bodies and boosting a determined and assertive mental approach.

Helpful, balanced discussion of cancer is often difficult because, for many people, the very word conjures up an image of pain and death. They shun the topic and shy away from learning more about it. But the term 'cancer' is used for many different sets of symptoms, some of them curable.

The causes, treatments and chances of a cure differ widely for the different forms of cancers. SMOKING, for example, is a cause of lung cancer; too much ultraviolet light a cause of skin cancer; and diet a cause of bowel cancer. The rigorous diet that may be appropriate in treating bowel cancer is quite unlike treatments which are recommended for dealing with skin cancer. While 98 per cent of people with skin cancer survive, only 7 per cent of lung cancer victims survive longer than five years.

Statistics about survival can be misleading. Death rates generally take no account of how late the condition was diagnosed and the treatment was started. In many forms of cancer, early diagnosis improves the success rate of treatment.

What is cancer? The one factor that all forms of cancer have in common is the growth and development of abnormal cells in some part of the body.

Body cells are constantly reproducing – more than 90 per cent of the body's cells are replaced every six months. Cells reproduce by dividing in two, each half taking its share of the nucleus (see illustrations below). Within the nucleus is the genetic code which controls what kind of cell develops and how it behaves.

A dividing cell sometimes produces mutant (abnormal) cells which are not properly coded and multiply uncontrollably, developing into a cancer. It is one of the tasks of the body's white blood cells to kill abnormal cells. A white blood cell has to make contact with a mutant to kill it, but the mutant will try to prevent contact by putting out a barrier of blisters on its surface.

Some research scientists believe that the production of mutant cells is not unusual, but that a regulating system in the body usually kills them off. When this regulating system breaks down or is swamped with more mutant cells than it can cope with, cancer is able to develop.

Certain mutant cells multiply much faster than others: cancer of the womb grows slowly, while cancer of the cervix (neck of the womb) is fast-growing. Mutant cells may also travel in the body and start other cancers – so-called 'secondaries' – away from the original site.

There are more than 200 forms of cancer, and doctors give them special names according to the part of the body or the body system mainly affected. The largest group are carcinomas – cancers of the external and internal linings of the body, its cavities and most of its organs, such as the lung and the breast. The second group, sarcomas, affect connective tissues such as

The orderly process that makes a matching pair of body cells

The stages in normal division of a human cell are shown in the series of photographs above. Magnification and staining with strong colour have made the process easier to see.
1 In a cell about to divide, the chromosomes (stained pink) of the nucleus, which carry the genetic code, are contained in an encircling envelope (orange). Cytoplasm (green) makes

up the rest of the cell. The chromosomes – each consisting of two matched chromatids – have begun to grow shorter and thicker.
2 The envelope around the nucleus has disintegrated and the chromosomes begin to move towards the midline – the 'equator'.
3 All the chromosomes have lined up along the equator, where the cell will divide.

muscles and bones. Individual cancers include LEUKAEMIA (cancer of the blood), lymphoma (cancer of the lymph glands), osteosarcoma (cancer of the bones), encephaloma (cancer of the brain) and melanoma (a form of skin cancer).

In South Africa, one in four people will develop some form of cancer in their lives. Currently, more than 36 000 new cancer victims are diagnosed annually. Although the incidence of cancer is increasing, today more and more people are surviving cancer – the National Cancer Association of South Africa quotes a figure of almost one in two cancer sufferers surviving.

About two-thirds of cancer victims who die are 65 or more years old. As the population avoids or survives infections such as diphtheria, scarlet fever and tuberculosis, which were the big killers of previous generations, more of them eventually die from cancer.

Causes of cancer Heredity may be a factor with certain cancers. For example, a woman is four times more likely than average to develop breast cancer if her mother, aunt or sister has had it. People who are only light smokers themselves are 15 times more likely than other light smokers to develop lung cancer if their parents have had lung cancer. People with fair or ruddy skin, red or light hair and blue eyes – all influenced by heredity – are more likely to develop skin cancer than dark-skinned people. Some leukaemias also run in families.

People who suffer from certain diseases, including ulcerative COLITIS, pernicious ANAEMIA and viral hepatitis B, also run an extra risk of developing cancer.

However, much more important than heredity or disease are environmental factors. We may take up the same occupation or adopt the same unhealthy diet or lifestyle as our parents and so develop the same illnesses – but not through heredity. The world we live in and the way we treat our bodies play a large part in the development of cancers.

Smoking, inhaling asbestos particles, excessive fat in the diet, heavy alcohol consumption, overexposure to sunlight or radiation from nuclear waste or leakage (as at Chernobyl) and contact with benzopyrenes (chemicals used in dry cleaning) are all known to increase the likelihood of developing various forms of cancer. See HEALTH HAZARDS.

We can avoid or limit our exposure to some of these so that they are not such a danger. Basking in the sun for an hour or two is unlikely to cause skin cancer, but frequent sunbathing without using a protective cream might – especially if you have a fair or ruddy complexion. The occasional alcoholic drink will not give you liver cancer, but frequent and excessive drinking, especially with heavy smoking, could well do so.

Psychological factors seem to play a part. People who bottle up their feelings are at a much greater risk than those who release them. DEPRESSION, GRIEF at bereavement or some other loss, and other forms of mental STRESS make people more likely to develop cancer.

What the therapists recommend

Most alternative therapies aim to stimulate a patient's life force, or will to live, and so bring to bear the body's natural defences. It is these defences that prevent cancers from developing in most people most of the time.

The mutant cells are regarded not only as the cause of cancer but as a symptom that the body's balance has been disturbed. Some practitioners concentrate particularly on diet to restore a proper balance; others give more emphasis to the patient's mind and emotions.

NATUROPATHY
The emphasis is on a healthy diet and lifestyle, not with the claim of curing diagnosed cancers, but of preventing cancer from developing and for use alongside or as a follow-up to orthodox methods of treatment.

The various regimes developed by alternative therapists have several recommended courses in common: a largely vegetarian or vegan diet (see VEGETARIANISM); a high proportion of raw, and preferably organic, foods; a low intake of sugar and salt; and the clearing of poisonous waste from the body – by FASTING or by enemas, for example.

Much medical research has shown that bowel, breast and stomach cancers in particular occur less in societies where the diet is low in fat and meat, and high in FIBRE. The benefit of fibre may be that it speeds up the movement of waste products

4 *Division has begun in earnest, with a deepening furrow forming around the cell. The matched pairs of chromatids have separated, with one from each pair moving to opposite ends of the cell. Two separate but identical groups now exist, each carrying the same genetic code.*
5 *Only a narrow neck of cytoplasm is left connecting the two parts of the cell. The chromosomes within each part of the cell start* *to lengthen again and there is the beginning of an envelope forming around each cluster.*
6 *The cells now have their chromosome clusters contained in envelopes. Before division starts again, the chromosomes will duplicate their genetic material so that matched chromatids exist ready for the next division. Cancer may begin when a fault occurs somewhere in the replication process, so that a cell receives a faulty genetic message.*

through the digestive tract so that any ingested cancer-causing substances do not linger for long in the body.

Both the Gerson diet and the Bristol diet, the best known of the regimes used to help cancer patients, are based on these principles.

Gerson Therapy The diet that is the basis of this treatment was devised in the 1920s by a German physician, Dr Max Gerson, to bring his own migraines under control. He recommended it to his patients and many benefited, including some with tuberculosis or cancer.

His treatment was designed to clear the body of various accumulated poisons, stimulate enzyme production to improve the digestion considerably, correct the body's balance of VITAMINS and MINERALS, and promote a positive attitude to the body – and to life in general.

Carrying out the strict regime is time-consuming. Every hour, 13 freshly made juices are taken, one made from oranges, four from leafy greenstuff, four from carrots and apples and four from calves' liver. All items must be organically grown or reared. Caffeine enemas and castor oil are taken regularly to cleanse the system. Meals are mainly based on salads, oats and baked potatoes.

For full details of the dietary treatment, contact The Gerson Institute, P O Box 430, Bonita, California 92002, USA. Patients may suffer from vomiting, diarrhoea and skin sores while the cleansing process goes on. Therapists support them with COUNSELLING.

Bristol Diet A strict diet which was devised by Dr Alec Forbes was an important part of the treatment originally offered by the Bristol Cancer Help Centre.

All the patients who chose this regime started off by eating a low-fat vegan diet, a high proportion of which comprised raw food. As they started to improve, the patients were slowly allowed to add small quantities of vegetable oil, eggs, poultry and fish.

In recent years, however, the centre has modified this regime and patients now adopt a basically vegetarian diet of fresh fruit and vegetables, whole grains and pulses, with a little fish, free-range poultry or eggs, or even organically farmed red meat for those who wish.

More of the food is cooked, and organically produced goat's-milk yoghurt is included for the friendly and useful bacteria that it supplies.

For cooking, cold-pressed or virgin olive oil is preferred, and herbs, spices and fruit juice replace salt and sugar. For the purposes of the diet, patients are strongly advised to cut down immediately on drinks such as tea and coffee, and to switch to readily available herb teas, fresh juices, mineral water, or various grain substitutes.

More information about the diet is available from the Cancer Help Centre, Grove House, Cornwallis Grove, Clifton, Bristol BS8 4PG, England.

Megavitamin Therapy This is an extension of the corrective diet therapies. Even with a healthy diet, cancer patients may not get enough of the vitamins and minerals they need because their bodies cannot absorb them properly. To counter this, much larger amounts than the usual recommended doses are given, to ensure that enough get through.

In this therapy, more than 1 000 times the usual daily 30 mg of vitamin C is prescribed, for example. Large doses of vitamins A, B and E, and of the minerals selenium, zinc, calcium, magnesium and molybdenum may also be given.

PSYCHOTHERAPY

Substantial evidence from studies of cancer patients shows that psychological factors play a significant part not only in causing their illness but also in their chances of survival.

People who have a positive outlook, are self-assertive, cheerful and able to express their feelings are less likely to develop cancer. Among people who do develop it, those who deny that they have a life-threatening illness and adopt a fighting attitude have a significantly higher chance of surviving longer than those who tend to accept their cancer stoically or feel helpless and hopeless.

Psychological therapies that are used to help cancer patients generally focus on shifting their mood and emotional state. They also give social support that can reduce patients' anxiety and depression to a large extent. The general assumption is that various thoughts, feelings and mental images that people entertain affect bodily states, particularly the IMMUNE SYSTEM.

Immunologists now believe that some cells in the immune system possess what is called natural killer activity. Stress and loneliness can lower natural killer activity while positive attitudes and a belief in one's well-being enhance it, so that the body's own defence mechanism will destroy cancer cells. Therapies to generate such attitudes include RELAXATION AND BREATHING, meditation, mental imagery or visualisation therapy, and HYPNOTHERAPY.

The best known therapy is Dr Carl Simonton's visualisation technique in which the patient is asked to see in the mind's eye a battle in which powerful immune cells seek out and boldly destroy confused cancer cells.

Signs to watch for

You should report any of the following signs and symptoms to your doctor at once. They are among the first indications of cancer, which is more likely to be treated successfully if it is discovered in the early stages.

These symptoms can also indicate a number of other, non-cancerous conditions, so do not be fearful and mistakenly assume that you have a serious illness if you notice one of the signs. Instead, find out its cause and have it treated promptly.
Persistent coughing; coughing up blood.
Skin sores (ulcers) that do not heal.
Blood in the urine or faeces.
Persisting changes in bowel habits.
Lump or puckered area in a breast.
Blood-stained vaginal discharge.
Indigestion with no known cause.
Persistent tiredness for no reason.
Vaginal bleeding between periods, after intercourse or after the MENOPAUSE.
Lump in the neck.
Unexplained weight loss.

Other alternative therapies

Immunoaugmentative Therapy In an attempt to boost the immune system, extracts from human blood known as 'immune protein factors' are injected into the muscle. Some of the blood is from healthy volunteers and some from people with cancer. Dramatic improvements have been claimed.

Acupuncture This has been used to combat the effects of radiotherapy for cancer of the cervix and has produced good results. It has also improved the number of white blood cells – responsible for destroying cancer cells – in patients after radiotherapy. It is mainly used, however, to relieve symptoms or minimise the discomforts that may be caused by the application of orthodox treatment.

An orthodox view

Surgery to remove tumours, radiotherapy to kill cancer cells by radiation, and chemotherapy to stop the multiplication of mutant cells with drugs are the treatments that orthodox medicine considers most effective. But these treatments do not constitute a complete answer to all forms of cancer.

It is becoming increasingly clear that by the time a tumour has grown large enough to be detected, the cancer cells will have been growing for several years and may have spread to other parts of the body, so that surgery may not remove all the cancerous tissue.

Nevertheless, removal of the cancer may be necessary to relieve symptoms caused by obstruction as well as to control local spread. Cancers of the breast, lung, bowel, womb and testicles are among those where surgery is most likely to be recommended.

Radiotherapy is often the first choice of treatment in skin cancer and early cancer of the cervix. Not all cancers are sensitive to radiation and the farther away from the skin, the more difficult is the treatment. The techniques which are used today in radiotherapy, as in surgery, have improved considerably but there may be unwelcome side effects. Their severity depends partly on the patient's level of well-being before treatment begins. Tiredness and nausea are by far the most common. Both can be alleviated by drugs. Depression is another frequent side effect. Many radiotherapy centres now employ counsellors to support patients during treatment.

In some cancers, chemotherapy is the preferred treatment, and the response can be excellent. Twenty years ago leukaemia was almost invariably fatal. Now many children are cured simply with chemotherapy. Chemotherapy is also used in treating Hodgkin's disease and for tumours of the testicles and of the bone marrow. More than 50 different drugs have been used for treating cancer, and the greatest success has come from giving drugs in combination as a 'cocktail'. In recent times, drugs have been developed which attack the cancer cells only. This reduces the side effects, but chemotherapy can still be an unpleasant form of treatment.

Although orthodox treatments do not guarantee a cure, they can halt the spread and should not be discarded out of hand. Alternative therapies are controversial and cannot replace normal treatment.

Many patients say that anticancer diets have helped by giving them some positive action they can take. However, there is no scientific evidence that they work. One recent study has even found that some patients who followed the Bristol Centre's programme in addition to receiving orthodox treatment had a poorer survival rate than those with similar cancers who had only conventional therapy, although the results of that particular study are still open to question.

Medical opinion in South Africa and abroad varies as to the worth of large vitamin supplements. Various clinical trials over the years have failed to show that there have been increases in survival time. However, there are doctors who recommend them for patients who have an increased risk of developing stomach cancer.

Herbal extracts are not regarded as effective, and one containing Laetrile (bitter almond) is dangerous because it contains cyanide. There are dangers also in injecting supposed immune factor extracts from blood: some extracts have contained the hepatitis B virus.

Orthodox doctors do not accept that visualisation therapy, hypnotherapy or meditation techniques have been proven to affect tumour growth or the survival time of patients. But they do recognise that individual and group psychotherapy can show an individual and group effect on survival time.

It is generally accepted in orthodox medicine that ongoing psychological support is a vital component in treating the various forms of cancer.

As with diet therapies, any benefit may be in taking positive steps that increase belief in one's power to recover. Such belief with its presumed effect on the immune system, may account for instances of 'spontaneous regression' (reduction of a tumour) by SPIRITUAL HEALING.

Monthly check for men

Cancer of the testicles is almost always cured if it is discovered and treated properly in its early stages. A simple, thorough check which you can carry out at home once a month will detect it.

Make the test just after you have had a warm bath when the skin is relaxed. If you find anything you consider to be unusual, be sure to consult your general practitioner as soon as possible.

Use the thumb and fingers of both hands to press gently all round the testicles one at a time.

After you have made a few regular checks you will be familiar with what is normal for you and notice any variation from normal. Don't be alarmed if one testicle seems a little larger than the other – this is quite normal.

The soft lump you will feel at the top and towards the back of each testicle is the epididymis, the sperm-carrying tube to which it is attached.

Check that the testicles are smooth and without swellings. They should be of about matching weight, and should not be harder or softer than usual.

CANDIDA

This is a fungal disorder more commonly called THRUSH. It is caused by an excess amount of the yeast-like fungus *Candida albicans*, which lives on the skin and vulva, and in the mouth, bowel and vagina.

Normally the fungus is quite harmless. However, it sometimes sets up an irritating infection which is characterised by sore white patches. These patches usually affect the mouth or vagina.

CARPAL TUNNEL SYNDROME

Tissues inside a space in the wrist called the carpal tunnel can sometimes swell, pinching a nerve and causing the painful condition known as carpal tunnel syndrome. There is a feeling of numbness, tingling and pain in the index finger and first finger of the affected hand, and also weakness in the thumb.

Middle-aged and pregnant women are the principal sufferers, especially those who use their fingers a lot, such as typists, housewives and pianists.

The condition is often worse at night, when the pain and tingling may spread up the forearm and interrupt sleep. Hanging the affected arm – or arms – over the side of the bed sometimes brings relief; a splint on the wrist may also help.

Without treatment, the symptoms will gradually worsen over the months or years. Anyone developing the symptoms should see an orthodox doctor before using any alternative treatment.

What the therapists recommend
NATUROPATHY

Self help The cause can be either fluid pressure on the median nerve within the carpal tunnel, or inflammation of the tissues making up the tunnel itself. When there is fluid build-up, vitamin B_6 is believed to be effective in reducing the local swelling.

Using cold packs for ten minutes twice a day can also help. However, in persistent cases surgery may be recommended, as in orthodox medicine.

An orthodox view
A doctor will usually prescribe painkillers – or, if the condition is particularly troublesome, he may inject the wrist with cortisone to reduce the tissue swelling. However, a minor operation on the wrist usually relieves the condition rapidly.

CATARACTS

One or both eyes can be affected by a cataract – a cloudy area in the lens which causes blurred or impaired vision. Cataracts usually appear in old age, as advancing years bring a deterioration in the blood supply to the lens. In many cases, one eye is affected more than the other, and most elderly people who have cataracts have little trouble with their vision. But if seeing becomes difficult they should consult a doctor.

What the therapists recommend
Naturopathy Some naturopaths believe that cataracts are partly the result of a deficiency of riboflavin (vitamin B_2), which must be rectified. Vitamin C is also thought to be useful in protecting the eye lenses against harmful effects of sunlight.

An orthodox view
In severe cases – especially if the sight in the 'best' eye is impaired – a doctor may refer his patient to an eye specialist. An operation may then be performed to remove the cataract or cataracts. The operation is simple and vision is restored with a contact lens or a plastic lens implanted within the eye. In South Africa, a common cause of cataracts is exposure to strong sunlight. Sunglasses should be worn to protect the eyes.

CATARRH

Any inflammation or irritation of the membranes that line the passages of the throat, nose and lungs can cause catarrh – a thick mucus. A little watery mucus is necessary to protect and lubricate the membranes, but too much and/or too thick mucus can cause a blocked or runny nose, COUGHS or earache. If the symptoms last more than a few days they may point to an infection (if the mucus is yellow or green) or COLDS, SINUS PROBLEMS, a poor diet or ALLERGY.

What the therapists recommend
NATUROPATHY

Self help Be sure to eat a nutritious wholefood diet including plenty of fresh fruit, salads, vegetables, fish, nuts, honey and wholegrain cereals.

Take regular outdoor exercise and get lots of sleep (see SLEEP DISORDERS). Avoid foods that encourage mucus production, such as milk and milk products, meat, eggs, animal fats, pulses, and those containing white flour, white sugar or FOOD ADDITIVES. A treatment which can provide effective relief is to add the juice of half a lemon to a cup of warm water in a bowl, and inhale the mixture gently through the nostrils, right up to the back of the nose. It may make you sneeze and splutter, but is a good way of clearing catarrh from the nose. Be sure to repeat this procedure several times a day.

Consultation Advice will be given about your particular diet, eliminating impurities from the body and treating bouts of CONSTIPATION – which naturopaths say is often associated with catarrh. Tests for allergies – especially milk and dairy products – may be done and, if necessary, a special diet will be drawn up.

Supplements such as the vitamin B-complex, vitamin C, bioflavinoids and zinc are sometimes prescribed. Initial FASTING or a RAW FOOD DIET may be suggested, but must be supervised.

HERBAL MEDICINE
Self help Infusions (see p. 184) of hyssop, slippery elm, marsh-mallow, elderflower, ribwort or catmint seeds are believed to help. Add honey or lemon juice if you prefer – they are also good for the mucous membranes. Some herbalists recommend a combination of equal quantities of hyssop, eyebright and yarrow taken as an infusion. Other helpful herbs include rosemary, *Echinacea*, white horehound, Irish moss and elecampane.

HOMOEOPATHY
Self help Homoeopaths recommend *Nat. mur.* for catarrh that has the consistency of egg white and causes sneezing; *Kali bich.* for stringy yellow or white catarrh; *Hydrastis* for continual dripping at the back of the nose and blocked ears; *Arsenicum iodum* if you feel run down and have a runny nose; *Graphites* for catarrh with constipation, skin irritation around the nose and a chill; *Pulsatilla* for a head cold and thick yellowish-white mucus, and *Euphrasia* for a cold with watering eyes and runny nose. In each case take one tablet (6C potency) every two hours six times, then three times daily until better.

Other alternative treatments
Aromatherapy Use basil, eucalyptus, black pepper, hyssop, lavender, lemon, marjoram, peppermint, thyme or cedarwood oil in a bath or steam inhalation. A gargle said to be effective can be made from one drop each of eucalyptus, lemon and tea-tree or cedarwood essential oils in half a cup of water; stir before each mouthful.

Biochemic Tissue Salts *Kali sulph.* and combination remedy Q are advised for all types of catarrh. In addition, *Ferr. phos.* and combination remedy H may help to get rid of nasal catarrh, and *Kali mur.* is recommended if the secretion is white.

Acupressure Pressure is applied to points at the back of the skull, on either side of the nose, and on the web of the hand.

Acupuncture Treatment usually involves acupuncture at points on the large intestine, stomach and lung meridians.

Massage Facial massage can help to drain the sinuses. If mucus is lodged in the bronchial tubes, superficial stroking massage of the upper back, vibratory petrissage (picking up) over the shoulder muscles and vibratory friction over the lower tip of the breastbone may help to bring it up.

Hydrotherapy Treatments such as mustard footbaths, hot and cold compresses, friction rubs and cold hip-baths may help. Nasal douches and gargling with a teaspoon of salt or baking powder dissolved in a glass of warm water may also give relief.

Reflexology Therapists recommend massage to the reflex areas relating to the nose and sinuses, plus areas relating to the head, eyes, upper lymph nodes and digestive system. See chart, p. 295.

An orthodox view

Catarrh is a symptom rather than a disease, so the orthodox view would support making an accurate diagnosis before resorting to any kind of treatment. However, most episodes of catarrh are self-limiting.

CELLULITE

The term 'cellulite' was coined by certain French doctors for what they believe is a form of fat that accumulates in women, causing the thighs, bottom, upper arms and stomach to look lumpy and dimpled. It afflicts women – even slim ones – mostly at the MENOPAUSE, and is difficult to get rid of.

The cause is believed by many European doctors and many health and beauty experts to be a build-up of waste materials in the body tissues, creating various pockets of water, fat and impurities, and encouraging the formation of a 'sludge' in the blood, leading to CIRCULATION PROBLEMS.

However, the theory is controversial, and most doctors in South Africa do not believe that cellulite is a special form of fat, and do not acknowledge it as a medical condition (see 'An orthodox view').

What the therapists recommend

NATUROPATHY

Self help A 75 per cent raw food diet is claimed to prevent cellulite forming, to eliminate existing cellulite and to prevent a further build-up (see EATING FOR HEALTH and RAW FOOD DIET). Eating about two or three pieces

of citrus fruit a day – including the pith – is also said to help.

These foods are also recommended:

Beetroot juice to help the liver to break down stored fats. Make fresh beetroot juice with an extractor, or buy it from health food stores, and drink 120 ml daily.

Celery to help remove excess fluid from the body. Eat it raw, or make a fresh juice cocktail with celery, beetroot and carrots.

Cucumber to make the kidneys eliminate more wastes. Extract and drink the juice or eat a large cucumber salad every day.

Seaweed contains minerals, proteins, vitamins and iodine. It is said to promote a smooth skin and to get fats moving in the body. Kelp (seaweed) tablets are available from health food stores and some chemists; other edible sea plants can be found in some health food stores and oriental food shops.

Spirulina is a blue-green algae plant, available as tablets or capsules from health food stores. It is held to be highly nutritious, while also suppressing appetite. It can be taken safely in doses of up to 8 g a day.

Watermelons are said to help remove excess fluid from the body.

Skin-brushing

This is a technique claimed to remove toxic wastes directly through the skin, and to stimulate the lymphatic system. Use a long-handled, natural-bristle brush or a friction glove – available from chemists – and follow a daily routine, brushing after getting up in the morning and before going to bed. Brush your whole body – except your face – starting gently, then using a firmer action as you get used to the feel of it.

Consultation Naturopaths believe that the underlying cause may be the typical Western diet, containing too much starch, fat, protein and sugar. A practitioner will prescribe a diet that includes lots of fresh raw vegetables.

He may also advise you to combine the diet with 30 minutes' general EXERCISE three times a week to improve circulation and general fitness. But check with your doctor first, to see if you are fit enough.

Finally, a skin-brushing regime (see illustrations below) and, if you are in good health, an occasional SAUNA BATH could be recommended, or alternating hot and cold sprays on the thighs and pelvis.

An orthodox view

Most South African doctors believe that cellulite is simply ordinary fat pulled downwards by gravity, and that when this is lost, so are the dimples. Because of its link with the menopause, doctors also believe that hormonal changes may be an important contributing factor.

However, research in France, Italy and Germany has revealed that CONSTIPATION, a poor lymphatic system, poor circulation and weak

1 Start at the feet, including the soles, then move up the legs, back and front, with firm sweeping strokes.

2 Brush from the hands up the arms and across the shoulders, then brush the back and buttocks.

3 Using a gentler action, brush your stomach with clockwise, circular strokes; then brush the chest and neck. Finally, take a shower: warm for 30 seconds, then cold for 30 seconds. Repeat, dry off and keep warm.

functioning of the kidneys and liver are all common in women prone to cellulite.

The orthodox approach locally is simply to lose weight. European commercial cellulite creams, which are massaged into affected areas, are available from most chemists, but the general opinion of the majority of health and beauty experts is that these cannot work on their own.

CEREBRAL PALSY

Damage to part of the brain – in the later months of pregnancy, at birth or in early infancy – is the cause of cerebral palsy, a disability that affects muscular activity and co-ordination in the limbs. Most cases can be ascribed to insufficient oxygen to the unborn child's brain during pregnancy.

It is a 'non-progressive illness' in the sense that it does not grow worse; and though a majority of sufferers are mentally retarded, some may be highly intelligent, and with skilled treatment be able to overcome some of their disabilities. Many so-called 'spastics' are the victims of cerebral palsy.

What the therapists recommend

Alternative therapists concede that this condition cannot be cured. Acupuncture and homoeopathy may be able to provide some symptomatic relief, however; and there is agreement with the orthodox view that physical therapy and speech therapy can do much to improve the sufferer's quality of life. Every effort must be made to develop the cerebral palsy sufferer's abilities to the full.

An orthodox view

With the help of physical exercises the patient can be taught to develop muscular control and balance. If speaking is a problem, a speech therapist should be consulted.

For details contact the National Cerebral Palsy Division of the National Council for the Physically Disabled in South Africa, P O Box 426, Melville 2109 (telephone 011-7268040).

CHAPPING

In cold weather, a number of people are troubled by chapped skin – especially if they have to wash their hands frequently because of their work. In some cases the skin tends to become inflamed and cannot tolerate soap and water at all.

Wind and cold may also affect the lips, which become cracked and inflamed.

What the therapists recommend

Traditional Medicine Mudpacks – especially those made from clay-rich earth – have been used to treat dry and chapped skin since the Middle Ages. They are said to soften the skin and, as the mud becomes harder and shrinks, to draw impurities in the skin to the surface, and to pull off the top layer of dead cells. They are available at chemists and health food stores. Do not use them if your skin is inflamed.

Glycerine mixed with rosewater is said to prevent rough and chapped hands even in the coldest weather. Rub the mixture well into the fingers and backs of the hands and then dry them with a paper towel. For very fine and sensitive skin, mix a little cocoa-butter with half its quantity of pure olive oil and rub gently into the skin.

Aromatherapy Benzoin and patchouli are strongly recommended, lavender and geranium are also useful. Add 15-20 drops of the chosen oil to 60 ml of base white carrier lotion and apply to the skin.

An orthodox view

Most doctors feel that there is no need to use anything more than the proprietary creams, lotions and lip salves from a chemist.

For housewives or kitchen workers, whose hands are often in water, a barrier cream applied in the morning, before starting work, can help. Otherwise, ordinary vanishing or cold creams should help (see also NATURAL AIDS TO BEAUTY).

Lanolin cream has also proved effective, but as it comes from wool fat some people may be allergic to it (see ALLERGY).

CHARISMATIC HEALING

The treatment of disease by charismatic healing is based on Christian faith and prayer. Meetings at which people pray for their own good health, as well as that of relatives and various friends, are held in churches of many denominations, and enjoy the participation of hundreds of thousands of believers throughout the world.

In Catholic churches they sometimes form part of a normal Sunday service. At any time during the week such meetings are sometimes held in the assembly places of Quakers and other religious groups.

The therapy – which comes from the Greek word *charis*, meaning 'grace' – dates back to Biblical times and Christ's miracles. Charismatic healing seeks to carry on this work

through the Holy Spirit. Healers may be laymen or priests, who appeal to the Holy Spirit to release healing forces and direct them at the sick – whether they are aware of it or not (see ABSENT HEALING). Prayer sessions can last from five minutes to several hours. See also HEALERS AND HEALING.

As well as praying for divine healing, many believers use personal prayer to help prevent sickness.

Who it can help Most believers in charismatic healing are practising Christians who go regularly to church. However, anyone who believes in God can pray at home for the blessing of good health.

An orthodox view

Although doctors recognise that so-called 'miracle cures' have sometimes occurred, they think of them as 'spontaneous remissions', in which the body heals itself.

CHICKENPOX

This highly infectious disease – with its irritating, itching rash and blisters – usually affects children. It is milder in childhood, so it is best not to keep children away from school during an outbreak, for catching chickenpox also brings immunity from it later in life, when its effects can be more serious.

Known medically as *varicella*, it is caused by the virus which also causes SHINGLES. Symptoms show between 12 and 14 days after infection, starting with a raised temperature and an itchy rash – usually on the body – which spreads to the limbs, face and head. The pink spots soon turn into watery blisters, then burst or shrivel and, after about five days, form scabs. Adult sufferers feel quite ill for the first few days.

The virus can be passed to people in close contact with the sufferer from about four days before the rash appears until the spots have gone. Although the sufferer becomes immune to the disease, the virus may remain in the system and cause shingles later.

What the therapists recommend
NATUROPATHY

Self help Raw fruit and vegetable juices are recommended: fresh orange and lemon juice, sweetened with honey if necessary, and a daily intake of about 600 ml of carrot juice, mixed with 150 ml of watercress juice to prevent dehydration. During convalescence, a modest wholefood diet (see EATING FOR HEALTH) is held to be beneficial.

Consultation Practitioners see the symptoms as the natural reaction to infection. A supervised fast may be advised, with the aim of raising the blood's white cell count – and in doing so, the temperature, to kill the virus and stimulate the IMMUNE SYSTEM. Sponging the spots with tepid water during the first few days may also be suggested.

HERBAL MEDICINE

Self help To soothe irritation, an infusion (p. 184) of elder flowers sponged on the spots is said to help. Alternatively, try tincture of comfrey, or essential oil of lavender on the spots, being careful to avoid the eyes. Aloe vera gel can reduce the itching.

To ease the fever for children between six and ten, try a dessertspoon of herbal tea four times daily: yarrow, lime blossom, camomile flowers or meadowsweet, with honey. For younger children give 2 teaspoonfuls.

Consultation A practitioner may advise taking GARLIC – either raw or in capsule form – and eucalyptus, as an infusion. Boil 30 g of eucalyptus leaves in 1 litre of water. Cover for ten minutes, strain, cool and give 1 teaspoonful three times daily.

Other alternative treatments

Homoeopathy At the onset of symptoms, *Rhus tox.* is said to soothe restlessness and ease the irritation. Other recommendations include *Antimonium tart.* if the child is irritable and has large blisters, a cough and cold symptoms; *Pulsatilla nigricans* if the child is weepy and not thirsty, and *Aconitum napellus* if there is fever, or the pulse rate increases.

Aromatherapy Try lemon tea, made with three drops of essential oil of lemon, one teabag and 900 ml of water. Drink a cupful three times daily.

Biochemic Tissue Salts *Ferr. phos.* is recommended to combat feverishness and restlessness; and *Kali mur.* once the fever has cleared and the spots blister.

An orthodox view

Many doctors feel that some alternative treatments may help and that they will not do any harm. However, they say that most cases can be treated at home by keeping the rash clean and dry, and easing itching with calamine lotion.

Avoid picking spots – this can result in permanent pockmarks. There is no immunisation against the virus.

Liquids are important, rather than solid food, and the patient should get plenty of rest. Consult your doctor only if the eyes are affected; if there is a high fever or excessive coughing and vomiting; or if the spots become overinflamed. If the lungs, skin or ears are secondarily infected, a doctor may then prescribe antibiotics.

Once the infection is overcome, recovery is complete – and the spots will leave scars only if they are scratched or become infected.

CHILBLAINS

Exposure to the cold can give people with sensitive skin or poor circulation chilblains – reddish-blue swellings that itch and burn. They occur when blood vessels shrink so severely that the skin's supply of blood and oxygen is severely reduced. Chilblains mostly break out on the toes and fingers, but they may affect the ears and other parts of the body. Never scratch chilblains – it only makes them worse.

What the therapists recommend

Traditional Medicine According to folklore even severe chilblains can be eased – if not cured – by a paste made of glycerine and honey. Mix a tablespoon of each with the white of an egg and a tablespoon of flour. Beat the ingredients into a fine paste and spread it over the swellings – first making sure they are clean and dry. Cover the sticky paste with a cloth or bandage and leave in place for 24 hours.

Naturopathy Many therapists believe the best cure to be a form of HYDROTHERAPY. First bathe your feet in warm water for about three minutes – then dip them in cold for one minute. Repeat for about 20 minutes morning or evening, always finishing with cold.

It may also help to massage your feet afterwards in a footbath containing 1 tablespoon of calendula or mustard oil to 2,3 litres of warm water. Vitamins E and C may also be prescribed for people particularly susceptible to chilblains.

Homoeopathy Recommended remedies involve rubbing the chilblains with *Tamus* ointment when the chilblains are cracked; *Rhus tox.* applied twice a day when chilblains are inflamed and itch; and *Agaricus muscaria*, applied every three hours when there is much burning, itching and redness. Use *Petroleum* when the skin is cracked and broken, with a tendency to ulcerate or chap, or where there are split fingertips. *Carbo veg.* is also for itching, burning, and when the chilblains feel worse in a warm bed. Apply the chosen remedy, in the 6th potency, three times a day for two weeks.

Nutritional Therapy Chilblains are said to respond well to a calcium-rich diet, particularly fresh green vegetables and oranges, almonds, yoghurt and sesame seeds. Vitamin supplements held to be beneficial include vitamin B-complex (500 mg a day).

An orthodox view

Doctors point out that, provided you do not expose susceptible areas to the cold, chilblains usually clear up without treatment in two to three weeks. However, they feel that alternative treatments may help. The best

way to prevent chilblains is to wear warm clothing – especially gloves, trousers and shoes. Do not smoke, as nicotine reduces the blood circulation in the skin (see SMOKING). People with poor circulation should take regular EXERCISE to stimulate the blood flow.

To soothe the burning and itching, doctors may prescribe suitable skin creams.

CHILL

A chill is often the first sign of a number of ailments but usually heralds COLDS or a FEVER – especially if accompanied by raised body temperature and alternating bouts of shivering and sweating.

Some people believe wrongly that a nip of brandy or whisky will 'take the chill off'. Alcohol dilates blood vessels just beneath the skin, bringing extra blood to the surface, causing you to lose body heat. An immediate feeling of warmth is soon replaced by an even greater chill – particularly if the 'nip' is taken outside. Better simply to stay indoors.

CHIROPRACTIC

Relieving pain by joint manipulation

By the skilful use of their hands, chiropractors set out to correct disorders of the joints, muscles and – particularly – the spine. Spinal problems can cause pain not only in the spine itself, but in other parts of the body – including the shoulder, arm, hip and leg. In addition, the disorders can also sometimes bring on SCIATICA as well as back problems such as LUMBAGO and SLIPPED DISC. In some cases they are even said to cause such diverse conditions as ASTHMA, ARTHRITIS, CATARRH, CONSTIPATION, MIGRAINE, PERIOD PROBLEMS and STRESS.

The techniques and approach of chiropractic around the world are similar in many ways to those of OSTEOPATHY. For example, neither therapy uses drugs or surgery to treat patients. But the major difference between them is that chiropractors make far greater use of X-rays and conventional diagnostic methods than osteopaths.

Who it can help More than 90 per cent of a chiropractor's patients suffer from some kind of musculoskeletal pain – especially low BACK PAIN and NECK PAIN. People with whiplash injuries from car accidents – in which the head has been abruptly jerked backwards or forwards – are also high on the list of those seeking treatment.

HEADACHES are another common ailment treated by chiropractic. In most cases treated the headache is caused by TENSION contracting the neck muscles – for example, those which help to balance the head on the neck joints at the top of the spine.

Sportsmen suffering from a range of injuries – including strained muscles, sprained joints, damaged ligaments, injured tendons, wrenched knees and TENNIS ELBOW – may also benefit from chiropractic. In some cases heat or ice applications are used, as well as specific joint manipulation.

There are no age barriers as far as chiropractic is concerned and anyone from babies to senior citizens can be treated.

Difficult births involving the use of forceps can injure a baby's neck or strain its spine, although this may not be apparent at the time of birth. Chiropractors say that it can, however, lead to neck problems or headaches later on in life.

Sometimes, in infancy or early childhood, a baby may fall from a cot, be accidentally dropped, or stumble against furniture when learning to walk. This can jar its spine, causing back pain to develop long afterwards. In some cases a baby's spine can adapt after a short period of pain only to prove troublesome later on. Many childhood or adolescent discomforts are wrongly attributed to 'growing pains', when the root cause may be musculoskeletal injury.

If a child has had any such accidents, or suffers from puzzling aches or pains, it could be that he or she needs to see a qualified chiropractor – ask your doctor's advice. In any

Daniel David Palmer (1845-1913)

Chiropractic's birth

In 1895 a 'magnetic healer' named Daniel David Palmer treated his office janitor for deafness. The man told Palmer that he had lost his hearing when bending down – he had felt a click in his back, and shortly became deaf. Palmer found that some small bones in the cleaner's spine were quite misaligned. He manipulated them and the janitor's hearing was restored.

The healer founded the Palmer School of Chiropractic – from the Greek *kheir*, meaning 'hand', and *praktikos*, meaning 'action'. 'Displacement of any part of the skeletal frame,' he stated, 'may press against nerves, which are the channels of communication, intensifying or decreasing their carrying capacity, creating either too much or not enough functioning, an aberration known as disease.'

case, chiropractors advise periodic checkups in childhood, to help to avoid spinal or pelvic problems later.

Many older people suffering from back or joint pain rely on painkillers to give them relief. However, this only deals with the symptoms – and the real cause of the pain is often not treated. Chiropractic, it is said, can often help these people considerably.

During pregnancy, women often suffer from backache due to the increased weight on the spine and difficulty in maintaining their balance.

And in childbirth itself changes occur in the pelvis and the sacroiliac joint (the joint at the base of the spine which carries the weight of the body to the legs). Again, this can cause back pain; and the spine can be further damaged after childbirth, when the baby is lifted and carried.

In all these cases chiropractors say that they can help to ease, if not banish, the pain.

Finding a practitioner Most people are recommended to chiropractors for assessment and possible private treatment by others who have benefited from the therapy themselves.

In South Africa, The Natal Technikon (P O Box 953, Durban 4000) offers a five-year programme leading to a master's diploma in Technology: Chiropractic. This must be followed by a one-year internship, required by the South African Associated Health Service Professions Board (P O Box 17055, Groenkloof 0027; telephone 012-466455), before registration with the board as a chiropractor can take place. For more details contact the Chiropractic Association of South Africa at 701 Poynton House, Gardiner Street, Durban 4001 (telephone 031-3044200).

Consulting a practitioner At the first consultation the chiropractor will inevitably take comprehensive details of your medical history, as well as the seriousness of the current problem. He will then examine you, feeling for areas of muscle spasm, pain and tenderness – and discovering which joints are moving properly and which are not.

The chiropractor may take an X-ray to determine the condition of the spine. This may also reveal signs of arthritis, bone disease or fractures. Finally, the practitioner will decide whether chiropractic treatment will help, or if a fracture or disease means that you should rely on a doctor.

A *chiropractor at work*

This 16-year-old patient suffered a whiplash injury, which seriously misaligned the vertebrae in her neck (top X-ray). Constant pain and the side effects of the drugs she took made her too ill to go to school. The chiropractor is shown manipulating the bones in the patient's neck. He was able to realign the vertebrae (bottom X-ray), and she made a complete recovery.

Once the diagnosis has been made, the chiropractor usually begins the treatment by asking you to strip to your underwear. Women patients may put on a robe. You will stand, sit, or lie on a chiropractic couch – specially designed for manipulative therapy, and various manual treatment techniques may then be used.

For example, to adjust (or manipulate) a painful lower lumbar or low back joint, the patient lies on one side. The chiropractor then manually rotates the upper spine one way, and the lower spine the other way. The rotation partially locks the joint to be adjusted. Usually, the patient's uppermost leg is flexed to help in the locking.

The chiropractor then feels the vertebra either just above or below the joint. The patient's position, plus slight pressure by the chiropractor's hand, now takes the joint to the end of its normal range of movement.

Next, the chiropractor makes a very rapid thrust to the vertebra, taking the joint slightly beyond its present range. This restores normal movement to the joint, and by suddenly stretching the muscles which are in spasm around it, helps to relax the deep spinal muscles that control the joint.

The adjustment should not be painful, and afterwards the patient is re-examined. The locked joint should now be moving more freely and, because the muscles have been relaxed, the area should be more flexible.

Some patients will feel relief from pain immediately; others may experience aching, soreness and stiffness later that day, or the day after. In certain cases four or more treatments may be necessary before the pain starts to go. Generally speaking, chronic (long-lasting) cases need more treatment than acute (severe and sudden) cases.

An orthodox view

Although there is little doubt in South Africa and abroad that chiropractic is of considerable help to a large number of people, including doctors, the orthodox view is that chiropractic is a collection of empirical techniques based on assumptions which have never been proved by scientific investigation.

Chiropractic's principal use is in the treatment of musculoskeletal disorders, but orthodox doctors would not support its use in general disease states, such as asthma or DIABETES.

CHOLERA

Like other infectious diseases of the intestine, cholera is acquired when contaminated water or food is consumed, and it is prevalent in areas of poor sanitation. The culprit responsible for the disease is the bacterium *Vibrio cholerae*, found in the faeces of patients and of carriers.

The severe symptoms of cholera may appear within a few hours of infection, or only after a few days: they include a sudden onset of watery diarrhoea, often accompanied by vomiting. The loss of fluid from the system is severe, and if not counteracted in good time may lead to death. Muscle cramps are a side-effect of the fluid loss.

What the therapists recommend

Homoeopathy Treatment will depend on the homoeopath's wider assessment of the patient's state of health.

Naturopathy Complete rest and warmth are priorities, with hot-water bottles or hot compresses applied to the abdomen. The patient can sip diluted, unsweetened lemon juice but must not attempt to eat for several days. Food should later consist of very simple, single-item meals, and then a diet high in protein and mineral salts but little carbohydrates.

Herbal medicine An infusion of buchu leaves, drunk as a tea, is an ancient traditional South African treatment for cholera.

An orthodox view

The doctor's immediate preoccupation is to replace body fluid, which he may arrange by means of an intravenous drip. Subsidiary treatment could include antibiotic injections or tablets. A cholera vaccine is available to travellers to lands where the disease is prevalent, but precautions must still be taken to avoid consuming contaminated food and drink. The vaccine is effective for only about six months.

CIRCULATION PROBLEMS

Poor circulation is a blanket term which is generally used to describe such diverse conditions as ANGINA, CHILBLAINS, CRAMP, DIZZINESS, FROSTBITE, VARICOSE VEINS and HEART DISORDERS.

What the therapists recommend

Naturopathy A diet which includes plenty of FIBRE and fresh green vegetables is recommended to avoid circulation problems (see EATING FOR HEALTH). A diet rich in fish and fish oils may be prescribed in certain cases. In addition, you should take plenty of EXERCISE – such as walking and swimming – and be sure not to let yourself become overweight (see SLIMMING THE NATURAL WAY). It is also advisable to stop SMOKING, as nicotine damages the arteries.

Many practitioners believe that vitamin supplements – especially vitamins C and E – can play a vital part in preventing the build-up of cholesterol in the body – see ARTERIES (HARDENING).

Herbal Medicine Practitioners recommend several remedies to improve circulation, including cayenne, hawthorn and prickly ash. They are normally prescribed in tincture form, amounts depending on individual circumstances. Advice on diet and exercise may also be given.

An orthodox view

In general, orthodox doctors think that diet, exercise, weightwatching and the giving up of smoking are key factors in preventing circulation problems.

CLAUSTROPHOBIA

The anxiety of confinement in small spaces

One of the most common forms of ANXIETY is claustrophobia – a phobia (exaggerated fear) of crowded places and being shut up in small spaces, such as lifts, tiny rooms or overcrowded buses.

When the sufferer feels confined, overwhelming symptoms of TENSION, HYPERVENTILATION, rapid pulse and SWEATING are experienced. Everyday life is often severely disrupted because the sufferer avoids the situations that make him tense, and his movements become limited. Very often this has a ripple effect on the people with whom he is living.

The condition is often an expression of an underlying mental problem of which the sufferer is not aware, such as STRESS, FEAR or an emotionally traumatic experience during childhood. It may also be hereditary.

What the therapists recommend
HYPNOTHERAPY

Consultation After discussing your problem, the hypnotherapist will place you in a trance, during which he will suggest changes that will affect your behaviour and the way you react to the world. These will be remembered by the unconscious mind. The hypnotist would also gradually take you out of your home in your imagination, and repeated sessions would eventually desensitise you to the problem. Hypnotherapy is said to be able to cure phobias, and to work faster than conventional psychotherapy.

NATUROPATHY

Consultation A naturopath will suggest a mainly raw wholefood diet (see EATING FOR HEALTH) and may use KINESIOLOGY muscle-testing techniques to find any food allergy that may be causing the problem.

Self help For the effective treatment of stress, high potency vitamin B complex tablets, available from health food stores, are usually suggested. You should take a dose of up to 50 mg two or three times daily, reducing gradually to one daily. Vitamin C is also said to help guard against stress – take 200 mg with each meal.

Zinc and magnesium mineral supplements may also be helpful for stress taken in a 100 mg zinc and magnesium combination.

In some cases, a naturopath will work alongside a psychotherapist and help in teaching specific relaxation exercises to combat stress.

Other alternative treatments

Acupressure You can help yourself to relax by gently massaging an acupressure point in the web of either hand – between the thumb and the index finger.

Autogenics This simple system of mental exercise can help the body and mind to relax, releasing you from stress and the abnormal pattern of behaviour it has been causing. Training is with a qualified practitioner and, once learned, autogenics is a technique you can use at home.

Homoeopathy A general remedy is *Argentum nitricum*, and *Aconite* is said to help people who are fearful and apprehensive before an ordeal, and fear closed spaces and crowds. Take the 30th potency every ten minutes until relief is found.

Reflexology The generally relaxing effect of this treatment may well be helpful, but professional treatment should be sought.

Bach Remedies Mimulus if the fear is well-defined; Aspen for vague apprehensiveness; Rock rose if it escalates into panic; Rescue Remedy for an acute attack.

An orthodox view

A careful case history is prepared by the doctor, and tests may be made to check whether the sufferer's problem is caused by anxiety or is inherited.

Medical treatment for severe anxiety may include COUNSELLING, with tranquillisers being administered to relieve symptoms and help the sufferer to relax and cope better in small, crowded spaces.

BEHAVIOURAL THERAPY may also be prescribed by doctors, and during it you are faced with claustrophobic situations for gradually longer periods. This may be combined with PSYCHOTHERAPY involving both the sufferer and his family. See also PHOBIAS.

CLINICAL ECOLOGY
Overcoming sensitivities to food and other substances

The idea that people are made ill by their environment – the basis of clinical ecology – is far from new. The father of medical science, Hippocrates, a Greek physician of the 5th century BC, knew of reactions to certain foods. Foods are the most common of the environmental factors that cause illness, but pesticides, fungicides, weedkillers, dust, pollen, petrol and diesel fumes, cleaning agents and many other chemical pollutants take their toll (see HEALTH HAZARDS).

Medical interest in patients' abnormally sensitive reactions to foods and chemicals swelled in the United States from the 1920s. In Britain, clinical ecology began to attract the attention of doctors in the 1970s. Many now accept that physical sensitivity short of ALLERGY does cause illness, but others find a major obstacle in the fact that no conventionally acceptable test for true allergy helps in diagnosing ecological illnesses.

Research into food and chemical sensitivity is slow. It is an unpromising area for the pharmaceutical companies that fund much medical research, since the treatments are unlikely to involve drugs that they could market. But investigations made so far suggest that patients have abnormalities in their IMMUNE SYSTEM.

People with true allergy have abnormally high amounts of a blood protein called immunoglobulin E (IgE). People with food and chemical sensitivities have increased amounts of the more common immunoglobulin G (IgG). The IgG molecules seem to lodge in certain parts of the body and produce inflammation. Depending on where they lodge, different symptoms are produced. If they lodge in the lining of the nose, they may cause a constantly streaming nose and frequent SNEEZING; in the intestine they may cause chronic DIARRHOEA; in the brain they can produce MIGRAINE.

The mechanisms that set off the abnormal reactions are of several kinds. The lining of the stomach or intestine may be irritated, especially by wheat, bran or spicy foods and especially when the lining is unsound. An enzyme deficiency may make a patient unable to cope with a food: insufficient lactase, for example, leaves the system unable to cope with milk, which then acts as a poison. In some people a psychological reaction to food sets off the abnormal immune response. Other patients can react almost like drug addicts in their continual craving for certain substances, for example the tyramine in chocolate or the caffeine in coffee.

Abnormal bowel bacteria cause sensitivity in a large number of people. The bacteria may be there as a result of taking antibiotics, which can kill friendly as well as harmful organisms. In the bowel, friendly bacteria are often not replaced, or the balance of bacteria is disturbed and too much of a yeast known as *Candida albicans* is produced.

In appropriate cases, a clinical ecologist identifies the foods or chemicals to which a patient is sensitive, to ascertain if possible what mechanism sets off the abnormal reaction, and to advise on treatment to avoid or reduce the reaction. Medical specialists, including doctors, involved in clinical ecology believe that ecological illness is affecting more and more people: at present 10-30 per cent of the population.

As a rule, the foods patients eat most are those to which they are sensitive. Milk and dairy products head the list, followed by sugar, then wheat, coffee, tea, chocolate, eggs, and lastly yeast.

But outside these commonly occurring items are many others that invariably trigger trouble in some individuals. Similarly with chemical triggers, the substances people are exposed to most are the likeliest sources of their intolerance.

The trigger items, whether they happen to be foods or chemicals, will occur not only singly, but often combined with others. Patients need to be aware of all the contents of prepared foods, household cleaning preparations and other products that could contain the source of their intolerance.

Who it can help Numerous symptoms may indicate ecological disease. Completely different symptoms are often triggered in different people by the same cause. Wheat, for example, will cause migraine in one person who is intolerant to it but COLITIS in another. In children, HYPERACTIVITY, disturbed sleep, stomach upsets, COELIAC DISEASE (a sensitivity in the bowel to gluten), ECZEMA, ASTHMA and migraine are among the symptoms. In adults, the symptoms include HEADACHES, DIGESTIVE PROBLEMS, night sweating, PALPITATIONS, RHEUMATISM, INSOMNIA, fatigue and BLADDER PROBLEMS.

People who suffer repeatedly from any of these symptoms, especially without apparent cause, may find a clinical ecologist able to pinpoint the source of the trouble. Sensitivity is increased after a prolonged viral infection such as GLANDULAR FEVER or INFLUENZA, and such cases can also be helped.

Finding a therapist Clinical ecology covers a large area within medicine. In South Africa, most cases would probably be dealt with by homoeopaths, but you can ask your doctor for the names of any clinical ecologists – or of alternative practitioners who have effectively treated cases similar to yours.

The methods used by clinical ecologists vary widely. Choose a therapist who is a skilled tester, not one who relies solely on the elimination diet.

A therapist who is experienced in KINESIOLOGY, electrical testing (see below) or the ACR technique (see below) would be cheaper than one using more time-consuming methods – and may give you a quicker solution to your problem.

Consulting a therapist Identifying the food or chemical to which you may be sensitive will be the first task. Give all the information you can about your diet and habits to help the therapist compile a list of suspect items. The list may be long and it could take time to establish an order of priority for testing. Often there are several items that cause illness, not just one. Eight techniques are in the repertoire of testers:

Radio-allergic solvents test This is the test most likely to be used in conventional medicine – a blood test that can show that IgE has been produced as an allergic reaction to a particular food. However, the RAST, as it is usually called, does not show whether IgG has been produced in people who are sensitive or intolerant to a substance rather than allergic to it.

Elimination diet In everyday life the patient has no distinct, obvious reaction to the substances that cause illness. The reaction becomes obvious after the patient has taken only fluids (usually as a hospital in-patient) for at least five days, and has then had suspect items reintroduced one by one. The fast puts the patient in a clinically hypersensitive state, in which there is usually a strong reaction within a few minutes to the offending food or chemical.

A similar but less drastic method of identifying food sensitivity is to spend five days on a diet unlikely to cause adverse reactions. This will most commonly be lamb and pears. The suspect foods are then reintroduced one by one. First, the less commonly eaten foods are reintroduced, with the initial meal consisting of one food alone.

If no adverse reaction (such as migraine or sweating, or whatever symptom is usual) occurs within ten minutes, then the next meal can consist of two foods. If the second food is cleared then a third can be introduced, and so on. The most commonly eaten foods such as wheat products, milk and dairy products, yeast and sugar are the last to be reintroduced.

Cytotoxic testing A blood sample is taken and carefully tested by introducing concentrates of substances to which the patient may be sensitive.

Changes occur in the white blood cells of patients who are sensitive. One drawback of this technique is that the findings are invariably difficult to interpret, as so many foods and chemicals appear to be implicated in each patient.

Sublingual drop testing The patient exists on fluids for five days, then one drop of a solution containing the suspect food is placed under the tongue. If there is a sensitivity to it, symptoms develop within minutes. This method also works for chemical sensitivity. It takes time to carry out all the necessary tests, so again the technique can prove expensive.

Intradermal testing Very small, diluted amounts of the suspect foods or chemicals are injected just under the skin. The troublesome symptoms will occur two or three hours after injection of a substance to which the patient is sensitive. The technique is very time-consuming and therefore expensive, but will no doubt be worth the trouble if the offending substance is identified.

Auricular cardiac reflex The ACR test, as it is generally called, relies on the movement of any pulse, most commonly the wrist pulse, when a food or chemical to which the patient is sensitive is placed within the body's electrical field. In skilled hands the test is believed to be about 80 per cent accurate, equalling the accuracy of other tests. Its principal advantages are that it is quick and cheap. Some 50 substances can be tested in a 15 minute consultation.

Electrical testing A small electrode is used to apply a low-voltage electrical current to the patient at an ACUPUNCTURE point, generally on the tip of the toe. The electrical reading is taken over the acupuncture point. A glass bottle containing a suspect food or chemical is then incorporated in the circuit. If the patient is sensitive to it, the reading over the acupuncture point changes. In skilled hands, this method is said to be about 80 per cent accurate and, like ACR, it is quick and cheap.

Kinesiology This is a muscle-testing technique. When a food or chemical to which the patient is sensitive is placed in the patient's hand or under the tongue, muscle power is affected – as a result of changing the body's electrical field, much as in ACR and electrical testing. In skilled hands, kinesiology is said to be about 80 per cent effective.

Treatment The simple treatment for ecological illness is to make sure that you avoid foods and chemicals that cause the trouble. Many people, however, are sensitive to several substances and where they are foods, avoidance can lead to serious nutritional problems. Either the patient has to be desensitised to the offending items or the underlying causes must be treated.

Desensitisation involves giving a patient different dilutions of the food or chemical as a drop under the tongue to find out what the body will tolerate without harm. This process probably works in a way similar to homoeopathy. Once a tolerance level has been established, the patient will usually be able to take limited exposure to the harmful substance without ill effect.

Treatment of an abnormal balance of bowel bacteria aims at replacing normal bacteria and treating an over-production of *Candida albicans*. This may simply involve the avoidance of sugar and yeast or, in more severe cases, the use of antifungal drugs.

An orthodox view

Many conventional doctors do not accept that sensitivity to foods or chemical pollution is a common cause of illness. Some would accept that there are true allergies to food, but many sufferers do not have allergic reactions when given a test acceptable to orthodox medicine. For example, there is no instant red weal on the skin as when pollen or a mould is injected under the skin of an allergy sufferer. Neurosis or emotional STRESS are seen as the likeliest causes of the symptoms presented by sensitive patients.

Some tests which produce results for clinical ecologists are, moreover, shunned by conventional doctors as having no scientific basis. But there is a growing acceptance among impartial doctors that a sensitivity that falls short of allergy can make people ill.

CO-COUNSELLING

A form of COUNSELLING pioneered in the United States during the 1970s, co-counselling is regarded as a tool for personal development. It pairs together people who want significantly to enhance their sense of identity and personal effectiveness. They take turns to be counsellor and client to each other, with the client choosing the subject and the depth of feelings he or she wishes to explore. The participants are given a short training course – Fundamentals of Co-counselling – after which they usually meet about once a week for a few hours.

COELIAC DISEASE

A dietary disorder of the bowel

Children are the most likely victims of this rather rare disorder of the small intestine, which usually strikes before they are three

Do's and don'ts for coeliacs

Don't eat bread, cakes, biscuits, and any food cooked or thickened with flour, such as meat or fish in batter or breadcrumbs, or oatmeal dishes such as porridge. Be sure to avoid foods containing wheat, barley or rye. Remember that gluten is usually present in frozen and tinned foods, and also processed foods, because flour is used as a thickener. Milk can also upset some coeliac disease sufferers.

Do eat fresh vegetables (including potatoes and other root vegetables for bulk), dried beans, fruit (either fresh or tinned), cream, nuts, eggs, bacon, fresh meat, plain fish (or fish in brine or oil), plain cheese, butter, honey, jam, plain marmalade, tea or coffee. Rice is also completely free of gluten, and gluten-free sausages are available.
Some health shops in South Africa carry a range of gluten-free foods.

years old. Symptoms are diarrhoea, with soft but bulky, foul-smelling stools and sometimes a stomach swollen with wind. The child gradually becomes weaker and weaker through malnutrition.

The cause is an inability to absorb gluten, a form of protein found in wheat, rye, barley and perhaps oats, and their products. Just why some children are unable to absorb gluten is not known, but the disease runs in families and sometimes occurs after a bowel infection. Some adults develop it after the age of 30, but are often found to have had it in mild form during childhood.

The remedy, a gluten-free diet, was discovered soon after the Second World War, when it was noticed that Dutch children with the disease became much better when they could not get bread to eat.

Medical researchers eventually pinned down gluten as the culprit. Once gluten has been removed from the diet (see box) coeliacs usually return to normal health within weeks or a few months.

What the therapists recommend
HERBAL MEDICINE
Consultation Many herbalists think there is a link between coeliac disease and bottle-feeding babies. But the treatment prescribed, which attempts to restore the imbalance of beneficial micro-organisms in the gut and of the IMMUNE SYSTEM that has led to the disorder, varies according to the person.

A detailed history of the patient's way of life, medical problems and diet will be compiled before arriving at a course of treatment. Herbs that are likely to be recommended to coeliacs include soothing agents such as marsh-mallow or slippery elm, or such anti-inflammatory remedies as meadowsweet or camomile.

An orthodox view
Long-term sufferers are immediately given vitamin and mineral supplements to help restore their health. Sometimes child coeliacs develop a tolerance for gluten by the time they are grown up, and consequently can return to a normal diet.

COGNITIVE THERAPY

Learning to believe in yourself

The aim of cognitive therapy is to boost people's self-confidence. It is a form of PSYCHOTHERAPY, and seeks to alter the perceptions, memories and thoughts of people who have a poor opinion of themselves, so that they feel and act in an outgoing and confident way. Therapists tend to believe that negative thoughts produce negative results – for example, if you believe yourself to be unattractive and boring, so will other people; their attitude strengthens your belief and you are trapped in a vicious circle.

The therapy reverses this process by teaching you to like yourself and to think and act positively. When people respond by taking an interest in you, your feelings about yourself are strengthened and you realise that you are likeable after all.

Cognitive therapy was introduced in the late 1960s by an American psychologist named Aaron Beck. It can be practised singly or in groups run in many cases by teachers of BEHAVIOURAL THERAPY.

COLDNESS

Apart from the obvious cause – exposure to cold, damp weather in inadequate clothing – coldness can be a general sign of poor health, particularly CIRCULATION PROBLEMS, and EXHAUSTION. Old people and those who are immobilised by illness are particularly

Do's and don'ts to guard against cold

Do wear a warm hat, especially if you are outdoors in very cold weather – it will keep your whole body warm, since a great deal of body heat can be lost from the head. A nightcap may help if you feel cold in bed.
Do wear warm woollen socks in winter. If it is particularly cold, you can wear bedsocks at night, and insulated inner soles in shoes (for cold feet).
Do keep your hands warm with a good pair of gloves and wear a scarf to protect your neck, particularly in cold wind.
Do check outdoor activity shops for jackets, hats, gloves, socks and thermal underwear which give maximum protection against cold and rain.
Don't try to get warm too quickly. If you get very cold, warm up slowly – take a bath that feels just slightly warm to the hand, because hot water may cause serious harm. Then take a warming drink such as hot milk or hot chocolate, and make sure that you wrap yourself up well in warm clothes.
Don't smoke – one of smoking's negative effects is that it constricts the blood vessels and causes poor circulation (see SMOKING).

susceptible, and need warm clothes and properly heated accommodation if they are not to become victims of HYPOTHERMIA, which can be fatal.

It is important not to stay cold for long periods, or you may develop a CHILL, CRAMP, CHILBLAINS or FROSTBITE.

What the therapists recommend
HERBAL MEDICINE
Self help Infusions (see p. 184) of ginger and prickly ash are thought to stimulate blood circulation, and increase the body's ability to withstand cold.

An infusion of cayenne is said to have a warming effect on the body and may also stimulate the body's circulation – to make it you should pour a cup of boiling water onto 1 teaspoon of cayenne powder, and leave for ten minutes. Drink 1 tablespoon of the infusion mixed into a cup of hot water as often as necessary.

NATUROPATHY

Self help The heart, circulation and nervous systems are believed to be strengthened by eating a diet high in magnesium-rich foods such as almonds, cashew nuts, Brazil nuts, whole grains, sweetcorn, spinach and bananas. Potassium may help by improving nerve functioning – it is found in fresh fruits such as bananas, grapes, melons and peaches, dried fruit, seeds and raw or baked (not boiled) vegetables.

EXERCISE can also help – regular running is said to be particularly good for cold feet. Cold showers, or swimming in cold water, can help to draw more blood into the capillaries under the surface of the skin, which warms the area.

HOMOEOPATHY

Self help *Arsenicum album* is recommended for those who suffer from anxiety, and have to sit next to a heater to stay warm; *Calcarea carbonica* for cold, clammy hands in those who tend to be overweight. *Hepar sulphuris* may help those who are very sensitive to pain and feel the cold severely.

An orthodox view

Doctors agree that warm clothing, exercise to improve circulation, and good heating are the most efficient ways of staying warm. In addition, have at least one good hot meal a day, and take hot drinks at regular intervals – especially at night. Patients with serious circulation problems may be given drugs called vasodilators to open up blood vessels that have become constricted by cold.

COLDS

That coughs and sneezes spread diseases is an old maxim, but a true one – especially in the case of the common cold. Colds are caused by VIRUS INFECTIONS and are highly contagious, particularly in enclosed places. Because the mucus in the nose and throat of cold sufferers is full of viruses, coughing, sneezing – and even breathing in a confined space – can easily spread the infection.

Cold viruses are in a constant state of change, so immunity acquired from one infection does not necessarily protect you from further attacks. Any run-down condition or general debility can leave you more liable to catch a cold. Babies and young children, the elderly, or those already ill are particularly at risk.

Symptoms include a runny nose, sore throat, headache, stuffed-up feeling, dry cough, sneezing, loss of appetite and a general lack of energy. These may last for up

Do's and don'ts when you have a cold

Do drink plenty of fluids – especially cool drinks – for a slight fever. This replaces fluids lost through sweating.
Don't take painkillers such as aspirin or paracetamol for headache, or other aches, unless you really need them.
Do inhale steam to relieve a stuffed-up nose: half fill a bowl with hot water, put a towel over your head to trap the steam and inhale for a few minutes at a time. Take care not to upset the bowl.
Do get some fresh air – take a gentle walk – as soon as you feel able.
Don't wrap up in extra clothes or blankets, do not overheat the room or sit in front of the fire – let the body lose heat naturally.

to three days, then die down over the following seven days, although the stuffed or runny nose may last for up to three weeks.

Being physically cold or getting wet does not cause a cold, but the chances of infection are heightened by STRESS, EXHAUSTION, DEPRESSION or chronic sickness, all of which lower resistance.

What the therapists recommend

NATUROPATHY

Self help The advice of naturopaths is to avoid all foods said to be mucus-forming, such as dairy products, eggs, starch and sugar. In the early stages of a cold, an Epsom salts bath (see box) is recommended. If the cold becomes feverish, either FASTING or a raw fruit and vegetable diet – including GARLIC and onions or leeks – for two to three days may help to reduce CATARRH. See also RAW FOOD DIET; EATING FOR HEALTH.

HERBAL MEDICINE

Self help Hot drinks and a good sweat seem to ease cold symptoms, and one recipe is: a pinch of cayenne pepper, the juice of a lemon, a minced clove of garlic and a gram of vitamin C, all mixed in half a cup of hot water. Be sure to sip it slowly. Both the garlic and cayenne should make you sweat; the lemon juice is rich in vitamin C and bioflavonoids, which are claimed to help your system to absorb the vitamin.

A variety of herbal teas are also said to be beneficial – including camomile, lemon

balm, boneset (especially for fever), coltsfoot (for coughs and congestion), elder, pennyroyal and vervain. Also recommended are infusions (see p. 184) of yarrow, peppermint, ginger and catnip.

HOMOEOPATHY

Self help Colds treated homoeopathically are held to occur less frequently, but prolonged ones should be treated by a doctor. However, for an occasional infection, the following preparations are recommended:

Early stages: *Aconitum napellus* will often stop a cold if taken on the first sneeze when feeling suddenly chilly. *Ferrum phosphoricum* is also useful at the outset, and *Arsenicum album* if there is much painful sneezing with watery discharge, which makes the skin sore, or if the patient is very chilly and thirsty. *Kali iodatum* is recommended for a cold due to exposure, especially damp, when the eyes smart and water, there is much sneezing and the nose is red and sore.

Persistent cold: *Sambucus nigra*; or *Teucrium marum verum* and *Wyethia* to relieve chronic catarrh and LARYNGITIS, and *Kali bichromium* or *Silica* for SINUS PROBLEMS. When the cold is severe, the chosen remedy can be taken hourly for up to 12 doses. Stop as soon as the condition improves.

Other alternative treatments

Acupressure To relieve nasal congestion and clear the sinuses, apply the thumb or index finger to two points, below the cheekbones, directly beneath the eye pupils when looking straight ahead, and about a finger's width from the end of the nose. Use a gentle, circular massaging motion.

Aromatherapy You are recommended to add six to eight drops of cinnamon oil to a warm bath, and rub the oil undiluted into the temples, the sinus area and chest four times

Epsom salts bath

Fill the bath with water as hot as you can comfortably bear and enough to lie in immersed to the neck. Dissolve two handfuls of unpurified Epsom salts in the water. Soak in the tub for as long as you can comfortably stay, with a compress wrung out in cold water on your forehead. On getting out, dab yourself gently dry, wrap yourself in a sheet and get into a warm bed.
Warning This treatment should not be used by the elderly, the very young, or those with high blood pressure.

a day. For a steam inhalation, put two drops of the cinnamon oil into a bowl of hot water and breathe in the steam for a few minutes, four times daily.

Traditional Medicine Chopped or crushed garlic taken in small amounts several times a day is said to help repel colds – especially head colds. If a cold has developed, you are advised to go to bed and drink the juice of a lemon in a glass of hot water with a teaspoon of honey. Two aspirins can also be added.

An orthodox view

Despite years of research, there is no effective cure for the common cold or any sure way of shortening its duration. Some people have great faith in the curative power of vitamin C (see MEGAVITAMIN THERAPY), but so far this has not been medically proved.

The general view among doctors is that colds should be allowed to clear up naturally at home – which they normally do after a week to ten days. But if the symptoms last for longer than that you should see your GP. There are, however, certain measures you can take to relieve the worst symptoms of a cold (see *Do's and don'ts* box on previous page).

COLD SORES
Irritating, recurring blisters

These small blisters usually appear on the lips and are caused by the *Herpes simplex* virus. The virus is common and infectious, and can also attack other parts of the face, the genitals and other skin areas.

It is usually picked up from someone during childhood, sometimes causing feverishness and sickness as well as blisters. The virus remains dormant in the body, sometimes without causing symptoms for years, but it can be reactivated at any time by FEVER, STRESS, exposure to cold, SUNBURN, lowered resistance – or even menstruation.

Warning Always see a doctor immediately for cold sores near the eyes – they can cause great pain if not treated quickly.

What the therapists recommend
NATUROPATHY
Self help Some supplements believed to help your body fight the virus include vitamins A, B₃, B₅, B-complex (which includes the previous two, plus five others) and C. Bioflavonoids, zinc, the amino acid lysine, and acidophilus tablets are also recommended. In addition to these general supplements, vitamins B₆, B₁₂ and E, folic acid, pantothenic acid, calcium, magnesium and selenium are favoured by some practitioners.

> ## Do's *and don'ts about* cold sores
>
> **Do** avoid all forms of skin contact – such as kissing – when others come close to the affected area while sores are still moist.
> **Don't** share towels, face cloths or pillowcases.
> **Don't** touch the blisters unnecessarily or more may develop. If you do touch them accidentally, or when applying a salve, wash your hands afterwards.

A mix of equal quantities of lemon juice and water may promote healing if applied directly to lip sores. To prevent further attacks, a wholefood diet which cuts out refined foods and sugar and includes plenty of FIBRE and alkali-forming foods such as fruit, vegetables, honey, milk and yoghurt is recommended (see EATING FOR HEALTH).

HOMOEOPATHY
Rhus tox. and *Natrum muriticum*, one or the other, morning and evening, are thought to help. Take the 30th or 6th potency every four hours for two days, then morning and night for two or three days.

An orthodox view

Chemists stock creams and lotions that can relieve the pain of the blisters and help them to heal. Doctors sometimes prescribe antiviral drugs to reduce the symptoms and shorten an attack. But once infected, there is no way of ridding yourself of the virus, and further attacks are always possible.

When the eye is affected, the doctor will put a drop of yellow dye in the eye to show up any ulcers (dendritic ulcers) that have formed. Antiviral drops and ointment will clear the attack, but corneal ulcers may recur. If you wear contact lenses, always moisten them with sterilising solution, never with saliva, which can cause reinfection.

COLIC

Parents with very young babies often have their nights ruined by loud, persistent crying. Often this is assumed to be caused by colic – spasmodic stomach pains – although this assumption has never been proved.

Breastfed babies do not often suffer from colic – provided that their mothers do not

---

themselves drink much milk. But whether bottle- or breastfed, babies generally grow out of colic attacks by the time they are three months old. If they do not, medical advice should be sought – especially if a baby suffers also from DIARRHOEA or vomiting, or if there is blood in the bowel motions.

In children colic may be brought on by fear of a coming event or 'ordeal'. In some cases going to school in itself can cause an attack; sometimes 'nervous colic' can strike when an examination is due, or – in older children – a career opportunity has to be discussed, or a job interview arranged.

Adults are affected less often by colic, but when they are, the intermittent pain comes and goes like a fist being clenched and unclenched in the abdomen, and can make them double up in agony. The pain occurs when an organ such as the bile duct or intestine contracts and becomes inflamed when trying to expel poisoned food (see FOOD POISONING), or to pass an obstruction such as GALLSTONES.

What the therapists recommend
HERBAL MEDICINE
Self help Babies' colic is said to be relieved by a teaspoon of warm herbal tea every hour. The infusions can be made from catmint, camomile or fennel seed. The mother can also take the infusion if she is breastfeeding.

Adult colic sufferers should drink infusions by the glass, three times daily. Seed tea is also recommended: mix a teaspoon each of aniseed, caraway and fennel in enough boiling water to fill a cup. Cover the cup and infuse for about ten minutes. Then strain and drink the tea while it is hot.

AROMATHERAPY
Self help For babies, use gripe water which already contains the essential oil of fennel – check on label. One drop of fennel oil mixed with a ½ teaspoon of honey can ease severe attacks, or gently massage the baby's stomach clockwise with two drops of fennel in a little carrier oil.

Several other oils which are said to help ease the pain for adults, and to aid digestion generally, include camphor, cinnamon, juniper, lavender and patchouli.

An orthodox view

For a child, a doctor will probably prescribe an antispasmodic medicine to relax the affected organs, which will work quickly. However, if the colic is severe or long-lasting the child may have to be examined in hospital. For adults, a painkilling drug may be prescribed, and the patient told to avoid rich foods and alcohol. Usually it is better not to eat at all during an attack and take only sips of water until the colic finally clears up.

COLITIS

Inflammation of the bowel

This disorder – known commonly as ulcerative colitis – is marked by chronic inflammation of the large bowel, which becomes ulcerated (see ULCERS).

The symptoms include pain in the abdomen and intermittent bouts of bloodstreaked DIARRHOEA which, in severe cases, can occur up to 20 times a day.

If the bouts increase in number and severity – or if the condition persists – you should seek medical advice.

What the therapists recommend

Acupressure Apply downward pressure to a point on the outside of the leg, immediately below the knee. This is thought to control the muscular movement of the abdomen and so relieve colitis. In severe cases, pressure should be applied on a point midway between the breastbone and navel.

Acupuncture The practitioner will concentrate principally on the gall bladder, the liver and stomach meridians. He may also pack warmed salt into the navel, and use MOXIBUSTION which is believed to relax the abdomen in general.

Naturopathy Diet is held to be the key to preventing or combating colitis. This involves cutting out milk and dairy products such as butter and cheese, and eating mainly moderately cooked vegetable broths and vegetable stews, and a mixture of slippery elm and mashed bananas. The disorder should clear up within a few weeks.

Colitis is often accompanied by STRESS – and a consultant may teach a patient relaxation exercises.

Herbal Medicine A favoured way of soothing inflamed or irritated intestinal walls is a twice-daily cup of slippery elm drink. Mix one part of powdered bark – available from health shops – in eight parts of water. Heat the water, pour on powder and drink warm.

An orthodox view

In general, doctors tend to view ulcerative colitis more seriously than do alternative practitioners.

In severe cases, the affected patient may be sent to hospital for a barium enema, X-rays and a bowel examination. Occasionally, an operation to remove part of the colon may be advised.

Usually, however, a doctor will prescribe medication to reduce the number and intensity of attacks. He will also probably recommend a suitable diet – avoiding vegetable roughage and raw fruits – and stress the importance of rest and relaxation.

COLOUR THERAPY

Casting light on your body's ills

The sun gives out a variety of electromagnetic rays with different wavelengths, some of them visible to the human eye as natural light. Light can be separated into its component wavelengths by a prism or filters, and the human eye then sees each component as a different colour.

The sun also emits wavelengths not visible to the human eye – infrared rays, ultraviolet rays, X-rays, for example. Although the eye is not sensitive to these invisible rays, the body is – and may be helped or harmed by them. Ultraviolet rays, for instance, enable the body to manufacture essential VITAMINS, but overexposure can cause severe burning and skin CANCER.

People are affected also by the visible rays – psychologically and physically. Red light has been found to speed up the circulation and raise BLOOD PRESSURE, while blue light is calming. The effect is the same even if the patient is blindfolded or blind. Colour can affect people's mood, perception of temperature and time, and their overall ability to concentrate. It is being used increasingly to produce desired responses in mental health clinics, hospital recovery rooms, prison cells and in work places.

Colour therapists attach even more significance to colours, and believe that specific ailments can be cured by adjusting the colour input to the body. They believe that the body receives the various electromagnetic components of light, absorbs them to some degree, and gives out its own aura of electromagnetism (which KIRLIAN PHOTOGRAPHY is believed to record) in a pattern of vibrations that the skilled therapist can pick up.

An unhealthy body is said to give out an unbalanced pattern of vibrations, and the colour therapist works to restore the balance. Colour, through light, food and surroundings, will work through the nervous system to stimulate the production of hormones that control the chemical and energy balance of the body.

Who it can help Colour therapists will treat any disorder be it mental, emotional, metabolic or physical, but they emphasise that their therapy is complementary to qualified medical treatment, not an alternative to it. Patients should always seek the advice of their orthodox doctor.

Therapists offer an extra means of promoting well-being which requires sustained effort from the patient. Sufferers from MIGRAINE, ECZEMA, ASTHMA, inflammation, rheumatic pain, ARTHRITIS, INSOMNIA, STRESS, high blood pressure, DEPRESSION and lack of energy have, according to therapists, benefited from treatment.

Finding a therapist Although colour therapy is still in its infancy in South Africa, the significance of colour is taken into account by many psychologists.

For details of specific therapies which are practised by psychologists, you should contact the Psychological Association of South Africa, P O Box 2729, Pretoria 0001 (telephone 012-3261981).

Consulting a therapist Diagnosis of your condition will occupy the first consultation and probably take well over an hour. The therapist will record details of your medical history, lifestyle, what you eat and drink, and your colour preferences. He will also make a careful study of your skin.

A skilled therapist will concentrate on these details and use extrasensory perception to tune in to your electromagnetic field and assess whether any imbalances exist there.

As an aid in deciding on treatment, the therapist dowses with a pendulum (see DOWSING) or strokes the length of the spine (or a chart of a spine) while concentrating on your condition.

In this manner he picks up certain vibrations from individual vertebrae which reveal where the colour balance is wrong. Each vertebra is related to an organ or part of the body, and also to one of the eight colours of the spectrum, which are repeated in sequence down the vertebrae, increasing in density of colour from the neck to the base of the spine.

The therapist compiles a detailed spine chart and uses it to explain to the patient which particular colours will be used for the therapy and why.

Seven or more weekly treatment sessions are required. A colour therapy instrument beams coloured lights on the patient through shaped apertures. A main colour and a complementary colour are used: the complementary pairings are red and turquoise, orange and blue, yellow and violet, green and magenta.

During the session the instrument gives increasing time to the main colour and decreasing time to the complementary colour in a carefully worked out irregular rhythm; a regular rhythm soon becomes ineffective. The total time before the instrument is just under 20 minutes per session.

Some therapists prefer to direct the colours at specific parts of the body instead of bathing the whole body in colour. As treatment progresses, the colours or their intensity may be adjusted to suit the patient's changing condition. Music or a particular range of notes may be used to reinforce the colour therapy.

The therapist also advises on what colours to wear and use for furnishings, and what colours of foods to eat to help in rebalancing the patient's energies. Patients are also taught to visualise the treatment colours.

An orthodox view

Few doctors doubt that colour does affect mood and can affect behaviour. Many accept that an individual's choice in colour points to personality traits. Psychologists attach more significance to colour and are engaged by some employers to make detailed assessments of job applicants by testing their colour preferences.

Although doctors have long known that the body is affected by radiation outside the visible spectrum (infrared, ultraviolet and X-rays), they see no scientific proof that visible colour rays affect particular parts and disorders of the body. However, the work of colour therapists is not regarded as harmful.

CONJUNCTIVITIS

The irritation of pink eye

A sensation of grittiness and irritation in the eye is usually the first symptom of this common condition. The conjunctiva – a delicate membrane that covers the white of the eye and inside of the lids – becomes inflamed, causing redness and pain. Sometimes the eye is also sticky and crusted, especially after a night's sleep.

Most cases are caused by bacterial or VIRUS INFECTIONS, but ALLERGY, foreign bodies in the eye and irritants such as tobacco smoke, aerosol sprays and some eye products can all be causes. In babies, blocked tear ducts are sometimes responsible, and in a few rare cases conjunctivitis may be a symptom of some more serious eye disorder.

Consult a doctor as soon as possible if you suspect another disorder, if the eye is very painful, particularly if the swelling and pain have not started to get better after two or three days, or if you have recently visited a tropical country where you may have picked up an eye virus.

What the therapists recommend
HERBAL MEDICINE
Practitioners recommend bathing the eyes with decoctions (see p. 184) of cornflower, marigold, elderflower, camomile, chickweed, eyebright or plantain, or using infusions to make compresses (see p. 184) for the eyes. Use separate eye baths and compresses for each eye. Do not bathe more than three times, to avoid irritation.

Do's and don'ts about conjunctivitis

Do stay away from cut grass, smoky rooms, dusty atmospheres or anything that irritates your eyes.
Do wear goggles if you work where metal is being cut or where there are wood shavings or other splinters that may enter the eye.
Do use your own towels and face cloths and don't lend them to others.
Do remove blockages from babies' tear ducts by gently massaging the bottom lid near the nose.
Don't cover a sore eye with an eye patch – this can spread infection.
Don't use eyedrops or eyewashes unless necessary – they can sometimes cause irritation.
If you get conjunctivitis Touch your eyes only when necessary, and wash your hands before and afterwards to prevent the infection from spreading.

HOMOEOPATHY
Self help Bathing the eye three times a day in a solution of one part Euphrasia mother tincture (see p. 184) in ten parts boiled or distilled water is thought to help. Ferrum phosphoricum is also recommended – take five tablets of the 6X potency dissolved in hot water four times a day.

Aconitum napellus is commonly recommended in the initial stages when the eyes are red, hot, gritty and swollen, and water after exposure to cold, wind and light; Apis mellifica when there is stinging pain, itching, blistering on the white of the eye and pus; Euphrasia officinalis when the eyes burn and water, causing blinking and dislike of bright light; Mercurius corrosivus when the lids stick together and there is pus in the eye; Pulsatilla nigricans when there is a thick, yellow discharge with itching, burning and a tendency to STYES; Arsenicum album when the eye is hot and waters.

NATUROPATHY
Self help Vitamin A is recommended for many eye disorders, but needs to be taken under supervision if large quantities are used or if it is taken for a long time, because in large quantities it can be poisonous. For safety, always take in combination with vitamins D and E – a total of 5 000-10 000 iu a day. Some therapists also suggest vitamins B_2, B_3, B_6 and C.

An orthodox view

Most conjunctivitis heals by itself within a week or two, but a doctor should be consulted to make sure that the right treatment is given and that the red, painful eye is not a symptom of a more serious condition, such as glaucoma.

CONSTIPATION

A typical Western diet does not usually contain enough of the FIBRE that the body needs to help rid itself of waste products. Constipation is the all-too-frequent consequence. The strain of passing hard motions from the bowel can lead to BOWEL DISORDERS, PILES – and even APPENDICITIS.

Bowel action varies from person to person – from three times a day to once every three days – but irregular and infrequent small, hard motions are the usual signals that you are constipated. If constipation lasts more than two weeks, see your doctor.

Apart from lack of fibre in your food, other causes include eating too much meat or dairy produce, not drinking enough fluids (fibre needs water to form soft motions), food ALLERGY, lack of EXERCISE, ignoring the 'call of nature', dependence on laxatives, the side effects of some medicines, PREGNANCY (when intestinal muscles often weaken), ANXIETY, STRESS and TENSION.

What the therapists recommend
HERBAL MEDICINE
Self help A herbal laxative should only be used as a short-term solution. Make one by crushing up to six senna pods (but start with only one or two per dose) into a cup of boiling water and adding a small piece of liquorice root. Leave to soak for ten minutes, strain and drink at night. Senna takes about eight hours to work and can cause a griping pain in the stomach – add a teaspoon of fennel seeds to relieve this.

Another strong laxative is cascara, which is believed to tone the bowel. You can make an infusion by soaking $\frac{1}{2}$ to 1 teaspoon of cascara bark in a cup of hot water for one hour. Strain and drink before bedtime.

Linseeds make a gentler laxative, acting to provide soothing bulk in the gut. Soak a tablespoon of seeds overnight in 150 ml of cold water and add to your breakfast cereal. Or soak a tablespoon of seeds in 150 ml of hot water for two hours, strain and drink sweetened with honey; eat the seeds. An infusion of dandelion leaves or chopped dandelion root has a gentle laxative effect. Take three or four tablespoonfuls daily.

NATUROPATHY

Self help A high fibre diet or RAW FOOD DIET is recommended; chew the food well and never rush meals. Get plenty of fibre from peas, beans, brown rice, wholemeal bread, jacket potatoes, raw vegetables, fresh and dried fruits; and drink plenty of fluids. Naturopaths believe it is far better to eat more food in its natural state than to sprinkle bran on top of food.

If possible, take regular exercise to condition your stomach and back muscles. This, in turn, aids bowel movement. If you are constipated through resisting the 'call', visit the lavatory regularly after a cereal breakfast and try to relax – read a book or magazine if necessary. Stay for ten minutes, whether or not a motion is passed, and your body should resume its regular habit.

TRADITIONAL MEDICINE

Bran absorbs up to nine times its own weight in water and so helps to form good motions. Added to food it helps to regulate the bowels, but you need to drink at least three glasses of water a day to make it work. Take 1 to 3 teaspoons of bran – always with some liquid – a day and slowly build up to a maximum of 15 g a day.

Do not rely on bran as a long-term cure, however, as it has been found to contain certain ingredients which prevent minerals being absorbed into the body. Bran may also cause WIND and a bloated feeling, but these effects normally pass within a week or two.

Prunes and prune juice work as a natural laxative, but should not be taken regularly in place of a fibre diet. Soak prunes in water overnight, and eat night and morning. A regular daily teaspoon of mineral-rich molasses is also said to help combat constipation.

Other alternative treatments

Homoeopathy *Alumina* is recommended for dry motions, when there is no 'call of nature' or movement of the bowels for days; *Nux vomica* if you feel the call but no motions are passed, or if poor bowel habits are due to laxatives (good for those who overeat and drink too much); *Plumbum metallicum* for long-term constipation with stomach pain; *Collinsonia canadensis* when hard motions are passed and when piles are present.

Reflexology Massage to the reflex areas relating to the small and large intestines, plus areas relating to the adrenal glands, solar plexus, liver and lower spine is recommended. See chart, p. 295.

An orthodox view

Bran is now approved by doctors for constipation. In general they will recommend a diet containing plenty of fluids and fibre. Laxatives or suppositories may be prescribed to help retrain the bowels, and an enema may occasionally be needed.

Change in bowel habit can be a serious symptom and should be investigated by a doctor.

For babies, a doctor may prescribe small glycerine suppositories and then recommend adding an extra teaspoon of sugar to every 180 ml of milk feed.

CONTRACEPTION

Throughout history, couples have tried to control their fertility – to have children or not as and when they wish. Modern medicine has developed a wide spectrum of highly effective means to prevent conception taking place, but many couples prefer traditional methods either for religious reasons or because they wish to avoid the side effects of drugs or other artificial contraceptives. See NATURAL FAMILY PLANNING, p. 96.

CONVULSIONS

Although not always dangerous in itself, a convulsive fit or seizure is frightening and disturbing for victims and their families, and if it happens while crossing a road or operating machinery the sufferer may be in danger of injury.

The cause is thought to be a temporary loss of control in the brain, leading to unco-ordinated and uncontrollable muscular jerking and twitching, often while the victim has lapsed into UNCONSCIOUSNESS.

Disorders that can induce convulsions include EPILEPSY, a high FEVER, injuries and reactions to some FOOD ADDITIVES.

Warning Convulsions are a serious symptom, and a doctor should always be seen so that the cause can be diagnosed and treatment given before using any alternative therapies. However, it is quite common for young children to suffer from 'febrile' convulsions as a result of a high temperature.

What the therapists recommend

NATUROPATHY

Self help Treatment depends on the cause of the convulsions. Some epileptics have found that supplements of vitamin B_6, vitamin D or calcium and magnesium prevent or lessen their convulsive attacks. Vitamin B_6 should be taken in large quantities only under the supervision of a doctor, or a naturopath who is also a doctor, since it may interfere with the effectiveness of other anti-epileptic medicines.

In other cases, convulsions may be an allergic reaction to artificial additives in processed foods, such as the flavouring agent monosodium glutamate which is used in some preserves and some Chinese foodstuffs, and the nitrates used to preserve many meat products.

It is often difficult to absolutely identify the exact ingredient that is responsible, but switching to a wholefood diet based on fresh fruit, vegetables and wholegrain cereals (see EATING FOR HEALTH) and excluding all processed foods may cure the problem.

Alternatively, keep a written record of everything you eat and the time you ate it, as well as the times of the convulsive attacks. If the cause is something in your diet, a pattern should soon emerge.

Consultation A naturopath will examine the patient to exclude the risk of a neurological problem. If one is found, the patient will be referred to a neurologist immediately.

An orthodox view

True epilepsy cannot be cured, but it can be controlled by drug treatment. Epileptics also need skilled counselling, as a diagnosis of epilepsy can have drastic and far-reaching implications on the person's lifestyle, employability and other aspects of life generally.

Natural family planning

There are many different ways of preventing pregnancy, but those which are favoured by most doctors and clinics involve taking drugs or using various chemical preparations and artificial devices which can cause a range of side effects. In South Africa and abroad many couples have become dissatisfied with these methods or prefer not to use them at all for religious reasons, and there is currently a growing interest in practising the more natural forms of contraception.

Recommended methods of natural family planning depend on charting the woman's menstrual cycle and avoiding intercourse on the days when she is likely to be fertile. There are three main ways of keeping track of your cycle.

The principles on which the methods of family planning work are given here, but more precise details of how to apply them to your particular circumstances should be sought from a doctor or family planning clinic.

Recommended methods

Calendar (or rhythm) method   Record the dates of your periods on a calendar for six to 12 months – the longer you do so, the more reliable the method will be. Then calculate the length of each menstrual cycle by counting the number of days from the first day of each period to the day before the first day of the next (inclusive).

Find the first 'unsafe' day of your cycle by subtracting 19 from the length of your shortest cycle, and the last unsafe day by subtracting 11 from the length of your longest cycle. Avoid intercourse between these dates. For example, if your shortest cycle is 26 days and your longest 33, your first unsafe day will be 26-19 = day 7, and your last unsafe day will be 33-11 = day 22.

Warning   The method may fail if something such as acute stress substantially alters the length of your cycle.

Temperature method   This involves taking your temperature to find the time when you ovulate – usually 12-16 days before your next period. Again, the more cycles over which you do this, the more reliable the method will be.

Take your temperature every morning at the same time for at least three minutes before getting out of bed, and record it on a chart. An ordinary thermometer can be used.

Printed charts are usually available from Catholic Church bookshops. In some countries special fertility thermometers are available.

From the first day of your period until around the day you ovulate, your resting temperature is 0,3-0,6°C (0,5-1°F) lower than from ovulation until your next period, so a 'step' will show on your chart (see sample chart below). You will be fertile for three

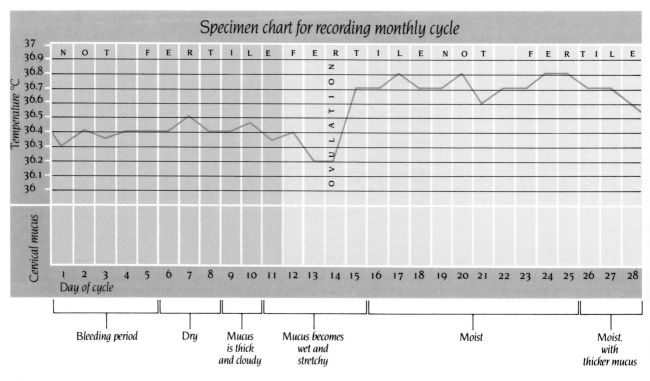

Specimen chart for recording monthly cycle

to four days before and after the temperature change, so avoid intercourse during this time.

Warning This method is unreliable if illness affects your temperature, or if your cycle is disrupted for any reason.

Cervical mucus method This depends on noting subtle changes that accompany ovulation, including changes in the mucus produced by the cervix. After a period, the vagina is usually dry for a few days, and then thick, cloudy mucus is produced. Before and during ovulation, the mucus increases in quantity and becomes thin and clear.

If you know how to locate it, the condition of your cervix can also be a guide. On unsafe days the cervix feels higher up in the vagina, softer and more open than on safe days. Some women also notice other signs of ovulation such as abdominal pains, tender breasts or slight vaginal bleeding.

Used in combination, the calendar, temperature and cervical mucus methods provide the best guide to ovulation and the safest form of natural birth control. The combination is known as the 'sympto-thermal method'.

Other methods

There are also two traditional methods of natural contraception. However, one is possible only for women who have recently had a baby, and the other is not always suitable.

Breastfeeding Nursing mothers who breastfeed their babies frequently and regularly – every two to four hours day and night, with no supplement feeds – are less likely to become pregnant than others. Even so, some may conceive.

Withdrawal ('coitus interruptus') This requires the man to withdraw his penis before ejaculating. Many couples find this method of contraception unsatisfactory, and care must be taken afterwards to prevent semen from coming anywhere near the woman's vagina. What is more, some sperm may escape from the penis before ejaculation.

Principal methods of contraception

METHOD	ADVANTAGES	DISADVANTAGES	EFFECTIVENESS
Natural methods			
Calendar	No cost; no side effects.	Needs long period of attention; long periods of abstinence.	Moderate when combined with other natural methods.
Temperature	No cost; no side effects.	Needs long period of daily attention; doesn't work when ill.	Moderate when combined with cervical mucus method.
Cervical mucus	No cost; no side effects.	Not reliable on its own; examining cervix not always easy.	Moderate when combined with calendar or temperature method.
Breastfeeding	No cost; good for baby; no side effects.	Not suitable for everyone; not a long-term solution.	Not completely reliable.
Withdrawal	No cost; no preparation needed; can be used at any time of cycle.	Can interfere with sexual fulfilment.	Unreliable.
Artificial methods			
Condom	Easy to use; no side effects; protection from sexually transmitted diseases.	Can interfere with spontaneous sex; diminished sensation for some men.	Very good, especially when used with spermicide.
Diaphragm and cap	Easy to use; no side effects.	Must be fitted by doctor or nurse and user taught to insert and remove it.	Very good when used with spermicide.
Spermicidal vaginal sponge	Easy to use.	Expensive.	Good.
Intrauterine device (IUD)	Needs no attention once fitted, except for occasional checks that it is still in place. Can be fitted up to five days after unprotected intercourse (eg, rape).	Must be fitted by doctor or nurse; may cause infections and heavy periods; not suitable for some women.	Excellent.
Contraceptive pill (various types)	Lighter, shorter periods: reduced premenstrual tension; protection from some disorders.	Requires daily attention; can cause weight gain; may increase risk of breast cancer and blood clots; prolonged use by smokers or other risk groups may be inadvisable.	Almost completely effective if taken as instructed.
Morning-after pill	Effective up to 72 hours after unprotected intercourse.	Not suitable for routine use; may cause nausea or other side effects.	Very good.

COPPER THERAPY

Traditionally, wearing a copper bracelet is thought to be an effective way of relieving the pain of ARTHRITIS and RHEUMATISM. Although doctors tend to dismiss the idea as an old wives' tale, research in Australia in the late 1970s showed that three out of every four volunteers who wore a copper bracelet for at least a month found their arthritic aches and pains considerably eased. It is said that traces of copper from the bracelet penetrate the skin and make up for any lack of essential copper in the body. See also MINERALS; BIOCHEMIC TISSUE SALTS.

CORNS

Badly fitting shoes are the most common cause of corns, which are formed by a thickening of the skin on toes or soles. Comfortable shoes which do not squeeze or rub the feet will prevent corns. Any already formed should go once the cause is removed.

What the therapists recommend

Naturopathy Wash your feet regularly and remove any rough skin with a pumice stone. Alternatively, bathe your feet for five to ten minutes night and morning in a small tub of hot water in which 120 g of Epsom salts is dissolved. Some practitioners recommend soaking the feet in sea water (or water to which sea salt has been added), for ten to 15 minutes, twice daily.

Herbal Medicine Paint the corns with fresh lemon juice, or crush a garlic clove onto the gauze patch of a sticking plaster and put it on the corn. Alternatively, soak the feet for five to ten minutes in a mixture of one-third vinegar and two-thirds warm water.

An orthodox view

A chiropodist will probably pare the corn with a sharp, sterile blade – and perhaps advise you to apply corn plasters and salicylic acid ointment or tincture. A change of footwear will usually help.

COUÉISM

In the late 19th century, a French apothecary named Emile Coué (1857-1926) developed a form of self-hypnosis based on repeating certain phrases, the most famous of which was: 'Every day, in every way, I am getting better and better.' His principles formed the basis of AUTOSUGGESTION.

COUGHS

The best way to treat a cough is to get rid of what is causing it, not to suppress it. Coughing helps to expel congested phlegm or inhaled dust from the lungs, bronchial tubes or windpipe.

A cough may be caused by infection or an irritant such as cigarette smoke or dust. A hoarse cough may be a symptom of LARYNGITIS or, in a child, CROUP. If a child is wheezing after a coughing spasm, the cause may be WHOOPING COUGH.

If the cough is persistent – lasting more than two or three weeks – or is accompanied by a high temperature, chest pains or blood in the sputum, you should consult your general practitioner.

What the therapists recommend
ACUPUNCTURE

Consultation A cough is believed by practitioners to be caused by an imbalance in the flow of energy to the lungs. An acupuncturist will treat it by inserting needles into points on the lung meridian in the arms. Needles may also be inserted in the meridian for another organ with a related rhythm in the body's 24 hour cycle – for example, the bladder meridian (see p. 14).

AROMATHERAPY

Self help In the early stages an inhalant is generally recommended to soothe the cough and help expel phlegm. Essential oils you should use include eucalyptus, thyme, cypress and sandalwood. Generally, two or three drops are added to a bowl of hot water and the steam inhaled for periods of about ten minutes, two or three times a day until the cough clears.

For a sore throat caused by a dry, hard cough, gargle with three drops of the same essential oils in half a glass of water.

BIOCHEMIC TISSUE SALTS

Self help Different salts are recommended for different types of cough: for a hard dry cough with FEVER, *Ferr. phos.*; cough with thick white phlegm, *Kali mur.*; cough with yellow phlegm and worse at night, *Kali sulph.*; spasmodic, painful cough, *Mag. phos.*; loose, rattling cough with watery phlegm, *Calc. sulph.* alternating with *Ferr. phos.*

Some of the salts are available in combined packs: Combination J, containing *Ferr. phos.*, *Kali mur.* and *Nat. mur.*, is a general remedy for coughs and colds.

The salts are taken as small tablets, and the recommended dose is given on the container. The tablets are generally taken three or four times a day, or every half hour in chronic cases.

HERBAL MEDICINE

Self help White horehound is one of the most highly recommended herbal cough remedies. Make an infusion (p. 184) of the dried leaves in a cup of boiling water, and take a teaspoonful three times daily. Liquorice can be added to offset their bitterness.

Other herbal infusions that can be used are: for hard coughs, mullein; irritating coughs, wild lettuce or, for children, wild cherry bark, which is a mild sedative; coughs with fever, yarrow or angelica; catarrhal coughs, elecampane or elder flower.

NATUROPATHY

Self help Recommended remedies include two garlic tablets three times a day, and vitamin A, B, and C supplements daily. Hot lemon juice with a spoonful of honey and glycerine added should soothe the throat. A towel soaked in three parts hot water to one of cider vinegar and applied as a compress to the throat and chest is said to help get rid of phlegm.

An orthodox view

If the cough is not a symptom of something more serious, a doctor will simply advise you to stay quiet in a warm room and take cough medicine, usually a linctus. These medicines may contain compounds such as codeine to suppress the cough, and expectorants such as triprolidine, pseudoephedrine and guaiphenesin, which help to get rid of phlegm. Linctuses also contain something soothing, such as syrup or glycerol.

COUNSELLING

When just talking to someone can help

There are times when we all need to talk over a problem that life has thrown at us. It may be a crisis of the moment requiring a decision – accepting a move at work, what to do after an exam failure, how to pay a debt. Or the trouble may have been deep or long-standing, darkening the whole of life – the threat of incurable illness, bereavement or splitting up with a partner, for example.

Because body and mind are inseparable, a physical cause can give rise to psychological symptoms and vice versa. Muscle pains or CONSTIPATION, for example, can result from severe STRESS and DEPRESSION, while loss of confidence and concentration may stem from a feeling of helplessness after an operation. Counselling is one way of coming to understand such problems and learning to manage them.

Although counselling is a treatment for the mind – a form of PSYCHOTHERAPY – it is not aimed principally at sick people, but at healthy people who want to deal with a crisis or improve their lives and relationships with others. Counselling does, however, form an important part of helping the terminally ill and their relatives to come to terms with impending death (see TERMINAL ILLNESS).

For people with mental illnesses, or who want extensive analysis and exploration of their own personality, different forms of psychotherapy are more suitable – for example, treatment by a psychologist, psychiatrist or psychoanalyst, all of whom have academic and often medical training in treating the mind. However, counselling may well form part of the treatment they offer.

Supportive counselling for clients who are basically healthy but are in crisis or at the end of their tether may be given by lay people who have had a course of training over a period of some months. The temperament of the counsellor is more important than academic or medical qualifications.

Many difficulties can be eased by a talk with a sympathetic friend or relation. Even a moan to a hairdresser or a letter to a magazine's advice column can lift the load. For more persistent problems, and when friends or relations are the problem, you may need professional help from an independent trained counsellor. But first be sure that you have made the most of your own resources.

Who it can help Anybody who feels that they have no one to turn to, or that they cannot cope with life, can benefit from counselling. Specific legal, educational or social problems can be taken to specialist counsellors. Even people with family and friends about them can receive more help from a totally objective, neutral 'ear' – and may find it easier or less embarrassing to talk to someone who is in no way involved.

Recently counselling has been offered to people who have been involved in a large-scale disaster such as a train collision, shipwreck or air crash. Uninjured survivors and members of the emergency services as well as the victims and their relations tend to suffer long-term distress after such events. Counselling and support groups have been of great help.

Finding a counsellor Spend some time thinking about what your problem really is. Do you want someone just to listen and sympathise, or do you want advice for a particular problem? If you need specific advice, a specialist counsellor is best – someone from a local law centre, careers office, student counselling centre or company personnel office, for example. Your local telephone directory will list such centres, or your local Life Line organisation will help you to find them.

Life Line was started in 1963 in Sydney, Australia, by Sir Alan Walker, to help the ever-growing numbers of people needing counselling for a wide range of problems. Today there are 17 Life Line centres in South Africa, and over 200 worldwide, in 14 different countries. Help is just a telephone call away, as all Life Line centres are listed in the telephone directory.

Although essentially a telephone counselling service, Life Line does also offer face-to-face counselling. The counsellors are trained volunteers from all walks of life and they man the crisis telephones 24 hours per day. All calls are treated confidentially and no problem is regarded as being too small. The counsellors will listen to you, and help find ways of dealing with your problems. They will also give you information and referrals, if needed.

A statistical breakdown of calls received by Life Line shows that many of them concern problems with relationships, STRESS and DEPRESSION. Other calls are made by people contemplating suicide, suffering from child abuse or experiencing SEXUAL PROBLEMS.

The importance of Life Line's existence in South Africa can be gauged from the fact that since its inception in 1968, the Western Cape centre has received over 198 000 calls – a monthly average of 1 900 or 63 calls a day.

Child Line and Rape Crisis are now incorporated in the general counselling. There are Rape Crisis centres countrywide as well, but not all offer a 24-hour service, and therefore work in co-operation with Life Line.

The South African Department of Health and Population Development has appointed Life Line as the official hot line to deal with any AIDS-related calls.

For more general counselling, you may find a sympathetic ear at your church, synagogue, mosque or temple. Or your doctor may be in a position to refer you to someone suitable.

Seeing a counsellor Listening is the chief role of a counsellor. A skilful one will quickly make you feel sufficiently at ease to talk freely. Your readiness to talk is vital. When you feel trust in the counsellor, you can reveal your thoughts and emotions fully, knowing that what you say will be in confidence. No judgment or criticism will be made, nor will you be cross-examined on matters you are not ready to deal with.

The counsellor may sum up and feed back to you what you have revealed, and point out important recurring patterns in your general behaviour. If a decision has to be made, the counsellor may outline the case for and against the various options, but any decisions are left to you.

Victims of disasters – such as the floods which devastated the Karoo town of Laingsburg in 1981 – can suffer psychological aftereffects that counselling can greatly help.

The opportunity to talk without interruption or contradiction is a beneficial release in itself. It boosts self-confidence, clarifies your situation and allows you to assess past actions and work out priorities for the future. The counsellor aims to help you gain insight into your motives and needs, but this will not of itself make your situation different or your future actions easier.

If you have gone to a counsellor for help with a specific problem, the counsellor may do more than just listen. Letter-writing skills, role-playing, practising new behaviour, discussing your problems and progress in a group or other useful techniques may be incorporated in the sessions.

Be prepared to give the counselling a fair trial, but do not persist if the counsellor is not right for you – go to a different one. It is vital to feel that the counsellor is genuinely interested in you and your situation.

Self help To get the most benefit from counselling, you must be prepared to back it up with your own everyday efforts. Eat a healthy, nourishing diet (see EATING FOR HEALTH) and cut down on coffee and tea, which can make you jumpy and irritable. Take some brisk EXERCISE and learn to calm yourself through RELAXATION and BREATHING exercises. Set aside time for hobbies or other activities you enjoy so that you can forget your problems for a time.

Do not bottle up your feelings between counselling sessions. Pour them out with a good cry, stamp your feet, punch a cushion – or express them in a diary. If writing about your anger and misery is not enough, talk to a discreet friend, an older relative or a priest.

An orthodox view

Doctors do not dispute the benefits of counselling, indeed many would like to have time enough to act as counsellors themselves. If there is no counsellor in their particular practice, they will readily suggest contacts for patients in need. Some, however, prefer not to be involved in what they regard as non-medical aspects of a patient's life. Or they may believe that patients come to them simply to be told what to do.

CRAMP

These agonising muscular spasms usually affect the legs, feet and (in writer's cramp) the hand. The muscles contract suddenly, causing severe pain that can last for several minutes. Various people involved in sports – such as running – and others who pursue outdoor activities, such as gardening, suffer from cramp, partly because they use certain muscles all the time.

Other causes of cramp may include swimming in cold water, poor circulation to the muscles (see CIRCULATION PROBLEMS), and salt or other mineral deficiencies. Period pains, which are often called cramps, are not caused by muscular contractions.

What the therapists recommend

NATUROPATHY

Self help A diet rich in VITAMINS and MINERALS is recommended, including leafy greens, soya beans, nuts, buttermilk and yoghurt, wholegrain cereals, and seeds such as pumpkin, sesame and sunflower. Some therapists advise avoiding high cholesterol foods such as animal and dairy fats, because the cramp may be a sign of poor circulation caused by 'furred' blood vessels.

Supplements of calcium, magnesium, potassium, iron, vitamins B, C and D, and kelp tablets may help if a deficiency is the cause. In addition, vitamin E is recommended for cramps after EXERCISE or during the night. If you sweat a lot at work or exercise, you may need salt tablets to replace salt lost with the sweat.

A practitioner may advise you to make time for relaxation as well as exercise, since

First aid for cramp

Cramp can often be relieved by stretching the cramped muscles from their contracted state. For cases of thigh cramp, sit down, straighten the knee and get a helper to lift the heel of the foot with one hand while pushing firmly down on the knee with the other. For cases of hand cramp, gently force the fingers to straighten, then spread them wide and push the fingertips firmly down on a flat, solid surface.

Cramp in the calf or foot
If help is available, lie down and get the helper to straighten the knee and toes, and push upwards under the ball of the foot. Otherwise, stand and push down with your full weight on the heel and toes.

TENSION can make cramp more painful. Some victims have also claimed relief from bandaging a magnet loosely to the affected area, and from a tonic which is believed to stimulate the flow of blood to the calves. Make it from a teaspoon each of lemon juice, honey and cloves, mixed with a tablespoon of ginger wine and half a cup of boiling water. Allow it to stand for 24 hours. Take 3 tablespoonfuls nightly before bed.

Other alternative treatments

Massage Treat the whole region, not just the affected muscles. Concentrate on stretching the muscles by using gliding and kneading movements (see p. 225) and finish off with chopping strokes, deep massage or effleurage to stimulate circulation to the affected area.

Homoeopathy *Cuprum metallicum* is used for severe cramp, especially in the fingers, legs and toes. *Colchicum* may help cramp in the soles of the feet, and *Nux vomica* is recommended when cramp occurs at night for no known cause.

People who also have cold feet or are overweight may find *Calcarea carbonica* useful, and those who suffer from a feeling of tiredness as well as cramp can be helped by *Arnica*.

Herbal Medicine Decoctions (see p. 184) of crampbark are said to have a relaxing effect on the muscles. Take one cup three times a day. For long-term treatment, decoctions of prickly ash and ginger are believed to improve circulation. Infusions (see p. 184) of ginger can also be used.

Biochemic Tissue Salts *Mag. phos.* is thought to nourish the nerves and muscles and to relieve cramp.

Hydrotherapy Mustard foot baths may help to relieve cramp in the legs, and applying hot and cold compresses is recommended for improving the blood supply to affected muscles.

Aromatherapy Three drops each of basil and marjoram and one drop of lemongrass essential oils are generally recommended for use in a bath.

Alternatively, mix them into 20 ml of carrier oil or lotion and rub it into the area immediately, twice daily if the problem is recurring. Regular aromatherapy treatment is said to be helpful for cramp.

An orthodox view

A doctor will advise rest as the best cure for overused muscles, and salt replacement for persistent cramp accompanied by sweating, diarrhoea or vomiting.

Sometimes doctors are unable to find the cause, and prescribe small amounts of quinine to relieve the symptoms. In general, they are not opposed to the application of naturopathic therapy.

CRANIAL OSTEOPATHY

Coaxing the skull bones into the right position

The dome of bone that protects the brain is not in one continuous piece. The eight separate bones that make up the skull – the cranium – have the finest of gaps between them. It was once thought that the bones are immovable after young childhood, but now it is known that they can move very slightly in relation to one another.

They move most during birth, and if they do not return to their proper position afterwards, they can distort the flow of 'shock absorber' fluid around the brain, cause pressure on parts of the brain or affect quite different parts of the body through nerves that originate in the brain. Later in life, blows to the head or dental work that displaces the jaw bones can cause the same problems.

Some practitioners of OSTEOPATHY aim to detect and correct pressures and displacements in the skull and facial bones, using the delicate form of manipulation called cranial osteopathy. The techniques were largely developed in the United States in the 1920s by William Garner Sutherland. While conducting experiments to test whether the bones of the skull could move, he devised various contraptions to squeeze his own skull bones out of position. His wife began to see significant changes in his behaviour while the pressure was on.

Who it can help People suffering facial NEURALGIA, MIGRAINE and other HEADACHES have been helped. Discomforts following blows to the head, whiplash injuries and dental work have also been relieved. Disturbances of balance and tinnitus resulting from slight displacement of the temporal bones at the sides of the skull often respond.

Slight pressure on the nerves in the brain can cause circulation and breathing problems, high BLOOD PRESSURE and stomach ULCERS – all of which, it is claimed, can be improved by cranial osteopathy.

Finding a practitioner There are few South African practitioners of cranial osteopathy. A qualified osteopath or chiropractor may be able to put you in touch with one. Or write, asking for a list of practitioners, to the Chiropractic Association of South Africa, c/o Dr Gert van der Walt, 701 Poynton House, Gardiner Street, Durban 4001.

Consulting a practitioner A careful assessment of your medical history and present symptoms will precede treatment. Manipulation is very gentle, some of it barely perceptible, consisting of tapping, moulding and holding the bones to coax them into the proper alignment. To correct wrongly positioned jaw bones, the osteopath may manipulate them from inside the mouth.

An orthodox view

Cranial osteopathy, like osteopathy in general, is far more widely practised and accepted in the United States than it is elsewhere. Many doctors who accept that osteopathy works do not agree with the fundamental concepts of cranial osteopathy. However, few of them would regard the treatment as harmful.

The only danger is that illnesses which could urgently need quite different treatment may not get it. This risk is avoided by consulting only a reputable osteopath, preferably one who is also a qualified doctor and who will not be too ready to give physical manipulation before checking whether symptoms are caused by a fracture, a tumour or an infection.

CROUP

A harsh, barking cough and strained, noisy breathing are symptoms of croup, which affects babies and children under five years old. It usually strikes in winter and is often accompanied by FEVER, irritability and restlessness. Croup is self-limiting normally, but if it persists – or if the child turns a pale grey-blue colour, or has difficulty in breathing – you should call a doctor.

What the therapists recommend

NATUROPATHY

Self help A hot, dry atmosphere is to be avoided, say practitioners, so lower or cut off any central heating in the child's bedroom, and see that the room is well ventilated. If you have room humidifiers, use them.

Consultation A naturopath will probably advise cutting down the child's intake of dairy foods such as butter, milk, cheese and yoghurt, which are believed to thicken mucus (see CATARRH). He may also advise supplements of vitamin C to build up body defences, and recommend garlic or onions in the diet. Soya milk or proprietary milk formula can replace cow's milk for babies.

HYDROTHERAPY

Steam inhalation can help to relieve croup symptoms. Shut all bathroom doors and windows, and fill the bath or basin with hot water. Since steam rises, sit with the child on your lap so that his head is held as high as possible. Do not leave the child alone, and take care to avoid scalding.

A therapist places glass suction cups mouth-down on the patient's back along the energy meridian lines. This aims to draw any 'bad energy' to the surface and bring relief.

Other alternative treatments

Herbal Medicine Camomile tea can help soothe croup, and so can an infusion of the leaves of horsemint (an indigenous herb, known in Afrikaans as 'balderjan'). Another soothing infusion said to ease croup can be made by adding a teaspoon each of coltsfoot and vervain to a cup of boiling water. Cover and leave for about ten minutes and then strain through muslin.

Aromatherapy Two drops each of eucalyptus and sandalwood essential oils added to a teaspoon of carrier oil and rubbed into a child's chest is recommended as beneficial for croup.

An orthodox view

As croup is usually a symptom, caused by a VIRUS INFECTION in the larynx, or voice box (see LARYNGITIS), a doctor may not prescribe antibiotics unless he establishes that there are complications – such as a risk of PNEUMONIA. However, he may give an analgesic to reduce fever, and recommend cool drinks of milk, fruit juice or water.

A baby or child in great pain or discomfort may be sent to hospital for observation, particularly if there is any difficulty in breathing.

CUPPING

Suction cups for removing 'poisons'

This technique was used by practitioners of Western medicine for many centuries to treat a range of maladies. It is still part of traditional Chinese medicine, and is most commonly used to relieve BOILS or abscesses, some cases of ARTHRITIS and RHEUMATISM, ASTHMA, BRUISING, COLDS and a CHILL.

Cupping involves applying suction 'cups' made of bamboo or glass in various sizes to the body. Alcohol-soaked cotton held in forceps and set alight – or simply a lighted taper – is held at the mouth of the inverted cup. The heat causes the air inside to expand, and some of it escapes. The cup is then placed mouth down on the patient's skin, and as it cools, the partial vacuum inside makes it stick on and draw the flesh into the cup. The skin becomes red with the increased blood flow that results.

To release the cup, pressure is exerted on the skin around it. The time the cups are left in place varies according to the age and constitution of the patient and the complaint.

Western doctors used to believe that the increased blood flow under the cup drew impurities away from nearby organs and tissues. Sometimes the skin under the cup was cut so that the 'poisons' flowed out of the body with the blood. Even in the early part of this century some doctors still used cupping to 'draw' boils.

The Chinese theory underlying cupping is that it gets rid of unwanted or 'perverse' Qi – energy, or life force – in the body. Practitioners believe cupping draws the perverse energy to the body's surface and disperses it.

CYMATICS

The healing effects of sound waves

Practitioners of this therapy compare the human body to a musical instrument which sometimes makes discordant sounds and needs to be 'tuned'. They claim to do this by directing high-frequency sound waves onto the affected area, restoring the body to a harmonious whole. The term cymatics comes from the Greek word *kyma*, meaning 'a billow' or 'great wave'.

Who it can help It is claimed that cymatics is particularly beneficial for people suffering from ARTHRITIS, BACK PAIN, bone FRACTURES, LUMBAGO, RHEUMATISM, SLIPPED DISC, and

forms of paralysis. The therapy is also given to people who are to have an operation such as a hip replacement (see HIP COMPLAINTS), to aid and accelerate the healing process.

Finding a therapist Though the term cymatics is generally unfamiliar in South Africa, physiotherapists routinely use ultrasound equipment. For further information, you can write to the South African Society of Physiotherapy, P O Box 47238, Parklands 2121.

Consulting a therapist Patients are treated mostly by means of a hand-held instrument called a sound-wave applicator, which is used in much the same way as a massage vibrator. There may also be a warm-water treatment pool into which sound waves are transmitted. This, it is said, greatly enhances the healing effect of the water. Special therapeutic music which incorporates sound waves aimed to relax and increase feelings of well-being may also be played.

An orthodox view

Doctors have confirmed that fractures heal quicker if sound waves are applied to the site of the fracture, and this therapy is now used in several orthopaedic centres. Research is currently directed at finding further uses.

CYSTITIS

Burning pain on passing urine; repeated trips to the lavatory, often to pass only a few drops; pain in the abdomen and back – the distressing symptoms of cystitis are well known to many women. The cause is an inflamed membrane lining the bladder – this is usually the result of bacteria passing through the urinary passage.

Food ALLERGY, chemical sensitivity, bruising during intercourse and vaginal THRUSH can also cause inflammation. Symptoms vary from mild to severe, sometimes disappearing within hours, sometimes dragging on for weeks. Many victims have only a single bout; others suffer repeated attacks. In all cases – especially if there is blood in the urine – it is advisable to see a doctor before seeking alternative treatments.

Men are rarely affected because bacteria have much farther to travel to reach a man's urinary passage and bladder (see also URETHRITIS). In children, cystitis is often associated with CONSTIPATION, which may cause pressure on the bladder.

What the therapists recommend
NATUROPATHY
Self help After urinating, rinse away any germs by pouring cool, boiled water over the

First aid for cystitis

Start home treatment as soon as symptoms begin. Attacks can often be cut short by taking the following steps immediately:

Drink 600 ml of water or mild ca-momile tea straight away, to flush germs out of the bladder.

Use hot-water bottles wrapped in towels to alleviate pain in the lower back or pelvic region.

Take a teaspoon of bicarbonate of soda in a glass of water every three hours. This makes the urine less acidic, which stops bacteria from breeding and relieves burning.

Warning Patients with high BLOOD PRESSURE or HEART DISORDERS should ask a doctor's advice before taking bicarbonate of soda.

If pain persists, take one or two mild painkillers (aspirin or paraceta-mol).

Apply live yoghurt to the affected area. The friendly bacteria it contains can help to fight invading germs.

Drink as much water or mild herbal tea as you can – at least 300 ml every 20 minutes – and go to the lavatory as often as necessary.

Lie down or sit in a comfortable chair, keep warm and relax. After three hours most attacks should begin to wear off. See your doctor if the symptoms persist.

Do not eat citrus or sour fruit, and avoid foods containing vinegar, and animal proteins such as eggs, fish, meat and cheese: they make the urine more acid and painful to pass.

urethral and vaginal openings while leaning back slightly on the lavatory seat. Wipe from front to back with toilet paper, taking care not to touch the anal area.

After passing a motion, make sure that you wipe as before, from front to back. Afterwards, gently wash the anus with warm, soapy water and then carefully pat dry with clean cotton wool.

A diet of mild, non-irritating foods may also help. Cut out any hot, spicy dishes, and replace tea, coffee and cola drinks with fresh herb teas, fresh juices or coffee substitutes such as chicory and barley extracts. Two or three glasses a day of mixed raw apple and carrot juice are recommended, and some sufferers have found relief by taking dolomite or propolis tablets.

Consultation The naturopath will make tests and ask questions to try to find out what is irritating your bladder. Allergy tests are often made, and a diet is drawn up to cut out any harmful foods. If you also suffer from thrush, the diet may exclude all yeast-containing foods such as bread, cheese, wine and beer.

HERBAL MEDICINE

Self help Single attacks of cystitis are said often to be cleared up by drinking large amounts of yarrow infusion. The following herbal mixtures may be used to treat more persistent cases: A decoction of equal amounts of marsh-mallow leaves, bearberry, sage and horsetail well mixed together: take one cup three times a day. An infusion made from corn silk, cherry stalks, bilberries and poppies in equal quantities: take two or three cups a day. An infusion made from equal amounts of corn silk, couch grass, bearberry and yarrow: take three times a day.

Barley water is also believed to have a soothing and mildly diuretic effect that can help. Put 120 g barley in enough water to cover it and bring to the boil. Strain it, then pour 600 ml of cold water over the barley, add the rind of half a lemon and simmer until the barley is soft. Leave until lukewarm. Now remove the barley, add 1-2 tablespoons of honey, and drink as required.

HOMOEOPATHY

Self help *Cantharis* is used to treat burning pains when passing urine, *Staphysagria* for cystitis due to bruising or injury, *Aconite* for the sudden onset of symptoms after exposure to dry cold, and *Sarsaparilla* when pain is felt only after urinating.

When the cause is a chill caught by getting cold and wet, *Dulcamara* is recommended. If you have a high temperature, try *Belladonna*.

BIOCHEMIC TISSUE SALTS

Ferr. phos. is recommended for early stages when there is frequent and burning urination; *Kali phos.* for a cutting or scalding pain, and *Mag. phos.* when there is a constant but unproductive urge to urinate.

Other alternative treatments

Aromatherapy Make a tea using juniper and eucalyptus oils and drink three or four cups daily. Also helpful are eight drops of essential oils in a warm bath lasting ten minutes once or twice daily. Other helpful oils include benzoin, bergamot, black pepper, cajuput, fennel, frankincense, lavender, naiouli, pine and sandalwood.

Hydrotherapy Spray the pelvic area thoroughly for about three minutes with warm water, followed by one minute of cold spraying, to relieve pain. Repeat over the upper part of the sacrum (between the two dimples in the lower back). Repeat three or four times in each treatment.

Reflexology Massage to the reflex area relating to the bladder is recommended, plus areas relating to the kidneys, ureter, lymph nodes of the pelvis, adrenal and pituitary glands and, in men, the prostate gland.

An orthodox view

Attacks of cystitis are usually treated with an antibiotic which often clears the infection within 48 hours. In cases of recurrent cystitis, a midstream specimen of urine may be taken to see which bacteria are causing the infection, and which antibiotics they are sensitive to. Alternative treatments may help the symptoms, but neglecting urinary infections could eventually lead to kidney damage.

Do's and don'ts for cystitis sufferers

Do maintain a high standard of personal hygiene.

Do avoid excessive vibration such as riding a motorbike for long journeys.

Do try alternative methods of CONTRACEPTION if taking the Pill or using a condom, cap or diaphragm seems to bring on attacks.

Do use sanitary towels instead of tampons.

Don't use perfumed soaps, powders or other toiletries on the skin or in your bath, and avoid vaginal deodorants.

Do wash underwear with hand soap or soap flakes, as some washing powders can cause irritation. Always rinse out soap thoroughly.

Do use a lubricating cream such as KY Jelly – available from chemists – or experiment with different positions if attacks occur after sexual intercourse. Passing urine immediately after intercourse can also help by flushing out any germs.

Do wear pure cotton underwear and loose-fitting clothes, and wear stockings rather than tights, to allow air to circulate freely.

Do go to the lavatory as soon as you feel the need. Holding back gives bacteria a chance to breed.

Don't expose the bladder to heat and cold: don't sit on icy ground or on radiators, and don't stand around in wet clothes or in a wind.

DANCE MOVEMENT THERAPY

Listening to the body's message

As small children we can readily express our feelings long before we learn to talk. One of the ways we communicate is through body movements. Once we can speak, we may forget that our bodies are still in touch with feelings that are worrying, embarrassing, or simply hard to talk about.

Dance movement therapy uses the connection between body movement and emotion in order to help us express and manage feelings too deep to recognise or too difficult to explain in words. Most tribal communities have recognised from earliest times the healing power of dance, but complex modern societies did not become aware of its relevance to modern ailments until the 1940s when dancers in the United States began to develop ways of using it to help those people who were suffering from various mental health problems. Dance movement therapy was initially introduced to South Africa only in the 1970s.

Who it can help Adults are generally referred to a therapist because of emotional problems, including ANXIETY and DEPRESSION, and difficulties with relationships. Therapy can also help in more serious illnesses such as SCHIZOPHRENIA, MANIC DEPRESSIVE DISORDER, ANOREXIA and BULIMIA, and in drug or alcohol ADDICTION. Adults with learning disabilities can benefit from it, as can people with certain stress-related physical illnesses – HEART DISORDERS, for example.

Dance movement therapy is particularly effective for children, especially those with learning or emotional difficulties, those with limited ability to concentrate and those who find it hard to get on with other children. Children with behaviour problems resulting from family stresses, including physical or sexual abuse, and even severely mentally handicapped children and those with AUTISM are successfully treated. Physically disabled children, such as the blind and deaf, may also benefit from the therapy.

Finding a therapist There are as yet very few qualified dance movement therapists practising in South Africa, nor is training in this therapy readily available here. For names and addresses of practitioners, write to the Professional Board for Occupational Therapy, c/o South African Medical and Dental Council, P O Box 205, Pretoria 0001. Alternatively, you can get in touch with the South African Association of Occupational Therapists, P O Box 17289, Hillbrow 2001.

Alternatively, consider curative eurhythmy – the nearest approach to dance movement therapy in South Africa. There are curative eurhythmists in Cape Town and Johannesburg. For more information, contact the Anthroposophical Society, P O Box 65119, Benmore 2010 (telephone 011-7268272), or Bonair, Price Drive, Constantia 7800 (telephone 021-7946445).

Consulting a therapist Treatment sessions may be individual or for groups. Before you join a group the therapist will usually wish to see you on your own. Some groups meet in the evening to suit people who work in the daytime. Others are run for hospital patients, day care clients or children at times more suitable for them.

Treatment varies according to the client's problems and the therapist's personal style, but some features are common. Clients need

Two members of the group, a man and a woman, became involved in moving together. When other group members join in, the man is shocked to discover how he suddenly feels inhibited. He realises that his problems in relating to women are connected to difficulties in coping with jealous and intrusive family members.

This young woman is going through a time when she feels overloaded by the claims life is making on her. She has asked for support from a group member while she struggles with a large bean bag. She is surprised to find support especially valuable as she rests between spells of more demanding activity.

The therapist is working with a non-speaking 14-year-old boy to build a relationship through their movements. It has taken a long time for the boy to develop enough trust to let his hands be touched. In earlier sessions the therapist moved at a distance, echoing the shape and rhythm of the boy's movements.

have no previous experience of movement or dance, nor is there any stress on competence in learning or carrying out sequences of movements. Instead, the emphasis is on exploring movements and expanding your vocabulary of movements as you discover resources within yourself.

You need not be young and active. Therapists are used to working with people who are anxious, elderly, frail or overweight. Sessions always begin with movements that everyone can manage.

If you begin dance movement therapy, always tell the therapist about any difficulties you may have, such as BACK PAIN or high BLOOD PRESSURE. The therapist may advise you to see your doctor before deciding on suitable treatment. However, while a therapist will always be alert to physical problems, the main focus of the work is understanding your feelings and working out how to deal with them. Although some people are helped by treatment that lasts only a few weeks, it is usually necessary to continue for longer.

Sessions start with a warm-up period to loosen muscles. Music may be used during the session, but not always – it can distract clients from what they want to express. The therapist may suggest movements but clients are not expected to follow the suggestions rigidly. They are encouraged to contribute ideas of their own.

A theme will usually emerge from the movements and this may be explored by clients working separately, in pairs or in a group. A theme that emerges might be, for example, the way in which one person always makes movements that are very fast and forceful at first but then fizzle out; or the way that, in a group, the members always move at arm's length, never coming closer to one another or getting farther apart.

To begin with, the therapist may need to step in, picking up the themes that clients have introduced and helping them to explore and resolve the problems they encounter. Eventually, clients may begin to identify important issues and learn how to work through a problem by themselves. Clients may discuss the feelings aroused by the movement and try to integrate their insights into further movements so that there is continuing interplay between feelings, talk and movement.

Therapists working with seriously disturbed or handicapped clients use their highly developed sensitivity to movement to establish a relationship that does not rely on words. The relationship enables the therapist to support the client through the experiences of excitement, sadness, frustration and fear that are part of normal development.

An orthodox view

There are no risks involved in dance movement therapy with a qualified therapist. Evidence is growing that it has psychological and emotional benefits. It serves as an effective non-verbal form of psychotherapy. The therapy helps, in particular, patients who are mentally ill or mentally handicapped, or who have severe behavioural problems.

DANDRUFF

The exact cause of dandruff has long been uncertain. Some general practitioners believe it is the result of either too much or too little oil being produced by sebaceous glands in the scalp.

However, some dermatologists suggest that it is caused by an infection, and a yeast fungus has been isolated that is believed to breed in a combination of sebaceous oil and dead skin cells. Antifungal shampoos are available in chemists and health stores.

What the therapists recommend
NATUROPATHY
Self help Yoghurt is recommended as a hair conditioner. Wash and rinse the hair, then rub yoghurt into the scalp, and leave for 10-15 minutes. Rinse, then wash again, using as little shampoo as necessary. An infusion (p. 184) of thyme, nettle or sage with 2 tablespoons of vinegar can be used as a final rinse.
Consultation A practitioner will tell you that dandruff may indicate poisons in the system or nutritional deficiencies and imbalances in levels of minerals and/or trace elements. He will recommend a diet of plenty of fresh fruit and vegetables, wholegrains and wheatgerm, vegetable oils and high-protein food, such as lean meat and nuts. To be avoided are: sugar and starch products, alcohol, and fatty or highly spiced foods.

Other alternative treatments
Herbal Medicine An indigenous treatment for dandruff is a paste made by mixing borax with an infusion in boiling water of the fresh roots of the wild scabious (or 'pincushion'), a common veld flower in midsummer. Rub the paste into the scalp once a week. For a scalp massage after shampooing, use infusions (p. 184) of rosemary or lavender.
Aromatherapy Mix essential oils of cedarwood (seven drops), cypress and juniper (each ten drops) in 50 ml of carrier oil. Rub well into the scalp and leave for one hour. To remove, rub neat, mild shampoo into the hair, then wash out with warm water.

To keep dandruff at bay, use the same quantities of the oils in 600 ml of warm water. Stir well and use as a final rinse.

An orthodox view

A doctor will probably recommend washing the hair only once or twice a week in a mild detergent shampoo available from chemists. You will also be advised to avoid harsh hair dyes and scented hair creams; also brilliantines and other oily dressings. In severe cases, a scalp lotion containing cortisone can be prescribed.

DEAFNESS

Some people are born totally or partially deaf; others become deaf gradually, after the age of about 50. Both conditions fall into one of two main categories: *conductive deafness*, which is mostly curable, and *nerve deafness*, which is not.

Conductive deafness is due to something hindering the transmission of sound waves to the cochlea, the sound-sensitive organ of the inner ear. It can have a number of causes including infections, earwax, sudden loud noises, foreign objects such as a bead in a child's ear, and otosclerosis – a fusion of the small bones in the middle ear, which mainly affects women aged between 20 and 40.

Nerve deafness occurs when the cochlea or the auditory nerve which carries stimuli from the ear to the brain is damaged. This is usually caused by viral infections such as MEASLES, MUMPS and German measles (rubella), which can damage the hearing of babies whose mothers contracted the infection during the first three months of pregnancy. It can also be caused by exposure to loud noises such as gunfire or disco music.

Never attempt to relieve deafness yourself. Poking about in the ear to remove wax or foreign objects can lead to perforated eardrums and possibly permanent deafness.

What the therapists recommend

NATUROPATHY

Consultation Practitioners believe that diet can affect the functioning of the ears, and may recommend a diet rich in VITAMINS A and B₁ (thiamine). Vitamin A comes in dairy foods such as cheese and eggs, as well as liver and carrots. Vitamin B₁ is found in brewer's yeast, wholewheat bread, potatoes and peanuts, and is said to help repair damaged cell tissue in the ear and to strengthen the auditory nerve.

Self help In straightforward cases of earwax, soften it with a few drops of almond or olive oil and lemon juice, heated in a cupful of warm water to body temperature. Apply with a small dropper two or three times a day, taking care not to poke your ear with the dropper. Do not probe the ear with a cotton bud, as this can make wax harder to remove and may cause damage.

ACUPUNCTURE

Consultation Some cases of deafness – those caused by, or associated with, CATARRH, DIZZINESS, MOTION SICKNESS, RINGING IN THE EARS and Ménière's syndrome – are said to respond to stimulating the nerves regulating the workings of the ear. Acupuncturists relate these workings to the kidneys and bladder, so the practitioner may treat points on the meridians for these organs. MOXIBUSTION may also be applied.

The bladder meridian extends from the eye, round the back of the head and down the spine and back of the left leg. The kidney meridian is down the left front of the body and the front of the left leg (see chart, p. 14).

Other alternative treatments

Chiropractic By manipulating the patient's neck, chiropractors can sometimes ease tinnitus (see RINGING IN THE EARS).

Biochemic Tissue Salts Practitioners recommend Kali sulph. for deafness caused by catarrh and Kali phos. for deafness accompanied by nervous exhaustion (see also NERVOUS DISORDERS). Normal recommended dosage is four tablets dissolved on the tongue three times a day for adults, two tablets for children and one for babies. In acute cases, adults can take one tablet every half hour. Do not eat or drink anything for 15 minutes before and after each dose.

An orthodox view

Where deafness is conductive, and therefore curable, most doctors do not object to the use of alternative remedies as a supplement to conventional treatments. They agree with naturopaths in using warm oil to treat earwax and are not opposed to tissue salts as an added aid. If these methods are not sufficient, they may syringe the ears.

However, a conventional doctor would send any patient suffering from any form of nerve deafness or other severe hearing loss to an ear specialist. In most cases – such as old-age deafness – a hearing aid may be fitted; in others, such as otosclerosis, the fused bones may be separated by surgery.

DEPRESSION

Depression is one of the most common psychiatric disorders, which can vary from a mild, self-limiting 'blue' period to a full-blown attack of life-threatening, suicidal depression.

According to psychiatrists, there are two kinds of depression: *exogenous*, becoming depressed as a result of outside factors such as divorce, job loss, money troubles, or the death of a loved one; and *endogenous*, resulting from internal biochemical sources – a medical form of depression. Sometimes, spells of euphoria and hyperactivity alternate with periods of deep depression (see MANIC DEPRESSIVE DISORDER).

With such a complex and serious illness it is hard to separate normal and therapeutic feelings of sadness and GRIEF from clinical depression. In some cases, symptoms of straightforward ANXIETY may mask a state of depression. Depression is more common among women than men, and tends to affect people of all ages – from young children to pensioners.

Symptoms include feelings of worthlessness, inadequacy, isolation and despair – and the belief that no one understands or sympathises with you. This may be accompanied by loss of interest in work or home life, inability to concentrate on anything, and, in

severe cases, sluggish thought processes and delusions (see also NERVOUS DISORDERS).

Physically, symptoms may include loss of energy, a sense of 'heaviness', difficulty or slowness in movement, a dryness in the mouth, INDIGESTION, sluggish bowel movements and CONSTIPATION. In some cases sufferers may lose weight and women may have PERIOD PROBLEMS.

Occasionally people may be prone to depression from birth due to irregularities in the biochemical make-up of the brain. With some patients depression is associated with ANAEMIA, hormonal changes, low thyroid activity (see THYROID DISORDERS), VITAMIN deficiencies or ADDICTION to drugs. Some women suffer from the so-called 'six-day blues' following childbirth, a depressive phase related to sudden hormonal changes.

Warning If symptoms – mental or physical – are severe or last for more than a few weeks, professional help should be sought.

What the therapists recommend

HOMOEOPATHY

Consultation A therapist should be consulted if bouts of depression are frequent or intense. For short-lived bouts, in which the sufferer is anxious, restless, or exhausted – especially in the small hours – *Arsenicum album* is recommended. To help overcome emotional upset or bereavement, try *Ignatia* immediately after the event. If the distress persists then take *Natrum mur.* All these remedies should be taken in the 6th potency, three times a day for two weeks.

If the sufferer feels suicidal, professional help must be sought without delay.

BACH REMEDIES

Self help If depression follows an illness or long-standing exhaustion, Olive is said to be helpful. For cases of sudden depression accompanied by repressed anger, Mustard is recommended; when depression is caused by resentment or bitterness, Willow. Gorse is said to be effective for constant feelings of hopelessness. Larch may help overcome lack of confidence.

People who are experiencing extreme despair, especially spiritually, are advised to take Sweet chestnut. Walnut is held to help victims of depression cope with major changes in life, and anyone who has all but lost interest in life, or is apathetic.

Other alternative treatments

Naturopathy Practitioners prescribe large doses of vitamin B to counteract depression. In particular, vitamin B₆ is recommended for mood swings associated with period problems. If the MENOPAUSE is thought to have caused depression, some therapists will advise the patient to have hormone replace-

Beating the blues

Everyone feels depressed from time to time, especially if things start to get 'on top' of them and they feel they cannot cope. If this happens, the following self-help measures may help solve the problem. If they do not, consult a therapist or doctor.

Taking exercise Try to increase your energy level by taking up an activity such as cycling, jogging, or swimming. Alternatively, you could join a BIOENERGETICS group.

Expressing your feelings Sometimes depression may be caused by pent-up anger or the inability to cry. If this seems to be so, release your anger and let yourself weep.

Making physical contact Feelings of loneliness and isolation may sometimes bring on depression. If this happens, you should make arrangements to have a MASSAGE or SHIATSU treatment.

Keeping a diary Writing down your thoughts each day is a good way of obtaining relief, especially if you are feeling overburdened and overwhelmed by life.

Talking things over Depression can often be lifted by simply talking over your problems with a friend, perhaps while taking a walk together.

Thinking positively Depressing situations may be relieved by making positive statements about yourself and your circumstances. For example, tell yourself, 'I am *not* a victim', 'I *will* overcome', 'Tomorrow *is* another day'.

Breathing deeply Taking full YOGA breaths, or bellows breaths, can be an effective means of overcoming feelings of gloom and despair.

Visualising peaceful images Imagining you are in a tranquil, comfortable place can assist in banishing depressing thoughts.

Creating artistically Painting, drawing, dancing, singing and playing musical instruments are all effective ways of combating depression.

trate on points on meridians associated with the liver, gall bladder, pericardium (the fibrous sheath around the heart), ren, du, spleen and stomach.

Aromatherapy Aromatherapy body massage is said to be most effective in relieving depression. Several oils are also held to be beneficial. They include basil, clary sage, neroli, otto, Roman camomile, rose and thyme. The oils should be inhaled deeply from a tissue at regular intervals, or six to eight drops of any one of them can be put into your bath.

Herbal Medicine One or two cups of borage or vervain tea are believed to raise your spirits. Alternatively, try a hot cup of rosemary tea each day with a pinch of valerian. A recommended nerve tonic is an infusion of four to five flowering lavender tops, with relaxing honey added to taste.

Autosuggestion and Hypnotherapy Therapists who practise both of these techniques have claimed success in the treatment of depressive cases.

Massage The pleasant and relaxing effects of massage are said to help relieve those suffering from depression.

An orthodox view

Although most doctors are not opposed to alternative remedies, they feel they should go hand-in-hand with conventional medical or psychological treatment. For example, in cases of mild depression, antidepression medication or sleeping pills will probably be prescribed. With more serious cases a course of antidepressant drugs – lasting for several weeks or even months – may be advised. Anyone who feels suicidally depressed should seek immediate medical help.

Sometimes a course of PSYCHOTHERAPY will be advised. This involves the patient seeing a psychotherapist at regular intervals, either individually or as part of a group. Alternatively, a GP may send a depressive patient to see a counsellor, who will try to help him to come to terms with his problems and so overcome them (see COUNSELLING).

DIABETES

Unquenchable thirst, weight loss and passing abnormal amounts of urine are among the first signs of diabetes. The disorder occurs when the pancreas, a gland situated behind the stomach, fails to produce enough insulin – the hormone that regulates the blood sugar level.

In some cases complications – such as ANGINA, blocked arteries (see ARTERIES [HARDENING]), CATARACTS and KIDNEY COMPLAINTS –

may eventually occur. But most diabetics learn to live fairly comfortably with their incurable – but controllable – condition. No one knows what exactly causes the insulin failure. Some doctors believe the disorder may be hereditary; others think that VIRUS INFECTIONS could be to blame.

Warning Since diabetes is a serious illness, medical advice is imperative, especially if the sufferer is a child.

What the therapists recommend

Naturopathy Most naturopaths consider that a high-fibre diet – including wholewheat bread, jacket potatoes, spinach, bran cereals, almonds and baked beans – reduces the body's need for insulin. It is also said to lower fat levels in the blood and lessen the risk of accompanying heart disease.

Some practitioners firmly believe that the complications which are associated with diabetes may be avoided by taking extra minerals and vitamins, including daily doses of vitamin C (1 g), vitamin E (250 iu), chromium (200 micrograms), manganese (4 mg) and zinc (15 mg).

Herbal Medicine As well as a strict, high-fibre diet, herbalists may recommend taking raw garlic. This is believed to help curb the increase of sugar in the blood, which otherwise causes the kidneys to produce large amounts of urine.

In addition, practitioners may offer the following herbs to ease the condition: burdock (to help the kidneys to work properly); gentian (to stimulate the working of the pancreas); and goat's rue (to cut down sugar levels).

Aromatherapy A body and bath oil containing a mixture of six to eight drops each of camphor, eucalyptus, geranium, juniper, lemon and rosemary is said to help to balance secretions from the pancreas. Back massage with four drops of the mixture in a teaspoon of vegetable carrier oil is also held to be beneficial for some people.

Yoga Some exercises in Hatha yoga are believed to balance the body's natural processes and so help relieve diabetes.

Homoeopathy Appropriate remedies are chosen according to individual symptoms – for example, *Phosphoric ac.* when exhaustion makes them worse, *Silicea* when the feet are cold and sweaty, *Uranium nit.* when there are digestive problems and weakness, and *Arg. nit.* when the victim feels depressed. In each case, 6C potency is recommended.

An orthodox view

Diabetes can be a serious, life-threatening condition which must be managed carefully by doctors with special skills – usually at a diabetic clinic. Once the condition has been brought firmly under control, then some of

ment therapy (HRT), the treatment that conventional doctors prescribe.

Hydrotherapy Therapists say that SAUNA BATHS and vigorous rubs have proved effective for some sufferers.

Acupuncture Depression is regarded as a LIVER DISORDER, and practitioners concenthe alternative therapies may well help to keep it under control.

However, daily insulin injections are necessary for children and most adults. These replace the loss when the pancreas fails to produce insulin. Some older people – whose bodies usually produce some insulin – need take only insulin tablets each day, and mild cases can sometimes be controlled by diet alone.

Diabetics using insulin will sometimes feel the effects of low blood sugar due to an accidental overdose. Symptoms include fainting, unsteadiness, sweating and disturbed behaviour such as incoherence and loss of memory. Most diabetics recognise these warning signs and can cut short the attacks by eating sugar. If they do not, they may appear intoxicated and are at risk of going into a coma. If this happens, call a doctor or an ambulance straight away.

People prone to such attacks should carry a card or wear a bracelet stating their condition and asking for immediate medical aid.

DIAGNOSIS

In any consultation, one of the first and most important tasks of a practitioner is to decide what the patient's problem is. This process is called *diagnosis*, and the ways in which it is done differ according to the kind of medicine practised. Having the problem diagnosed is obviously very important to the sick person, for it helps a patient to understand the situation and feel more in control.

However, not all practitioners make a formal diagnosis before beginning treatment. Some alternative therapists simply accept whatever reason the patient gives for the visit, since they view all illness as coming from the same source – the individual's separation from divine or natural healing forces (see HEALERS AND HEALING).

Conventional doctors generally view each illness as a separate problem with its own particular causes, symptoms and treatment. Their diagnosis is basically a scientific process of making observations of the patient and then using logical reasoning to identify the illness.

In practice, however, many doctors tend to offer some sort of treatment *before* they make a formal diagnosis, and admit that they do not always use purely scientific methods. Like many alternative practitioners, they use their accumulated experience and subjective impression of the patient's condition to form an opinion. They recognise a pattern in his symptoms or behaviour, and feel able to see the whole picture from just a small part.

All practitioners begin by asking about the problem and the patient – a process known as 'taking a history'. A physical examination and, sometimes, tests follow. Here are some of the diagnostic methods that are used by alternative therapists:

Taking a full history Questions are asked about the problem, how long it has been present, and how it began. The patient may also be asked for background information about family, work and past illnesses; also about personal habits and way of life – for example, patterns of sleep (see SLEEP DISORDERS) and any ADDICTION, such as SMOKING. The practitioner will listen carefully to the answers, and also hear the patient's own views regarding the problem.

Other specific questions are also asked by particular types of therapists.

Homoeopaths need to know about personality traits which they call 'mentals' – for example, whether you are anxious or easily upset – and also about unusual symptoms such as if pain is worse on one side of the body than the other, or if there is numbness or discomfort in an apparently unconnected area. Cravings for certain foods and responses to changes in the weather are also deemed important, as is your vaccination and immunisation record.

Naturopaths are more interested in diet and way of life. They will ask about sleep patterns, and the appearance of the urine and motions, as well as your sexual and, for women, menstrual history.

Oriental medicine considers weather factors and emotional states to be of particular importance. The practitioner – in ACUPUNCTURE, ACUPRESSURE or SHIATSU – will probably want to know how the changing seasons affect you, and how you respond to heat, cold, wind, dampness and dryness.

Chiropractors will ask about injuries and accidents, and will be interested in your posture and how you sit, walk, stand and sleep.

Physical examination Some of the alternative therapists also make different kinds of physical examinations.

Oriental medicine views taking pulses and examining the tongue as most important. The practitioner will also listen to your breathing, observe the brightness of your eyes, and consider the colour and texture of the skin. Acupuncturists measure 12 different pulses – six in each hand – each of which is held to reflect the health of a different organ or bodily system.

Chiropractors carefully examine the spine, ask you to perform some simple movements, measure your legs to see if one is shorter than the other, and examine the working of your joints.

Tests As well as blood tests, X-rays and other conventional means, many alternative

therapists use HAIR DIAGNOSIS to reveal any shortage of VITAMINS, MINERALS or other nutrients; KINESIOLOGY to test for ALLERGY; electronic instruments called biometers to show if there are ENERGY blocks; and KIRLIAN PHOTOGRAPHY to check the state of the aura. Cranial osteopaths, spiritual healers and some acupuncturists diagnose mainly by passing their hands over the patient's body to sense his aura and feel for blockages in the flow of vital energy (see AURA THERAPY).

The diagnosis To a practitioner who adopts a holistic approach, the diagnosis is seen as a way of understanding the patient as a whole person, rather than just labelling his illness. Nevertheless, most patients want to know what is wrong with them, and the practitioner may tell them that they have a particular condition, such as ASTHMA or ARTHRITIS, or say that the symptoms show that their systems are 'out of balance' and need to be restored.

Instead of treating the illness as something specific that happens to the patient and has to be treated in its own right, the illness is considered to be a sign that something is wrong with the person's *overall* health, and treatment should help them become wholly well again. The patient, and not the illness, is diagnosed and treated.

DIARRHOEA

Some cases of diarrhoea occur after eating infected food, others are often caused by a viral or bacterial infection. The resultant inflammation of the large intestine normally clears up within a day or two. More prolonged attacks can be serious, and babies and elderly, frail victims are particularly at risk, as the resultant fluid loss can cause dangerous levels of dehydration.

If the diarrhoea lasts for more than 48 hours, call a doctor. See also DYSENTERY.

What the therapists recommend
NATUROPATHY

Consultation Practitioners tend to feel that diarrhoea is the body's natural reaction to unwanted substances – and should not be dealt with by suppressants such as kaolin for at least 36 hours. But they emphasise the importance of avoiding bodily liquid loss by keeping up the fluid intake.

Self help Victims are advised to avoid food for 24 hours, taking only mineral water or 2 tablespoons of apple juice at regular, 15-30 minute intervals. When symptoms subside, the advice is to eat boiled rice and water, vegetable juices or soups.

It is claimed that live yoghurt helps the large intestine to restore its protective bacteria in cases where they have been destroyed by the infection.

Return gradually to other nutritious solid foods such as steamed carrots, bananas, hard-boiled eggs and toast, then slowly resume a normal diet. This dietary procedure is claimed also to be particularly effective for children, but the advice is to first purée the food in a blender.

HOMOEOPATHY

If diarrhoea is caused by food poisoning, especially meat, take *Arsen. alb.*, or *Carbo veg.* if bad fish is the culprit, or if the attack occurs before a big event. Take the 6th, 12th or 30th potency every half hour for six doses, then hourly. Stop taking the treatment as soon as a definite improvement is felt.

For symptoms caused by sudden fright, or aggravated by cold, dry weather, try *Aconitum napellus*. For particularly severe attacks, with cold sweats, *Veratrum alb.* is advised, and *Arg. nit.* if worry or stress is the cause.

AROMATHERAPY

One drop each of peppermint and cypress oil on a sugar lump every two hours has been known to bring relief in attacks of diarrhoea. Or make a tea as in the advice for WIND, using one drop each of peppermint, cypress and sandalwood or camomile; drink a cup two- or three-hourly until symptoms subside.

Nervous diarrhoea should be treated with oils that are beneficial for stress. They include camomile, geranium, juniper, lavender and sandalwood. Use three to four drops in a tea. Alternatively, the same amount in a teaspoon of carrier oil or lotion should be massaged gently into the abdomen twice a day. Six to eight drops in the bath are also regarded as beneficial.

HERBAL MEDICINE

Herbalists advise taking a garlic oil capsule once or twice a day if the cause is a mild infection, and 3-4 tablespoonfuls three times daily of an infusion of agrimony, plantain, geranium, camomile, sage, thyme or yarrow, with a pinch of powdered cinnamon, ginger or crushed caraway seeds. Use 600 ml of water to 30 g of chopped herbs. Cover, allow to stand for 15 minutes, then strain.

An orthodox view

A doctor will probably recommend rest and plenty of fluids, allowing the attack to subside naturally. However, in severe cases antibiotics, codeine or a suppressant may be prescribed. If the attack lasts longer than three days, the doctor will seek other causes. Diarrhoea in babies can be rapidly fatal, and they must be given oral rehydration therapy. Special salt and glucose rehydration mixtures can be bought from chemists.

DIETS AND DIETING

Taking a close look at what's on the menu ...

Alternative practitioners consider nutrition and diet to be one of the most important factors in health and disease, and in addition to the specific therapies they practise, most also offer very specific dietary advice. Usually, they recommend that you follow a basic wholefood diet (see EATING FOR HEALTH), which consists mainly of fresh fruit and vegetables, unrefined grains, pulses such as beans and peas, and small quantities of dairy products, fish, lean meat and poultry. Depending on the patient's needs, special adaptations may be made.

Cleansing diets Some therapists, particularly those who practise NATUROPATHY, recommend highly restricted diets when they think the system needs to be cleansed and purified. These include FASTING and the RAW FOOD DIET.

Non-mixing diets Diets that separate certain food groups, particularly starch and protein, all stem from the original HAY DIET, which was formulated by a well-known American doctor, William Howard Hay, earlier this century (see p. 164).

Diets based on particular beliefs Certain diets are based on special beliefs or nutritional theories. Vegetarians avoid meat, while vegans will eat no animal products at all (see VEGETARIANISM). MACROBIOTICS depends on balancing so-called YIN AND YANG foods. Religions such as Islam and Judaism have their own strict dietary rules, based on hygienic considerations.

Slimming diets Anyone who follows a sensible, wholefood diet should avoid putting on weight (unless he is underweight). If you are overweight, you will find that you gradually become slimmer, but if the process seems too slow, see SLIMMING THE NATURAL WAY, for safe, healthy ways to lose weight.

Therapeutic diets Although the wholefood diet is believed to help in curing or preventing many illnesses, more specialised diets are also used to treat particular problems. LOW-FAT DIETS are often recommended for patients with ANGINA, hardening of the arteries (see ARTERIES [HARDENING]) or HEART DISORDERS; and high BLOOD PRESSURE may be helped by SALT-FREE DIETS.

A diet which contains plenty of FIBRE is regarded as high on the list of priorities for those people who suffer from various BOWEL DISORDERS. Furthermore, several rigorous, specialised diets have also been used in the treatment of CANCER.

DIGESTIVE PROBLEMS

Stomach aches, feeling too full, WIND, nausea and acid regurgitation are just some of the uncomfortable symptoms associated with digestive problems. The most common complaints are ACID STOMACH, HEARTBURN and INDIGESTION, usually caused by overloading the stomach, too much rich, fatty food or too much alcohol.

Treatment depends on individual cases, but simply sticking to a more sensible diet (see EATING FOR HEALTH) generally solves the problem. Allergy to certain cereals (see COELIAC DISEASE) and to dairy products (see LACTOSE INTOLERANCE) can also interfere with digestion.

In rare cases, symptoms such as stomach pains, vomiting (see NAUSEA AND VOMITING), DIARRHOEA or CONSTIPATION may indicate more serious conditions such as APPENDICITIS, ULCERS, FOOD POISONING or GALLSTONES, which need medical attention.

See a doctor immediately if pain is severe. Otherwise, seek medical advice if any digestive problem or abdominal pain persists for more than 48 hours, or if it is accompanied by loss of appetite or weight.

See also IRRITABLE BOWEL SYNDROME and COLITIS.

DIZZINESS

In most cases the spinning sensation and feeling of faintness brought on by a dizzy spell are caused by a slight change in BLOOD PRESSURE or posture – such as rising quickly from a chair, or jumping out of bed in the morning. The attacks are usually over in less than 30 seconds.

However, if they last for longer than that – and are accompanied by recurring HEADACHES with NAUSEA AND VOMITING – see a doctor as soon as possible: the symptoms could indicate a brain tumour (see CANCER).

What the therapists recommend

Acupressure In straightforward cases of dizziness, two main pressure points can be used – in the foot and neck. The foot point is located between the metatarsal bones about 50 mm from the angle between the big and second toes. The neck pressure point is immediately below and behind the bottom of the ear lobe.

To use the foot points, press down hard with your thumb and massage in small circles for one to three minutes about six times a day. For the neck, use your index finger to massage in the same way.

Naturopathy Many practitioners attribute dizziness to low blood-sugar levels, and advise patients to change their eating habits. White sugar, white flour and all fatty foods are to be avoided, but lean meat, fresh fruit and vegetables, and whole grains are recommended (see EATING FOR HEALTH).

Chiropractic Chiropractors can sometimes help attacks of dizziness, which may be due

Using acupressure to treat dizziness

Firmly massage the foot point – about 50 mm from the angle between big and second toe – moving the thumb in small circles for up to three minutes. Repeat six times daily.

In the same way, massage the neck point – immediately below and behind the bottom of the ear lobe – with an index finger.

to misalignment of the upper neck joints. These joints contain nerves which balance the head, so that the eyes are level for vision. If the upper neck joints are not correctly aligned, faulty nerve signals may give rise to dizziness. Manipulation of the upper neck, and often further down the spine, can be used to correct this.

An orthodox view

As dizzy spells can accompany many complaints and illnesses, a doctor will want to know what – if any – other symptoms you have had. For example, if someone staggers or is unable to stand up, the doctor may suspect VERTIGO or poor circulation (see CIRCULATION PROBLEMS).

Most dizzy spells have a simple explanation, but if they occur more than once or twice will need a thorough investigation.

DO-IN

Massaging your way to health

This ancient form of Chinese self-massage – pronounced 'dough-in' – aims to prevent disease, rather than cure it. A series of exercises is said to strengthen 'energy channels' called MERIDIANS, linked to the heart, lungs, liver, gall bladder and other organs, keeping them in a healthy condition.

As a stimulant Do-In is best done first thing in the morning when you wake up. And it can help to relax you when you get home from work and last thing at night before you go to bed. However, it can be practised at any time of the day, except after eating. You can spend as much or as little time on it as you like – and, as with SHIATSU, with which it is closely related, age and infirmity are not necessarily a barrier. Providing you are fit and mobile, all you need is a tracksuit, or loose, comfortable clothing, and a reasonable amount of free space.

Although Do-In is essentially a self-help technique, it is a good idea to attend some classes before attempting the exercises on your own, to make sure that you are on the right lines.

DOUCHING

This is a form of HYDROTHERAPY in which a jet or jets of water are hosed onto parts of the body. Douching is believed to have many therapeutic benefits, including stimulation of the circulation, sedative effects and easing

Six basic Do-In exercises

The exercises are designed to make the organs involved stronger and healthier – and so help to ward off ailments such as stress, tension, rheumatism and arthritis. Before commencing the exercises you should limber-up for about five minutes.

Prelude to exercises
Start by sitting on the ground with your back rounded and holding your knees with your hands. Rock backwards and forwards. Finally, loosen your body by crossing your legs and briefly holding your toes.

Heart – small intestine
Sit with your legs open and the soles of your feet touching. Put your hands around your toes and breathe in. Then bend slowly forward, keeping your back straight and bringing your forehead down towards your toes. Breathe out, pause and repeat.

Liver – gall bladder

Sit up straight with your legs extended and as far apart as possible. Breathe in, stretching your arms along your left leg until you can grasp the sole of your foot. Be sure to keep your right buttock on the floor. Stay in position and take two deep breaths. Then repeat on the right side.

Circulation – pericardium

Sit with your legs and arms crossed. Hold your knees and bend forward, slowly trying to press your knees to the floor with your hands. Cross your arms and legs the other way and repeat the exercise.

Stomach – spleen

Face the wall and stand as close to it as you can. Raise your left arm as high as you can and place the palm of your hand against the wall. With your right hand, hold up your right foot and press the front of your thigh against the wall. Bend your head and neck backwards, stretching the whole of the front of your body. Stay in position and take two deep breaths. Then repeat on the other side of your body.

Lung – large intestine

Stand straight with your feet hips' distance apart. Put your arms behind your back and lock your thumbs together. Breathe in. Breathe out, stretching your arms out and up. Bend forward and straighten up.

Completing exercises

End by lying flat upon your back and relaxing. Open your legs to hips' distance and let your feet flop sideways. Stretch your arms by your side, palms up. Raise your head and look at your feet. Then gently and slowly lower your head. Gently shake your body and head to loosen your neck, arms and legs. Finally, close your eyes and rest for about five minutes.

Kidney – bladder

Sit up straight with your legs extended and your toes flexed upwards. Stretch your arms up and breathe in. Breathe out, bending your upper body forward and down, and grasp your toes. Stay in position and take three deep breaths. Then repeat.

of muscular and other PAIN. The temperature and pressure of the water varies, as does the length of treatment, and there are several kinds of douche.

In a Scottish douche, hot water is directed at the body for up to five minutes, followed by cold water for up to 30 seconds. It is said to be a circulation stimulant, good for the body as a whole, and to help in cases of SCIATICA, LUMBAGO and related skeletal pains. An underwater douche, in which the patient stands in a pool or bath, is held to have a similar effect to deep finger kneading MASSAGE – another circulation stimulant and muscle and ligament relaxant. For muscular and joint pains, the Vichy and Aix douches – in which massage is applied under warm water sprays – are considered beneficial.

DOWN SYNDROME

Children with Down Syndrome (sometimes known as 'mongolism') have a chromosomal abnormality . In 95 per cent of cases this takes the form of an extra chromosome: 47 instead of the usual 46. The remaining five per cent of affected children have the normal complement of chromosomes in each cell, but a portion of one chromosome has been transferred to another (a process which is known as 'translocation'). Defective formation of the egg in the mother's womb is the likely cause. About one in every 660 babies is affected by the condition, but the chance of it occurring increases when the mother is 35 years old or more.

The affected child is mentally retarded, but is likely to have an affectionate, friendly nature. Conspicuous physical characteristics include narrow eyes, a broadly ridged nose, flattening of the back of the head and of the neck, and short, broad hands. It is usual for about one in four such children to be born with a heart defect.

Over the years modern medicine has greatly increased the average life expectancy of people who have Down Syndrome to 60 or 70 years.

What the therapists recommend

Anthroposophical Medicine This system takes a holistic view, aiming to improve the person's whole lifestyle by a range of activities including artistic therapies (art, music, dancing) and more conventional occupational therapies. The overall aim is to give the Down Syndrome child a measure of independence.

Homoeopathy Long-term treatment by various homoeopathic means can be used to strengthen the immune system of persons suffering from Down Syndrome, to prevent infections and prolong life. The immune system of those people affected by the syndrome is impaired.

Traditional divining-rods came in a variety of shapes and sizes and could be used in many different ways, as these French dowsers of the 17th century demonstrate.

An orthodox view

No treatment or cure is available for the Down Syndrome child. However, medical and surgical techniques may be used to alleviate congenital defects – which may take a number of forms in addition to those which are mentioned above – and to prolong life expectancy.

For more information you should write to the Down Syndrome Forum of South Africa, 87 Waterfall Avenue, Craighall 2196. The Forum will gladly put you in touch with local Down Syndrome Associations. Alternatively, consult your telephone directory.

DOWSING

Diagnosis by rod and pendulum

In the 1920s a French priest, the Abbé Mermet, claimed to have extended the ancient art of dowsing, or water divining, into a means of effectively locating and diagnosing illness. He firmly believed that if dowsers could find water under the ground and assess its freshness, then healers could 'dowse' the human body to locate and treat diseased and faulty organs.

He was particularly impressed by the claims of medieval dowsers that they could find underground 'black streams' containing currents of 'evil energy', which brought illness to anyone living along them. Further, the dowsers claimed that they could destroy this evil power by driving their divining-rods into the ground.

Most dowsers use divining-rods and forked hazel twigs, but some use a pendulum suspended by a silk thread, and this was the diagnostic tool used by Mermet.

His theory was that all substances, including those making up the human body, emit 'good' and 'bad' radiation waves which can be picked up – much as a radio picks up sound wave frequencies – and identified. Once a diagnosis was made, the patient could be treated with appropriate herbal, homoeopathic or other remedies.

Finding a therapist Practitioners occasionally advertise in alternative health magazines, although they mostly find their clients by word of mouth. The Wellstead Resource Centre, 1 Wellington Avenue, Wynberg 7800, may be able to put you in touch with a dowsing therapist.

Consulting a therapist To diagnose and treat disease, practitioners may dowse a lock of the patient's hair, or a sample of blood.

Holding a pendulum over the specimen – or, in some cases, the patient himself – the practitioner may, for example, ask aloud if there is any organic or glandular imbalance. The way the pendulum swings is interpreted as either a 'yes' or a 'no' answer, and treatment is then given accordingly.

An orthodox view

Doctors point out there is no evidence that dowsing can correctly diagnose disease. Attempts to show that bodies emit 'radiation waves' have proved inconclusive, and the claims made by practitioners are unacceptable to orthodox medicine. Patients may also be lulled into a false sense of security if dowsing reveals nothing wrong, and may delay seeking help for serious illness.

DRUGS AND THEIR DANGERS

Since earliest times man has sought drugs – external substances that affect the composition or function of living organs – to relieve distress, discomfort and pain. Herbs – fresh, dried, cooked or pounded – infusions, liniments, ointments, balms, poultices and linctuses were all known to the ancients.

The Egyptians thought they had the 'ultimate cure', the golden pill: medicines were wrapped in gold (or silver) leaf – thus ensuring, in fact, that they were not absorbed at all by the alimentary tract and so had little or no effect!

The great expansion of knowledge in the European Renaissance augmented the contemporary physician's array of drugs with those of the ancients and the Arab and Asian worlds. By the 17th century, the apothecary – one who specialised in the preparation of drugs – was firmly established alongside the physician, traditional folk healer, quack and white witch.

The modern drug industry began with the invention of gelatine capsules by French apothecaries in 1834. At last, unpleasant medicines could be delivered in palatable form. Their effects lasted longer too, for the drugs were released slowly into the intestine as the gelatine dissolved. Traditional remedies began to lose their appeal, and by the end of the century the travelling quack peddling his elixir ('Beneficial for Rheumatiz, Ladies' indispositions, Colic, Stones and Baldness – and preserving saddles') gave way to the pharmaceutical or drug representative. He visited doctors and tried to convince them that his firm's drug for a particular ailment was superior to all others on the market.

Modern advances Even during the earlier part of this century, medical knowledge of drugs was limited. Before the discovery of the sulpha drugs in 1935, possibly only a dozen or so drugs had a clear medical value. Most of these were the extracts of plants, while other drugs, such as aspirin, were chemically closely related to plant extracts.

In the past 50 years that picture has changed dramatically. Not only is an impressive variety of effective drugs now available for medical use, but scientific knowledge in the drug field has virtually exploded.

Today's doctor understands far better than his or her predecessors the complexity of drug actions in the body and the wide range of effects drugs can have on it.

He or she can also recognize that some drugs interact harmfully with other drugs, or with certain foods and alcohol.

While the exact workings of some drugs are not fully understood, medical science provides clear knowledge as to what most of them do once they enter or are applied to the human body. Drugs, of course, serve different purposes, sometimes curing a disease, sometimes only alleviating symptoms.

Today, most of the drugs in use have been developed in the laboratory and are manufactured through various chemical processes. Many drugs, however, are synthetic forms of naturally occurring substances – chemical copies indistinguishable from the original. Nevertheless, a few important drugs are still obtained from botanical or animal sources. For example, belladonna, which is used for certain gastrointestinal disorders, is derived from deadly nightshade.

The opiate drugs, including morphine, ultimately rely on a certain type of poppy. Many vaccines, thyroid hormones and (until recently) insulin depend on animal sources.

Pharmaceutical manufacturers find new products in a variety of ways. New drugs are usually developed for one purpose but quite commonly a variant will be found that will be useful for something entirely different.

When a new drug is discovered the manufacturer often undertakes a programme of molecular tincturing, or elaboration. This refers to investigation into variants of the drug to see if the substance can be made more effective or more free of side effects. Sometimes that experimental process has unexpected and useful results. The elaboration process, for example, transformed some sulpha drugs, originally valued for their antibacterial properties, into widely used diuretics, oral antidiabetics and anticonvulsants.

The hidden dangers Doctors and patients increasingly have come to believe that treatment requires prescription of one or more drugs. But this does have dangers. Some result from bad medical practice, others from misunderstandings between doctors and drug companies, some from patient error,

'Hidden functions' of prescriptions

Apart from its therapeutic value, a medication may be prescribed as a:
Visible sign of the doctor's power to heal.
Symbol of the power of modern technology.
Sign that the patient is 'really ill'.
Concrete expression that the doctor has fulfilled his or her contract.
Reasonable excuse for patient contact with the doctor.
Satisfactory termination of a consultation.
Sign that modern humans can control their own destiny.
Expression of the doctor's control of the relationship or patient.
Indication of the doctor's concern.
Medium of communication between doctor and patient.
Way of forestalling lengthy discussions.
Source of satisfaction to the doctor.
Means of identifying the clinical situation as legitimately medical.
Way of legitimising sick role status in employment.
Means of satisfying one of a patient's goals.

and a few from lack of adequate trials before drugs are released for general use.

Some practitioners over-prescribe. When 50 000 prescriptions in an American teaching hospital were analysed, one in eight revealed over-prescription – too much or too frequent use or both. Doctors' handwriting is not always legible, and incorrect copying of repeat prescriptions by receptionist staff sometimes occurs. The introduction of computers in general practice has been seen as a way of minimising errors, but the wrong medicine for the wrong person continues to be prescribed. Occasionally, pharmacists fail to tell patients all they should know.

Once patients are prescribed drugs, they may fail to have them dispensed; some 10-15 per cent of prescriptions are not fulfilled. Other patients obtain their medicines and then fail to take them. More commonly, patients do not complete the course of treatment, usually because they note some improvement and think they are 'cured'.

The volume of hoarded drugs suggests that the true figures may be higher. During a 'drug amnesty' some 200 000 tablets were surrendered in Dudley, Hereford and Worcester in the United Kingdom in 1976. The figure for a similar operation in 1979 was about 300 000, and in 1982, 740 000. Other patients misunderstand prescription instructions, some continuing with one medication after beginning a new one.

Drugs are extensively tested before being put on the market. However, very occasionally the tests fail to reveal harmful side effects, sometimes with tragic results. The sedative thalidomide, which resulted in foetal abnormalities when taken in pregnancy, is an example. Other medicines produce harmful effects when taken together.

Occasionally, a practitioner may have a difficult choice and resorts to the risk/benefit ratio: the risk of taking the drug against the benefit derived from it. For example, in cases of serious infection such as typhoid fever, the doctor may give the antibiotic chloramphenicol despite the fact that it may cause bone marrow damage, less toxic drugs being useless in such cases.

DYSENTERY

There are two forms of this bowel infection, which causes severe DIARRHOEA. The most common type is bacterial dysentery; the other form is amoebic dysentery. In both cases, the disease is spread by poor hygiene, infected food and contaminated water.

Symptoms include FEVER, frequent bowel movements (up to 20 a day in children), griping stomach pains, WIND and vomiting. Both conventional and alternative practitioners stress the importance of personal hygiene and scrupulous cleanliness in handling, preparing and cooking food. Always wash the hands after using the lavatory.

Bacterial dysentery sometimes occurs in epidemics in schools, but usually passes within about a week. If it persists, or becomes worse, medical advice must be sought. Amoebic dysentery, often accompanied by blood, mucus or pus in the stools, should always be treated by a doctor.

What the therapists recommend

Moxibustion For bacterial dysentery, the practitioner (usually an acupuncturist) will probably treat points on the abdomen.
Naturopathy A practitioner would advise the patient to take plenty of liquids – particularly those such as milk and vegetable juices that are rich in minerals and salts – to replace lost body fluids. He would also advise him to avoid solid foods and eat bland dishes such as semolina, tapioca, porridge and pasta, or plain boiled rice with a little butter. These are believed to absorb much of the poisonous matter in the bowels.

Traditional Medicine Simmer 3,5 litres of fresh milk containing 30 g of cinnamon, 30 g of oak bark, two nutmegs, 20 cloves and 20 white peppercorns. Strain the mixture, allow it to cool and pour into four equal measures. Drink one measure every six hours for 24 hours.

An orthodox view

Dysentery can kill, particularly the young, the old and the chronically sick. Before treatment with antibiotics and other medication, it is essential to make an accurate diagnosis by sending stool specimens to the laboratory for examination.

DYSLEXIA

Coping with learning difficulties

Children who have difficulty recognising words and letters when they are being taught to read and write are victims of dyslexia, a learning disorder once misleadingly called word blindness. It affects about one person in ten to some degree, and one in 25 are significantly troubled by it.

Dyslexic children can be diagnosed early in life – at the age of six or seven, after starting school, when teachers discover that they are finding it hard to read.

Often dyslexic children have some difficulty in learning sequences, such as the order of the days of the week, or the months of the year. In addition, they generally tend to have trouble in distinguishing different sounds in words and in identifying the different letters.

Sometimes the victim also suffers from dyscalculia, or difficulty in learning numbers – for example, when giving his address, the child may write 27 instead of 72.

Learning disabilities are quite independent of a person's intelligence. Many specialists believe that they are genetically determined, but others attribute them to environmental factors. The problem lasts throughout the person's life, but much can now be done to help dyslexics live with their disability – and sometimes to overcome it, at least in part (see box, *Do's and don'ts for parents of a dyslexic*).

In suspected cases of dyslexia it is important initially for the children's vision and hearing to be carefully tested, in case the learning fault lies there.
Finding a teacher Discuss the problem with your child's teacher. The teacher will confer with the school principal, who in turn should be able to refer you to a school clinic in your area. School clinics, which are state-subsidised, employ remedial teachers.

Do's and don'ts for parents of a dyslexic

Do read to a dyslexic – even a teenager. He needs all the help and encouragement he can get – at home and school.
Do show an interest in the child's school notes and homework – and go through them with him.
Do try to get tape or video versions of books needed for English Literature lessons, and encourage the child to watch any required plays that come on television, or listen to them on radio. Tape-recordings can be obtained from Tape Aids for the Blind.
Do praise any particular achievements or improvements in the child's performance.
Don't scold the child if he has trouble tying shoelaces or a tie – encouragement is the key.
Don't lose patience if the child has difficulty with the calendar – help him to work out the weeks and days.

Other useful starting points are your GP or a psychologist. The favoured approach to the treatment of dyslexia is multi-disciplinary: the problem should not be seen as merely educational, but also one that a variety of specialist therapists can help to solve.

Despite attempts in the past to form a national dyslexia association, no such body at present exists in South Africa.
Consulting a remedial teacher Teaching depends on the degree of each child's disability. Dyslexic children need a programme based upon learning the structure of words.

What the therapists recommend

Naturopathy Food intolerances are often experienced by dyslexics. Food chemicals, sugar, and dairy and wheat products are among the foods that may be implicated. Once a diagnosis has been made, the naturopath can formulate an appropriate diet.

An orthodox view

Dyslexia is best managed through skilled remedial teaching and a sympathetic approach by teachers and parents. However, a firm diagnosis must first be made by an experienced educational psychologist. The role of the doctor is usually confined to excluding physical disease such as deafness or visual defects. Drugs can be of help in selected cases, but tend to be overused.

EATING FOR HEALTH

Getting the balance right is the first essential of healthy eating. No matter how much you spend or to what lengths you go in shopping for or growing your own food, it will be to little purpose if the proportion of the various nutrients is not correct.

The body needs carbohydrates, fats and proteins in varying quantities, plus smaller amounts of vitamins, minerals and fibre to function well and to maintain itself. All are essential, but too little of one and too much of another can lead to poor health. See CHOOSING THE RIGHT FOODS FOR VITALITY AND WELL-BEING, p. 116.

EATING PROBLEMS

These generally fall into three categories: ANOREXIA and BULIMIA, which are psychological illnesses, and OBESITY.

Anorexia usually affects teenage girls or young women who refuse food due to a morbid fear of gaining weight, or, in some cases, of growing up. In bulimia, bouts of compulsive eating are followed by self-induced and ultimately involuntary vomiting.

Obesity is the condition in which excess fat accumulates in the body. It is caused by overeating and is cured by adopting a diet of healthy, wholesome food (see EATING FOR HEALTH).

See also SLIMMING THE NATURAL WAY.

ECZEMA

An eczema victim's skin not only becomes inflamed, but usually develops a persistent itchiness – often with blisters that weep and then form dry scabs and crusts. Mostly it strikes during childhood and clears up after PUBERTY AND ADOLESCENCE (p. 292). However, many people are affected in later life – especially housewives with an ALLERGY to bleaches, detergents, wax polishes and so on, who get eczema on their hands.

The two most common forms are *contact eczema*, which develops within minutes and is caused by reactions to anything from rubber shoes to metal watch straps, and *atopic eczema*, which usually affects people with a family history of ASTHMA or HAY FEVER, and can take months, or even years to develop, appearing at any time.

Self help To relieve skin irritation, try putting two tablespoons of sodium bicarbonate in your hot bath.

What the therapists recommend
ACUPUNCTURE

Consultation Traditionally, acupuncturists believe that eczema is associated with exposure to heat, damp and wind. Treatment is therefore based on counteracting the effect of the elements – and also by trying to correct any blood and ENERGY deficiencies that may occur as a result.

Meridians treated would be those corresponding to the large intestine, lungs, spleen and stomach. If the practitioner believes that the liver is not functioning properly, and is failing to expel the eczema, he will probably advise that you follow a special diet. This involves avoiding all alcoholic drinks, coffee, fats and dairy products.

HOMOEOPATHY

Consultation Practitioners view eczema as an outward sign of an underlying disorder. Treatment would depend on the individual case and requires expert help – especially if steroid creams have been prescribed by an orthodox practitioner (see below).

If the eruptions exude a sticky, honey-like fluid, *Graphites* is said to be effective. *Petroleum* is recommended if the eruptions itch at night and ooze a watery discharge in people with a tendency to chapped skin and cracked fingertips. If the itching gets worse with heat and the desire to scratch becomes irresistible: *Sulphur*. Only a few doses of the 6th potency are advisable – and the effect should be closely watched.

AROMATHERAPY

Self help Essential oils recommended include fennel, German camomile, geranium, sandalwood, hyssop, juniper and lavender. If the eczema is dry, use calendula oil as the carrier for the essential oils. If moist, use carrier lotion. The ratio should be 12 drops to 50 ml of carrier. Apply to the affected area every morning and night.

Consultation Therapists will advise on diet and use the creams and lotions which do not contain lanolin – an oil derived from wool, which is a frequent cause of allergy, as are milk and milk products.

NATUROPATHY

Consultation Naturopaths, like conventional doctors, believe allergy to be a prime cause of eczema. They will recommend a diet of raw fruit and raw vegetables, washed down by mineral water, herbal teas or fresh fruit drinks. You will be advised to keep to it for a week, then fast for two or three days.

Warning Do not adopt the naturopathic diet or fast without first getting a doctor's advice. The diet is unsuitable for anyone who is either weak or run down.

Other alternative treatments

Herbal Medicine Since eczema is a complex condition, a practitioner should be consulted and careful treatment of individual cases is required.

Marigold tea has long been recommended to relieve symptoms of itching, blisters and flaking skin. It is also said to help ward off eczema. Add 30 g of marigold flowers or petals to 600 ml of boiling water, let it soak for five to ten minutes, then strain and drink as required. In addition, marigold ointment can be obtained from some chemists or health food shops.

To treat infantile eczema, you should apply each day to the affected parts a lotion made from the juice of sour-fig leaves, and mixed with water.

Traditional Medicine Fresh green cabbage leaves – well washed and well pounded – are said to relieve even bad cases of eczema. Warm the leaves and use a bandage to hold several layers of them in place on the affected areas every morning and night. To soothe the pain of eczema, add to a hot bath a handful of twigs of the wild dagga plant (also known as the 'minaret flower' or 'lion's ear').

Bach Remedies Therapists believe that Crab apple tends to decrease any feelings of embarrassment about eczema – and Clematis and Mimulus both help to combat oversensitivity. If eczema sufferers experience irritability about their condition, Impatiens is said to help. Rescue Remedy cream is said to bring relief when rubbed on the affected areas.

Reflexology Massage to the reflex areas relating to the areas of skin affected, plus the areas relating to the solar plexus, adrenal and pituitary glands, liver, digestive areas, kidneys and reproductive glands is recommended. See chart, p. 295.

An orthodox view

For all types of eczema, a doctor may prescribe a corticosteroid cream or antibiotics to help heal the skin. Sedatives may also be prescribed. If unsure of the cause, the doctor may send you to a dermatologist, who will make patch tests by applying suspected irritants to the skin. If contact eczema is identified – caused by a woollen jumper, perhaps, or a certain after-shave – you will be advised to avoid it.

Coal tar preparations can also be helpful in eczema; as can preparations of oatmeal used for bathing.

Some doctors believe that eczema also has psychological causes – that it can be triggered by, for example, an unhappy marriage or unpleasant atmosphere at work. If so you may be sent to a psychiatrist to discuss your problem and find a way to resolve it.

Choosing the right foods for vitality and well-being

There is no need to make sacrifices or go without anything to eat a healthy diet. Hearty and wholesome meals, simply cooked – or not cooked at all – can be varied to include all your favourites. It is only the balance you need to check. With plenty of bread and cereals, as much fresh fruit and vegetables as you can eat, and a moderate amount of protein, you will give your body all the nutrients it needs. Fuss, fads and extravagance are out, simple enjoyment is in.

Healthy eating means choosing food that gives all the nutrients your body needs to grow, repair itself and carry out vital chemical processes. A good diet must also provide you with enough energy to stay fit and active. People's needs differ, depending on their age, way of life and metabolic rate (how fast their bodies perform these functions), but there are certain nutrients that everybody needs.

Carbohydrates, proteins and fats are needed in relatively large quantities to provide energy and build body tissue. VITAMINS and MINERALS are needed in much smaller amounts to help the body to function properly. Lastly, a good diet must contain FIBRE to keep the digestion healthy.

Alternative practitioners and nutritionists both recommend a diet based on unrefined and unprocessed foods such as fresh fruit and vegetables, wholewheat bread, lean meat and salads. This is called a wholefood diet, meaning that as little nutritional value as possible is removed from food during preparation. For example, wholemeal (not wheat-meal) flour is used because it is made from the wholewheat grain, including the outer shell which contains valuable vitamins and fibre. Whole-

foods should not contain FOOD ADDITIVES such as preservatives, colourings or flavourings. Wherever possible, they should be organic foods – crops grown without the use of chemical fertilisers and pesticides, and meat from free-range poultry and animals reared without antibiotics or artificial hormone supplements.

Immediate source of energy

Carbohydrates, especially in their natural, unrefined forms, are highly nutritious and are our most immediate source of energy. They should therefore be eaten in substantial quantities, especially by sporting enthusiasts and by those whose work is physically demanding.

The body eventually breaks carbohydrates down into the simple sugar glucose. This is then either used immediately to provide energy or stored for a short time in muscles and liver as glycogen or animal starch, whose molecules comprise branched chains of glucose molecules. A longer-term excess of glucose is converted and stored as fat, and can lead to OBESITY.

Carbohydrate molecules contain carbon, hydrogen and oxygen atoms only, and include starches and sugars. Thirty years ago, more of our carbohydrates came from starches than now. Refined cane and beet sugar is now our major source of carbohydrates and an important source of energy. It consists mostly of the sugar sucrose, and is the sweetest of the natural carbohydrates in our diet.

However, refined sugar does not make you feel full as easily as other carbohydrate foods, so it is easy to eat far too much, with the possible danger of obesity. It can also cause tooth decay. You should eat sugar and honey (mostly sugar) only in very small quantities, and only as a small proportion of any meal so that it is absorbed more slowly.

Starch molecules comprise chains of glucose molecules which the body must break down with digestive juices before it can absorb them. Although the process begins in the mouth, most of it occurs farther down the gut, so in the final analysis starchy foods are less likely than sugary ones to cause tooth decay. They also tend to contain more fibre, vitamins and minerals than sugary ones, so they are more bulky and eventually provide the body with less glucose per gram.

The hormone insulin is necessary for the oxidation of glucose – the process that produces energy for the body. When not enough insulin is produced in the body, DIABETES results. Starchy foods are therefore an even more important component of the diet for diabetics than they are for other people.

Honey and many fruits such as figs (and some vegetables including carrots and beetroot) contain the sugar fructose, which is also known as fruit sugar. Metabolism of fructose does not require insulin, so the sugar is especially useful for diabetics. These foods contain other valuable nutrients too.

Do's and don'ts at mealtimes

Do sit down while you eat.
Do eat slowly and chew thoroughly, giving your body a chance to digest the food.
Do maintain regular mealtimes.
Don't get stuck in a rut, eating an unvaried daily diet.
Don't watch television.
Don't use food to cope with emotional problems.

Starches should make up most of your daily carbohydrate intake. The best sources are breads, oats, rice and other grains, beans, peas and potatoes. Because the message has been stressed that wholewheat bread is good, it has been assumed that white bread is bad. In fact white is good, but wholewheat is even better. To make our diet better balanced, we should be eating more of the old staples bread and potatoes, and less red meat, fat and refined sugar. Whether bread is white or brown matters less than eating more of it. Some of the white flour used for bread is 'fortified' – calcium and several vitamins have been added to it. So white bread has about the same carbohydrate, protein, vitamin and mineral content as wholewheat – but it has only about half the fibre.

Occasional helpings of cakes, biscuits and puddings made with white sugar and flour do no harm, but should not form a regular part of the diet. Such foods are also usually rich in fat, so it is easy to consume too many kilojoules if you eat them. Replace them with vegetables such as carrots, or a low-fat sandwich, when you feel the need of a snack. Many conventional recipes work successfully with wholemeal flour instead of white flour; and if fresh or dried fruit is used, less sugar (or none at all) may be needed.

Vital roles

Body-building proteins form the basic structure of muscles, tendons, bones and other tissues. Without them the body cannot repair damaged tissues and generate new cells for growth and to make good the bodily wear and tear of daily life. Equally vital is their role as hormones and enzymes, which regulate the body's chemistry and functions.

A protein molecule contains carbon, hydrogen, oxygen and nitrogen atoms, and sometimes phosphorus and sulphur atoms too. It comprises a chain (or chains) of amino acids, which are built up by the body from the amino acids obtained by the digestion of the protein in food. Any excess of protein that the body does not need is converted into glucose to provide energy or be stored as fat. Proteins can give the same energy as carbohydrates, but their prime value is as 'building materials'.

Proteins are needed in smaller quantities than carbohydrates – some 40-60 g a day is enough for most adults. Since meat is about one-fifth protein (the rest is water and fat) this would mean eating about 25 g a day, if meat were the only source of protein. Bread, which is less

than one-tenth protein, would have to be eaten at the rate of about 450 g a day.

Many people think – wrongly – that red meat is the best protein and that other forms are second class. In practice, most people in the West eat a variety of protein-containing foods which more than make up the daily need: meat, fish, eggs, cheese, yoghurt, milk, bread, peas, beans, oat-based or wheat-based breakfast cereals, nuts – even potatoes give a little protein to the diet. However, a lot of protein is not recommended; this is because the human body is unable to store surplus protein in its original form, and so the protein molecules are converted and stored as fat.

Right combinations

The amino acids in proteins have to be present in certain combinations before the body can use them. Many animal foods, such as meat, eggs, cheese, milk and fish, have the right mixture, but many of them also contain much fat, so plant protein is to be preferred.

Pulses (beans, peas, lentils), oats, wheat and many other vegetables contain protein and starch with little fat, but need to be combined to provide the right mixture of amino acids. Particularly good combinations are vegetable proteins with small amounts of animal proteins – bread and cheese, or fish and rice, for example – and pulses with grains in dishes such as beans on toast or a lentil curry served with rice.

Vegans should take special care to include pulse-and-grain combinations in their diet as sources of protein, since they exclude all animal products (see VEGETARIANISM). However, in practice those who eat a wide variety of vegetable foods will get plenty of protein without worrying about combinations.

A healthy diet must contain some fats for they form vital parts of the structure of body cells. They are the main insulating material beneath the skin and around organs such as the kidneys. Fats are also necessary for the absorption into the body of the fat-soluble vitamins – A, D, E and K – from the gut. They make foods tastier and easier to swallow. However, fats must be eaten in only small amounts for they are the most concentrated form of food, giving more than twice as much energy for their weight as either carbohydrates or proteins. Excess fat leads to obesity.

Fats are made up of fatty acids – substances containing hydrogen and oxygen atoms attached to chains of carbon atoms, edible fats having an even number of carbons in

Reducing sugar intake

White sugar contains no vitamins or minerals, and brown sugars and honey contain a very small amount of no nutritional importance. In large quantities sugar and honey are fattening, cause tooth decay and even become addictive, yet most of us still eat too much. Here are some ways to cut down:

Reduce sugar in hot drinks gradually until you no longer need it. As they get used to it, many people find that the taste of the drink is improved.

Cut out proprietary soft drinks. Have water or diluted freshly squeezed fruit juice instead.

Read the labels on packaged foods and drinks such as fruit juice, tomato sauce, breakfast cereals and peanut butter, and buy only those brands without added sugar.

As a rule finish meals with fruit or cheese, and break the habit of having sugary desserts.

Do not use sweets as presents or rewards for children, or they will come to associate harmful foods with happy occasions – fruit and small toys are good alternatives.

Do not keep sweets, chocolates or biscuits in the house.

If you want something to nibble between meals, try olives, raw vegetables, fruit – even cheese or nuts, in small quantities because of their fat content. These are more nutritious and may help cure your sweet tooth.

the chains. Fatty acids in which all the possible chemical bonds are used up are known as saturated (or hydrogenated) fatty acids. Monounsaturated fatty acids have one unused bonding site for a hydrogen atom in the molecule, and polyunsaturated, several. Animal fats are mainly saturated and are generally solid at room temperature. Vegetable fats are mostly unsaturated; they are generally liquid at room temperature, and like all such fats are usually known as oils.

Saturated fatty acids seem to make the body form too much cholesterol. Some cholesterol is needed for a healthy brain and nervous system and for the production of hormones. However, any excess can cause GALLSTONES and coat the inside of the arteries, eventually impeding blood circulation, causing heart attacks and strokes (see ARTERIES [HARDENING]). To avoid this danger, we should eat far less fat and try to make sure that the little we do eat is mainly unsaturated. In a diet where fat consumption is already low, however, the occasional cake, fried food or slice of buttered toast presents no danger.

Cut down on meat, dairy products (especially cream and hard cheeses), eggs, hard margarines, some soft margarines, peanuts and peanut butter, and products containing palm or coconut oil; these are all rich in saturates. Olive oil and some fish oils are monounsaturates. Sources of poly-unsaturates are oily fish such as maasban-ker, mackerel, trout and salmon, and oils from sunflower seed, maize (corn), wal-nuts, safflower seed, sesame seed and grapeseed. Eating oily fish and peas and beans is now thought to help appreciably in clearing cholesterol deposits already formed in arteries.

Whenever possible, buy oils that are la-belled 'cold-pressed', 'virgin', or 'extra vir-gin' – other oils will have been treated with heat or chemicals, which can convert un-saturates to saturates. Never eat oils that have a rancid smell or taste.

Virgin olive oil is excellent for salad dressings. The traditional Mediterranean cuisines that use it so much are among the world's healthiest. Also suitable, but with less flavour is corn oil (not readily avail-able). Walnut and sesame oils are more ex-pensive but give a distinctive flavour.

Olive oil is also suitable for gentle shal-low frying – as are other cold-pressed or virgin vegetable oils except coconut or palm oil. For the occasional deep-fried food, for which a high temperature is needed, use sunflower oil.

Many people now use soft margarines for spreading and in sauces and cakes. Although such margarines are made largely from unsaturated oils, they have been through heat or chemical processes which alter the unsaturated structure of the fat mole-cules or leave chemical residues in the margarine. There is no way of knowing whether good-quality oils have been used in the manufacturing pro-cess. Both margarine and low-fat spreads usually contain preservatives and other chemicals. It is better to use sparingly a natural food like butter. In baking, butter gives the best flavour and in a well-bal-anced diet where cakes and biscuits are not eaten often it will do no harm even though it is rich in saturates. Its advantage is that it is a natural food, not processed or high in additives. Choose a slightly salted or unsalted variety. Those who must avoid butter altogether, because of a heart condition for example, could use a soft margarine high in polyunsaturates, but would do better to cut out all cakes and biscuits.

Giving protection

The body requires many different vitamins and minerals to function efficiently. They are needed in small amounts only – the total daily requirements amount to about 7 g of minerals and only about one-tenth of a gram of vitamins. However, they play essential roles in all bodily processes and provide protection in the fight against in-fection and disease.

The best sources of vitamins and mine-rals are fresh or frozen unprocessed fruit and vegetables, dairy products, cereal foods, meat, eggs and fish. Many of these nutrients dissolve in water or are de-stroyed by too much heat, so it is import-ant to use good cooking methods and eat raw fruit and salads as much as possible. Many vegetables can also be eaten raw; try finely chopped broccoli, spinach, peas, carrots, cabbage and mushrooms sprin-kled on salads.

Steaming, stir-frying, baking or adding vegetables to casseroles does not waste their nutrients so much as boiling can. If you do boil them, add the vegetables to a little rapidly boiling water and cook them for the shortest time, keeping them crisp. Add the cooking water – which contains some of their nutrients – to a soup or stew.

How to cut down on saturated fats

Read the labels on oils and tinned, packaged or processed foods, and avoid those which list saturated or hydrogenated fats or oils.

Buy lean cuts of meat and trim off any visible fat. Poultry has little fat with the flesh, but the skin is fatty; remove it before sautéing, grilling or casseroling it. Game such as springbok, which is available in mid-winter, is lean meat.

Avoid fried food. Grilling, roast-ing, stewing and baking use a mini-mum of fat. If you do fry chips or other foods, cut them into large pieces to reduce the total area of fried surface. Use corn or sunflower oil at a high temperature – but not so high that the oil begins to smoke – so the food develops a crisp crust quickly and absorbs less oil. Pat off the excess oil with kitchen paper.

Eat more fish. White fish is low in fat and oily fish such as pilchards, mackerel, trout and salmon are rich in an unsaturated oil not widely available in other foods, and which helps to combat cholesterol. Try to have two servings of an oily fish every week.

Cut down on meat. Even the lea-nest beef is about 15 per cent fat and a juicy steak about 30 per cent. Replace meat with vegetable or fish dishes for a few meals a week.

Use yoghurt instead of cream, which is rich in saturated fat. If you want cream occasionally, use single rather than double or clotted cream.

Before serving meat casseroles, curries, soups and stews, remove surface fat with absorbent kitchen paper.

Look out for low-fat sausages, cheeses, milk and yoghurt. Try and cut down on chips – although they are generally cooked in unsaturated oil, they contain as much as 38 per cent of it.

Watching salt intake

Be sure to cut down on the salt you use in cooking, or omit it altogether. Most people tend to eat more than they need and those suffering from high BLOOD PRESSURE have to avoid it altogether (see SALT-FREE DIETS). Salt makes the body retain water and certain waste products. You should season food with GARLIC, herbs, spices, freshly ground black pepper or lemon juice instead. Your taste for salt will soon dwindle and disappear, but if you want an alternative to salt, there is a vegetable salt made from vegetable extracts.

Vitamins and minerals are needed in complex combinations by the body, but anyone who eats a balanced and varied diet of wholefoods, including plenty of fresh fruit and vegetables, will receive enough. It is rarely necessary to take vitamin or mineral supplements, nor are people who take them ensuring that their diet is healthy. They can still be eating too little fibre, for example. See pp. 361 and 242 for the food sources of vitamins and minerals.

Fibre adds bulk

Plant foods – bread, rice and other cereals, leafy and root vegetables, fruits, salads, beans, peas and other pulses – provide dietary fibre, especially if they are unrefined. Fibre has no nutritional value. The body cannot digest or absorb it, but it adds bulk to our diet which pushes waste products through the system faster, and absorbs dangerous substances. It keeps the digestive tract healthy and carries the waste away. Eating sufficient fibre prevents CONSTIPATION and helps to reduce the risk of CANCER of the bowel. Fibre also makes us chew food longer and fills the stomach, making meals more satisfying.

Until the last few years, people were relying less on bread as a staple food and eating fewer vegetables. Of the vegetables we do now eat, far more are frozen or processed and fewer are fresh and leafy. There is now a marketing drive to promote foods to which fibre has been added. However, to get enough fibre it is not necessary to add bran to foods or to eat special breads, crackers or muesli. Simply eat a variety of wholefoods that are naturally rich in fibre. Bread, white or brown, and oats are good sources of fibre. The skin of potatoes is another, but it contains the natural pesticide solanine, which you may wish to avoid. Daily helpings of bread, porridge, fresh vegetables, raw and dried fruits and pulses will carry you to the daily fibre target of 30 g.

Balancing your diet

Making up a balanced wholefood diet is not difficult and gives you plenty of choice. Whatever your age, you should have three servings a day of meat, fish, poultry, nuts, beans, peas or lentils; one serving of milk, cheese or yoghurt; four servings of bread, brown rice, muesli, potatoes or wholewheat pasta; four servings of fresh fruit, vegetables or salads; and as little fat, oil and dressing as possible. The small amount of fat needed comes from the rest of the diet. Breastfeeding mothers and growing children need an extra daily serving of milk, cheese or yoghurt to provide the calcium they need.

Three meals and a mid-morning or evening snack will provide all you need. Adjust the size of servings to match body weight. Generally about 63 kilojoules a

*Healthy drinking ... **Top shelf:** grapefruit juice, white wine, tomato juice, rose-hip tea. **Second shelf:** pineapple juice, decaffeinated coffee, pear juice, apple juice. **Third shelf:** mint tea, peach juice, fennel tea, pawpaw juice, beer. **Bottom shelf:** grape juice, orange juice, water and carrot juice.*

day per 0,45 kg of body weight is needed to maintain that weight. Thus someone who weighs 63,5 kg – and leads a moderately active life needs about 8 820 kilojoules (140 x 63) a day. Those who use more physical energy need more kilojoules, those whose lives are sedentary need less. Protein and carbohydrates provide 16,8 kilojoules per gram and fat 37,8 kilojoules per gram.

Many shops – particularly health shops – and supermarkets now sell organically produced foods. They are usually more expensive than similar non-organic products.

Besides the wholefood diet, many special diets are used for a variety of medical reasons. People who are suffering from HEART DISORDERS or ANGINA or who have hardening of the arteries are usually advised to adopt LOW-FAT DIETS, and salt-free diets can help to lower high blood pressure. NATUROPATHY and nutritional medicine use diets to treat a range of illnesses – for example, therapists sometimes recommend highly restrictive regimes such as the RAW FOOD DIET or FASTING to cleanse the system.

Other diets are based on special nutritional theories. Vegetarianism maintains that meat is not necessary in man's diet, and veganism that all animal products should be avoided. Balancing so-called yin and yang foods is the basis of the way of eating known as MACROBIOTICS, and the HAY DIET shuns proteins and starches in the same meal.

You should be wary of extreme and restrictive diets. Concentrate instead on eating moderate amounts of wholesome unprocessed foods free as far as possible from chemicals. Variety, with more emphasis on fruits, vegetables and grains, less on meat and dairy produce, and avoidance of animal fats, will make the greatest contribution to your health. Enjoy your varied diet, eat your food slowly in relaxed surroundings, and savour to the full its colour, taste and texture.

'Part of the secret of success in life,' wrote the well-known American humorist Mark Twain, 'is to eat what you like and let the food fight it out inside!' Twain was playing devil's advocate, of course, and it goes without saying that his advice should not to be taken too seriously by anyone who has a genuine interest in maintaining a daily balanced diet. Remember, however, that while it is important to eat healthily you should never allow your emphasis on correct food habits to become a humourless and mechanical obsession.

Choose a wholegrain breakfast cereal free of refined sugar or honey. Add sweetness with the natural sugars of fruit. This meal can double as a snack instead of biscuits.

Pastas in strands, butterflies, hoops or nests are a base for quick and healthy meals. The darker wholewheat or buckwheat pastas have more flavour.

Brown breads contain protein, vitamins and fibre as well as starch. White is good too, just lower in fibre.

Starches for ready energy

Bread and potatoes were once the staples of many people's diet and should be restored to pride of place. Their value is as starches — complex carbohydrates which satisfy the appetite, produce glucose to fuel the body's activities, and come in a package with other valuable nutrients. They can be varied now with many other starchy foods, including cereals, crispbreads, pastas and rice. Four substantial helpings a day of these foods are needed in a healthy diet.

Choose breads with distinctive tastes — black rye or rolls with poppy or sesame seeds — and they will not need spreading with fat or jam.

Rice, brown or polished, is a base for curries as well as a good substitute for the hard-working potato.

121

Melons, grapes, mangoes, strawberries, apples, citrus fruits, pineapples and bananas are among the wide range of home-grown fruits that are familiar fare to most South Africans.

Vitamins, fibre – and protein too

In a balanced diet we should enjoy four ample helpings a day of fruit and/or vegetables. Their value for most people is in the vitamins, minerals and fibre they contain, but vegetarians and vegans may also obtain sufficient protein from them. There is always a wide variety in season so that you can buy fresh foods rather than processed ones. Eat them raw for maximum food value, or cook for the shortest possible time.

Sweet golden pawpaw, knobby little lychees and tangy juice from dark green limes can add extra flavour to fruit salads.

Beans – a valuable protein source for vegetarians.

Sweet peppers, red or green, are becoming as common in salads as the traditional radishes, lettuces and tomatoes. Baby marrows have largely ousted their older relatives marrows, from vegetable stalls.

Fresh garden peas – a source of vitamins and protein – have become harder to find in young and perfect condition, but their flat-podded cousins, mangetouts, are more common. Eat pod and all, raw or lightly cooked.

Look for okra in farm stalls or in neighbourhood shops with a cosmopolitan spread of customers.

Fresh asparagus is still largely an early summer luxury.

The familiar mainstays such as cabbage, carrots, leeks, cauliflower, red cabbage, onions, parsnips and turnips have been joined for much of the year by varieties of broccoli and glossy purple eggplant.

Spring onions, celery and young broad beans add bite when used raw in salads, but artichokes need careful cooking and preparation.

123

The protein in pulses such as peas, beans and lentils is absorbed more easily when combined with a cereal food such as bread or rice.

Trim the fat from meat such as pork chops and do not eat the fatty skin of chicken.

Offal, such as kidneys, is low in fat.

Red meat is a valuable source of iron. Reduce its fat by casseroling it and skimming off the fat that rises to the surface.

Nuts are rich in protein – and also in high-kilojoule fat, but it is unsaturated. Peanuts and coconut are also rich in protein and fat, but their fat is largely saturated.

Limit your intake of
dairy foods and choose
those with reduced fat,
such as skimmed
milk, low-fat yoghurt,
cottage cheese or
such soft cheeses as
camembert.

In need of care and control

Our protein requirement is much more
limited than generally thought. Just three
helpings a day of meat or fish and one of
dairy produce is quite enough – and the
helpings should be small. Although these
foods provide the protein we need for body-
building and repairs, and contain several
vitamins and minerals, many of them are
high in the saturated fats that clog arteries
with cholesterol. Nuts and pulses are rich
vegetable sources of protein.

Eat more fish, a low fat form of protein.
Mackerel and sardines and other oily fish
contain unsaturated fat that helps to clear the
body of cholesterol.

125

ELECTROTHERAPY

Stimulating the body against pain

The idea of using electrotherapy to alleviate pain originated when a Roman doctor treated GOUT by placing a patient's swollen foot on a live electric eel. In the 19th century, when it was possible to store static electricity, it became fashionable for doctors to discharge electric currents through their patients' bodies to relieve various aches and pains. Later, dentists used the same method to reduce the pain when extracting teeth.

Today, electrotherapy's most widely accepted form is transcutaneous electrical nerve stimulation (TENS), which activates the nerves that block out pain. To do this, a small, battery-powered machine sends weak electrical pulses – machine output varies but is only in milliamps – through the skin by means of a pair of rubber pads. The pads are coated with jelly and taped around the area to be treated.

Who it can help The therapy is mainly used in physiotherapy to treat LUMBAGO, SCIATICA and SPORTS INJURIES. Many hospital maternity wards overseas use TENS machines specifically designed to relieve pain in childbirth. As an alternative to drugs, TENS is also offered for non-painful conditions such as CIRCULATION PROBLEMS.

However, TENS merely reduces the level of pain, and does not cure the underlying cause of it. It is important, therefore, that a problem is medically diagnosed before any treatment is given.

Warning People with a heart pacemaker should *not* use the machines, as they can affect the pacemaker's action.

Self help Although TENS machines are not that common in South Africa, they can be hired or bought from local distributors, provided you have the approval of a doctor or physiotherapist, who should be able to give you the distributors' addresses.

The treatment is safe and effective, as long as proper instruction is given as to where the pads should be placed and how the machines are operated.

Small, hand-held electrical stimulators can also be bought. With these, the current is applied by a probe to a specific point on the body. However, they are less effective than proper TENS machines.

Some practitioners offer a similar form of therapy to TENS called electro-ACUPUNCTURE. This is also used mainly to treat pain and sports injuries. The machines employed pass electrical pulses into the body from up to eight needles, and they must be operated by a fully qualified acupuncturist. Before undergoing electro-acupuncture you should always consult your GP, as a more orthodox treatment may be advisable.

An orthodox view

As far as slimming is concerned, most doctors believe that EXERCISE is a more effective way of losing weight. However, the use of TENS is now a standard feature in many pain clinics, and electro-acupuncture is used in some special units. Surgeons also use a form of electrotherapy to destroy nerve tissue in cases of severe pain.

EMPHYSEMA

The gradual breakdown of the lungs

Heavy smokers and people living or working in polluted atmospheres are at risk from this progressive and incurable disease. It occurs when tiny air sacs in the lungs become distended and rupture. This damages the lungs' elasticity, making them less efficient and slowing down their flow of blood. As a result, the heart has to work harder to pump blood through the system, and the added strain can lead to heart failure.

The main symptoms are breathlessness and blueness of the lips. People with ASTHMA and chronic BRONCHITIS are also at risk. The disease is far more common among men than women.

What the therapists recommend

Acupuncture Although the disease cannot be halted, acupuncturists claim to have brought relief in certain cases, allowing the patient to breathe more easily and improving blood circulation in the lungs. But this can only be done in less advanced cases where the lungs are not too distended and the chest has not taken on a beer-barrel appearance.

Acupuncture points treated are similar to those for asthma and bronchitis.

Chiropractic Some breathing difficulties are believed to be the result of slight spinal problems which affect nerve impulses to the lungs. Chiropractors can treat these problems and sometimes ease difficult breathing.

Naturopathy Practitioners claim that vitamin and mineral supplements have helped long-term patients. For example, 7 500 iu of vitamin A taken daily is said to strengthen lung tissue; and 200 iu of vitamin E taken three times a day to make breathing less arduous. Many emphysema victims also suffer badly from mucus; practitioners will advise them to avoid dairy products (milk, butter, cheese and so on).

Herbal Medicine Always discuss your health problem with a herbal practitioner before taking any teas or using liniment rubs. He will probably offer the same treatment as for bronchitis. However, a drink he may recommend specifically for emphysema is made from 15 g each of liquorice root and comfrey, added to 600 ml of water. Simmer for about 15 minutes, allow to cool and take 4 tablespoonsful four times daily. Both herbs are relaxing, soothing expectorants to loosen and remove phlegm. Other remedies are also used, but these depend on individual consultation.

Aromatherapy A number of essential oils are said to make breathing less laborious for emphysema victims, including basil, cajeput, eucalyptus, hyssop and thyme. The best way to use the oils is in a diffuser, or an essential oil burner – six drops in water – in the bedroom at night. Or they can be inhaled from a kitchen tissue.

An orthodox view

Bronchodilator drugs are often prescribed to widen the bronchi. Patients with severe breathing problems may be given oxygen, and antibiotics may be prescribed to control secondary infection in asthma and bronchitis – which aggravate the condition. A doctor will certainly advise a sufferer to stop SMOKING, take regular but moderate exercise in fresh air, and avoid polluted atmospheres.

Alternative therapies may help by encouraging patients to focus their minds on a more healthy lifestyle, and may also give psychological support. However, the unpalatable truth is that once lung tissue has been damaged, it cannot be repaired. Emphysema is irreversible, and no amount of therapy, alternative or orthodox, can replace it.

In these cases, prevention is far better than cure. Stopping smoking, or even better, never starting, and avoiding heavily polluted atmospheres could make emphysema a thing of the past.

ENCOUNTER GROUPS

Learning to know yourself and others

The principal aims of encounter group therapy are to raise self-awareness and improve an individual's ability to get on with others and form fruitful relationships. This is done by making people aware of their own feelings – of ANXIETY or aggression, for example – and of the true feelings of other people.

Layers of behaviour can build up over years to hide feelings which people think make them unacceptable to others, and also to protect themselves from being hurt by other people's expression of feelings. Encounter group members are helped to discard these layers to reveal their true feelings freely within the group, and to become aware of and accept the feelings of others.

The American psychologist Carl Rogers was among the principal developers of the therapy, in the 1940s. He moved away from earlier methods, in which a medical expert had face-to-face meetings with a patient, and towards a freer group in which people used here-and-now, face-to-face interactions to help each other to uncover their problems and learn how to deal with them.

This type of therapy has now been taken out of the world of psychiatric clinics and developed by non-medical bodies into courses that ordinary people can use to develop their own self-awareness and self-esteem, and to move closer to fulfilling their own potential as human beings.

Who it can help Besides helping people receiving mental health care – sometimes in hospital or as outpatients – encounter group therapy can encourage confidence in people who find personal and business relationships difficult. Working out their feelings in the group has also been found to benefit some who have suffered distressing upheavals in relationships.

Finding a group The counselling service, Life Line – address in your local telephone directory – conducts self-awareness encounter groups as Part One of its two-part course primarily intended for prospective counsellors (there is no obligation to pursue the course to the end).

Attending a group The numbers and activities in encounter groups are very variable. Some groups hold several short sessions on successive days, some have weekly sessions, while some have one continuous session lasting 24 or 48 hours.

Group members will have an initial period of getting to know each other, and may use simple exercises to help the process of 'letting go'. These may include physical contact, eye contact, communication exercises, group games and 'trust' exercises. As the group unfolds, members will be encouraged to be as honest as possible with one another about their feelings, thoughts and reactions.

The emotional climate may at times become intense. Anger and frustrations can well up and are voiced openly, and members will be encouraged to resolve conflicts as they arise. When they discover something about their own behaviour that is destructive or limiting, they will be asked to try more effective alternatives. For example, a quiet, with-drawn person may be given encouragement to speak out and to express himself openly to the group.

There should always be a balance of challenge and support within a group. Usually there are regular pauses to review what has happened so far, and the therapist or group leader makes sure that the group concentrates on what the members are feeling there and then about each other. Problems involving people not in the group are dealt with by group members playing the role of the absent person.

An orthodox view

Many qualified psychiatrists and trained counsellors lead encounter groups, but there is no scientific proof that the therapy gives lasting help. Group courses to promote more skilled handling of colleagues at work rarely do harm, but allowing too much challenge and release of aggression can result in some members feeling humiliated and gaining no benefit. Some people can even be pushed towards mental illness by untrained probing of their mental scars.

Advice should always be sought from a doctor before joining any such group.

ENERGY

Some alternative practitioners believe that energy – also known as Qi or chi, prana, vitalism or life force in different healing traditions – circulates through the body in channels called meridians (see also ACUPUNCTURE). At certain points – called chakras in YOGA – the energy becomes concentrated, affecting you both physically and mentally. Disease is thought to be the result of a 'blockage' or 'imbalance' (too much or too little) in the energy flow, which alters the molecules and cells of particular organs; also that this happens before any effects detectable by orthodox means occur.

Healers (see HEALERS AND HEALING) and Chinese practitioners say that they can often tell that something is wrong long before conventional doctors can. Some therapists believe that technical methods such as KIRLIAN PHOTOGRAPHY can also show the flow of energy in the body.

It is not fully understood how – or even whether – this view of energy is related to scientific definitions of physical kinds of energy. When spiritual healers talk about energy flowing between them and their clients, or Yoga teachers describe it circulating through the chakras of the body, no scientifically measurable changes have been shown to occur. Nevertheless, attempts continue to be made to find some objective evidence for these forms of energy.

Self help Alternative therapists say that good health does not mean being continually in a high-energy state – this would exhaust both body and mind and deprive us of time for relaxation, reflection and rest. It is also necessary to allow ourselves to feel sad and depressed at times; to live fully and healthily means accepting both positive and negative, high-energy and low-energy states of both body and mind. In a healthy person, energy should flow naturally and freely among all four of these states.

Different therapies offer a variety of ways to encourage the free flow of energy. Here are some simple self-help methods:

Exercise and self-expression These are said to increase low-energy states and reduce high-energy ones. Regular rhythmic EXERCISE of the 'aerobic' type – JOGGING, swimming and skipping, for example – releases physical and mental TENSION and encourages the production of chemicals in the brain which have a painkilling and uplifting effect. If practised regularly, this can help even long-standing DEPRESSION.

Expressing feelings by shouting, laughing, pummelling a punchbag or cushion, or crying also helps many people to relieve tensions. Crying, for example, has been shown to alter the breathing pattern and reduce high levels of STRESS hormones.

Diet Stimulants such as tea and coffee have the effect of increasing energy levels, as do sugary snacks such as sweets and chocolates. Many people who suffer from ANXIETY find that simply avoiding these foods reduces the problem considerably. Fasting decreases adrenal hormones in the blood, which may help to calm people who are in a state of agitation or tension. And in India, Ayurvedic practitioners use certain foods, such as milk, fats and FIBRE, to achieve this effect; other foods – meat, spices and sweets, for example – are prescribed to increase the energy levels of depressed patients.

Breathing One of the most immediate ways of altering the energy state is through special breathing exercises (see RELAXATION AND BREATHING). To aid relaxation, therapists recommend diaphragmatic breathing (see p. 299), which slows down the pulse rate and decreases BLOOD PRESSURE. The Full Yogic Breath practised early in the morning helps to get your system going and keep you wide awake. Even in the lowest energy state, the 'shining skull' exercise – rapid in-and-out diaphragmatic breathing – should rouse and invigorate body and mind.

An orthodox view

The concept of energy, in the scientific sense of the word, forms part of certain orthodox treatments such as radiotherapy and isotope medicine, used against CANCER. The body receives energy beamed at it, altering the structure of targeted cells.

Conventional doctors today tend to reject alternative theories of energy because of a lack of scientific explanation and evidence for them. Recently, however, experiments with certain traditional healers seem to have demonstrated a transfer of energy between living things and between people and various inanimate objects.

The techniques for measuring this energy are still quite primitive and most orthodox scientists do not accept the evidence of methods such as Kirlian photography and intuitive DIAGNOSIS. However, although proof remains uncertain, the possibility of this kind of energy is now more widely acknowledged by doctors.

EPILEPSY

People with epilepsy suffer periodic CONVULSIONS, or fits, during which they lose consciousness for anything from a few seconds to several minutes, depending on the type of epilepsy involved. The two most common forms are called *grand mal* and *petit mal*.

Grand mal normally affects adults, who sometimes froth at the mouth and are in danger of swallowing their tongue. An attack, with its accompanying BLACKOUT, can last for up to ten minutes. Petit mal affects youngsters who are aged between about four and their late teens.

These attacks are usually so brief and undramatic that the victim is often not even aware of them. He loses consciousness for only a few seconds, during which time his eyes may flicker or blink rapidly.

The main cause of epilepsy is abnormal electrical discharges among some of the brain's nerve cells. Head injuries or, in some adults, brain tumours (see CANCER) can also be causes. But in many cases the cause remains unknown. Rarely, a baby under six months may have an epileptic fit which is sometimes mistaken for COLIC.

Epilepsy sometimes runs in families and affects about four people in 1 000. Sufferers should always carry a card or tag stating their problem, in case they collapse in public.

What the therapists recommend

Naturopathy A well-balanced wholefood diet is favoured by practitioners, who say that it reduces the frequency and intensity of epileptic attacks. Mixed salads and raw fruit are said to be particularly effective (see EATING FOR HEALTH).

Bach Remedies Rescue Remedy may be used during a sudden attack of epilepsy, with Olive to help afterwards. Clematis may assist the victim regain normal consciousness. In addition, certain remedies may help to control various mental and emotional states which may herald an attack. For example: Holly if hatred or anger brings on an attack; Rock water if the victim tends to be hard on himself; Mimulus for fear of the condition itself; Hornbeam if the victim easily becomes mentally exhausted; Clematis for feelings of vagueness, dreaminess and lack of interest.

Aromatherapy Practitioners believe that relaxation is one of the keys to combating epilepsy. A cup of camomile tea at bedtime promotes a good night's sleep. And one drop of Roman camomile essence on a cube of sugar, taken three times a day between meals, is said to aid general relaxation. Basil, cajeput, rosemary and thyme are helpful oils, but hyssop, sage and possibly fennel should be avoided by anyone prone to fits.

Cranial Osteopathy Practitioners claim to have relieved symptoms by cranial massage.

An orthodox view

There is no evidence that any alternative therapy can reduce the frequency or severity of fits.

Effective orthodox medications are available which allow many epileptics to live a virtually normal life. However, it is essential that cases of epilepsy should be fully investigated for underlying causes, particularly in cases of late onset.

EURHYTHMY

This system of rhythmical body movements is performed in harmony with the rhythm of the spoken word. The vowel and consonant sounds each have their own type of movement. Eurhythmy was devised by Rudolf Steiner as part of the system of ANTHROPOSOPHICAL MEDICINE, which he pioneered, and information about eurhythmy classes can be obtained from any Waldorf School.

The body movements are said to be especially helpful for children as aids to developing suppleness and rhythmic sense.

The Cape Town School of Eurhythmy at 37 Columbus Road, Claremont 7700, offers a four-year diploma training course.

EXERCISE

Taking sensible, regular exercise can aid slimming, improve fitness and help the body resist many diseases and disorders. Exercise also has great psychological benefits, and is known to help alleviate symptoms of stress. See IT'S YOUR BODY – USE IT OR LOSE IT, p. 130.

EXHAUSTION

Extreme and seemingly unshakable feelings of weariness and general depletion are the telltale symptoms of exhaustion. The condition has many causes and may take many different forms. ANXIETY which develops into STRESS is often responsible for people becoming weary and depleted.

However, exhaustion may also be brought on by heat stroke (in which there is profuse sweating leading to the loss of body salt and causing muscle cramps and general weakness); extreme coldness leading to HYPOTHERMIA; various NERVOUS DISORDERS, including the depressive phase of MANIC DEPRESSIVE DISORDER; or intense TIREDNESS.

EYE DISORDERS

Threats to healthy vision

The most frequent disorder affecting the eyes is a foreign object in the eye. If such an object enters the eye, do not rub it as this will only increase the pain and cause swelling.

Homoeopaths may recommend washing the affected eye in an eyewash made by mixing 150 ml of lukewarm water with four or five drops of *Hypericum* mother tincture, obtainable from most health shops. Blink repeatedly while washing to dislodge the object. If this fails, wet a small, clean piece of cloth or gauze with the eyewash and gently try to clear the eye. It may help if you pull the eyelid upwards or downwards.

If the object remains lodged, see a doctor or go to a hospital casualty ward. Never try to remove a loose or embedded foreign object by force – this could cause serious damage. And never even touch a foreign object that is embedded in the eye.

Other fairly common eye disorders apart from EYESIGHT PROBLEMS and EYESTRAIN include: CATARACTS (a misting of the eye's lens, affecting elderly people); CONJUNCTIVITIS (inflammation of the conjunctiva, the thin transparent membrane across the front of the eye); glaucoma (a gradual loss of vision which, if left untreated, can lead to blindness); and STYES (small boils near the base of the eyelashes).

A minor disorder is the appearance of floaters, black threads or dots that seem to float in the field of vision. They are caused by

Eye injuries

An injury to the eye, including a foreign object under the eyelid, is potentially dangerous and needs expert medical attention – as well as on-the-spot first aid. Never rub or touch an injured eye or eyelid.

A homoeopathic treatment for a foreign object in the eye is to wash the affected eye in an eyewash of 150 ml lukewarm water containing about five drops of Hypericum mother tincture. Blinking helps to dislodge the object.

First aid: stand behind the victim and examine the injured eye (left). Prepare to carefully and gently remove any loose foreign object from it.

Tilting the head right back, gently grasp the lashes of the upper or lower lid and pull the lid back. Now carefully remove the object with the point of a clean handkerchief or piece of gauze.

tiny amounts of blood leaking into the eyeball. They are not serious and usually disappear in a few weeks without treatment. If they persist, see a doctor.

EYESIGHT PROBLEMS

Among the most common eye problems are short-sightedness (myopia), in which only nearby objects are clearly focused, and long-sightedness (hypermetropia), in which the eye can focus only on distant objects. Shortsightedness often runs in families, affecting about one person in five. Long-sighted people often

Another method is to press down on the eyelid with a matchstick to pick up the object on the inner surface of the lid. The lid is then pulled up against the match and the object removed from inside the lid using a clean cloth.

have blurred vision and EYESTRAIN through overusing the eye muscles.

Long-sightedness is also a natural consequence of the ageing process, when it is known as presbyopia. Most people experience it by the age of about 45. Apart from wearing spectacles or contact lenses, both conditions are said to be helped by the BATES METHOD of eye exercises.

Another common eyesight problem is ASTIGMATISM, or distortion of vision. This occurs when the eye lens has different curvatures in different directions, so that the image on the retina is irregular. It can be corrected by the aid of specially made spectacle lenses. The Bates method is believed also to help.

EYESTRAIN

The growing use of visual display units (VDUs) at work and at home is one of the major causes of eyestrain. The eyes ache and feel tired, and the condition is often worsened by a HEADACHE. Eyestrain can also be caused – or aggravated – by working in artificial light, reading in poor light, and watching hours of television in the dark.

Self help People using VDUs should spend no more than two hours at a time in front of the screen, followed by at least one hour away from it. When reading, make sure that sufficient light falls onto the pages, and when watching television at night, always have a side light on in the room. In either case, relax your eyes by looking away from the page or screen for a few seconds at least once every half hour.

What the therapists recommend

Homoeopathy Bathe the eyes with four drops of Euphrasia mother tincture in 150 ml of lukewarm water. If the trouble persists, seek medical help.

Bates Method Practitioners recommend a series of basic eye exercises; they claim that these dispense with the need for spectacles.

Naturopathy Try a daily intake of vitamin A (7 500 iu) and vitamin B_2 (10 mg).

Acupressure Relief may be obtained by massaging a few key points on the face. Use the thumb and index finger of one hand to massage the bridge of the nose with an up-and-down motion.

Use both thumbs to massage the top of the nose on both sides, keeping the other fingers flat on the forehead. Use the index fingers to massage beneath the eyes, just below the cheekbones.

Herbal Medicine Herbalists recommend various compresses – including cucumber, eyebright and marigold petals – to combat eyestrain. Immerse a clean piece of cloth in an infusion (see p. 184) of the herb. Let the cloth cool and then hold it to your eyes. It is best to do this when sitting or lying down. Alternatively, cut thin slices of fresh cucumber and place them on the eyes. Leave the compress in place for about ten minutes.

An orthodox view

In cases of straightforward eyestrain a doctor will probably agree with bathing them in water. However, he is more likely to advise the use of a proprietary brand of eyedrops.

If reading presents problems – such as having to hold the reading material close to the eyes – he may send you to an optometrist for an eye test. If long- or short-sightedness is diagnosed (see EYESIGHT PROBLEMS) you will be advised to wear glasses or contact lenses.

It's your body – use it or lose it

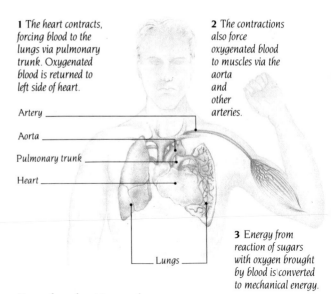

1 The heart contracts, forcing blood to the lungs via pulmonary trunk. Oxygenated blood is returned to left side of heart.

2 The contractions also force oxygenated blood to muscles via the aorta and other arteries.

Artery

Aorta

Pulmonary trunk

Heart

Lungs

3 Energy from reaction of sugars with oxygen brought by blood is converted to mechanical energy.

Sitting behind desks or minding machines, we in the West become less fit as we get older. But does it matter? It does, because with your body it's a case of use it or lose it. Good health – life itself – is put at risk by inactivity.

Physical activity is a natural part of human life – like sleeping or eating. Nobody who sees how children rush around can doubt it. But as adults, our inclination and capacity for exercise become gradually eroded by sedentary jobs, readily available transport and home-based leisure activities such as watching television.

So it becomes necessary to take planned exercise. For not only does the body simply deteriorate if it is not used, the health hazards of a sedentary life – such as high BLOOD PRESSURE and cholesterol build-up – need to be offset. Perhaps just as important, exercise simply makes us feel better. Getting fit relieves TENSION and STRESS, which boosts mental as well as physical health.

What getting fit means

Many people think mistakenly that fitness training is designed to develop a bigger heart or lungs. However, the amount of air an adult's lungs can hold is largely an inherited capacity, which cannot be changed much. Nor does a healthy person's heart get bigger through exercise – indeed, any such increase is a warning signal of possible heart failure (see HEART DISORDERS). What fitness training does is make our lungs, heart, blood and muscles work more efficiently.

All human activity depends on moving muscles. The energy for this comes from the breakdown of sugars (and indirectly fats) in muscle tissue; the amount of energy produced there depends on how much oxygen reaches the muscle cells through the bloodstream.

If we exercise a group of muscles over and over again – say, by raising an arm overhead once every second – it soon becomes painful. This is because we have used up the available oxygen and the muscle is now working without any. It can still produce energy, even without oxygen, but the process leads to a build-up of lactic acid in the muscles, which causes painful muscle CRAMP.

Physically fit people can transfer large amounts of oxygen from their blood to their muscles, allowing the muscles to work for longer than those of unfit people before cramp sets in. The large amount of oxygen results partly from increased carrying capacity in the blood. This capacity has been improved through improved

Power from heart to muscle

When you exercise, your muscles need extra oxygen and nourishment. The heart beats faster and more strongly to meet the demand, and in this way is itself exercised. The diagram shows how oxygen reaches a muscle, in this case the biceps muscle of the arm.

oxygen exchange in the lungs and more efficient expulsion of carbon dioxide. The muscles also extract oxygen more efficiently from the blood, because physical training increases a muscle's number of mitochondria – microscopic parts of cells that exchange oxygen and sugar for energy.

The effect is that a fit muscle is capable of more work – and does not have to work as hard to do a particular task as it did before getting fit. It can work for longer and produce more energy before lactic acid builds up and causes cramp.

The heart is, of course, a major muscle. One effect of an exercise programme is to train the heart muscle along with others. The heart's job is to pump blood all over the body – first to the lungs where it picks up oxygen, and then back to the heart to be pumped out to organs and tissues. Each squeeze of the pump is felt as a heartbeat or the throb of a pulse with each fresh surge of blood through the body.

The amount of blood reaching, say, the legs during one minute depends on how frequently the heart beats and also on how much blood it pumps out at each beat. Exercise makes the heart muscle more elastic, so at each beat it contracts more efficiently, forcing out more blood. This means that fewer beats are needed to supply the same amount per minute of oxygen-bearing blood to the legs. The heart can therefore afford to slow down.

You should be able to measure how much it does so. After a few weeks of training, your heartbeat – and consequently your pulse rate – should slow. A pulse rate of perhaps 65 beats a minute would come down to only 60 or less (see p. 132, *Test your fitness*). In highly trained athletes it often comes down into the 40s. This more efficient heart pumping also means that when your muscles are working hard – to run for a bus or climb stairs, for example – your pulse rate does not go as high as before.

Choosing your exercise

Many people are now taking up weight training to get in better shape. The repetitive exercising they do with light weights works the heart and increases oxygen consumption – and so is a form of aerobic exercise (see p. 134). But not all forms of exercise are like this. People interested in getting strong lift heavy weights to build large muscles. They exercise in short bursts, exerting very high effort – which does little to train the heart.

However, people often combine the two – weights for strength, and aerobic exercise to make the heart more efficient through regular and repetitive routines. It is important to know the difference between the two, especially for unfit middle-aged people. Lifting heavy weights causes muscles to contract fiercely and puts pressure on the blood vessels – which can raise blood pressure quite dramatically. *This is a danger that would-be weight trainers should consider.*

When people who have not exercised for years decide to take up an exercise programme they are often confused about which kind it should be and whether they need their doctor's advice (see box, *Do's and don'ts about exercise*). Although you will often read and hear the advice that you should ask for your doctor's approval before beginning, you should remember that your doctor can only examine you for any obvious problems – no collection of tests can prove that you are immune to every problem that exercise could cause.

The best advice is to find a form of exercise that you like and can do easily. If you are unfit, you might decide first to introduce more physical exertion into your everyday life. When you move about, do it briskly. In shops and offices, walk upstairs instead of using lifts or escalators. Walk to the local shops or station instead of driving. Get off your bus one stop before your destination and complete the journey on foot. Unwind at the weekends by walking or gardening instead of sitting all the time.

When you are ready for exercise routines, start slowly and never push yourself to the point where you are uncomfortable – you should, for example, just be able to carry on a conversation with someone exercising next to you. Only if you are a professional sportsman and your living depends on winning is there any need to force yourself through the pain barrier. You can achieve a training effect well before that moment arrives.

The idea of a training zone – a heart rate that develops increased elasticity in the heart and greater oxygen uptake in the muscles – is the basis of all exercise programmes. Such programmes try to make the body work close to its maximum rate of absorbing oxygen. This absorption rate is linked to heart rate, and consequently to pulse rate, which is easily measured and tells whether you are working hard enough to train the heart and other muscles.

Measure the rate by taking your pulse immediately you stop exercising, before the rate begins to drop. The simplest way is to take your pulse for just 6 or 10 seconds while the rate is at its highest – and multiply the number (by 10 or 6 respectively) to get the rate per minute. If you take your pulse for a full minute, the figure will be misleadingly low since the rate will drop rapidly during that minute. As you gradually get fitter, your heart and pulse rate should drop from exercise to normal level more quickly, and this *recovery time* should eventually level out at approximately 1½ minutes.

Remember that any activity uses *some* energy, but much of it does not use enough to produce a training effect. The exercises that use large muscle groups such as the arms and legs – running, cycling, skiing or rowing, for example – are those that give a training effect and so increase fitness. Generally, exercise has to require 6-10 METs (metabolic units) to give a training effect. The MET is a unit for measuring the body's metabolic rate – that is, the rate at which energy is used to maintain structure and activity. One MET is taken to be the body's metabolic rate when it is at rest. Carrying out everyday tasks multiplies this rate according to the amount of effort needed. It is only quite energetic activities that raise the rate enough to give a training effect – that is, above 6 METs.

Brisk walking, cycling at 17,5 km/h, competitive badminton, social tennis singles and water-skiing are among the activities that require 6-7 METs. Jogging at 8 km/h, cycling at 19 km/h, galloping on horseback, swimming, mountain climbing, canoeing, football and disco dancing require 7-8 METs. Activities requiring 8-10 METs include running at 9 km/h, cycling at 21 km/h, social squash, basketball, rowing and competitive tennis.

Running and JOGGING are undoubtedly the most popular forms of exercise in the Western world. You can do them more or less anywhere and with little equipment other than well-cushioned running shoes. But they still have drawbacks – apart from traffic and pollution hazards, they can be plain boring. Also, running on hard roads can cause muscle problems, SPRAINS and sometimes knee damage.

Do's and don'ts about exercise

Do ask your doctor's advice if you suffer from high blood pressure, DIZZINESS, BLACKOUTS, any HEART DISORDERS, DIABETES, BACK PAIN or ARTHRITIS.

Don't exercise for more than 20 minutes at a time at first. If you cannot manage 20 minutes, then build up your sessions slowly.

Do stop and rest if you become breathless or feel pain or discomfort. You should always be able to hold a conversation while exercising.

Don't exercise when you are tired, ill or feverish.

Do wait at least two hours after a meal before exercising.

Don't choose a competitive sport if you suffer from stress or tension.

Do warm up properly before strenuous exercise, to reduce the risk of strained muscles or ligaments.

Do wear loose, comfortable clothes for your exercise session, cotton if possible because this material absorbs sweat better than synthetic fabrics and allows air to circulate more freely.

Do buy well-made, comfortable training shoes for exercising, to protect yourself from injury.

The second most popular exercise is aerobics (a term coined in the 1960s in the United States by Dr Kenneth Cooper). Essentially, this consists of movement to music, either alone, using exercise tapes now available, or with a teacher in a group.

Recently the value of walking has been rediscovered. Many doctors have recommended patients to walk more instead of going by car or bus, but sports specialists have doubted whether walking would put the heart rate up into the training zone. In the mid-1980s, a group of doctors in Massachusetts asked several hundred people, both young and old, to walk 1,6 km briskly. Most of their heart rates rose enough for a training effect.

Walking also avoids many of the problems posed by more energetic exercise. However, it does not do much for the flexibility of the joints and muscles, so it should be combined with some form of stretch exercise, such as a hamstring stretch or a calf stretch. For a hamstring stretch, bend at the waist and clasp the backs of the calves with your hands, holding the position for 10 seconds and repeating it five times. For a calf stretch, stand 46 cm away from a wall and press your hands against it while you push your pelvis forward (repeat three to five times).

How much exercise should we take?

Somebody unaccustomed to exercising – especially if in poor physical condition – should start cautiously, feeling out how the body reacts to exertion. You should not exercise for longer than you feel comfortable, even if this is only five minutes at first. Aim at building up steadily to three sessions a week, each of about 45-60 minutes. By the time you have become used to that amount, about half of each session should take you into the training zone, so that oxygen intake is increased and your heart rate is slowed.

A ten-week programme is usually required to reach this stage, and the effects of training will not show for the first few weeks. However, once you are fit, two exercise sessions a week are sufficient to maintain fitness. With less than that, you will quickly begin to lose fitness again.

Some people take exercise only occasionally, then do it as violently as they can in the hope of getting increased benefit. In fact, the opposite happens. For example, one game of squash every few weeks does little to improve fitness but increases the danger of injury. Getting into an exercise programme slowly and taking short, regular sessions is far more effective and far less risky than trying to achieve instant fitness in violent bursts.

Most exercise injuries involve muscles and the ankle, knee and hip joints. Muscle injuries can be avoided by not driving yourself too hard, and by following a planned programme that makes sure you warm up properly and build up gradually to a peak effort. Joint injuries arise from constantly pounding the feet down on a hard surface, and they are a particular problem in running and aerobics.

A well-cushioned pair of training shoes is one answer to the problem – always buy the best you can afford. Many aerobics teachers provide another answer by specialising in 'low impact' aerobics, where students learn how to move their feet up and down without jarring the rest of the body. A third development

is to work against taut rubber belts that take the impact of feet and hands. These increase the effort you have to make against the resistance of the rubber, so you work harder but with reduced risk of injury.

There are more serious health problems to look out for. Occasionally newspapers carry stories about middle-aged businessmen who take part in violent exercise and then drop dead. Some years ago doctors in Scotland investigated the deaths of 29 men who expired after playing squash. All but six showed evidence of previous heart disease which they had chosen to ignore. This spotlights the need for a medical check for obvious

Test your fitness

A simple way to gauge your fitness is to take your pulse for a minute before you get out of bed in the morning. It is normal for individuals to have different pulse rates. In general, women have a slightly higher resting pulse than men. The fitter you are, the slower, stronger and more regular your pulse will be. A resting pulse rate higher than the 'unfit' level indicates that you should see a doctor as soon as possible.

FITNESS LEVELS FOR RESTING PULSE RATES

Age	20-29	30-39	40-49	over 50
Men				
Very fit	59	63	65	67
Fit	60-69	64-71	66-73	68-75
Fairly fit	70-85	72-85	74-89	76-89
Unfit	86	86	90	90
Women				
Very fit	71	71	73	73
Fit	72-77	72-79	75-79	77-83
Fairly fit	78-95	80-97	80-98	84-102
Unfit	96	98	99	103

If your resting pulse rate is slower than the 'unfit' level, you can test your stamina – but first read the *Do's and don'ts* box.

Step up with one foot after the other onto the bottom step of an ordinary staircase (with the step about 20 cm high), then step down again with one foot after the other. Keep on doing this at the rate of twice every five seconds for three minutes. If you begin to feel dizzy, sick or uncomfortably out of breath, stop at once. After you have rested for 30 seconds, take your pulse again to assess your fitness for exercise.

FITNESS LEVELS AFTER EXERCISE

Age	20-29	30-39	40-49	over 50
Men				
Very fit	74	78	80	83
Fit	76-84	80-86	82-88	84-90
Fairly fit	86-100	88-100	90-104	92-104
Unfit	102	102	106	106
Women				
Very fit	86	86	88	90
Fit	88-92	88-94	80-94	92-98
Fairly fit	99-100	95-112	96-114	100-116
Unfit	112	114	114	118

Do the step test again after a few weeks of your regular exercise routine – you should see quite a difference.

signs of disease before taking up vigorous exercise. But, since no medical tests can spot an individual's risk of potential heart or other disease, it emphasises even more the need to listen to your body and *never exercise beyond a comfortable limit*.

The same Scottish doctors found that a third of squash players who died had been very aggressive, driving themselves to win at all costs. The investigation did not prove that squash is dangerous – only that some people find dangerous ways to play it.

Benefits of exercise

Combined with a sensible diet, fitness training can reduce your weight – one of the main reasons for overweight people to take exercise. There are no instant results – running a kilometre burns off no more kilojoules than you get from a small piece of cake. In the long term, however, exercise increases the rate at which the body breaks down foods, so less of your intake is stored as fat reserves. And this remains true despite the fact that prolonged strenuous exercise is apt to increase the appetite considerably. (Moderate exercise, by contrast, actually tends to decrease the appetite, not enlarge it.)

Exercise also affects cholesterol, the fatty substance in the blood that can build up inside arteries, blocking circulation and leading to the possibility of heart disorders or a stroke. Choles-

The right training zone for you

An exercise session should raise your heart rate to between 70 and 90 per cent of maximum. Below that, there is little training effect, nor is there any point in pushing yourself above it into exhaustion. The fastest your heart will go is about 220 beats a minute, minus your age; the maximum rate declines as you get older. At 35 your maximum is about 185; by 50 it has fallen to about 170. If you are 40, your maximum is about 180 and the 70-90 per cent training rate you should be aiming for is 126-162 beats a minute.

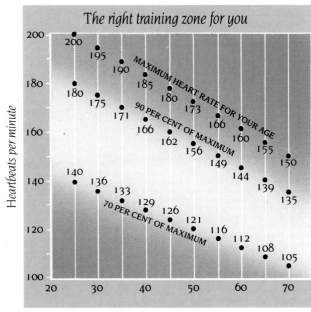

The right training zone for you

terol exists in two forms. LDL (low density lipoprotein) cholesterol increases the risk of a heart attack, while the HDL (high density lipoprotein) form actually reduces it. Exercise is believed to increase the proportion of HDL in the bloodstream, and so should have a protective effect. At first it was thought that HDL increased only in people who took vigorous exercise – for example, running at least 10 km a week. Now it seems that lower exercise levels may also increase HDL.

Exercise may reduce the risk of heart attacks in other ways as well. It may contribute to lowering blood pressure, if only by helping to reduce body weight. Some smokers find that exercise helps them to give up the habit (see SMOKING). It may also help by encouraging people to 'think healthy'. They start to see being fit as just one part of a healthy lifestyle that incorporates watching their diet and their weight, giving up smoking and trying to reduce stress.

Links between fitness and mental health are also emerging. The effect goes beyond lifting the mood of people in normal health. It certainly does that, but medical research in the USA in 1978 showed that exercise can be as effective as PSYCHOTHERAPY in treating patients with mild DEPRESSION. Patients with quite severe depression have also been helped by exercise that achieved a training effect.

Just why exercising makes people feel better about themselves remains a mystery, however. One theory is that it releases chemicals in the brain that give a sensation of pleasure. For example, many distance runners say that after a number of kilometres, their pain and fatigue suddenly change into a feeling of great well-being.

Scientists are now learning something about these brain changes, which may be due to the body's own tranquillising, painkilling group of hormones called endorphins. However, endorphins disappear from the body in a few hours, whereas the exerciser's feelings remain boosted long after the session has come to an end.

Another theory is that exercise simply distracts the mind from problems – that having got away from them briefly, the mind is refreshed and ready to face them again. Exercising in a group is particularly beneficial – a social activity in which people get to know one another. As physical fitness improves, so does self-confidence, and the whole personality becomes more open and relaxed.

Never assume that you are too old or too infirm to take exercise. Indeed, a moderate exercise programme tailored to your particular needs can actually help to slow down the ageing process. With continued inaction the muscles become weak and flabby, the joints feel stiff and the sense of balance decreases. Physical exercise can alleviate these problems – and the risk of falls, which is comparatively high among the aged, is reduced.

At the very least, exercise gives a feeling of accomplishment – a sense of mastery over at least one aspect of your life. You see your weight going down progressively, and your body shape starting to improve; you move more easily, can do more, and keep going longer: all satisfying proof of what you can do if you put your mind to it.

Aerobics used wisely to achieve fitness

Working in a group is generally more enjoyable than exercising on your own — although there are many books and tapes that offer programmes planned to suit the age and fitness of anyone who cannot get to an aerobics class. One slight problem in a group is to avoid competing with others and pushing yourself too far. A good teacher will prevent this and keep students aware of their pulse rates. A well-planned class has three essential parts. First, the warm-up uses movements such as those shown on these two pages to accustom your muscles to exercise and reduce the chance of injury. Next, the most active part of the class progressively raises your heart rate into the training zone. Finally, a warm-down and stretch period allows your heart and pulse rate to return to normal.

Confident teachers will let you watch a class in action before committing yourself to one. Once you join, the teacher will advise you how to start slowly and build up if you are a beginner. Your age — whether it be 30 or 70 — will also be considered when a programme is worked out. People who take up exercise in their 40s or later can greatly improve their fitness, but usually they are not able to work as hard at it as younger people — nor should they try.

Shoulder warming
Standing erect with feet apart and hands hanging loosely at your sides, raise your left shoulder towards your ear while the right shoulder drops. Then raise the right one and drop the left. Repeat another three times.

Neck loosener
Start your gentle warm-up of cold muscles by stretching the neck muscles. Drop your head first towards your left shoulder, then towards the right. Repeat three or four times.

Star jumps
Swing your arms out sideways and over your head while you jump and land with feet apart. Jump again to land with feet together and swing your arms out as you lower them to your sides. Do the jumps ten times.

Quicken the pulse
Now warming up more energetically, run on the spot making 40 landings. Each time land on the ball of your foot then let the rest of the foot touch down before the other foot lands.

Twist and jump

As you jump, swing your arms to the right and your body to the left. Land like this, then jump again with arms going left and body right. Repeat another nine times. Be sure to take steady deep breaths during the exercises to give your muscles the extra oxygen they need for the work.

Swing a leg

As you jump, swing your right arm and leg sideways and then land on your left foot. Then swing out your left arm and leg to the side as you jump and land on your right foot. Do these jumps 20 times.

Side stretches

Stand with feet apart, knees slightly bent, and hands on hips. Raise your left arm fully with the palm turned out (far left) and reach sideways to the right. Breathe out as you bend and hold the position for 6-10 seconds before returning to the starting position. Repeat the stretch (left) with right arm raised and bending to the left. Then clasp your hands above your head (right) with palms up and push upwards. Hold the stretch for 6-10 seconds before relaxing. Now you are warmed up enough to start on more strenuous exercises.

FAINTING

Although books and films give the impression that it is ladies who swoon, in fact anyone can suffer the brief loss of consciousness which is generally called a faint. In medical circles the term syncope may be used. Lack of oxygen in the brain is the immediate cause of fainting, but there may be various reasons for that lack of oxygen.

Standing up too quickly is the commonest cause, especially in older people. In the short delay before the blood vessels adjust to the new position, blood (which carries the oxygen supply) is not circulated to the brain. When someone stands in one position for too long, blood tends to collect in the legs and circulation to the brain is slowed.

Fatigue, pain, emotional distress or SHOCK can all slow down the heart rate, and again the result can be a failure of circulation to the brain.

A slow heartbeat – and consequent reduced oxygen supply to the brain – is quite common in people with heart disease or DIABETES, and in those who have been given certain drugs or anaesthetics.

A very rapid heartbeat, when the heart circulates blood that is inadequately supplied with oxygen, is characteristic of several conditions, including ANAEMIA, heart failure and some THYROID DISORDERS. It can also be the result of drinking too much coffee or alcohol, or of HYPERVENTILATION.

Self help Many faints can be prevented if you take the following precautions: If you have to stand in one place for a long time, tighten and relax your calf and thigh muscles from time to time and flex your toes to pep up the circulation.

Do not stand up too quickly after lying down or slumping in a chair; first sit erect and then perch on the edge for a time before standing. Take care not to jerk your head to the side or tilt it back quickly to reach a shelf or peg; such movements can compress the arteries in the neck.

If you get the warning sensations that often precede a faint – weak legs, a feeling of lightheadedness and pale, cold skin – lie down for a time and get up slowly when the feelings have passed.

Anyone who faints frequently should seek medical advice to find out about the cause. If the fainting follows an injury or happens without any apparent cause, medical advice is certainly needed.

Where the victim recovers in a minute or two and the cause is clear – heat, cold, fatigue, distress or shock, standing still for too long, or standing up too quickly – medical help is not necessary. Prompt first aid is sufficient for recovery.

In both orthodox and alternative medicine the procedure is the same. Lay the victim down flat and prop up the legs slightly. This will quickly restore the blood supply to the brain. Make sure there is no tight clothing round the neck or chest and nothing in the mouth to block the airway. Turn the victim on one side and send for medical help if breathing seems difficult.

What the therapists recommend

Homoeopathy *Aconite* is given after a faint from fright, *Arsenicum album* after a faint from exhaustion or cold, and *Carbo vegetalis* after one from lack of air.

Bach Remedies A few drops of Rescue Remedy taken on the tongue, in water or in tea are given as the victim comes round. Do not give anything by mouth to a person who is unconscious; it can cause choking.

Acupressure A fingernail is used to stimulate strongly the point that is on the midline two-thirds of the way up, between the victim's top lip and nose.

An orthodox view

Prompt first aid (see above), without any other remedy, is the conventional treatment. The victim may like to take a sip of water and some fresh air after he has come round.

FAITH HEALING

The basis of faith healing is a belief in positive or 'right' thinking, which, it is held, can cure or relieve any one of the wide spectrum of illnesses. This is particularly so when practised within a religious system such as Christian Science, which preaches healing through spiritual means.

In one form or another, healing – using a reliance on the subject's faith, either in a deity or the healer's own powers – has been practised for centuries in many parts of the world (see HEALERS AND HEALING).

In the early 1890s a French neurophysiologist, Jean Martin Charcot, asserted that his form of faith healing could cure most organic diseases, including CANCER. 'This', he stated, 'is commonly known in medical circles as miracle healing. However, in the majority of cases, it is shown to be a natural phenomenon which occurs throughout history at all times at most levels of civilisation, and among most religions, however they may otherwise differ.'

In medical theory, faith healing activates and enhances the body's natural defences through reducing the body's response to STRESS. It may produce health-giving hormones – substances carried by the bloodstream which modify the structure and function of organs and tissues, promoting growth and so on.

It may also strengthen antibodies – proteins in the blood which fight infection and disease. In addition, it can strongly reinforce the mental attitudes of patients, so that they feel much better – even if their actual condition is not improved.

FASTING

A deliberate and controlled abstinence from solid foods for a certain period – fasting – should never be undertaken without your doctor's consent. Naturopaths are probably its keenest advocates in alternative medicine. A leading practitioner, the British naturopath Leon Chaitow, has described fasting as 'the oldest therapeutic method known to man', adding that 'primitive people stop eating instinctively when not feeling well … drinking as much as is needed and eating nothing, until health returns'.

The theory is that fasting makes the body concentrate its resources on ridding itself of disease and poisons rather than using them to digest food. However, naturopaths stress that it must be done under the supervision of a qualified therapist or dietitian.

The length and strictness of a fast is worked out in accordance with the person's age and the condition being treated. From middle age onwards, the system does not react to fasting in the same way as that of younger people – instead of using up body fat to keep going, it is thought to use up protein matter, the basic materials of skin, muscle and other tissues.

A practitioner may recommend short or extended fasts – from perhaps one or two days a week up to periods of 40 or even 50 days. Longer fasts are usually supervised in a residential clinic, health farm or spa. Patients are warned that their early reactions to an extended fast can be unpleasant: DIARRHOEA, HEADACHES, vomiting and BAD BREATH during the first days. However, these symptoms should then gradually disappear, along with pangs of hunger.

An orthodox view

Doctors have tended to dismiss fasting as a healing process, but it has recently begun to earn some acceptance. Claims have been made that it has been effective in treating ARTHRITIS, high BLOOD PRESSURE, certain types of food ALLERGY, and RHEUMATISM. Fasting has also been used to treat SCHIZOPHRENIA, with encouraging results, at hospitals in Moscow and New York.

FEAR

It affects us all at times ...

Walking through a deserted car park at night or facing a large, unfriendly dog – many common situations can arouse feelings of fear in even the most confident and capable people. The response is natural, normal and useful, because fear sharpens the senses, gives extra strength and quickens reactions, helping you to respond to danger.

Sometimes, however, fear seems to have no obvious cause, or to be excessive for the circumstances. Occasionally it continues long after the danger has passed, or becomes almost a way of life. In these cases, fear itself and not the frightening situation becomes a problem. People who suffer from this sort of unreasonable fear have difficulty coping with the demands of everyday life and work, and find it hard to relax or enjoy themselves. If the fear continues for any length of time, they experience physical and emotional STRESS.

Irrational fear takes many forms. When it is provoked by particular objects or situations such as spiders, heights or flying, it is known as a PHOBIA. In some cases the victim experiences sudden, severe panic attacks in crowded or closed-in public places, CLAUSTROPHOBIA, or finds it hard to leave the house, AGORAPHOBIA.

Often, however, there is just a vague, persistent feeling of ANXIETY, or dread, which either has no apparent cause, or has its roots in some forthcoming event – an interview or examination, for example.

Sometimes the causes of these irrational or exaggerated fears stem from events far in the past – even from such childhood terrors as fear of the dark and 'bogeymen' – which have been forgotten, or which may not even have made much of a conscious impression at the time. Repressed feelings or NERVOUS DISORDERS also play a part.

Mild attacks of fearfulness can be dealt with at home, but more severe or long-lasting feelings need to be treated by a doctor or qualified psychotherapist.

What the therapists recommend

Bach Remedies Rock rose is said to relieve extreme fear or intense panic which has reached crisis level. Mimulus is suitable for known fears, such as getting CANCER, being rejected, finding yourself alone in the dark, and dread of spiders, snakes, or heights. For feelings of foreboding, or of being punished for no good reason, try Aspen. Cherry plum may help with fear of insanity, of losing total self-control, or feeling paralysed with fright. Fear of being alone may be helped considerably by Chicory or Heather.

Relaxation and Breathing; Meditation Both these therapies offer help in overcoming fears. Practitioners consider meditation an effective way of strengthening people's resistance to fear and anxiety. In addition, relaxing and breathing in an even and natural manner will help to prevent panic and the heightening of fear.

An orthodox view

Doctors see fear as a normal human emotion which can help to protect us from irrational behaviour and dangerous situations. When fear gets out of hand and becomes a phobia, doctors usually refer patients to a behavioural psychologist for 'desensitising' treatment (see BEHAVIOURAL THERAPY). The success rate is good for fears of specific things such as snakes or confined spaces, but less effective when the person has a generally fearful or timid personality.

FELDENKRAIS METHOD

Learning new patterns of movement

'A body that is organised to move with minimum effort and maximum efficiency' – this was the purpose for which Moshe Feldenkrais devised his lessons for helping people to learn how they are moving and methods of improving the way they move. Trained in engineering and applied physics, he took a practical scientist's approach to making the 'machinery' of his own body – and then others – work properly.

He came to believe that, in infancy or later, the brain develops an image or pattern of how movements should be made and that the body 'obeys' this image when it moves. He further theorised that this brain image could turn out to be less than ideal for some of the movements, instructing the body to move in ways that eventually would cause it pain and damage.

His lessons aim to develop new patterns in the brain, so that movements are made more efficiently. Two techniques were developed. AWARENESS THROUGH MOVEMENT, taught in classes, is intended to make people aware of their habitual patterns and of new possibilities. FUNCTIONAL INTEGRATION uses gentle manipulation to do the same on a one-to-one basis.

Who it can help The gentle lessons which are given in awareness through movement classes have been found to help a large number of people who suffer recurring pain in

Learning to free a shoulder

The student lies face-down as shown, with head turned towards the stiff left shoulder. The teacher holds the left elbow and shoulder, and moves them in relation to one another.

Then, with the student's left arm resting on the head, the Feldenkrais teacher raises and rotates the entire upper torso.

By rotating the left leg the teacher shows the student how the hip joint and entire spine are related to the left shoulder.

their muscles and joints. The lessons are generally designed to improve your posture and therefore breathing, circulation and overall well-being. Athletes, dancers and other people whose lives involve them in a great deal of movement can, it is believed, lessen the risk of injury by learning efficient muscle use.

A functional integration lesson with a trained teacher aims to restore or control movement in stroke victims and people with cerebral palsy and spinal disorders, as well as easing ARTHRITIS, chronic BACK PAIN and muscle injuries.

Finding a teacher While there are as yet no teachers of the Feldenkrais Method in South Africa, you can contact the Feldenkrais Guild in Britain by writing to 188 Old Street, London ECIV 9BP. The British guild will be able to give you detailed advice on how to obtain lessons on tape. Alternatively books are available on the subject at some specialist libraries. Senior teachers who were trained by Moshe Feldenkrais himself are now con-ducting popular professional training pro-grammes in England and elsewhere in the world. The training is concentrated in periods of three to five weeks, and is undertaken twice a year for four years.

Consulting a teacher At classes in aware-ness through movement the teacher leads students through sequences of movements. None of these movements is strenuous. The students usually lie down at first, in order to free them of the usual efforts involved in sit-ting and standing.

Pelvic clock

The purpose of the sequences of rotations known as the pelvic clock is to explore the possible range of movement of the pelvis. By becoming more aware of the possibilities students are able to improve the relationship of the pelvis to the spine, head and legs, create new patterns of action and develop a wider range of movement.

Copying the moves

The head naturally rotates in the same way as the imaginary dial – the pelvis (see below) – mimicking its movements.

6 o'clock

12 o'clock

3 o'clock

9 o'clock

Imaginary dial

Students imagine that fixed on the back of the pelvic girdle there is a clock dial (which from the front would appear to be reversed). On the dial, 6 o'clock is at the lowest point (the coccyx), 12 o'clock at the highest point (where the spine meets the pelvic girdle), 3 o'clock at the right hip joint and 9 o'clock at the left hip joint.

1 *Lying as shown, the student lifts the lower back from the floor, arching as much as possible and putting the pressure on the 6 o'clock point. The weight is shifted to the 12 o'clock point, the arch disappears and the coccyx lifts from the floor. The student then rocks the pelvis from one position to the other several times, making the movements smooth and easy and breathing normally throughout.*

2 *The movement is repeated, paying attention to how the head copies the pelvic movement.*

3 *The pelvis is tilted to 3 o'clock, with the pressure on the right side while the left lifts. Then the weight is moved to 9 o'clock and the left side lifts. The sideways rocking is repeated several times.*

4 *Starting with pressure at 12 o'clock, the pelvis is moved to 1 o'clock and back, then to 1, to 2, and back, and so on until the pelvis is rolling smoothly to 6 o'clock and back. The head will again copy the movement.*

5 *The movement is repeated but this time on the left side.*

6 *With 3 o'clock as the starting point, the student rolls the pelvis back and forth, first to 2 o'clock, then to 4, and adds an hour at a time until rolling to 12 in one direction and 6 in the other.*

7 *The movement is repeated with 9 o'clock as the starting point.*

8 *The pelvis can then move all round the clock, first clockwise, then anticlockwise, with smooth movements every time. The student notices each time how the head moves in unison with the pelvis.*

Between sequences, the student rests on his or her back with legs stretched out and feels the different sensations in the area of the pelvis just moved.

The lessons can be varied, sometimes with one leg drawn up and the other straight; with both legs straight; with one leg crossed over the other; in a sitting position with knees bent, leaning back on the hands.

After the lesson the pelvis feels flatter and the lower back closer to the floor while lying down. On standing, a change of position of the pelvis in relation to the spine and legs is felt.

They repeat the gentle movements over and over until they become easy and smooth, then students can concentrate solely on developing awareness of what they are doing. They quickly become sensitive to tiny adjustments made to the way they organise themselves for movement. More comfortable habits are easily learned – and can affect the way students think and feel.

At a functional integration lesson the teacher sees only one student and uses touch and manipulation to suggest new ways of organising movement.

An orthodox view

Posture, breathing and circulation have been improved by the method, as have muscle and joint disorders. The ALEXANDER TECHNIQUE and ordinary MASSAGE may be equally effective for these problems, as well as for STRESS and serious loss of muscle function.

FETAL ALCOHOL SYNDROME

Alcohol, like tobacco, affects the normal development of an unborn child, and so it makes sense for any mother-to-be to give up alcoholic drinks (and smoking) completely for the duration of her pregnancy. Even quite small quantities of alcohol may prove harmful – and so can the occasional drinking binge indulged in by someone who is usually abstemious. Certainly any pregnant woman who consistently takes two or more alcoholic drinks a day is running a risk, not only of harming her offspring but of miscarriage.

Fetal alcohol syndrome is the term given to the combination of defects at birth that result from the mother's alcohol abuse. They may include a cleft palate, heart defects, deformities of the joints, and a low IQ; in addition the baby is usually abnormally short, with small eyes and jaw. Victims of fetal alcohol syndrome tend to be irritable and to sleep badly; and as many as one in five of them fail to survive beyond infancy.

What the therapists recommend

An assortment of therapies is available to alleviate the symptoms of this syndrome and, so far as possible, enhance the child's quality of life. The holistic approach of ANTHROPOSOPHICAL MEDICINE may be an appropriate choice with its use of EURHYTHMY and access to the network of Camphill villages (where the mentally handicapped are cared for). Speech therapy may be necessary for those individuals with a cleft palate (even after it has been treated by surgery).

An orthodox view

There is no 'cure' for fetal alcohol syndrome. The doctor will try to ensure that the child receives good parental support. A proper diet and, as the child grows older, a healthy exercise schedule are important. A cleft palate can be effectively repaired by surgery after about one year.

Sadly, mothers of babies with fetal alcohol syndrome are sometimes unaware that their offspring have this disability.

The condition is often identified by the doctor only when the child is brought to the surgery because of some other ailment, for example pneumonia.

FEVER

The onset of a fever is a symptom, rather than a particular illness. It is a sign that the body is fighting infection. Most people's body temperature is normally 98,6°F (37°C), although a few individuals may be 1°F (0,6°C) above or below this. At the outset of many childhood infections, temperature can rise up to 104°F (40°C), while among adults it generally rises to a lesser extent.

However, elderly people may suffer infections and yet their temperature stays normal. This is a sign that the body's ability to fight infection has lessened.

If the patient has severe shivers, shakes and chattering teeth – a condition known as rigor – call a doctor immediately. These can be symptoms of PNEUMONIA, pyelonephritis (kidney infection) or malaria.

What the therapists recommend
HERBAL MEDICINE
Self help A variety of herbal teas is recommended for fevers – here are three:
Cayenne The hot, red, powdery pepper may be added in small quantities to warm milk, water or tea. Alternatively, swallow a gelatine capsule of cayenne, washed down with a glass of water.
Willow bark This is also said to be helpful in lessening fever. The ancient Greeks used it, as did American Indians. The inner bark is boiled and the 'tea' is drunk in strong doses. Willow bark contains an ingredient which the human system converts into salicylic acid – a basic ingredient of aspirin.
Boneset Another American Indian herbal remedy: 1 or 2 teaspoons of the dried herb are infused in a cupful of boiling water for 10-15 minutes, and drunk every half hour until the fever subsides.
Consultation Like most alternative practitioners, a herbalist tends to regard fever as

Other herbal remedies for fever

To induce heavy sweating, drink an infusion of yarrow hourly. The dried herb – 1-2 teaspoonfuls – is infused for about 10-15 minutes in boiling water.

To relieve a feverish cold, make a herbal tea of elderflower and lime-blossom in equal proportions.

To ease fever during influenza or a cold on the chest, drink a tea made from lavender flowers.

To clear mucus from the lungs, hyssop tea is recommended. Most herbal teas can be drunk every one to two hours, as hot as possible, in 3-4 tablespoon doses until perspiration subsides. However, take only 1 tablespoon of hyssop.

Catnip, camomile and feverfew are fever-reducing herbs, and a tea made from any of these can be drunk either hot or cold.

the process of the body 'burning up' poison wastes in the system. Intense sweating is taken as a good sign that the unwanted matter is being ejected, so treatment does not necessarily aim to suppress the fever.

A practitioner may recommend various preparations, depending on the intensity and stage of development of the fever. In addition to those already outlined, the herbalist may also advise – as an infusion, decoction or tincture – borage, German camomile, eucalyptus or marigold.

NATUROPATHY
Consultation Practitioners regard fever as a kind of 'healing crisis' – a process by which the natural protective functions of the body are attempting to help it recover from some infection. They advise avoiding solid foods and suggest taking four to six glasses of natural unsweetened vegetable juices a day.

If the patient is feeling weak, but still has an appetite, a broth of mixed vegetables may be allowed. Once the feverishness dies down and normal appetite resumes, solid foods can be taken, beginning with natural yoghurts and fresh fruit.

If the patient is a child under five, sponging the neck, face and limbs with tepid water is advised, with the body covered to prevent chill. For older children and adults, a trunk or abdominal pack – that is, a blanket soaked in tepid water placed over the body, then covered with a second, dry blanket – may be applied for three hours or even overnight. Alternatively, regular cold compresses are placed on the forehead.

Other alternative treatments

Homoeopathy *Aconite* is prescribed for the first signs of fever, accompanied by restlessness and intense thirst which is worse after midnight; *Belladonna* for a 'burning up' feeling, with a hot, flushed face and dilated pupils; and *Bryonia* for a dry mouth, intense thirst for large amounts of water at long intervals and irritability. If a child is restless, cries a lot and constantly seeks attention, *Pulsatilla* may be prescribed. *Nux vomica* if the patient is extremely irritable, over-sensitive and feels chilly. If the condition is accompanied by oversalivating and there is bad breath, particularly worse at night: *Mercurius solubilis. Gelsemium* when there is lack of thirst, chills up and down the spine and headache, and the patient is worse at the least movement, has a feeling of heaviness in the eyelids and limbs, and wants to lie in the dark.

Biochemic Tissue Salts *Ferr. phos.* is recommended when there is a rapid pulse, flushed face, with chilliness and vomiting of undigested food. Take every half-hour until the fever subsides. For fevers associated with nervous conditions and general weakness, *Kali phos.* is recommended.

An orthodox view

Like alternative therapists, general practitioners consider fever as a symptom of the body fighting infection. A doctor would first advise rest in a warm – but not hot – room, with plenty of liquids. Aspirin-type painkillers or an anti-infective medicine may also be prescribed – and an attempt would be made to find out the cause of the fever.

FIBRE

An essential part of healthy eating

For thousands of years, mankind was largely vegetarian, so roughage or dietary fibre formed an integral part of our diet. Cellulose, the main component of fibre, is found in all plant cell walls, while lignin supports the plant's cellulose structures. Pectins, the third component, are found in most ripe fruits.

However, with the increasing affluence brought by the Industrial Revolution, and especially after the lifting of food restrictions following the Second World War, preferences for white bread (from which much of the fibrous bran has been removed) grew, and meat gained a much larger place in the diet

---

Ideal fibre intake

The average adult should aim at a total daily intake of about 30 g of fibre. This could be made up in the following way on an average day: bowl of muesli or wholegrain cereal (3,5 g); slice of wholewheat toast (2,5 g); wholewheat sandwich (5 g); piece of fruit or handful of nuts and raisins (2 g); helping of wholewheat pasta or of lentils, beans or peas, or medium jacket potato (7 g); two helpings of vegetables (4 g); fresh fruit salad (4 g) – total 28 g.

---

than vegetables. Fatty, sugary foods such as biscuits and cakes were preferred to fresh, raw fruits – especially as snacks.

Many nutritionists blame all this for the increase in BOWEL DISORDERS and HEART DISORDERS in the last two centuries. During that time, the number of reported cases of CONSTIPATION, PILES and CANCER of both the upper and lower bowel multiplied apace. People became overweight and developed high BLOOD PRESSURE, placing undue – even fatal – strain on the heart.

Both conventional and alternative practitioners believe that a high-fibre diet helps to combat these disorders (see also EATING FOR HEALTH). Fibre is the part of the food intake that is not digested and absorbed by the body to produce energy. It comes in two forms: insoluble and soluble.

Insoluble fibre is mostly found in wholegrain cereals and bran. The indigestible cellulose and other components in the fibre give bulk to the body's waste products and speed their passage through the bowel. It is held that the less time that cancer-causing waste stays in the bowel, the less chance there is of tumours forming.

Soluble fibre is contained in most ripe fruits and in vegetables, particularly beans, lentils and peas. It slows up the absorption of nutrients in food and delays the intake of sugar into the blood.

It is believed to help people with that form of DIABETES which is caused by too much blood sugar. In some cases diabetics on high-fibre diets have been able to reduce – and even forgo – their daily intake of insulin.

Soluble fibre also binds with cholesterol in food and helps in its elimination from the system. It is therefore thought to reduce the risk of heart attack and to cut down the likelihood of GALLSTONES. Excluding meat, almost any food which has not been processed or refined should provide enough fibre for most people's needs. However, if desired, fibre in

---

the form of bran or special high-fibre or high-bran biscuits, breakfast cereals, breads and other products can be obtained from health stores and some food stores, and taken as a supplement.

FIBROSITIS

Not strictly speaking a medical term, 'fibrositis' refers to stiffness and pain of the fibrous tissue of muscles, especially those around the joints and in the lower back. Sometimes small, hard nodules can be felt in the muscle. Inflammation is normally present, though it may be hard to detect in a medical examination. Causes of the affliction vary from tension and anxiety to bad posture, lack of exercise and damp living conditions or damp weather. The pain is accompanied by tenderness in the affected muscles.

What the therapists recommend

Acupuncture The nature of the fibrositis, and which muscles it affects, will determine where the acupuncturist inserts his needles. He may stimulate bleeding by applying an instrument that has a number of sharp points at its head; this is known as 'plum-blossom therapy'. ACUPRESSURE, MOXIBUSTION and MASSAGE, all closely related to acupuncture in Chinese medicine, may also be used to treat fibrositis.

Herbal Medicine An infusion of an anti-inflammatory herb such as devil's claw, yarrow, meadowsweet or celery seed will provide relief. If the painful condition makes sleep difficult, drink a vervain (wild verbena) or passiflora (passion-flower) tea before retiring. Other herbal sedatives include camomile, lavender, lemon balm and sage; a strong infusion of any of these, poured into a hot bath, is another way of promoting proper sleep.

Homoeopathy *Rhus tox* and *Ruta* are among general remedies that can be used to treat fibrositis.

Naturopathy An over-acid state of the body tissues contributes to fibrositis. The body can be cleansed by means of fasting, followed by a balanced diet that excludes highly acid fruits, high proteins, and excessive amounts of salt, tea and coffee. Green, leafy vegetables are recommended.

An orthodox view

Anti-inflammatory medication and pain-killers may be prescribed for the patient's immediate relief. Heat treatment (including hot baths), massage and relaxation exercises are longer-term remedies; and damp conditions must be eliminated in the home.

FLATULENCE

Gas building up in the stomach and intestine causes WIND, or flatulence. It can result in considerable discomfort – and can find embarrassingly audible means of announcing its presence and making its escape.

FLOATATION THERAPY

Total relaxation of mind and body and relief of STRESS are the basic aims of floatation therapy, but it can be combined with other therapies to treat a variety of problems. It is a form of Restricted Environment Stimulation Therapy (REST), in which the client is left in a state of relaxed awareness.

The client lies in an enclosed tank of water, which is 25 cm deep, in total or semi-darkness and silence. The water is kept at skin temperature, around 34,2°C (93,5°F), and a blend of Epsom and other mineral salts is dissolved in it.

The therapy evolved from experimental work in the 1950s by John C Lilly, an American doctor, psychoanalyst and neurophysiologist. Dr Lilly set out to discover how the brain reacted when it did not have to deal with normal outside sensations – not even with gravity. Lilly and another doctor named Jay Shurley observed each other as they took turns to float in a tank, and by the early 1970s

Buoyancy in a floatation tank is assisted to a great extent by salts dissolved in the water.

they had pioneered a floatation tank similar to those now in therapeutic use.

They believed that once the brain did not have to cope with outside sensations it turned inwards.

Then by becoming more aware of the many inner mental and biological processes, a person could possibly be able to control them consciously.

Who it can help Therapists claim that floatation can help to relieve STRESS or stress-related problems such as INSOMNIA or ANXIETY.

Finding a floatation centre Floatation is a therapy that has not yet become established in South Africa, and float tanks are few and far between. To find one, watch for advertisements in alternative health magazines; or if there is a health hydro in your neighbourhood, ask the supervisor for information.

Going to a floatation centre Sessions last for one to two-and-a-half hours. You take a shower before entering the tank, and then insert ear-plugs as a protection against salts and minerals in the water. Once the door is closed, you float in complete or semi-darkness.

An orthodox view

This technique is used more as a research method than a treatment, and most doctors would not recommend it unless it is supervised by a well-qualified practitioner. It is potentially dangerous in certain psychiatric conditions (psychosis, severe DEPRESSION and PHOBIAS) – and people undertaking this form of 'treatment' should consult their doctor if they have any doubts.

FLOWER ESSENCES

Health-giving vibrations from petals

The holistic aim of this therapy is to harmonise the mind, body and spirit – and so encourage people to express feelings of love and peace. The bottled flower essences, some of which are imported from as far afield as Alaska and California, are said to contain vibrations of the sun's energy, absorbed by the flowers' petals when immersed in sun-warmed water.

The essences are on sale in shops selling natural remedies, and at some homoeopathic pharmacies. They range from Aloe vera (said to increase sensitivity to others), to Zinnia (believed to promote laughter as a potent form of self-healing).

The flower essences are not in any way meant to replace any form of medical treatment. However, therapists claim that by working on a mental and emotional level, their vibrations are calculated to relieve a number of common conditions such as ANXIETY, DEPRESSION, NERVOUS DISORDERS and TIREDNESS.

A few drops of the essences, placed on the tongue, or in a glass of water, should be taken regularly until the condition eases.

Finding a therapist This is essentially a self-help therapy, although practitioners of some alternative remedies do treat their clients with flower essences. See also BACH REMEDIES, to which flower essence therapy is closely related.

An orthodox view

Smell and emotions are well known to be closely linked and in so far as this approach is used with caution, most conventional doctors would not object to it. The dramatic claims made for the essences, however, should be viewed cautiously.

FLUORIDATION

Controversy rages among both conventional and alternative practitioners over the question of adding soluble fluorides to water supplies in order to reduce tooth decay (see TOOTH AND GUM DISORDERS).

Fluorides are chemical compounds containing the element fluorine. Those who support their use as water additives claim that fluoride ions prevent tooth decay (dental caries) in children.

Those opposed to using fluoride in this way point out that there has not been a single laboratory study proving that fluoridation alone prevents or reduces tooth decay, and is safe for human consumption.

Fluoride occurs in the human body, in animals, most foods, particularly fish, and in some plants.

Fluorides are contained in volcanic gases and are released by man in various industrial processes, including the steel and aluminium industries, oil refining, the manufacture of phosphate fertilisers and in nuclear power generation. Those who object to fluoridation argue also that industrialists see it as a convenient and lucrative way of getting rid of their waste fluoride.

However, the amount of fluoride put into drinking-water supplies is comparatively very small: usually one part fluoride to one million parts of water. Excess fluoride can permanently stain children's teeth, and a high intake of fluoride can be dangerous.

Will chemicals make us safe or sorry?

Tiny amounts of chemicals are added to what we eat, for safety or to improve the appearance or extend the shelf life of convenience foods. But now they are causing anxiety. In the Western world 75-80 per cent of the food people eat has been processed, and in South Africa we eat more food additives than ever before. Buyers should always be fully aware of what they are, what they do, and whether they are safe or to be avoided.

An additive is any ingredient that you would not eat as food on its own. In more detailed parlance, as defined by the Food and Agriculture Organisation of the United Nations, a food additive is any substance not normally consumed as a food by itself, and not normally used as a typical ingredient of a food, whose use with other foods for technological reasons results in it becoming a component of, or otherwise affecting the characteristics of, those particular foods. The term, 'additive' does not include 'contaminants' or substances added to food for maintaining or improving nutritional qualities. In South Africa there is one Food Act – the Foodstuffs, Cosmetics and Disinfectants Act (Act No 54 of 1972). All individual laws and legislation subsequent to this Act are referred to as regulations.

An additive is considered necessary if it will keep food wholesome until it is eaten, or make it look and taste good, or make it easier to prepare, store and pack.

The aim is to make it possible for people to have a nutritious diet all the year round. Without additives our food would be less varied in winter and would cost more. Food poisoning would be more common. Whether we do ultimately benefit from the system is a tricky question. Few people dispute that preservatives are necessary to keep meat products safe to eat and antioxidants to prevent fats from going rancid. Many, however, believe that colours and flavour enhancers are not necessary even though grey margarine, khaki tinned peas and brownish strawberry yoghurt would result from leaving them out.

There is no evidence that the great majority of South African residents have been harmed by food additives, but some certainly have. These are people who have been made abnormally sensitive by some defect in body chemistry. Many have suffered one of a range of ailments – skin rashes, dermatitis, ECZEMA, breathing problems (including ASTHMA), MIGRAINE, BOWEL DISORDERS and PALPITATIONS. Lumps and blotches on the skin are the commonest bad reactions. HYPERACTIVITY in children has also

been blamed on food additives, but no properly controlled study has been able to confirm this theory, which has resulted in much controversy in many countries. Food additives have also been blamed for causing cancer in some instances, but the factors causing cancer are so complex that there are no clear answers yet. It is difficult to estimate the number of people with a true food allergy, but in general it is thought to be between one and four per cent of the population. Milk, eggs, wheat, shellfish, nuts, oranges and strawberries are among the many known to cause reactions. Without food preservatives even more people could be affected by food poisoning.

For most people, convenience outweighs the slight hazard of additives. A public that works more, travels more and eats a greater variety of foods at home and in restaurants demands attractive-looking food that is cheap, quick to prepare and has a long storage life. Manufacturers and retailers are anxious to provide this. Now that there is some public pressure for fewer additives, manufacturers and retailers have responded, cutting colourings from some crisps and some preservatives from bread, for example. The swift distribution of foods, fast turnover in supermarkets and strict control of hygiene and temperature throughout production and retailing should allow manufacturers to reduce the amounts of preservatives used, and under pressure from customers no doubt many of them would. There would then be a greater onus on the customer to store food safely and cook it properly.

Long-term worries

A large number of buyers would gladly accept that onus. It can be assumed that the container of milk or the loaf of bread that we buy daily is not going to endanger our lives, but the process of evaluating food safety is far from perfect. It is not yet so effective that it can determine the precise risk associated with the cumulative effects of absorbing a range of additives over many years, or of the possible interactions between the different additives approved for use in South Africa.

Some people assume that all additives are bad but nevertheless use the long-familiar bicarbonate of soda or baking powder in home baking. Some substances approved as additives are a natural, desirable part of foods. There is some carotene and monosodium glutamate in tomatoes, for example, but the colouring carotene and the flavour enhancer monosodium glutamate are viewed in a much less favourable way when they are added to processed foods.

The use of natural extracts rather than synthetic additives – which allows a manufacturer to claim a product is free from artificial additives – does not lessen the worry. If you suffer ill effects from a particular chemical substance, the effect will be the same when you eat it whether it has occurred naturally or been man-made.

People who are concerned to eat a healthy diet without being cranks balance the uncertain risks of additives against those of food being contaminated by bacteria. They reduce the risks by making up their diet from foods that have been interfered with as little as possible and by avoiding the additives that are suspected of causing bad reactions in sensitive individuals. Above all, consumers need accurate information on all the contents of foodstuffs so that they can make the choices that suit them.

Identifying foods containing additives

Ingredients of processed foods are listed on the wrapping or package in order of the amount used. Thus, a product labelled as containing 'vegetable fat and butter' in that order would have more vegetable fat than butter. Additives are present only in tiny amounts and so they appear at the end of the list. They are grouped under category headings – for instance, thickening agents, emulsifiers, colouring, flavouring, preservatives and so on. In South Africa all products containing a preservative must carry the appropriate label. The majority of other additives need not be documented.

The outcry against tartrazine, a yellow dye, also had an effect on food labelling. According to our labelling regulations, tartrazine must be declared in letters 2 mm high on labels.

If you know you are sensitive to a particular additive, it is important to examine ingredient labels carefully, and to consider only those products whose ingredients have been fully listed. Reputable food manufacturers label the contents of foodstuffs accurately, but there are food producers that do not.

Foods often contain traces of substances that are not listed. These are substances that are not ingredients of the product but have previously been added to one or more of the ingredients to keep them in good condition – for instance, enzymes used to tenderise meat for pies and other meat products.

Sulphites prevent fruits and vegetables from turning brown, and are also used as antioxidants. They are used extensively at salad bars and on fruits and vegetables, as well as in fruit juices. Sulphites are also commonly used in dried fruit, dehydrated vegetables, vinegar, beer and wine. Common reactions to sulphites include wheezing, shortness of breath, a tight chest, tingling sensations and stomach irritation.

There are strange quirks in the labelling regulations. Butter, cheeses and cream list only the ingredients not essential to making them. Thus the colour in some cheeses is listed but not rennet, the enzyme that makes the milk coagulate. In South Africa wines, spirits and other alcoholic drinks do not have to list their ingredients – despite the fact that several controversial additives are used. Some items such as vinegar and lemon juice are listed but not among the additives, because they are considered to be foods with nutritional value even though they act as preservatives in the product (vinegar has now replaced 'artificial' preservatives in some wrapped breads). Vitamins and minerals are not generally classed as additives but sometimes vitamin C or E is used as an antioxidant and is listed.

What additives are for

There are 17 categories of local additives, grouped according to function. An additive may be in a product to do more than one job but will be listed only under the main one – which is not necessarily the one for which it was originally tested and approved. The categories are: acids, acidity regulators, anticaking agents, antifoaming agents, antioxidants, artificial sweeteners, colours, emulsifiers, flavour enhancers, flavourings, flour improvers, gelling agents, glazing agents, preservatives, raising agents, stabilisers and thickeners. The table on pp. 146-7 lists the main additives and their uses.

Preservatives are the most necessary of the additives. Food sellers have a legal duty to the consumer to make sure that food stays uncontaminated up to its 'sell by' or 'best before' date. Most, but not all, preservatives are man-made. They slow the development of bacteria and other micro-organisms that would make food go off and cause food poisoning.

The nitrates and nitrites are preservatives used in meat products, and in Edam, Gouda and some other cheeses – but not in Cheddar, Cheshire or Parmesan. They protect against botulism, a dangerous (often deadly) form of food poisoning. There is concern that we may be getting too much of them because of the multiplicity of sources. Tap water and fresh vegetables may contain more of these substances than processed foods because of residues from agricultural dressings. They are thought to have caused nausea, headaches and dizziness in some sensitive people. In laboratory animals they have produced reactions that could lead to cancer – but only rarely and only after massive doses beyond the possible intake in real life. Vitamin C (from citrus fruits, for example) eaten at the same time as the preservatives gives some protection from their harmful effects.

The labels of some food products reveal their additives, although most additives do not have to be documented.

INGREDIENTS:

Cornflour, Milk Solids, Maltodextrin, Salt, Chicken Fat, Flavouring Agent, Monosodium Glutamate and Colourants (including TARTRAZINE)

410g

Benzoates are preservatives that can cause skin problems, hay fever and asthma. Sulphites can cause problems for asthmatics too. They are added to some frozen seafoods, fish products, fruit and vegetable products, dried fruits and vegetables. You should go for foods in which lactic acid acts as the preservative instead. This is made by fermentation of the sugar occurring in milk. It is the natural preservative in yoghurt and is widely used in cakes and prepared meat dishes.

Some additives aid manufacturing. Antifoaming agents prevent liquids from boiling over or from frothing when they are bottled. Anticaking agents keep fine powders, such as salt, flowing freely. Flour improvers help to make bread rise.

The mineral hydrocarbons are used as glazing agents to seal and give a gloss to fresh citrus fruits, dried fruits and cheese rind. However, they can impede vitamin A, D, E and K absorption and can also cause itchiness of the anus. Cellulose, gums and gels are not harmful but are used to add bulk to foods and allow them to retain more air or water. In this way, they act like dietary fibre.

Antioxidants prevent oils and fats from going rancid and some fruits from going brown when air gets to them. Butylated hydroxyanisole (BHA) and butylated hydroxytoluene (BHT) are synthetic antioxidants used in many breakfast cereals, cheese spreads, margarines, ice-creams, chewing gum and soft drinks. They may trigger hyperactivity in children.

Some of the colour additives can cause problems – for example, hyperactivity – and a host of other disorders: rashes, blurred vision, respiratory problems, asthma and the allergic reaction of people sensitive to aspirin. The azo dyes, derivatives of coal tar, are responsible for many bad reactions. Chief among the suspects is tartrazine, a yellow colouring used in desserts, drinks, sauces and crumb coatings. About half the permitted colours are extracts from natural sources: chlorophyll for green, beetroot for red, and carotene, xanthophylls and turmeric for yellow.

Emulsifiers and stabilisers are added to prevent oil and water from separating. Without them, salad creams, ice-creams, margarine and many made-up dishes would disintegrate into separate liquids and be quite unrecognisable.

Emulsifiers and stabilisers are usually extracts derived from natural foods and include lecithin from egg yolks or soya beans. Carob (or locust) bean gum is another natural extract which is used as an emulsifier and gelling agent. It is also a cocoa substitute commonly used in confectionery and drinks and, unlike cocoa, it contains no caffeine.

How to avoid additives

If you are worried about additives because of controversies about particular dangers or possible long-term cumulative effects, adapt your eating habits to avoid them. Eat more fresh foods and cut out processed ones to reduce your additive intake. Remember that foods without preservatives are more liable to bacterial contamination. Extra care is needed to store and cook them so as to avoid food poisoning.

Learn how to store fresh foods and read your refrigerator handbook again. You may have to spend more time or money, but not necessarily. Extra money spent on freshly grown vegetables can be saved by cutting out cakes, biscuits and prepared dishes.

Time spent on shopping more often for fresh ingredients with a shorter storage life can be recouped by turning to foods that can be eaten raw, so reducing cooking time. Using fresh fish and cheap cuts of meat trimmed of fat costs less than buying made-up dishes, and you can enhance their flavour with spices and fresh herbs.

Apart from fresh meat, fish, fruit and vegetables, you can buy additive-free tinned fruits and vegetables, cereals and biscuits for the store cupboard.

Rice, pulses and pasta are usually additive free, and so are many cheeses and yoghurts. There are also additive-free beefburgers, canned fish and frozen meals on sale.

The growing interest in organic foods and healthy living has made more manufacturers seek alternatives to disputed additives, so a wider range of acceptable goods is available. Retailers, especially the large supermarket chains, are also keen to provide what an increasing number of customers want and to carry lines free of particular categories of additive – sausages free of preservatives, for example.

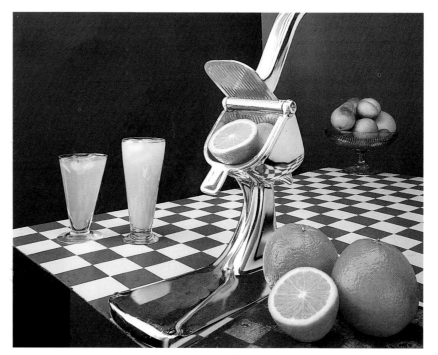

Processed juices and squashes may contain colouring, preservatives, flavourings and artificial sweeteners. To enjoy juice at its freshest and purest, squeeze your own with a hand press – or invest in an electric juicer to deal with hard fruits and vegetables.

The lists of ingredients on processed foods give you another means of avoiding additives. Note down names of substances you want to avoid and take your notes when you go shopping. It will take some time to work out your own list of acceptable goods. In any one visit to a supermarket or store you will probably be able to deal with only one or two types of food. If you shop mostly in one supermarket, find out the company's policy on additives and ask for any booklets they produce, some of which are very useful. But remember, the company's policy may apply only to its own brand-name products.

Identifying the additives – a checklist of those to watch out for

Only a few people have unpleasant reactions to food additives. Most of us never suffer the slightest ill effect. But for the unfortunate few, tracking down and learning how to avoid the offending ingredients can bring welcome relief from alarming asthma attacks or the maddening itch of a skin rash. These are among the worst effects of additives. Although the people affected are few, the symptoms they suffer are numerous and the additives that might trigger them make a long list. Other ill effects include fever, blurred vision, hay fever, stomach upsets, breathlessness, nausea, dizziness, headaches and heart palpitations.

Those people who suffer from allergic reactions to certain foodstuffs have defects in their metabolism – the chemical and physical processes within the body, whereby food constituents are broken down to produce energy, and complex substances are built up to form tissues and organs. The defects make them allergic or intolerant to minute amounts of food additives which are no problem to the vast majority with normal metabolism.

Listed on the next two pages are the additives that are commonly suspected of causing various ill effects in sensitive people, and typical foods they are used in.

ADDITIVE	FUNCTION AND USES
ACIDIFYING AGENTS	
Acetic acid (vinegar), Citric acid (lemon juice), Malic acid (apples), Calcium hydroxide, Potassium carbonate, Calcium lactate	Used to control taste, for example the flavour of cooldrinks, jellies and sweets.
ANTICAKING AGENTS	
Magnesium carbonate, Sodium ferrocyanide, Silicon dioxide	Prevent powder from clumping and food from sticking to bags. Used in most dry powders as well as in crisps.
ANTIOXIDANTS	
Butylated hydroxytoluene (BHT), Butylated hydroxyanisole, (BHA) Tertiary-butyl-hydroxy-quinone (TBHQ)	Prevent food from spoiling when in contact with the oxygen in the air, and thus prevent fatty foods such as crisps from going rancid. Also used in biscuits, sweets, breakfast cereals, ice-creams, soft drinks and prepared fried foods.
L-ascorbic acid (Vitamin C)	Used as an antioxidant in fruit products, soft drinks, dried potatoes and beer.
BLEACHING AGENTS	
Chlorine	Used as a bleach in white flour and so found in bread, cakes and biscuits.
Chlorine dioxide	Used in the same way as chlorine and also to purify water.
Potassium bromate	Used to bleach flour and so found in bread, cakes and biscuits.
COLORANTS: NATURAL COLOURING	
Annatto	Widely used in dairy products, such as butter, cheese and margarine, to give a yellow or orange/red colour.
Anthocynanin	Gives the red or blue colour to foods with strawberry and blackcurrant flavouring, such as jellies, dairy products, cooldrinks, confectionaries and soups.
Beetroot red	Used in jams, jellies, sauces and soups.
Caramel	Used in breadcrumbs, meat analogues, confectionary, wines and spirits.
Carotene	Orange/yellow colour from carrots and pumpkin. Used in bread spreads, baked goods and cooldrinks.
Chlorophyll	Colours food green and comes from leaves. Used in chewing gum, ice-cream and soups.
Cochineal	Used in pie fillings, biscuit creams, icings and bakery products.

ADDITIVE	FUNCTION AND USES
Curcumin	Golden colour used in savoury rice, processed cheese, fish fingers and curry powders.
Flavones	Yellow colour, used in fish fingers, breaded chicken pieces, sauces and preserves.
Riboflavin	Colours food yellow and occurs naturally as vitamin B_2. Used in milk products, processed cheese and sauces.
COLORANTS: SYNTHETIC COLOURING	
Azo dyes include:	
Tartrazine	Used in yellow/red/green foods, from soft drinks and biscuits to sauces and sweets.
Carmoisine	This red/purple colour can be added to raspberry and chocolate-flavoured desserts, jam, bottled sauce and various breaded meat products.
Ponceau 4R	Red hue used to give colour to tinned strawberries, jam, jelly, ice-cream, tomato soup and cheesecake mix.
Green S	Used to make tinned peas green; also added to asparagus soup, lemon or lime drinks, jellies and mint sauce.
Coaltar dyes include:	
Erythrosine	Gives a cherry pink-to-red colour to tinned strawberries, packet trifle, stuffed olives, some processed meats and biscuits.
Patent blue V	This dark blue-violet colour is used to deepen shades in such foods as Scotch eggs.
Quinoline yellow	Used in Scotch eggs and smoked haddock.
EMULSIFIERS AND STABILISERS	
Agar	Thickener and stabiliser used in ice-creams, frozen trifles and meat glazes.
Carrageenan	This emulsifier, thickener and gelling agent which is extracted from seaweed, is used in desserts such as ice-creams, jellies and frozen trifles, as well as spray creams, cake decorations and cheeses.
Tragacanth	Emulsifier, thickener and stabiliser extracted from the gum in the trunks of certain trees. Used in processed cheeses, cake decorations, sherbet and salad dressings.
Gum arabic	Thickener, emulsifier and stabiliser from the gum exuded by the branches of some acacia trees. Used in some packet cream cheeses.
Mannitol	Texture improver and sweetener extracted from seaweed and certain ash trees. Used in sweets and ice-creams.
Polyoxyethylene (8) stearate Polyoxyethylene stearate	Emulsifiers and stabilisers used in baked goods.

ADDITIVE	FUNCTION AND USES
FLAVOUR MODIFIERS/ENHANCERS	
Potassium chloride	Salt substitute and gelling agent.
Ammonium chloride	Used for flavour in yeast goods.
Monosodium glutamate (MSG) Monopotassium glutamate	Usually extracted from sugar beet but also occurs in seaweed. Used as flavour enhancer in meats, soups, savoury snacks and many prepacked meals.
Calcium glutamate	Used in the same way as monosodium glutamate.
Sodium guanylate Sodium inosinate Sodium-5-ribonucleotide	Flavour enhancer used in savoury snacks, packet soups, gravy granules and precooked rice dishes.
FLOCCULATING AGENTS	
Aluminium sulphate	Used to absorb solid particles which would discolour vegetable oil or cause an 'off' flavour.
PRESERVATIVES	
Sorbic acid	Preservative to slow the growth of moulds and yeasts. Used in yoghurts, cheese products, wrapped cakes, cake fillings and toppings, sweet sauces, soft drinks and frozen pizzas.
Benzoic acid	Preservative that occurs naturally in tea and raspberries but is made synthetically for use in fruit products, pickles, marinated fish, salad dressings, beer and coffee essence. Also used as an antioxidant.

ADDITIVE	FUNCTION AND USES
Sodium benzoate	Preservative used in bottled sauces, soft drinks, sweets and prawns.
Potassium benzoate Calcium benzoate Hydroxybenzoate salts	Uses as for benzoic acid.
Sodium hydrogen sulphite	Preservative used in wine and beer. Also used as a bleaching agent.
Sodium meta-bisulphite	Preservative used in sausages and bottled sauces, pickled onions, packet mashed potato and orange squash.
Potassium metabisulphite	Preservative used in home-bottled fruit and homemade wine, and also in brewery beer.
Calcium sulphite	Preservative used in cider.
Calcium hydrogen sulphite	Preservative used in beer.
Potassium nitrite Sodium nitrite	Preservative used in cooked and cured meats and sausages.
Sodium nitrate	Used in the same way as potassium nitrate and also in some cheeses.
Potassium nitrate	Used for curing and preserving meat.
Lactic acid	Preservative which is commonly used in margarines, baby milks, salad dressings, confectionery and soft drinks.

Additives are used as colouring agents, flavour enhancers and preservatives in a wide range of consumer products. These include such items as jams, jellies, sauces and soups, and a whole spectrum of seasonings, tinned fruits and vegetables.

FOOD POISONING

Symptoms of food poisoning are vomiting (see NAUSEA AND VOMITING), DIARRHOEA and cramp-like abdominal pains, which are often worse just before diarrhoea (see COLIC). Victims may also be feverish and sweaty.

The usual cause is germs that inflame the lining of the stomach and intestines. Reheating or only half cooking food encourages the growth of bacteria such as *Salmonella* and *Staphylococcus*, which are among the commonest causes of food poisoning. *Lysteria*, another bacterium, can be caught from soft cheeses and paté, but has little effect on most healthy adults – though unborn children are at risk. *Campylobacter* can be caught from contaminated poultry, fish or unpasteurised milk – and may cause bloody diarrhoea.

Other causes include rotaviruses, which are spread by direct contact with either vomit

or diarrhoea – not necessarily via food. They cause outbreaks of food poisoning in families, schools and at work.

Vomit and diarrhoea contain a lot of water, so the main danger of food poisoning is fluid loss – particularly in babies and the elderly. In any case, consult a doctor if abdominal pain is severe, if the patient is not passing much urine – a sign of dehydration – or if symptoms are severe or prolonged.

What the therapists recommend

Homoeopathy If there is severe diarrhoea resulting from tainted food, particularly meat, *Arsen. alb.* is recommended when there is also vomiting, acute prostration, chilliness and ANXIETY, which is worse between midnight and 2 am. If, after eating bad fish, the flatulence and bloatedness are marked, the patient feels cold and clammy, collapses or needs air, take *Carbo veg.* For upsets from too much, or unripe, fruit, when there is weakness and colic, vomiting and painless diarrhoea, use *China off. Phosphorus* is advisable when there is diarrhoea, vomiting and a craving for iced cold water, which is vomited as soon as it warms in the stomach. In each case, try one tablet of 6th or 30th potency every hour for up to 12 doses.

Herbal Medicine In mild cases, taking three or four GARLIC capsules a day may help to fight infection, while camomile tea three times a day is said to reduce inflammation. Hot spices such as cayenne may help to give protection in tropical countries.

An orthodox view

A sufferer can rest the stomach and intestines by avoiding all solid food, and replace lost fluid by drinking small amounts of water or diluted fruit juice regularly. Recovery is usually complete within a few days.

Drinks of sugar and electrolyte solution such as Rehidrat, available from chemists, help to replace chemicals lost through vomiting and diarrhoea and are particularly effective for children and the elderly or infirm. Anti-diarrhoea medicines, such as kaolin, soothe the stomach and reduce diarrhoea.

FOOT PROBLEMS

Ill-fitting shoes are the cause of the most common foot problems, such as CORNS and BUNIONS. But there are other complaints with various different causes:

Ingrowing toenails These usually affect the big toe and cut into surrounding skin, becoming painful and sometimes infected. Apart from being caused by tight shoes, they can also occur from cutting down the side of

the nail instead of across, so that when the nail grows, skin and nail are competing for the same space.

Flat feet This is a condition that tends to occur in small children and in older people whose ligaments are generally slack. Almost anyone who can bend back their fingers more than average or who is 'double-jointed' will flatten out the arches of the feet when standing. If the feet ache, arch supports worn in shoes might help; otherwise no treatment is necessary.

Verrucas Also known as plantar warts, these are contagious and often picked up in school changing rooms, showers or swimming baths. They are painful warts that grow into the skin of the sole of the foot. They sometimes disappear within 18 months without treatment.

What the therapists recommend

Aromatherapy You should try dabbing undiluted lemon essential oil on a verruca three or four times a day, avoiding the healthy skin.

Hydrotherapy Cold and swollen feet and sprained ankles may benefit from cold baths and ice packs at first, followed by hot ones. Practitioners will advise on treatment and exercises for other disorders such as weak or flat feet, or getting over a FRACTURE.

Massage Try these simple techniques for problems such as tired, aching feet, flat feet and poor circulation or coldness. Hold the foot firmly and with flat fingers or the palm of your hand apply firm effleurage strokes (see p. 225) along the sole of the foot from toes to heel; then use the same techniques across the instep to strengthen the arch. Next, by kneading and friction with the thumbs and fingers, massage the foot muscles with deep upwards pressure to the sole, particularly the instep and inner edge of the foot. Finish off with finger kneading and effleurage to the top of the foot, thorough kneading of the calf muscle, and stretching petrissage to the front lower leg and ankle.

A useful exercise to loosen the joints and flex the big toes of bunion sufferers involves looping a large, thick rubber band across both big toes. Sitting with heels together and legs outstretched, move the feet outwards so that they form a 'V'. Gentle manipulation by a qualified practitioner may also help to relieve other painful conditions.

An orthodox view

For ingrowing toenails practitioners suggest properly fitting shoes and advise that nails should be cut straight across only. Antibiotics would be prescribed in the case of infection and, if severe, part of the base of the nail would be removed, or chemically destroyed, so that the nail would be narrower and therefore less likely to grow into the skin.

Do's and don'ts against food poisoning

Do always wash your hands carefully before handling food, before meals and after using the toilet.

Do keep kitchen work surfaces clean, cook meat thoroughly and don't eat anything which you suspect to be 'off'.

Do keep all waste materials well away from food in firmly lidded bins.

Do cover any cuts or sores on your hands with waterproof sticking plaster when working in the kitchen.

Do wash all your dishes and kitchen utensils thoroughly, being careful to rinse off any detergents.

Do make sure you defrost frozen food – especially meat and meat products – thoroughly before preparing.

Do cook food thoroughly at a high temperature if you are reheating it.

Do make sure your kitchen is well ventilated; extractor fans or carbon filter extractors take out fumes.

Don't handle cooked meat after handling raw meat unless you have washed your hands in between.

Don't keep cooked meat near raw meat – it is a frequent cause of food contamination and poisoning.

Don't leave hot, cooked food in a warm place, such as a cooling cooker – it promotes bacterial growth.

Standard treatment is to pare the dead skin from the surface of a verruca, then destroy it either with salicylic acid in collodion, in ointment or in paint form, or by heat (cauterisation) or cold (cryotherapy).

See also ATHLETE'S FOOT and CHILBLAINS.

FORGETFULNESS

After the age of about 50, many people have difficulty in remembering dates, names, telephone numbers and so on. In some cases, sufferers are unable to recall them at all; in others their MEMORY of them returns after some thought. Forgetfulness should not be confused with AMNESIA, which has physical or emotional causes. See also GROWING OLD.

What the therapists recommend

Autogenic Training This form of therapy, it is claimed, frequently results in a spontaneous improvement in memory. There have been cases of sudden flashes of recall during a session, resulting in articles that were mislaid weeks previously being found.

Hypnotherapy Treatment consists of producing relaxation, then taking the patient back in time and getting him or her to relive the period.

FRACTURES

Cracked or broken bones are usually caused by injury, and are more likely to occur if the bones are thin or porous. For example, elderly women with OSTEOPOROSIS are particularly prone. A bone broken into several pieces is called a comminuted fracture. In a compound fracture there is an open skin wound over the broken bone through which infection may enter.

What the therapists recommend

Cymatics The practitioner holds an instrument called a sound-wave applicator over the site of the fracture. Patients may also use a warm water treatment pool through which sound waves are passed.

Herbal Medicine Comfrey, also known as Knitbone, has long been used to treat fractures. The ointment helps to heal broken bones and tissues. The roots can be pounded into a sticky paste and bound around a fracture. When dry, this paste binds the bone.

An orthodox view

First aid immobilises the broken limb to prevent further damage and relieve pain. If possible, the joints above and below the fracture are supported. The patient can support a fractured arm with the other hand, and a sling provides support for a broken collarbone. The patient should then be taken to hospital immediately. There X-rays will reveal the extent of the fracture so that appropriate treatment can be given.

Practitioners have confirmed that broken bones heal faster if sound waves are applied to the broken limb, and CYMATICS is now used in several orthopaedic units overseas.

FRIGIDITY

Understanding a difficult, personal problem

Men often say of a woman who is sexually unresponsive, 'She's frigid'. It is a derogatory and hurtful term, and is used less and less as understanding of sexual difficulties and their causes increases. The problem is properly called *general sexual dysfunction*. See also SEXUAL PROBLEMS.

Like IMPOTENCE in men, frigidity in women is when sexual excitement fails to occur or does not develop into arousal and responsiveness. The woman feels unresponsive to her sexual partner.

Sexual arousal in women results in an increased blood flow around the vagina, a swelling of the tissues surrounding it, and the production of vaginal lubrication. In frigidity, this lubrication hardly appears or is absent altogether. Production of lubrication is also dependent on an adequate supply of oestrogen, the most common cause of deficiency being the MENOPAUSE.

Psychological factors may also be involved, and they are usually related to conflict or fear about intercourse, or about the particular partner.

The conflict may stem from early sexual abuse, or it may be caused by an insensitive or sexually aggressive man. If a woman tends to feel uncertain about engaging in sex, then her body sends out signals based on the conflict or fear. Even though she feels loving towards her partner, she is unable to let it be expressed in her physical reactions, and frigidity is the distressing result.

What the therapists recommend
BEHAVIOURAL THERAPY
The aim would be to produce an atmosphere in which lovemaking is relaxed and enjoyable. Sexual contact is withdrawn, then progressively reintroduced, perhaps over a couple of weeks. This may start with an embrace, then kissing, caressing, oral stimulation and, finally, intercourse.

Contact may gradually become more intimate, moving from the face to the neck, shoulders, back, thighs, breasts and finally the vagina. When each stage has been mutually enjoyed, then the partners move onto the next one.

AROMATHERAPY
Self help Several oils have been found helpful. One of the best ways of employing them is for the partners to give each other a relaxing back massage as an introduction to lovemaking, using jasmine, ylang-ylang, and clary sage.

Another way is to sprinkle a few drops of the oils on kitchen tissue and place it in the bed, just on and below (but not under) the pillow about an hour before retiring. It is also an excellent idea to use the oils in a room burner, in both the bedroom and rooms used before retiring.

Other alternative treatments

Acupuncture The aim of treatment is to remedy any hormonal imbalance and mental and emotional conflicts. The best results occur when acupuncture is combined with dietary changes and homoeopathic or herbal remedies. MOXIBUSTION can be applied to points governing the kidney, bladder, stomach and conception meridians.

Bach Remedies The following are recommended: Crab apple for feelings of disgust with the body; Impatiens for impatience with oneself; Rock water for those who have repressive Victorian attitudes to sex and find it hard to relax; Pine for feelings of guilt and shame; Mimulus for fear of being rejected because of frigidity, and fear of physicality in general; Honeysuckle for those who idealise the past and cannot appreciate the present; Star of Bethlehem for shock; Rock rose for intense fear; and Holly for anger.

An orthodox view

A doctor will investigate and treat any physical conditions that are inhibiting or are likely to inhibit sexual arousal and response, such as vaginal dryness or pain during intercourse. He may, for instance, prescribe hormone replacement therapy (HRT; see p. 238) for vaginal dryness at the menopause.

A doctor will help a woman experiencing mental conflict about intercourse or her partner to work out for herself the nature of the conflict(s), and what she is going to do about the situation.

He may also refer her to a specific therapist, who may give behaviourally based treatments. In non-threatening circumstances, the senses are encouraged to respond sexually, so that arousal takes place and not only becomes a pleasure, but also acts as an inhibitor of fear.

FROSTBITE

South Africa is generally regarded as a hot country, but there are parts of the country that get extremely cold in winter. Ice crystals form in the body tissues when their temperature falls to about -5°C (23°F). They damage the tissues, restrict blood circulation, and eventually cause blood clotting. Without immediate treatment the frozen tissue will die, causing gangrene, and amputation may become necessary.

Good circulation and warm clothing usually keep body temperature above such a level, but areas of bare skin are at risk, and if circulation is impeded, body temperature may fall dangerously low (see HYPOTHERMIA).

Susceptibility to frostbite can be increased by an injury with bleeding and SHOCK, over-exertion that causes fatigue or dehydration, clogged arteries or beta-blocker drugs (see ARTERIES [HARDENING]; HEART DISORDERS). Take special care if prone to CHILBLAINS.

Fingers, toes and the face – especially the nose and ears – are most likely to be affected. Frostbitten parts first feel cold and stiff, and prickle slightly. Then the skin goes hard and white, later turning blue. Soon it becomes numb and the victim feels neither cold nor pain – a dangerous stage.

To prevent frostbite, wear several layers of light, warm, loose clothing with a waterproof and windproof layer on top. Make sure socks, boots and gloves are not tight. Protect ears with muffs, keep your head warmly covered and wear a face mask. Do not go out in unusually severe weather unless it is essential, and do not risk getting stranded.

What the therapists recommend

Traditional Medicine For the early phase of minor frostbite apply slices of peeled cucumber dipped in warm water, slices of raw onion, or cold salted mashed potato.

Naturopathy Therapists aim to improve the circulation by regular EXERCISE, friction rubs, and making sure hands and feet are warmly wrapped in cold weather. It can help to bathe the feet in warm water for two to three minutes, then in cold water for 30 seconds, dry them thoroughly and put on warm, dry socks. People susceptible to chilblains may be prescribed vitamins E and C.

An orthodox view

Once frostbite has set in, swift treatment is essential. Both alternative and conventional first aid aims to restore circulation quickly but gently with indirect warmth. When this is achieved, the frostbitten area often blisters. Reddish blisters reaching to the tip of the area are a good sign of returning circulation – but the area may be left scarred and numb because of damaged nerves.

Do's and don'ts for frostbite

Do take immediate first aid measures if medical help is not within immediate call, or while waiting for it to arrive.

Do seek shelter, in a hut, car, sleeping bag or plastic survival bag. Remove any wet clothing from the affected part, and anything that can slow its circulation – gloves, rings, wristwatch, boots, socks.

Do warm the damaged area gently by placing a warm hand on it or tucking it into your (or a companion's) armpit. Do not squeeze or rub it. Do not heat it by a fire or radiator, or with hot water.

Do bathe or soak the area in water at blood heat, if available – just comfortably warm to your elbow.

Do cover the area loosely with a clean cloth and then a light rug or sweater, once feeling and normal colour return, showing that the circulation is restored.

Do get medical help quickly to prevent infection, and to deal with any blistered and scabbed skin.

Don't touch a hot mug with frostbitten fingers (although warm drinks may improve circulation), or let hot steam reach a frostbitten face.

Don't drink alcohol or anything that can make you less alert.

Don't walk about. If possible keep the frostbitten part above chest level. Lie down and prop up affected legs or feet.

Don't burst, or put any lotion on blood blisters that develop during thawing.

FROZEN SHOULDER

Reaching up to brush your hair, fastening a zip at the back of a skirt, or taking a wallet from a hip pocket can be agony – even impossible – if you have a frozen shoulder. The condition usually starts with inflammation of the tendons that move the shoulder joint, or inflammation of the fibrous capsule of the joint, or swelling of the soft sac that cushions the joint (see BURSITIS).

The shoulder joint has an unusually wide range of movements because of its complicated mesh of muscles and bone. This and its almost constant use make the shoulder vulnerable to damage and slow to mend.

If you avoid using the shoulder because of discomfort, it may become stiff and even more painful to use. If it is not treated, the pain and stiffness may spread to the neck and upper arm, making lying down so uncomfortable that sleepless nights result.

The pain will ease after some months, but by then scarring of the joint capsule and prolonged immobility may mean that the full range of shoulder movements never returns.

What the therapists recommend
ACUPRESSURE
Self help The shoulder must be properly treated before stiffness develops. Apply pressure as in the illustrations on the opposite page. You may find this pressure to be uncomfortable at first but it should soon induce numbness.

In addition, press downwards midway down the front of the fibula (outer bone of the lower leg), then downwards midway down the back of the tibia (shinbone). Use a fingernail or a matchstick to stimulate the outer rim of the ear just above the point where the rim rises out of the lobe.

Other alternative treatments

Chiropractic Treatment is given after an examination and probably an X-ray. In the acute, very painful stage, gentle manipulation will be applied. In many cases, there is a spinal neck lesion contributing to the problem and treatment of this may help considerably. In the later stages, when stiffness and restricted movement are the main symptoms, chiropractic manipulation may shorten recovery time significantly.

Herbal Medicine Gently exercise the joint to stimulate the circulation. Avoid possible build-up of deposits in the joint by cutting out acid fruits, white sugar, alcohol, tea and coffee. Eat plenty of celery.

Aromatherapy Take hot baths with ten drops of essential oil of rosemary or pine added, or rub the shoulder gently with warmed oil of thyme or rosemary.

Homoeopathy Try Rhus tox. if the pain lessens with continued movement of the shoulder, and Bryonia if it increases.

An orthodox view

Keeping the joint moving is the main aim in conventional medicine, so physiotherapy will be recommended. If the shoulder is very painful, manipulation under anaesthetic or a steroid injection into the inflamed tendon or joint capsule may be preferred. Infrared heat treatment, painkillers and anti-inflammatory drugs will ease discomfort and allow more use of the shoulder.

Your doctor may diagnose calcium deposits in one of the tendons and advise surgical removal.

See also HYDROTHERAPY

FUNCTIONAL INTEGRATION

This is one of the two methods used in the FELDENKRAIS METHOD for retraining muscles in the body to work properly. It involves gentle manipulation of muscles that have been injured or do not work because of either brain or spinal damage. A trained therapist uses the technique, which is aimed at introducing new brain patterns in the recipient and with them, new habits of moving his or her muscles.

FUNGAL INFECTIONS
Keeping them at bay

The warm, moist areas of the body, such as the armpits, groin and beneath the breasts are ideal places for fungi to grow, and there they cause RINGWORM. If between the toes, it is called ATHLETE'S FOOT, and if in the groin, dhobie itch. Ringworm of the scalp (*Tinea capitis*) is most common in children, and there is also a variety that affects the fingernails and toenails. Thrush is a fungal infection of the mouth or genital area. Some diabetics are prone to ringworm when there is more sugar in the system to feed the fungi.

Ringworm infections are highly contagious, and can be caught from cattle or pets. They occur as raised, inflamed patches with a definite ring around the edge – hence the name – and glow under ultraviolet light.

What the therapists recommend

Naturopathy Excluding white bread, cakes, biscuits, sweets and other refined sugars and starches, as well as alcohol, from your diet may help, since yeasts and fungi tend to thrive on these foods. You should seek qualified help to increase resistance to recurring infections.

Homoeopathy Recurrent infections are treated by boosting the IMMUNE SYSTEM. For ringworm, particularly on the scalp, *Sulphur* may help, or *Tellurium* if it is on the trunk only. Treat brittle, painful and inflamed nails with *Graphites* four times a day for three weeks. If the skin at the base of the nail is red and inflamed, try *Thuja*, and if there is brittleness with horny thickening, *Antim. tart.* Try *Ranunculus scleratus* three times a day for three weeks for athlete's foot.

Herbal Medicine Thrush in the mouth may be helped by gargling several times a day with tincture of myrrh. For all fungal skin infections, try three or four GARLIC capsules a day or one clove of fresh garlic. Apply tea tree essential oil to the area several times a day. For recurring infections, seek treatment by a qualified practitioner to strengthen the immune system.

An orthodox view

Fungal infections can be slow to go and may recur. Antifungal ointments usually help, and antifungal powders are of particular benefit in moist areas. Hydrocortisone creams relieve itching, but can cause the fungus to spread. All are available from chemists without prescription. Sometimes antifungal tablets such as griseofulvin are prescribed.

Acupressure for a frozen shoulder

Allow 20 minutes daily for these treatments plus those given in the text. Use thumb or fingers to apply strong, deep pressure in the direction shown for two to three minutes at each point.

Press upwards at the top and front of the humerus – upper arm bone – (above), and then at its back and top where it engages with the shoulder blade (above right).

Press upwards at the innermost point of the elbow joint (left).

Press downwards midway between neck and shoulder, on the ridge above the collarbone.

Do's and don'ts for fungal infections

Do shower or bath at least once a day, and dry thoroughly. Wash feet twice a day, and pat dry, never rub.

Do keep your towels and face cloths separate from those of the rest of the household.

Do wear cotton socks and underwear, and change them frequently.

Do wear leather shoes, not trainers as they encourage sweating.

Don't machine-wash linen and clothes at low temperatures; the fungus could survive and infect the whole load.

Do wear slops or takkies to protect your feet when using facilities in public bathing or showering places.

GALLSTONES

Small, hard, coloured pebbles known as gall-stones form from liquid bile in the gall bladder, or in the bile ducts, which drain bile from the liver. These ducts join the duct from the gall bladder to form the common bile duct, which carries the liquid to the small intestine, where it is essential for fat digestion.

Sometimes a stone gets stuck in a duct and causes biliary colic – severe pain in the upper abdomen which may radiate into the back. Blockage of the common bile duct causes jaundice.

If the gall bladder becomes inflamed, fever with pain in the upper abdomen and tenderness under the ribs on the right side may result. Occasionally gallstones block the flow of fluids from the pancreas, again causing inflammation and pain.

Warning Gallstones are only one of many possible causes of severe abdominal pain. If such pain persists for more than four hours, see your doctor immediately. Do not follow alternative remedies without his approval.

What the therapists recommend

Acupuncture After determining the cause of the symptoms by questioning and examination, the practitioner stimulates points on the liver, stomach, bladder, gall bladder, spleen and conception meridians.

Herbal Medicine Bitter herbs are used, aimed at encouraging the flow of bile and reducing any inflammation of the gall bladder. Herbalists have a number of remedies to choose from, depending on the exact nature of the problem; marshmallow root, gentian, barberry bark, boldo, golden seal and dandelion are typical examples, taken as tinctures. Since some liver and gall-bladder stimulants may also stimulate the muscles of the uterus, pregnant women should always seek medical advice before using any of them.

Naturopathy A very low fat diet with no dairy products and no animal fats is advised, along with plenty of fresh vegetables and whole grains. Increased intake of polyunsaturated oils such as sunflower and safflower is also recommended, with extra vitamin C aimed at reducing cholesterol levels in the bile. Fresh lemon juice is held to be particularly beneficial, also bitter salads such as chicory, endive and globe artichoke.

An orthodox view

Small gallstones sometimes disappear without treatment; they simply enter the intestine and pass out of the body with the faeces. Others remain in the gall bladder for years, causing neither harm nor pain.

Stones that do cause pain or inflammation are removed surgically, together with the gall bladder. Occasionally small stones – particularly those that are difficult to see on X-rays – can be dissolved by drugs. In some hospitals the stones are broken up by sound waves.

GALVANISM

In this early form of ELECTROTHERAPY, direct electric current (rather than alternating current) is passed through the body by way of electrodes attached to the skin. It was once widely used to treat SPORTS INJURIES such as sprains, strains and contusions, the aim being to improve circulation in affected parts and reduce inflammation. It was named after the 18th-century Italian anatomist, Luigi Galvani, who discovered that a severed frog's leg twitches when an electric current is passed through it.

GARLIC

The oldest herbal cure-all?

Without doubt, garlic is the herbalists' and naturopaths' favourite remedy – and has been used medically for something like 5 000 years. It is regarded – with some scientific and medical approval – as one of the most versatile and effective plants in the entire herbal cornucopia.

Variously known as *Allium sativum* (its botanical name), 'poor man's treacle' and – to the ancient Greeks – the 'stinking rose', garlic is a member of the same group of plants as the onion, chive and leek.

The list of ailments for which garlic has been prescribed – as an oil, in soups or inhalants, eaten raw, crushed and applied to affected parts or, more recently, taken in tablet or capsule form – is extensive. Complaints treated range from ACNE, ASTHMA and ARTHRITIS to high BLOOD PRESSURE, various BOWEL DISORDERS, BRONCHITIS, DIGESTIVE PROBLEMS, KIDNEY COMPLAINTS, RHEUMATISM, insect stings, TENSION, toothache, tuberculosis, warts (see WARTS AND WART CHARMING), WHOOPING COUGH and WORMS.

Garlic is known to contain the VITAMINS A, B_1, B_2 and C, along with various natural antibiotics, antiblood-clotting agents and cholesterol-controlling ingredients.

Among the many beneficial effects claimed for garlic are: its ability to destroy harmful bacteria (pathogens) in the intestines, without any effect on the natural, beneficial organisms and fungal infections which help digestion; its power to break down cholesterol, the fatty substance which causes furring of the arteries and can lead to HEART DISORDERS; its effectiveness against bacteria which may be unaffected by other antibiotics; its capability for improving resistance to viral infections; and its use as a general preventive against many illnesses, especially those that people suffer in winter, such as COLDS, chills and INFLUENZA, SINUS PROBLEMS and bronchial complaints.

Garlic also apparently has the ability to lower blood pressure. A specialist working at the University of Geneva has claimed that it causes blood vessels to widen, so reducing the pressure inside them.

Home help with garlic

Garlic can be used in numerous ways to protect against, or to treat, many ailments. Here are a few preparations you can make at home:

To ward off colds Take one garlic capsule three times a day on a regular basis to keep you generally fit and healthy.

For coughs and bronchitis An old folk remedy is to make a garlic syrup. Pour 600 ml of boiling water over 60 g of finely chopped garlic. Allow to stand in a sealed container for ten hours. Then add honey until a syrupy consistency is formed. Take a teaspoonful up to three times a day.

For sickness or diarrhoea Two garlic capsules a day are recommended – especially for those going abroad – to protect against stomach upsets caused by change of diet and climate.

For a sore throat or voice loss Try eating a single clove of garlic three times a day.

To reduce blood pressure Take between one and three capsules of garlic three times a day with water. However, make sure that you also seek qualified medical treatment for the condition.

Many people are embarrassed by having the odour of garlic on their breath. Capsules, which dissolve in the stomach and intestines, are less pungent than raw garlic. Another way to reduce the aroma is to chew fresh parsley after eating garlic.

Caution If you are already consulting a general practitioner, always seek his advice, or that of a medical herbalist, before using herbal alternatives.

A herbal of 1385 shows the cultivation of garlic, which had been used for centuries. Clay models of garlic bulbs were found in an Egyptian tomb of 3750 BC, and when their garlic ration was cut, slaves building the Great Pyramid are believed to have gone on strike in the world's first industrial dispute.

GEM ESSENCE THERAPY

Stone vibrations that care for the emotions

Physical, emotional and spiritual well-being can all be helped by this therapy, according to its practitioners, who believe that it strengthens and speeds up other, more conventional treatments. Naturally occurring crystals – which include precious and semi-precious stones – are thought to contain 'positive energy', which can be channelled through healer to sufferer.

The various techniques include contact healing (in which the crystals are placed on body parts in need of treatment), and pressure-point healing (in which the crystals are placed on relevant ACUPUNCTURE points). Or the sufferer is simply asked to wear the gemstone prescribed for his ailment.

A wide variety of stones is used. For example, rock crystal is said to reinforce all the body cells and to be particularly useful in treating heart and eye conditions. Aquamarine may be prescribed for throat problems and sinusitis, while tourmaline soothes nerves, and haematite prevents cramps.

In a related – though in South Africa little-used – therapy, bottled essences of gemstones are made by immersing the stones in pure water and leaving them in the sunshine. The sun's energy percolates through the stones into the water, taking the gem's vibrations with it.

The essences are said to be most effective if taken in a relaxed state at least 30 minutes before or after eating. A few drops are poured directly from the bottle into the mouth (under the tongue).

Finding a therapist For names and addresses of practitioners, write to The Wellstead, 1 Wellington Avenue, Wynberg 7800.

An orthodox view

There is as yet no scientific basis to these therapies, and many doctors would regard them as beyond the fringe.

GENITAL HERPES

The virus that causes genital herpes is very closely related to the one that causes COLD SORES. Both are types of *Herpes simplex*. A different herpes virus, *Herpes zoster*, causes CHICKENPOX and SHINGLES.

It is usually *Herpes simplex* Type II that causes genital sores. The virus is caught only by direct contact with active sores. These may be quite visible on the genital area or buttocks. Alternatively, they may be hidden in the vagina or anus. The virus can also be passed from around the mouth to the genital area and vice versa.

After an incubation period of 2-12 days, the infected area feels itchy and prickles. Painful blisters develop which burst and leave ulcers. These usually heal within three weeks, but sufferers may feel feverish or generally unwell during the attack.

After the first ('primary') infection, the virus lies dormant in a nerve root. At times of stress or other illness it may become active again and produce new crops of painful blisters at the original site of infection.

In rare cases, *Herpes simplex* can cause inflammation of the brain. The patient develops severe headaches and confusion and may be very ill.

Self help To avoid infection, do not have sexual intercourse with a partner who has active sores. Use condoms if in any doubt.

If you develop sores, ease the discomfort by sitting in a shallow bath of gently warm water with half a cup of salt added. Try dabbing on witch hazel to dry up the sores – but only if it does not sting too much. Wear loose cotton pants instead of synthetic ones. Do not wear wool against your skin.

To help avoid a flare-up of a dormant virus, ensure that your diet is adequate in VITAMINS A, B and C. Get enough rest, and start YOGA or RELAXATION AND BREATHING exercises to reduce stress.

What the therapists recommend

Naturopathy Naturopaths consider that outbreaks of dormant genital herpes are triggered by a lowering of vitality. Naturopathic advice is aimed at correcting this imbalance. The amino acid L-lysine seems to help reduce an attack, and may be supplemented with vitamin B to support the IMMUNE SYSTEM. Lysine is found in lamb, chicken, fish, cheese, milk, brewer's yeast, beans and beansprouts, as well as in most fruits and vegetables. Salt washes or baths can reduce the irritation.

Aromatherapy Try a mixture of eucalyptus, thyme and geranium in the bath, and apply a lotion made from three drops of each of these oils in a tablespoon of carrier lotion.

An orthodox view

Doctors endorse the self-help preventive measures outlined above. They may prescribe anti-viral drugs such as acyclovir to clear up an attack. While these drugs can be effective during the primary infection, they are not able to prevent further attacks and are less effective during them.

GEOPATHIC STRESS

How the earth's energy may affect your health

Electromagnetic fields and other forms of radiation from the earth are believed by some practitioners – both orthodox and alternative – to have potentially stressful and unhealthy effects on people. This is called 'geopathic stress' and may contribute to illnesses ranging from INSOMNIA and MIGRAINE to RHEUMATISM and CANCER.

The idea that physical and geological features can affect people's health and well-being is not new. The Chinese have long practised *Feng-Shui* – a way of positioning objects and structures such as houses, furnishings, roads and wells so that they are in harmony with what is seen as the natural flow of energy in the earth. Some people in the West believe that prehistoric standing stones such as those at Stonehenge and elsewhere in Britain were placed to protect dwellings from lines of geopathic stress. Many different factors are thought to cause geopathic stress. Among those considered important are so-called 'ley lines' – lines of energy that are said to correspond to underground streams of water or small electrical currents produced by pressure on quartz crystals in the ground. Man-made structures such as railways, overhead power cables, large buildings and quarries may all interrupt the natural pattern of ley lines and cause further geopathic stress.

Another factor is the effect of magnetic storms on the surface of the sun – 'sunspots'. When sunspots are particularly active, they disturb the earth's magnetic field and these periods also appear to coincide with human disasters such as wars and famines. Heart attacks, too, are said to become more common during sunspot activity.

Certain minerals and rocks such as granite contain radioactive substances or release radioactive radon gas which can cause illnesses such as lung cancer. In the USA, some houses have had to be vacated where they were found to have high levels of radon gas, probably caused by using concrete which contained radioactive material which released radon.

Generally, geopathic stress is thought to affect city dwellers less than people in country areas, where there are fewer people to 'soak up' earth radiation. It is also said to be stronger inside buildings than outside, since electrical wiring systems can enhance the effect of other electromagnetic fields. This may be the reason why people sometimes feel better outside their homes than inside.

The most serious danger of geopathic stress is believed to be its weakening effect on the IMMUNE SYSTEM, which increases vulnerability to disorders such as cancer, MYALGIC ENCEPHALOMYELITIS (ME), ARTHRITIS, INSOMNIA, migraine, MULTIPLE SCLEROSIS, LEUKAEMIA and AIDS. Many alternative practitioners also believe that geopathic stress can contribute to problems such as DEPRESSION, high BLOOD PRESSURE and ALCOHOLISM. In addition, certain types of geopathic stress have been associated with particular effects: underground water may disturb sleep, while strong electromagnetic fields have been related to higher rates of suicide and leukaemia. Sharply increasing or decreasing fields – such as are found close to overhead power lines – have been associated with migraine and depression.

What the therapists recommend

If a practitioner – of any sort – suspects that a patient's problems are caused by geopathic stress, he will probably call in a trained dowser (see DOWSING). Alternatively, the practitioner may use electronic equipment to examine the sick person's home.

Dowsers are thought to be particularly sensitive people who can detect small changes in the earth's magnetic field – whether caused by ley lines, underground water, sunspots or other factors – by holding a willow or hazel twig, dowser's rod or a pendulum over a suspected stress zone. Depending on how the instrument responds, the dowser is able to say where the energy lines are strongest.

This is thought to work because the twig, rod or pendulum exaggerates small muscle reactions caused by the field in the dowser's body, and makes them observable. Dowsers say that they can tell the difference between healthy and harmful energy lines, and some even claim to alter them by using objects such as crystals and electrical coils.

The first spot that is checked for geopathic stress is over a patient's bed, since vulnerability is thought to be greatest during sleep. A picture is drawn up of the field around the bed and, if necessary, the patient is advised to change its position or even move to another bedroom.

Sometimes simply switching to a foam rubber mattress or one without metal springs is enough – mattress springs are thought to reinforce the strength of electromagnetic fields in the bed.

Other parts of the house are also checked if necessary, and dowsers will offer advice on how to reduce geopathic stress in areas where electromagnetic fields are found to be strong. An IONISATION machine in the room is also believed to help.

An orthodox view

Although most conventional doctors still reject the idea that geopathic stress can cause illness, it has gained support in Germany, where research is being done into its connection with cancer and accident 'black spots'. Cancer specialists have known for years of certain 'cancer houses' where the disease occurs much more frequently than usual, and some think that geopathic stress may offer an explanation. On the other hand, other environmental factors, which have not yet been identified, may also be implicated.

Signs of geopathic stress

The history of a house and its particular location are said to be a guide to levels of stress within it. Homes that change hands frequently are believed to stand on stressful sites, while those in more tranquil spots tend to have occupants who stay for many years.

Stunted or deformed trees may indicate the existence of stress zones, and roses, celery, onions and corn are said not to do well. Also held to be badly affected are apple, pear, ash and nut trees; while oaks and firs, plum and cherry trees appear to do well. Asparagus, mushrooms, mistletoe and some medicinal herbs are also said to thrive in these areas.

Animals are also said to provide a clue: horses, dogs, cows, sheep, pigs and mice are believed to be unwilling to settle in areas of geopathic stress, but cats, ants, wasps, beetles and termites – as well as viruses and bacteria – are thought to do well.

Intuitive feelings and the different parts of a house you are drawn to or wish to avoid are also considered a guide to geopathic stress. It is said that four out of five people are sensitive enough to learn how to dowse – at least for water – but short of this, even ordinary feelings are believed to be an accurate indication.

GESTALT THERAPY
Doing your own thing

A way of promoting personal growth through self-awareness, similar to but gentler than ENCOUNTER GROUPS, was developed by Friedrich (Fritz) Perls (1893-1970). The former Berlin psychoanalyst was practising in America after the Second World War when he worked out his Gestalt therapy. It is based on the view that a person's ideas, feelings and actions are related aspects of his whole personality. (Gestalt comes from a German word meaning an organised whole.)

Gestalt therapists generally argue that if someone's response to any event is not experienced by all aspects of their personality, that experience is incomplete and inner conflict results, which in turn causes distorted behaviour patterns.

Blocking out one aspect of your responses may have been learned in childhood – perhaps to please an adult – but may eventually leave your inner needs unsatisfied.

Gestalt therapy tries to remedy a distorted way of responding by teaching you not to analyse your past, as other psychotherapies may do, but to be aware immediately of thoughts, feelings, actions and gestures aroused by what is happening around you.

The aim of Gestalt therapy is to become fully aware of yourself, so that you see your life clearly, realise what you want from it, appreciate your own worth and feel free to be yourself.

Perls summed up his theory as: 'I do my thing, and you do your thing. I am not in this world to live up to your expectations and you are not in this world to live up to mine. You are you and I am I.'

Who it can help People who suffer from ANXIETY and TENSION, or who spend too much time explaining and judging what they have done, can benefit. Gestalt can also help those who repeatedly have difficulties in getting on with other people or in forming close relationships.

Finding a therapist For a list of therapists, contact the T A Gestalt Therapy Institute of South Africa, c/o Professor Diana Schmukler, Psychology Department, University of the Witwatersrand, 1 Jan Smuts Avenue, Johannesburg 2001. Therapists can train here on a yearly basis. Prospective therapists must have an appropriate professional qualification (for example, in psychology or social work), and be registered with the South African Medical and Dental Council.

The period of therapy is discussed before weekly sessions start. It is usually a few months, but some people choose to continue treatment for longer. Group therapy and marital therapy are also available.

Consulting a therapist Most therapists use whatever means they think best for helping people to self-knowledge. MOVEMENT, ART THERAPY and BIOENERGETICS may play a part. Sessions may be on a one-to-one basis with the therapist in private; in a group using special self-awareness exercises; or in groups working in pairs.

Early exercises may include focusing on your opposite number's hands and feet and then describing exactly what you notice.

An orthodox view

With a skilled therapist, individuals who seek personal growth will come to no harm. However, relationships with others do not invariably improve since the emphasis is on being more aware and demanding of life – and this may work against forming safe and stable relationships.

See also HUMANISTIC PSYCHOLOGY.

GINGIVITIS

The gums are known as the gingivae, and gingivitis is inflammation of the gums caused by dental plaque – a layer of bacteria and other organic matter that forms on a tooth, usually at the neck, where it narrows into the root. Regular brushing – particularly after meals – and use of dental floss help to prevent plaque. But if untreated, it leads to dental caries (decay) and periodontitis, which loosens the teeth, and is probably a greater cause of tooth loss than decay itself. See TOOTH AND GUM DISORDERS.

GINSENG

For some 5 000 years, the Chinese and Koreans have used the root of the ginseng plant – and credited it with many beneficial effects. The botanical name of this Asian variety – *Panax ginseng* – derives from the Greek word *panacea*, meaning 'all-healing', but it is largely regarded as a supplement and all-round tonic as well as a curative.

The plant belongs to the Araliaceae family, which includes ivy and American spikenard. It is cultivated in China, Korea and other parts of eastern Asia in damp, cool, wooded soil, rich in humus.

Ginseng is generally claimed to relieve such physical problems as HEADACHES, TIREDNESS, EXHAUSTION and AMNESIA, to slow down the ageing process (see GROWING OLD), and to be a complementary aid in the treatment of various HEART DISORDERS, DIABETES, tuberculosis, KIDNEY COMPLAINTS, NERVOUS DISORDERS and CIRCULATION PROBLEMS.

The root has also been held to have aphrodisiac properties, particularly in the East (see APHRODISIACS), but most practitioners now feel that any such effects are a natural result of its inherent tonic value. In any case it is relatively harmless, but is believed to help the body regain normality if stress or damage strikes.

Active constituents Ginseng contains so many different ingredients that researchers have found difficulty in determining which ones, or what combinations of them, are responsible for the effects attributed to it.

Some of the main constituents and what they are thought to do include: various oils, such as sapogenin and panacen, that are believed to stimulate the central nervous system; a group called the saponin glycosides – plant substances that break down to produce sugars, and known as ginsenosides to the Japanese and panaxosides to the Russians – that are believed to influence the IMMUNE SYSTEM, increasing resistance to infection, to reduce blood clotting, and help to balance the body's internal systems; panaxans – chemically called steroidal glucosides – that reduce blood sugar levels; and various plant phenols, in particular maltol, believed to help to protect the tissues, possibly reducing damage caused by ageing.

In addition, ginseng contains a range of hormones, VITAMINS (B_1, B_2 and D) and other substances, all of which are believed to com-

Ginseng is usually available to consumers in Western health food shops and in some pharmacies in various forms: as a root to be chewed, in powdered form in tablets or capsules, or as loose powder or extracts to be made into decoctions or herbal teas.

Ginseng tablets

Ginseng tea

Ginseng extract

Ginseng tea powder

Ginseng powder

Dried ginseng root

Ginseng extract powder

Ginseng capsules

Sliced ginseng

bine with the above ingredients to result in the complicated overall effect.

Using ginseng Opinions vary among herbalists and those who take ginseng as to which type is most beneficial. Apart from the Asian variety, there is also an American type (*Panax quinquefolium*), and a root called *pfaffia*, which is known as Brazilian ginseng.

Herbalists suggest different doses, depending on the patient's general condition. However, the usual recommendation for those taking a month's course, simply as a tonic to improve their general well-being, is 60 mg of the powdered root each day, taken as tablets, capsules or decoctions.

An orthodox view

Many conventional doctors now accept some of the claims made for ginseng both as an overall tonic and a stimulant.

GLANDULAR FEVER

Children and young adults are most prone to glandular fever, which is caused by a virus infection and is passed on by close contact, such as kissing.

After an incubation period of up to seven weeks, the patient develops a sore throat with white seepage on the tonsils, FEVER and swollen lymph glands in the neck, armpits and groin (see IMMUNE SYSTEM). Sometimes the spleen is enlarged so that a doctor can feel it in the upper left abdomen when the patient takes a deep breath. There may also be a rash similar to that in German measles, and sometimes the liver is affected and the patient develops JAUNDICE. Diagnosis can be confirmed by a blood test.

Once the disease has manifested itself, the patient may be unwell for two to eight weeks or even more.

What the therapists recommend

Naturopathy During the feverish state, herbal infusions of yarrow and elderflower aim at inducing sweating and regulating temperature. A light but nourishing diet is prescribed – home-made soups, for example – until appetite and strength begin to return. High levels of vitamins B and C may also be given, aimed at boosting the immune system and maintaining a healthy nervous system.

Herbal Medicine Infusions of yarrow and elderflower taken three or four times daily are aimed at controlling the fever, inducing sweating and maintaining an even temperature. Afterwards, the common problem of tiredness is tackled with tonics – two or three

cups daily of yarrow or rosemary tea are recommended; also plenty of porridge.

Homoeopathy For a high fever with painful glands, *Belladonna* is prescribed; for a late-developer child with very swollen glands, *Baryta carb.*; and for dark red tonsils, with pain extending to the ears, *Phytolacca*.

Constitutional treatment is advised if the condition drags on. Other members of the family are said to be protected by taking Glandular Fever Nosode (available from homoeopathic pharmacies) daily for a week to ten days.

Biochemic Tissue Salts Practitioners prescribe *Ferr. phos.* hourly in the early stages of fever. If glands are affected, *Kali mur.* is advised – again hourly. If at a low ebb after infection, try *Calc. phos.* three times daily.

An orthodox view

As with most infectious diseases, doctors advise rest, plenty of liquids and a painkiller such as aspirin to relieve discomfort and reduce fever. The liver may be inflamed, so avoid alcohol. Children under 12 should not be given aspirin without advice.

GLAUCOMA

Glaucoma is a serious eye condition in which the pressure of the fluid within the eyeball is abnormally high. This results in pain and blurred vision. There are two principal types. Chronic glaucoma, the commoner form, seldom affects anyone under 40, and it tends to be hereditary. It progresses slowly, the outflow of fluid from the front compartment of the eyeball being gradually blocked, and it is often undetected until blindness is quite far advanced – the characteristic loss of peripheral vision is so slow as not to be noticed.

Acute glaucoma is more sudden. It is caused by a blockage of the drainage channel running around the inside edge of the iris; the blockage is aggravated when the pupil dilates, as it does in darkness and during excitement. Typically the sufferer from acute glaucoma notices rainbow-like rings around lights at night.

Other, rarer glaucomas are caused by eye injury or disease.

What the therapists recommend

Homoeopathy What the therapist prescribes to alleviate chronic glaucoma depends on his broad assessment of the patient's condition.

Naturopathy While acute glaucoma needs immediate specialist treatment (preferably in hospital), the slow-acting chronic variety may be alleviated with daily doses of vitamin

C, which reduces inner-eye pressure. To restore better circulation around the eyeball, the blood needs to be cleansed, and this can be achieved by fasting, followed by a blood-cleansing diet in which Vitamins A, B_2, C and D in their natural forms predominate.

An orthodox view

If your general practitioner suspects chronic glaucoma he will administer eye-drops in an attempt to reduce the pressure within the eye (and to keep the pupil small). Drugs may be prescribed for the same purpose, and also to relieve pain. You will almost certainly be referred to an eye specialist for further treatment; if medication fails to relieve the eye pressure, a drainage operation may be necessary.

Acute glaucoma is an emergency, and the patient should be hospitalised, to be treated with eye-drops, drugs and whatever else is needed to relieve the painful condition. A drainage operation known as an 'iridectomy' may have to be performed at the periphery of the iris.

GLUTEN INTOLERANCE

For most people, gluten – a protein found in grains such as wheat, barley and rye – is a nourishing food. But people with a digestive disorder called gluten intolerance cannot absorb such food. See COELIAC DISEASE.

GOITRE

Swelling of the thyroid gland in the front of the neck is known as goitre. It may be caused by insufficient iodine, which the gland needs for the production of hormones. If there is insufficient iodine, less hormones are produced, and the gland swells in an effort to produce more (see THYROID DISORDERS).

GOUT

Contrary to popular belief, gout is not usually caused by overindulgence, although excess alcohol and some medicines, such as diuretics (which encourage urine excretion), increase the risk. It is a disorder of the body chemistry in which too much uric acid and its compounds accumulate in the blood.

Acid and urate crystals collect in one or more joints, causing attacks of severe PAIN, swelling and redness (see ARTHRITIS). The joint at the base of the big toe is often affected. Repeated attacks can damage the bones of the joints. The crystals can also collect in the kidneys, causing kidney stones, kidney failure and high BLOOD PRESSURE, and in the skin where they form hard lumps, most commonly on the ears, fingers and toes. Diagnosis of gout is made by a blood test.

What the therapists recommend

Herbal Medicine Wash the leaf of an arum lily, warm it in hot water and apply it to the gout-affected area for soothing relief. Buchu or camomile tea – or a combination of these two – also relieves gout.

Naturopathy A largely vegetarian diet with plenty of salads is advised to counter excess uric acid production. Red meat, coffee, alcohol and refined carbohydrates such as sugar are particularly to be avoided. During a severe attack cold compresses may help.

Homoeopathy When the pain feels like a bad bruise and the patient is frightened of the affected area being touched, *Arnica* is prescribed; and *Belladonna* when the joint is hot, red, swollen and unbearably tender. *Colchicum* is recommended when pain shifts from joint to joint and the patient is angry and irritable. *Urtica urens* is for intense itching, burning and swelling during a severe attack.

Acupuncture The points on the liver and spleen/pancreas meridians are stimulated.

An orthodox view

The usual treatment of gout is to relieve pain and inflammation by prescribing anti-inflammatory drugs. Further attacks can be prevented by avoiding excess alcohol and medicines that raise the blood urate level. Drugs that increase urate excretion may be prescribed. Allopurinol, also available only on prescription, reduces urate production and the risk of further attacks. It normally has to be taken daily over a period of years.

GRIEF

Coping with the shock of losing loved ones

Our greatest suffering frequently comes with the death of people we love – an experience for which modern society gives us little training. Death is not talked about and is rarely witnessed, as the severely ill and the elderly are taken into professional care.

Previous generations saw more of death. Children and adults gathered in the family home at the bedside of aged grandparents, fevered infants, tubercular adolescents and others, as they neared death. The dead person lay at home until the funeral. Rituals of

mourning were observed, with the bereaved wearing black and avoiding company.

Now our first sight of death may be when someone very close dies in a laboratory-like ward. Within days, the normal routines of life are apparently restored, with acquaintances shunning mention of the person who has died and the bereaved often forced to carry on almost as if nothing has happened. Even so, the emotional progress of those who are bereaved follows a general pattern which they have to work through before they can face the future.

Obstructing this emotional progress leads to psychological and physical problems. Without a sufficient period of grieving, the survivor of a close partnership can become ill: widows seem to show an increased tendency to develop breast cancer and widowers to have heart attacks.

Self help Do not try to numb yourself to the pain of bereavement by blotting it out with tranquillisers or sleeping pills. Let the process of grieving follow its course, remembering that it may take many months.

Do not be afraid to talk to family and friends about your feelings. Often they avoid mentioning the dead person for fear of upsetting you, but will gladly listen and reminisce when they know this is what you want. You may feel a need to talk again and again about what has happened; perhaps feel guilt for what you did or did not do, and anger at your loss.

Do not let everything from your relationship with the dead person be lost. Remember happy times and shared achievements. Look at photographs and other mementos that remind you of the value of the life that has ended.

Mourning other losses Death is not the only loss that we need to mourn, although it is likely to be the greatest. Women who have had a miscarriage, stillbirth, hysterectomy or mastectomy suffer a deep feeling of loss. Equally a person who loses a limb may be stricken by the loss. Being made redundant or uprooted – even evicted – from one's home can cause similar feelings.

Getting help Coming to terms with the permanence of loss is at the heart of grieving. COUNSELLING can play a significant role here, offering a sympathetic ear and time to listen. You have an opportunity to recount what has happened and how you feel, over and over if necessary, without worrying whether you are imposing on a friend, and without the counsellor showing impatience or losing interest.

Gentle questioning may lead you to explore feelings you find hard to acknowledge. The general pattern of emotions that develops when people are grieving is familiar to counsellors. Denial of the death is a typical first reaction – 'I can't believe it; it's not true!'

Usually this stage passes quickly, but sometimes it is prolonged.

Often the next stage is anger – perhaps directed against a doctor for not working miracles, against relatives for still being alive, or against the dead person for taking risks or deserting you.

Some people are spurred to raise funds or agitate for laws or safety devices that would prevent similar deaths. Such hectic activity helps to pass the time but also staves off the essential painful stage of sadness and depression, where the extent of loss is acknowledged and accepted. This stage has to be worked through before normal zest for life begins to return.

The many organisations that offer counselling for the bereaved include: Compassionate Friends Support Group, whose head office at P O Box 29182, Sandringham 2131 (telephone 011-7284451 or 7283723) will supply addresses of branches in other centres; Widows & Widowers Caring Service, 502 CTC Building, Plein Street, Cape Town 8001 (telephone 021-453500) – Monday, Wednesday, Friday, 10 am-2 pm; Cancer Care & Resource Centre, c/o National Cancer Association of South Africa (with branches in all major centres); St Luke's Hospice, 92 Harfield Road, Kenilworth 7700; Cot Death Society, P O Box 15306, Vlaeberg 8018; Life Line (in your telephone directory).

What the therapists recommend

Homoeopathy *Arnica* 30 is prescribed for sudden shock when the person insists that he is all right, and wants to be left alone and not touched; *Ignatia* 30 for someone who is hysterical with grief.

When the person is cold, shaky and frightened, try *Aconite* 30; and a few doses of *Pulsatilla* if weepy and emotional. For shock, the medicines can be taken hourly for up to 12 doses, then morning and night for two to three days if necessary.

A homoeopathic doctor should be consulted for problems in the later stages of grief, but three self-help remedies are offered: *Natrum mur.* 6 when tears result if sympathy is offered, or the sufferer prefers to hide his feelings; *Ac. phos.* 6 for depression and apathy; *Nux vomica* for those who become angry and critical. Take three times daily for up to three weeks.

An orthodox view

It must never be forgotten that grief is a perfectly normal emotion which manifests itself after the loss of someone we love, so it is important to accept the painful symptoms. Any therapy which attempts in any way to deny or avoid the process of mourning is likely to result in long-term, health-threatening problems for the bereaved.

Making the most of our autumn years

Scientists now believe the potential human lifespan to be between 110 and 120 years – yet very few people live to this age. True, the proportion of elderly people in the developed world is at a record high, but this is mainly due to comparatively low birth rates and a general improvement in the standard of medicine and living conditions.

While people in their forties no longer consider themselves 'middle aged', and expect to still look and feel good in their fifties and early sixties, the current retirement age of 60 for women and 65 for men is still associated by many with the spectre of boredom and inactivity, loss of independence, and ultimate loneliness through bereavement.

But are these really inevitable? Our way of life and circumstances clearly affect how quickly we age, but many psychologists maintain that state of mind plays a significant role – that if we expect to go into a decline in our seventies, it is likely to happen.

Gerontologists (experts in the phenomenon of ageing) have found that the process is a combination of many significant changes – for example, internal 'body clocks' tend to switch off functions, slowing the production of a number of important hormones; and the IMMUNE SYSTEM weakens and we become less resistant to illness.

There is also general wear and tear on the body from the sun's ultraviolet light, pollution, drugs, pesticides – and the physical exertions of a lifetime. All these factors cause the formation of highly active atoms or atom groups which react with others to damage body cells and collagen (protein fibre). This in turn leads to 'cross-linking', which causes the protein fibres to become tangled and the skin to lose its suppleness. Wrinkles develop, veins and arteries harden, muscles soften and limbs stiffen.

However, research has shown that some primitive peoples living on sparse diets of natural foods such as fish and grain live to advanced ages and feel healthy and energetic, little troubled by the Western diseases of degeneration such as ARTHRITIS and HEART DISORDERS. Nutrition may therefore play an important role in longevity. Several alternative therapies are particularly concerned with countering the ageing process.

What the therapists recommend

HERBAL MEDICINE

Russian scientists believe that GINSENG strengthens the body's resistance to illness, TIREDNESS, STRESS and ageing. Siberian ginseng roots are a mild stimulant and are believed to improve memory and protect against cell and collagen damage and cross-linking. Korean ginseng is thought to help rid the body of poisons, and to ease tiredness and DEPRESSION. (However, some Western doctors feel that people with high BLOOD PRESSURE should not take ginseng.)

Mexican herbalists claim that sarsaparilla (available from specialist herb shops) has the same restorative effect as conventional hormone replacement therapy (HRT; see MENOPAUSE), but with none of the potential side effects. This herb also helps to restore the function of the reproductive system, especially in men. It is less potent than pure hormone treatment and therefore less disturbing to the system.

Make a sarsaparilla infusion by putting 25 g of sarsaparilla root in 600 ml of water and boiling for 25 minutes. Then strain and drink. Herbalists believe that this herb is best taken by 40- to 50-year-olds for a period of two to six weeks: two tablespoons (40 ml) twice a day. But it is advisable to consult a herbal practitioner, since dosage depends on the individual.

NATUROPATHY

Too much protein, lack of exercise and being overweight are all thought to speed up the ageing process. People in the West eat an average of about 14 700 kilojoules a day. Naturopaths believe that about 7 560 kilojoules are sufficient, with little salt, fat or refined sugar and mainly consisting of raw food, with wholegrain cereals and bread, pulses and seeds, and moderate amounts of protein (see EATING FOR HEALTH). This type of diet is believed to strengthen the immune system, slow the ageing process and keep you mentally alert. Avoiding highly processed foods, FASTING for a maximum of 24 hours about once every three months, and taking EXERCISE are also advised.

Various special vitamin and mineral-rich foods that are recommended include liver, egg yolks, sunflower seeds, blackstrap molasses, seaweed (available as kelp tablets from health stores), GARLIC, cabbage, raw green vegetables and wheatgerm (sprinkled on salads and wholegrain cereals).

It is important to eat a variety of the foods. Unless there is gastric irritation, garlic can be eaten quite freely, and unless otherwise prescribed one kelp tablet should be taken each day. Fresh pineapple and pawpaw fruits eaten raw once a week, on an empty stomach, are said to improve the skin and promote fresh skin protein fibre.

A naturopath may also advise you to take nutrients known as 'antioxidants', which are said to prevent, among other things, the destruction of vitamin C and to slow down the destruction of body cells. Antioxidants are also said to strengthen the immune system. The naturopath will advise you on personal daily dosages, or you can buy combination formulas as tablets from health stores.

The following nutrients are said to complement each other and can be taken in a good-quality multivitamin and mineral tablet with breakfast each day: vitamin A, aimed at stimulating the immune system; vitamin C, said to boost the immune system and stimulate production of interferon (a natural antivirus chemical); zinc, believed to rebuild skin proteins; bioflavinoids, said to promote strong, smooth, unlined skin; vitamin E, aimed at slowing the ageing of body cells, and warding off infection and damage from air pollution; and a mixture of B vitamins to prevent a range of deficiencies from loss of appetite to tiredness.

Naturopaths also recommend aerobic exercise to stimulate the endocrine glands (which produce vital hormones, such as those for growth), to improve circulation, and to help prevent cross-linking, high blood pressure and depression. Or go walking, dancing or swimming for at least 30 minutes, three to five times a week.

Although you may not be as mobile or flexible as in past years, the more you exercise, the more mobile you will remain. Even those people who have physical handicaps – including disabilities which confine them to a wheelchair – can, with their doctor's advice, do certain exercises.

Warning Elderly or middle-aged people should always consult a doctor before embarking on a new exercise routine, particularly if it will include strenuous activities.

VISUALISATION THERAPY
Therapists believe that the more you expect the future to hold for you, the more likely you are to resist illness and grow old gracefully. They recommend that you take ten minutes a day for regular relaxation and MEDITATION, visualising an image of yourself feeling healthy, happy, playful, active, creative and full of love and hope. You can also use COUÉISM and each day repeat to yourself positive thoughts such as: 'I am well and will continue to be so as the years pass.'

Other alternative treatments

Acupuncture Regular acupuncture sessions, four or more times a year including at the change of the seasons, are said to help keep you young. The therapist will give your entire system a tune-up, aimed at promoting health and energy. Acupuncture is also said to relieve diseases of ageing such as arthritis and RHEUMATISM.

Alexander Technique Bad posture adds years to people's appearance. This technique improves posture and is said to give agility, energy, a feeling of well-being and relief from BACK PAIN.

Aromatherapy Therapists believe that ageing involves a slowing down of the body's natural 'rhythm', and that essential oils can stimulate and restore rhythm,

delay the ageing process of the skin and help promote regeneration of cell tissues which are out of balance and cause arthritis and SINUS PROBLEMS. Certain aromas are believed to sharpen the mind, improve perception and aid MEMORY.

Biorhythms A personal biorhythm chart claims to tell the ups and downs that you are likely to face in the near future. Older people can use it to work out which days are best for conserving energy, and which are best for activity – so preserving mind and body for a longer and more rewarding life.

T'ai-chi Ch'uan This Chinese daily meditation routine, which involves slow and continuous movements, is suitable for every age, and is said to make the elderly feel young again. It aims to promote good posture, flexibility, balance, energy and general well-being.

Yoga Yoga postures are said to relax the mind, ease TENSION and help people grow old stylishly. Some aerobic or health centres in South Africa are now holding regular Hatha yoga classes for all age groups.

An orthodox view

Scientists have been able to double the lifespan of some laboratory animals using fasting and low-kilojoule diets, and believe that these nutritional approaches can also rejuvenate and protect the human immune system. They believe, too, that if they could fully understand the nature of our internal 'body clocks', which begin switching off our vital functions as we grow older, it might be possible to reprogramme them in such a way as to slow down the process of ageing.

An orthodox science called psychoneuroimmunology (PNI), which studies the connections between mind and body, has shown that your state of mind affects your immune system. The immune system of someone who constantly feels helpless and depressed does not work as well as that of a person who generally feels happy and hopeful. So it is possible that techniques such as meditation and visualisation, which can alter a person's mental and emotional states, could be used to encourage immunity.

It has been noted also that artistically creative people lead longer and healthier lives – perhaps because they remain mentally active and open-minded.

A substantial number of people in South Africa are of pensionable age and are spending the last quarter of their lives in retirement. Increasingly, these people are in good health and enjoying the opportunity to make new friends and to take up fresh interests. Instead of being the twilight of a busy and purposeful life, retirement is a time of freedom in which there is at last the leisure to follow pursuits that earlier responsibilities ruled out.

Do's and don'ts for staying young

Do exercise for 30 minutes, three to five times a week.
Do eat a fresh, mainly raw diet with ample vegetables and wholegrain foods for vitamins and minerals.
Do go easy on alcoholic drinks.
Do practise relaxation techniques such as meditation to combat everyday stress and promote well-being.
Do take up a hobby or other interest that keeps your mind as well as your body active after retirement.
Don't overeat.
Don't smoke.
Don't take drugs unnecessarily.
Don't drink too much non-decaffeinated coffee or tea.
Don't expose yourself to the sun for too long, or use a sunbed.

HAIR CARE

Keeping your head healthy

The basic character of your hair depends on four features that are due to heredity: density, texture, pattern and colour. But its condition depends largely on variable factors, including your general health, hair hygiene, care in choosing shampoos, conditioners and any other treatments, and the use of grooming equipment – combs, brushes, curling tools and so on.

Along with skin, hair is one of the fastest-developing cellular constituents of the human body. On average, hair grows about 13 mm a month – more at night than in day-time, and faster in summer than winter. When healthy it should be supple, and shiny from a thin coating of sebum – a natural oily substance secreted by the scalp's sebaceous glands, near the root of each hair. Sebum keeps the outer layer of the scalp supple, helps to prevent skin moisture evaporating, lubricates the hair itself, and is thought to prevent bacteria breeding on the scalp.

To maintain a healthy head of hair – provided there are no obvious HAIR PROBLEMS – simply keep the scalp clean by washing and adopt a balanced and adequate diet.

There are no hard-and-fast rules about washing your hair: whenever you feel it necessary – which differs from person to person – is a good rule. Those with particularly greasy hair, because of overactive sebaceous glands, obviously need to wash the hair more often – even daily. However, people with a dry scalp may need pre-shampoo treatment with natural oils (see box).

Hair can be damaged by the wear and tear of over-grooming. If you wash your hair frequently, use a mild shampoo – preferably non-detergent – and avoid using heated, spiky rollers, plastic brushes and sharp metal combs, which can all cause damage. Do not use elastic bands to tie up your hair – they can tear it and damage the roots. Also to be avoided are electric tongs, strong sunshine and chlorinated or sea water, all of which can dry the hair and scalp.

Hair can also be damaged by dyeing, bleaching, perming and massage. Perming at home should be done strictly according to the instructions on the package. Temporary dyes and rinses are not harmful, but permanent dyes can damage the scalp and penetrate the hair shaft, creating harmful chemical compounds there. The scalp may become swollen and inflamed as a reaction. **Warning** Always test a hair dye by dabbing a small amount on the scalp behind your ear. If there is any sign of inflammation within 48 hours, do not use the dye.

Repeated bleaching with hydrogen peroxide-based preparations can make the hair rough, dry and brittle, with split ends. It can also become thin or shortened. The ends split because they are short of sebum and divide into a Y-shape; and the farther the ends are from the scalp, the drier they become – although greasy hair can also split. Mid-length fractures are also common, causing the hair to break off.

To avoid split ends, snip off the ends cleanly every couple of weeks. Otherwise the split may travel back along the hair towards the scalp. Ragged ends that prove difficult to remove may be treated temporarily with conditioner applied only to the ends.

Going grey Your hair colour is determined by the ratio of two pigments in the hair – brown-black and red-yellow. As you grow older, less pigment is deposited in hair shafts as they grow, and grey hairs appear. These usually start appearing at the temples, then gradually spread over the rest of the scalp. However, the speed and extent of greying depends much upon hereditary factors.

Loss of hair Some loss of hair is quite normal; a hair drops out because a new one has grown under it. However, there are some ailments (see BALDNESS; HAIR PROBLEMS) which can cause abnormal hair loss. Women sometimes lose hair due to hormonal changes after childbirth, or after giving up using the contraceptive pill. Some drugs given to CANCER patients can also cause loss of hair. Though such cases can be distressing, gradually with time the hair tends to grow back in all of them.

Women's hair tends to thin – and remain so – during the menopause. Other causes of hair loss include tight hair styles, such as a pony tail, tight and too frequently applied hair rollers, repeated, vigorous massage and over-zealous brushing.

Never use sharp combs or brushes, which may tear the hair, do not brush or comb vigorously when the hair is wet and always towel it dry gently. Never hold a hair dryer too close to the head – at least 15 cm away is best – and set the heat control on low or medium, rather than high.

As a measure against mild cases of DANDRUFF, halve a lemon and rub the two halves into the scalp. Leave for ten minutes, then wash the hair. Alternatively, carry out a similar procedure with sour milk. Try each treatment – and decide which one you feel is most suited to you.

Olive oil for dry hair

Put 2 tablespoons of olive oil into a cup, warm it in a pan of hot water, then massage the oil thoroughly, but gently, into the scalp, using your fingertips.

Steep a towel in hot water, wring and wrap it around the head. On cooling, immerse the towel once more in hot water and make sure you repeat the process two or three times, until the scalp is completely saturated. Finally, shampoo in the normal way.

If this does not clear up the dry condition, see your doctor for a checkup. He may wish to refer you to a dermatologist (skin specialist), if any scalp disorder is present.

HAIR DIAGNOSIS

Laboratory tests on a lock of your hair – preferably taken from the nape of the neck, where hair grows quickest – are used in hair diagnosis to detect whether your body contains any harmful mineral imbalances.

Hair is made of a type of protein called keratin, which contains large amounts of sulphur. Practitioners believe that the sulphur attaches itself to minerals – both harmful and beneficial – and holds them in the hair. Poisonous minerals such as aluminium, arsenic, lead and mercury can, in excess, give rise to disturbed behaviour – such as acts of violence. In addition, mineral imbalances can cause a variety of ailments, including ALLERGY, DEPRESSION, DIGESTIVE PROBLEMS, HYPERACTIVITY and TIREDNESS.

Hair analysts say they can determine mineral deficiencies or excesses by putting hair samples in a chemical solution for 36 hours and then examining them by a sophisticated electronic procedure called atomic absorption spectroscopy. This will reveal what, if any, harmful minerals have been absorbed into the body from such things as hair dyes, perm lotions, shampoos and sprays. Air pollution – which can affect city joggers and cyclists – is another potential cause of mineral imbalance. In addition, the minerals absorbed from aluminium cooking utensils may also prove harmful.

But before any analysis is undertaken, patients must get their doctor's approval and co-operation. The results of the tests – which are printed out on charts – are interpreted by the laboratory, which also usually supplies the treatment.

An orthodox view

There is much scepticism among doctors and some dermatologists (skin specialists) as to the reliability of hair analysis, and many will not accept the readings as valid. However, some doctors will use the tests as a guide, and advise patients about diet, work and leisure environments, which can have a bearing on the balance of essential minerals that we need to help us to stay healthy.

HAIR PROBLEMS

Only the skin on the palms of the hands, soles of the feet, ends of the fingers and toes, umbilicus and parts of the genitals is without hair. Hair conserves heat by trapping air to form an insulating layer. It has no nerve endings, so although the skin hurts when hair is pulled, there is no pain when it is cut. Hairs eventually fall out; eyelashes and armpit hairs have the shortest life (about four months) and scalp hairs have the longest (four years).

This is why there is a limit to the length hair will grow, and why dead hairs frequently appear on hairbrushes and combs. Healthy adults normally shed between 50 and 100 hairs each day. However, the number of hairs on the average head varies between 90 000 and 100 000.

The condition of the hair and scalp reflects the general well-being of the body and mind (see HAIR CARE). Almost any illness or emotional stress can cause lifeless, dull hair; ANAEMIA, lack of VITAMINS and thyroid hormone deficiency (see THYROID DISORDERS) can result in hair loss.

BALDNESS of the scalp, beginning with a receding hairline and thinning of the crown, is normal in many men, and so is thinning of the hair in older women. Most women experience a thinning of the hair two or three months after giving birth, but there is usually improvement over the following months.

Alopecia – a sudden and generally temporary, patchy loss of hair – can occur in men and women, boys and girls, sometimes at times of STRESS. The hair usually regrows, but the colour may be different. This form of alopecia may occur as a side effect of cytotoxic (anti-cancer) drugs and radiotherapy. Generalised alopecia, in which all the hair drops out and does not regrow, is rare.

DANDRUFF – scales of dead skin from the scalp – commonly occurs in teenagers and young adults. Severe cases are sometimes caused by a type of ECZEMA called seborrhoeic dermatitis.

Highly contagious lice can infest the hair, leaving nits – tiny, white eggs – stuck to individual hairs. Lice thrive in clean hair and they often spread among family members and in schools.

What the therapists recommend

NATUROPATHY

Self help Gently massaging the scalp will stimulate circulation. Try using plain YOGHURT as a conditioner, rinsing off with an infusion of rosemary, nettle or thyme to combat dandruff.

However, practitioners regard hair condition as an early warning indicator of lowered vitality and ill health, and see any disorders as signs of a possible underlying imbalance. Taking more EXERCISE and adopting a wholefood diet (see EATING FOR HEALTH) are held to be useful measures to take, but individual consultation is advised.

HERBAL MEDICINE

Self help To encourage the hair follicles and promote growth, try massaging a few drops of oil of rosemary into the scalp, then rinse; or use a strong infusion of nettles to rinse off shampoo. For an itching, flaky scalp and dandruff, try massaging it with infusions of rosemary, thyme, lavender or juniper, as cleansing and antiseptic treatments.

Herbalists regard hair and scalp problems as often reflecting inner disorder, and may prescribe camomile as a relaxant or a skullcap to counter STRESS.

To enhance the colour of fair hair, rinse with a strong infusion of either camomile or rhubarb leaf. The colour of dark hair can be enhanced to some extent with an infusion of rosemary and sage. Greying hair can be treated by the same means.

AROMATHERAPY

Self help For lank, lifeless hair, try regular rinsing with 600 ml of water containing five drops each of lemon, rosemary and lavender oils. Therapists warn, however, that poor health may be the underlying cause and that this, too, should be treated.

For thinning hair, the prescription is three drops each of rosemary and ylang-ylang oils in a teaspoon of vodka or other strong alcohol, made up to a tablespoonful with orange-flower water. Apply a few drops to the scalp daily and massage firmly for two to three minutes.

Dandruff may be treated with a mixture of three drops of cedarwood and two drops each of rosemary and lemon oils in a tablespoon of carrier oil or lotion. Apply sparingly to the scalp and leave for two hours or overnight before shampooing and rinsing.

TRADITIONAL MEDICINE

Self help For hair loss, use a bay rum and jaborandi lotion, following the manufacturer's instructions. Alternatively, massage the scalp with castor oil at night, shampoo in the morning, and repeat the process once

or twice a week. Safflower oil or wheat-germ oil may be used in the same way.

To reduce dandruff, cut a lemon in half and rub the juicy sides liberally over the scalp. Leave for about ten minutes, then rinse off thoroughly with plenty of cold water. Repeat this treatment weekly.

An orthodox view

Doctors sometimes prescribe minoxidil solution, which when rubbed into the scalp daily for at least four months produces a temporary improvement in male baldness. The baldness returns when the treatment is stopped, and minoxidil is not suitable for treatment of hair loss in women.

Small areas of alopecia sometimes respond to steroid injections or creams. A steroid scalp lotion often benefits sufferers from seborrhoeic dermatitis.

Hair lice can be killed by rubbing in malathion or carbaryl lotion – but *not* garden insecticides containing these – and leaving it for 12 hours before washing it out. The whole family and, ideally, school classmates should be treated at the same time.

HAKIMS

This is the name given to Indian and Muslim herbal therapists, who generally tend to work only in their own communities. The word comes from the Arabic for 'learned' or 'wise'. Treatment is similar to that used in AYURVEDIC MEDICINE. However, instead of preparing herbal mixtures for each patient's needs, Hakims use ready-prepared patent mixtures. See also HERBAL MEDICINE.

HAND CARE

Simple measures to keep hands in trim

For housewives and manual workers especially, the hands are the most overworked part of the body, and yet they are often the least cared for. The back is covered with soft skin, with fine hairs and sebaceous (oil) and sweat gland openings. The palm has tougher skin, no hairs or sebaceous glands, but plenty of sweat glands, which are often set into action by heat or stress to produce sweaty palms.

The exposed parts of the fingernails – the nail plates – are made of inert keratin. They grow throughout life, not always at the same rate, the average time for a nail to grow from quick (base) to tip being 16-20 weeks.

Self help Constant pressure or friction may cause calluses – small patches of thickened skin. Use a dry-skin remover according to the maker's instructions, and rub in hand/body lotion or night cream.

Sometimes the top layers of nails separate and flake off, or the nails split easily due to contact with detergents, solvents and other preparations; using an emery board that is too coarse or a metal file; too little protein in the diet; or extreme old age. Keep the nails short and follow the *Do's and don'ts of hand care* and remedies (right) for very dry hands.

Alternatively, rub nail cream or oil into the nail bases each night and increase your protein and vitamin intake. Eating two cubes of concentrated jelly or a dessertspoon of gelatine a day helps the problem in some people. Nail varnish will act as a 'splint' for broken nails, but do use a moisturiser base coat. Avoid using nail-varnish remover as much as possible; add more coats of moisturiser and/or varnish instead.

If nails become dry or brittle, immerse them in warm olive oil for 30 minutes daily.

For minor ridges and furrows on the nails, use a ridge-filling base coat. The problem will eventually 'grow out'. More serious ridges and furrows may result from an injury or cyst near the cuticle. The furrows may split and become infected. If there is any inflammation or swelling, see your doctor.

Constant immersion of hands in water may cause hangnails – splits where the outer skin has come away from the cuticle, often allowing infection to enter. Carefully snip off the hangnails with scissors and apply a proprietary antiseptic cream. To prevent hangnails, apply hand cream nightly.

A heavy blow or pressure will cause bleeding underneath a nail and turn it black. With minor injuries, the problem will grow out. If the nail falls off, is very painful or the bleeding continues, see your doctor.

Some nail varnishes, especially if used without a base coat, turn nails yellow. Again, the condition will grow out, and so will white spots or flecks.

What the therapists recommend

Traditional Medicine For dry hands, soak 3 tablespoons of linseed in 600 ml of warm water overnight. Boil, strain and retain the gel. Add 600 ml of white vinegar and 60-90 g of glycerine. Heat to boiling, remove from the heat, beat for one minute, and then bottle the mixture while still warm. Store in a cool place and rub a little into the hands as required. Alternatively, apply an unperfumed hand cream (a perfumed one may cause further irritation).

For very dry hands, soak them in warm olive oil for 30 minutes. Alternatively, apply vitamin E, either as wheat-germ oil, or by cut-ting open a vitamin E capsule and rubbing the contents in well. Cod liver, safflower or sunflower oil will also help. Either rub it into

Do's and don'ts of hand care

Do avoid all detergents and highly alkaline soaps (over pH 7,5).
Do wet your hands as little as possible.
Do wear rubber gloves when doing wet jobs, preferably cotton-lined ones. If you are allergic to rubber, use plastic gloves instead. If the job cannot be done in gloves, apply a barrier cream first.
Do wear cotton gloves for dry tasks.
Do brush your nails once a day with a soft brush and warm, soapy water.
Do have a manicure at least weekly.
Do buff your nails as often as possible, working in one direction only.
Do use a nail moisturiser as a lacquer base and top coat.
Do use an emollient at night, if necessary wearing cotton gloves in bed.
Do dry your hands thoroughly and apply hand cream after each wash.
Do eat a healthy, well balanced diet, with plenty of calcium, vitamin B_1, iron and fresh fruit and vegetables (see EATING FOR HEALTH).
Don't expose the hands to harsh sunlight, extremes of hot and cold or very dry atmospheres.
Don't use creams and lotions containing lanolin if you think you may be allergic to it.
Don't bite your nails.
Don't pick at the cuticles, or push them back too hard.
Don't cut your cuticles; if it is necessary, have a professional do it.
Don't cut your nails except when they are soft and pliable after a warm bath.
Don't use nail varnish/lacquer remover containing acetone unless it also contains oil to prevent over-drying.
Don't use base and top coats containing formaldehyde; they are too drying.
Don't apply nail-varnish hardeners containing formaldehyde too near the cuticle, as this will cause drying.

Do-it-yourself manicure

You will need: cotton wool; emery boards; a hoof stick with a blunt point at one end for cleaning, and a rubber 'hoof' at the other for easing back cuticles; nail or cuticle cream; chamois-covered nail buffer, and some oily nail-varnish remover.

1 Remove any nail varnish: put some oily nail-varnish remover on a swab of cotton wool, hold it on a nail for a second or two, then gently rub until all the varnish is removed.

2 Shape the nails with an emery board, using the fine side only. Movements should be from side to centre only. Do not file down the sides so far that strength is impaired.

3 Massage nail or cuticle cream all over the nails, and wait two minutes.

5 Gently ease the cuticles back from the nails using the rubber end of the hoof stick.

4 Soak the fingers in warm soapy water for two minutes, and dry thoroughly.

6 Wrap a little cotton wool around the pointed end of the hoof stick, dip it in the soapy water, and run it around under the tips of the nails to clean them. (If you are not going to apply a highly coloured nail varnish, run a white nail pencil under the nail tips.)

7 Buff the nails, using strokes in one direction only.

8 Massage cream into the hands (and wrists, forearms and elbows, if desired). Run nails along a piece of fabric to find any snags, and smooth with the emery board.

9 If you are going to apply nail varnish, dip a piece of cotton wool in soapy water, squeeze almost dry, and gently rub each nail to remove traces of cream.

10 Apply one coat of base coat or moisturiser, two coats of varnish and one top coat. Use long straight strokes from base to tip, one in the centre and one on either side. If necessary, remove any smudges of nail varnish on the skin by wrapping a little cotton wool around the pointed end of the hoof stick, dipping it in oily remover, and running it around the nails and under the tips. Allow at least 20 minutes to dry.

the hands at night, or drink a teaspoon of oil before retiring. See also CHAPPING.

To remove discoloured areas such as the stains acquired by smokers, rub the hands with the juicy side of half a lemon. Leave for one minute, rinse off thoroughly, dry carefully and massage with hand cream.

An orthodox view

Extreme cases of chapping may lead to EC-ZEMA. If this happens, or if there is an allergic reaction (see ALLERGY), consult your doctor immediately.

Sometimes a whitlow – a small, painful abscess – forms at the side of a nail if the hands are in water a great deal. The skin becomes abnormally soft and infection enters. This too needs the attention of a doctor, who will lance it to drain out the pus. Antibiotics may be prescribed, and patients should keep their hands as dry as possible, and not handle food or dress wounds.

Sometimes the skin around the nails becomes cracked, usually because of an allergen. If a doctor cannot find the cause, he may prescribe supplements of vitamin C and cod liver oil (vitamins A and D).

Children and young people are especially prone to WARTS on the hands. They are caused by a virus and are therefore contagious. If they persist, see a doctor.

Liver spots – large brown spots on the backs of the hands – are the result of the ageing effects of climate. Mild bleaching creams are available from most cosmetics counters. If the spots appear before old age, have them checked by a doctor immediately, for in rare cases they can be malignant.

Excessive sweating of the palms may cause embarrassment at times. Try to remain calm, and avoid stimulant drinks such as coffee and cola. If the problem becomes very severe, a doctor may prescribe a cream or lotion to reduce sweating, or even sedatives or tranquillisers for important occasions.

HANGOVER

Remedies for the morning after

Drinking too much alcohol usually results in a hangover. If the overindulgence takes place in the evening, the hangover may not be apparent until the next morning. A person with a hangover is suffering from dehydration – or loss of fluid – and the symptoms include NAUSEA AND VOMITING, thirst, TIREDNESS and HEADACHES.

Often the hangover is heightened by a group of substances called congeners. These are formed during fermentation, especially in drinks such as red wine, brandy and lager, and irritate the lining of the stomach. In addition, smoking usually adds to the severity of a hangover.

Self help One of the best ways of helping to prevent a hangover is to make sure that you do not drink on an empty stomach, and to drink plenty of water – up to 600 ml of it – beforehand. Some people find a glass of milk to be an effective substitute, while others swear by a dessertspoon of oil. A sure way of avoiding a hangover is to drink slowly, and to alternate alcoholic drinks with non-alcoholic ones.

Having got a hangover, water – litres of it – is probably the best drink to replace lost fluids; and eating something light, such as a slice or two of dry wholewheat toast will help to replace the blood sugar which the alcohol has destroyed, and so help reduce weakness, dizziness and trembling. A walk in the fresh air should also help to clear the head.

Activated charcoal is known to absorb congeners, and is available in tablet form from most chemists and health shops. Take several tablets as directed before you go to bed after an evening's drinking.

To 'cure' a hangover some people drink black coffee. This is a mistake, for like alcohol, coffee itself is a diuretic (a substance that increases the flow of urine) and only prolongs the discomfort.

What the therapists recommend

Herbal Medicine After drinking, take plenty of water before going to bed to prevent dehydration. Some herbalists suggest that throughout the next day you drink peppermint, nettle, camomile or yarrow tea to help settle the stomach and liver.

Naturopathy If you are going to drink, then you are advised to make sure to eat something at the same time. This will slow down the absorption of alcohol. Then drink at least a litre of water just before going to bed. If you still get a hangover afterwards, have a glass of water or a peppermint tea to help settle the stomach.

Traditional Medicine One of the oldest and most popular folk remedies is 'the hair of the dog that bit you' – that is, more alcohol. Although this will not cure a hangover, it may make the victim feel slightly stronger. But if more than just a 'nip' is taken it could lead to another and even worse hangover.

A 'prairie oyster', made of a raw egg immersed in liquid – usually Worcestershire sauce or vinegar – and swallowed whole is another supposed cure. Honey is also a remedy of long standing: try 12 teaspoonfuls, either neat or in a little warm water. The honey will help to replace the blood sugar lost, and its potassium content is also said to be beneficial.

An orthodox view

Although doctors are not opposed to alternative hangover cures, they mostly agree that time is the best cure. If you are able to, stay in bed, keep warm, and take painkillers such as soluble aspirin or paracetamol. (Ordinary aspirin tablets may cause nausea or sometimes, with a severe hangover, bleeding in the stomach.) If you must drink, it is safer to take white wine, vodka or gin, as they contain comparatively few congeners.

HAY DIET

Avoiding the foods that fight

An American doctor, William Howard Hay (1866-1940), devised a diet aimed at combating DIGESTIVE PROBLEMS. He recommended that carbohydrates (starches and sugars) should not be eaten with proteins and acid fruits at the same meal. He pointed out that protein stimulates the production of acid in the stomach, and that the acid interferes with carbohydrate digestion, which needs an alkaline medium.

While many foodstuffs contain both protein and carbohydrate, virtually all of them are 20 per cent or more one or the other, and can be classified as such. The exceptions are peas, beans, lentils and peanuts, and these Hay excluded from his diet. However, modern vegetarian proponents now include them as proteins.

Hay's foods for a protein meal include meat, poultry, game, fish (including shellfish), eggs, cheese, yoghurt, milk, and acid fruits such as apples, apricots (both fresh and

Do's and don'ts of the Hay diet

Don't eat any carbohydrates together with proteins and acid fruits in a single meal.
Do make vegetables, salads and fruits the major part of your diet, and cut down on proteins, starches and fats.
Don't eat refined or processed foods, including white flour, white sugar, margarine, or things containing them.
Don't eat a meal of one type within four hours of eating a meal of the other type.

dried), gooseberries, oranges, pears and prunes. His carbohydrate group includes bread (whole grain), flour, rice, sweet fruits such as ripe bananas, dates, figs, currants, raisins and sultanas, and potatoes and Jerusalem artichokes.

Hay's third group of 'neutral foods' combines well with either of the other two. Nuts (excluding peanuts), butter, cream, egg yolks, olive oil, safflower oil, sunflower and sesame seeds and oils, salads, herbs, and all green and root vegetables except potatoes and Jerusalem artichokes belong to this third neutral group.

Hay did not ban alcohol. He recommended dry red or white table wine or dry cider with protein meals, and ale or beer for carbohydrate meals. Whisky or gin may be drunk with either type of meal. Of course, all must be taken in moderation.

An orthodox view

Tests by the Russian physiologist Ivan Petrovich Pavlov (1849-1936) proved that meat mixed with starch takes twice as long – or more – to pass through a dog's stomach as either of them does alone, and that sluggish digestive action continues through the rest of the alimentary canal. Hay's diet therefore gives some relief to people suffering from indigestion, stomach and duodenal ulcers and constipation.

Any well-balanced diet, taken in moderation as Hay recommended, promotes good health, avoiding obesity and related heart disease, diabetes and arthritis. See also DIETS AND DIETING; EATING FOR HEALTH.

HAY FEVER

In spite of the name, hay fever is neither caused by hay nor associated with fever. It is usually an ALLERGY to pollen released by grasses, flowers and trees in spring and summer. The pollen causes cells to release histamine and other chemicals, resulting in a running, itchy nose; blocked sinuses; SNEEZING; redness, prickling and watering of the eyes, and/or a sore, itchy throat; and sometimes ASTHMA.

But allergic rhinitis, as it is medically named, may also be caused by allergy to things such as house dust, mites, the fur or feathers of animals or birds, or by moulds, plants or chemicals.

What the therapists recommend
NATUROPATHY
Consultation A practitioner may prescribe vitamin B as a preventive in late spring and early summer. He will also recommend that you cut down on dairy products (cheese, milk and so on) and refined carbohydrates such as sugars. These are all held to encourage excess mucus, and a sensitivity to dairy foods is believed to exacerbate the pollen reaction itself. Large doses of vitamin C – 1 or 2 g daily – are prescribed for an antihistamine effect.

HOMOEOPATHY
Self help *Allium cepa* is prescribed for an acute attack, with running eyes and nose, sneezing and sore lips and nose, which is worse indoors and towards evening. For violent, painful sneezing, with a ticklish spot in a running nose, try *Arsen. alb.*; *Sabadilla* may be a better choice for an itching, stuffy or running nose, red eyes and frequent sneezing spasms. A practitioner may offer individual treatment in winter to reduce the tendency to hay fever later.

Other alternative treatments
Acupuncture The therapist stimulates points on the large intestine, governing, lung and spleen meridians.

Hypnotherapy The patient is put in a relaxed state, then instructed in appropriate breathing techniques. Suggestions are made under hypnosis which take effect at times when the patient needs them. Hypnosis has been used to prevent attacks in people susceptible to certain allergies, even though skin tests remain positive (see ALLERGY).

Traditional Medicine Use small lumps of honeycomb as a chewing gum all through the winter and spring. Brewer's yeast tablets taken according to the manufacturer's instructions are said to be beneficial.

An orthodox view

Doctors often prescribe or advise their patients to take antihistamine tablets during the hay fever season. Drowsiness may be a side effect of these and, if so, patients should not drive a car or operate machinery. The regular use of cromoglycate eyedrops, nasal sprays and/or inhalers, available on prescription, can also prevent or reduce the allergic response of the body.

Cortisone inhalers and nose sprays can help to reduce inflammation and swelling of the sensitive membranes of the lungs and nasal passages. In severe cases, or when hay fever might interfere with a critical event such as an important examination, a course of cortisone tablets or a long-acting cortisone injection can relieve hay fever symptoms dramatically.

However, steroids such as cortisone should not be used as a routine treatment because of long-term side effects, such as bruising and bone thinning. The side effects depend on how long the particular substance has been taken.

Courses of desensitising injections need to be used with great care because patients can die from anaphylactic shock, a severe allergic reaction to protein in the injection.

HEADACHES

Almost everyone experiences headaches at times. Most are caused by TENSION in the muscles of the scalp and neck after periods of concentration or STRESS. Some result from EATING PROBLEMS or alcohol abuse (see HANGOVER). Others are the forerunners of COLDS or INFLUENZA. MENSTRUATION can be another cause.

EYESTRAIN only rarely produces headache, despite popular belief, and if it does, it usually arises from ASTIGMATISM. MIGRAINE can cause severe headaches, often on one side of the head only, and sometimes associated with numbness or weakness down one side of the face or body. Headache is common after head injury (concussion), and it can also be caused by SINUS PROBLEMS or problems involving the lower jaw muscles that may result from TEETH-GRINDING.

A sudden, severe headache, which feels like a blow to the back of the head, often followed by unconsciousness, may indicate internal bleeding underneath the brain known as a subarachnoid haemorrhage. Meningitis produces a headache aggravated by bright light, and accompanied by fever and neck stiffness. The headache caused by a brain tumour is worst in the mornings or when lying down, and may be associated with nausea and mental disturbances. However, all of these are very rare complaints.

Warning If a headache persists or recurs frequently, see your doctor at once; do not attempt to treat yourself.

What the therapists recommend
NATUROPATHY
Consultation The cause of the headache should always be sought. A consultant will therefore inquire about the patient's way of life to try to discover any factors which may aggravate the problem. Diet can also be a trigger, especially in cases of migraine. Cheese, chocolate, alcohol or coffee can all be causes, but each case will be assessed on its merits.

Hot and cold compresses to the forehead and neck, depending on the type of headache, may also be applied.

BEHAVIOURAL THERAPY
Consultation For a stress-induced headache, the aim is to relieve tension in the muscles of the body. This can be done through progressive muscular relaxation, in which all

Demons with corkscrews, red-hot pokers, trumpets and mallets torture a headache victim at his fireside in this cartoon by George Cruikshank published in 1835.

the muscles are tensed, and then relaxed in turn starting with the toes and working up the body.

The patient becomes aware of the tension and relaxation of the muscles and can then aim at maintaining relaxation as much as possible. Particular emphasis is placed on the muscles around the shoulders, neck, jaw and face.

Other alternative treatments

Acupuncture Headaches are held to be due to an energy blockage in the yang channel of the head. Those that do not respond well to conventional medicine are thought to respond best to acupuncture. Depending on the type of headache, points on the meridians relating to the gall bladder, large intestine, stomach, small intestine, governor and bladder are treated.

Massage Certain kinds of headaches – particularly those which tend to start at the back of the head – may be helped by firm effleurage strokes down the back of the neck, and gentle petrissage and kneading of the muscles over the upper part of the shoulders. Follow by deep friction with the thumbs over the tight muscle band on either side of the spine of the neck, and friction with the fingers behind the ears.

Then apply firm stroking across the forehead, from one temple to the other. Make sure that you use the ends of the fingers. Finish with more firm stroking down the neck towards the shoulders, avoiding completely any contact with the front part of the neck and the throat.

Osteopathy Many headaches these days are believed to be caused by accumulated muscle tension, which can result from generally poor posture, eyestrain and the ongoing pressures of everyday living. Osteopaths may therefore try to free the contracted muscles

at the base of the skull, and improve the mobility of the neck joints.

An orthodox view

The main role of the doctor is to reach a diagnosis and treat serious causes of headache. Orthodox painkillers such as paracetamol and aspirin are of only limited value in the treatment of tension headaches.

HEALERS AND HEALING

Summoning inner powers to fight disease

For at least 3 000 years healers throughout the world have been seeking to cure people of illness – physical and mental – by various non-physical means. By concentrating their attention solely upon their patients, healers claim that they can sometimes relieve pain, soreness and tiredness within minutes – and so help the body to heal itself. For example, swellings may quickly diminish, wounds rapidly get better, and infections speedily clear up; patients are also said to spend less time recuperating.

Very occasionally healers are said to achieve so-called 'miracle cures', in which the blind are able to see again and the crippled able to walk. But although these 'miracles' are often widely reported in the popular Press, they are generally viewed with scepticism by many doctors and scientists (see FAITH HEALING).

Some healers believe that their powers of healing are channelled through them by an outside 'spiritual' source. This often results in a spirituality developing in the patients, which is thought to speed up the cures and make them more effective. Even so, belief in the healer and his particular therapy does not

always seem to be necessary as in some reported cases infants, unconscious patients, animals and plants are said to have responded positively to healing. By observing their growth patterns, it has even been demonstrated that healing has had a beneficial effect on bacteria and yeasts.

In the late 1980s controlled experiments in healing were conducted at London University by two lecturers in physiology, Dr David Hodges and Dr Tony Scofield. They scientifically tested the curative powers of a psychic healer and medium who claimed he could take 'sick' organisms such as cress seeds – whose ability to grow had been hampered by soaking them overnight in salty water – and make them 'well' again.

The healer held half of the seeds in his hands and directed 'healing energy' at them for a couple of minutes. The treated and untreated seeds were laid on wet filter paper and placed in a laboratory for almost a week. A series of tests then showed that the 'treated' seeds grew at a significantly faster rate than those which the healer had not touched. From this, Dr Hodges and Dr Scofield concluded that the healer was somehow able to transmit a healing power which enabled the sick seeds to throw off any ill effects and grow almost normally.

Some medical experts dismiss the work of healers and say that unexplained cures are due to 'spontaneous remission', in which the body heals itself (if only temporarily), or AUTOSUGGESTION, whereby patients heal themselves by self-hypnosis. The experts also suggest that healing is similar to parapsychology, in which clairvoyance (the supposed power to see things not present to the senses) and telepathy (the awareness, even at a distance, of someone else's feelings and thoughts) play a significant part (see PARANORMAL THERAPIES).

In some cases, it has been suggested that the healers go into medium-like trances in which they are possessed by the spirits of the dead, who do the healing for them. In addition, the sick have reportedly been cured by ABSENT HEALING, in which healers apparently project their powers from another room or even another continent – and some patients are not even aware that they are being treated. Other healers use the LAYING ON OF HANDS and THERAPEUTIC TOUCH, whereby powers appear to be activated through their hands. In some cases this is done simply by making a series of 'passes' around the patients' bodies without physically touching the affected areas.

Finding a healer Most people contact a healer through the personal recommendation of a friend or relative. The advertising columns of alternative health magazines (or magazines that aim to promote a 'more conscious style of living') usually carry the names and addresses of a variety of healers. The South African Federation of Spiritual Healers will also be able to help you. Federation addresses are: Cape branch – 10 Corvette Avenue, Sun Valley, Fish Hoek 7975; Natal branch – 18 Ebony Drive, Glen Anil, Durban 4051; Transvaal branch – 6 Roos Street, Monument, Krugersdorp 1739.

Consulting a healer Healing is generally regarded as a two-way process, and the first thing a healer will do is talk calmly and soothingly to a patient to induce relaxation and open his mind to the possibility of getting well again.

Once a mutual bond has been established the healer will focus his mind on his powers, allowing them to flow freely from – or through – him and onto his patient. He may also instruct the patient to visualise projections of white or coloured light, which are said to aid the healing process (see Colour Therapy and Visualisation Therapy).

During healing sessions – usually held once a week until improvement is shown – the patient should gradually become less tense and nervous. He may have sensations of heat, cold and tingling (like small electric shocks) – especially on the skin over the site of an illness, such as the liver or kidneys. This is taken as a sign that a beneficial form of energy is being transferred from the healer to the patient – although no known form of energy or healing power has so far been scientifically identified. However, even if such sensations do not occur, healing may still be taking place.

Some patients begin to feel better as soon as healing begins, or shortly after. Others do not feel any benefit until hours or days later. Occasionally healing may take weeks or months before it has any effect. Frequently symptoms which the patient has omitted to mention are cleared up – while the original illness remains unchanged. In such cases, further healing may be carried out.

Generally healers do not charge a fee for treatment, although a small 'donation' may be requested. Make sure that you know what the situation is about payment before you agree to treatment; and avoid any healer who demands an exorbitant fee.

An orthodox view

Spiritual healing, significantly older than Western medicine, is still widely practised throughout the world. No scientific basis to the claims made for healing has been identified, but many doctors believe that faith and hope are important ingredients in recovery. Insofar as spiritual healing encourages these factors, it can do no harm.

However, doctors are justifiably concerned if false hopes are raised and if patients do not seek orthodox treatment for complaints of a serious nature because they are seeing a spiritual healer.

HEALTH FARMS

People visit health farms (health resorts) for a tone-up, or for naturopathic cures for ailments such as Arthritis and Back Pain. See Getting Fit – Away from it All, p.170.

HEALTH FOODS
Balancing fads and true food values

It is tempting to expect extra benefits from eating what we call health foods and from increasing our intake of Vitamins and Minerals. They are today's equivalent of the elixirs of bygone days. But is there not as much nutrition – equal magic – in ordinary fresh foods if they are chosen and combined wisely?

Some foods have a powerful health image. Wholegrain cereals and pulses, nuts and seeds, dried fruit and honey, natural yoghurt and cottage cheese are among the goods people seek out in health food stores. They are there in abundance – and with them is a bewildering array of pills and potions promising convenient bottled health: vitamins, minerals and oils to supplement your diet, Ginseng, Royal Jelly and amino acids to act as tonics or lift your mood. Some shops also have a pharmacy selling herbal, homoeopathic and other remedies.

What are you to do faced with such a wide choice and with that persuasive 'health' tag backed by potent advertising? Are these special foods, supplements and tonics necessary for your health?

How healthy are they?

Cereals and pulses Wholegrain cereals and pulses are undoubtedly valuable foods that play an essential part in a healthy diet (see Eating for Health). Indeed, they sustain much of the world's population. They have a similar nutritional content – protein, starch, dietary Fibre, vitamins and minerals – in differing permutations and amounts. You should eat a wide variety of them to ensure that you get a supply of all essential nutrients. It is best to eat a cereal and pulse at the same meal since the usable proteins in them are enhanced in combination.

Pulses (seeds from pods) such as beans and lentils have, when dry, more protein than meat, but you cannot eat them dry. Once they have been soaked, washed and thoroughly cooked (which removes the poisons most beans contain), they have far less protein than meat but still make a useful protein contribution to the diet: they contain about the same amount as bread.

Fresh and frozen peas also have a similar protein content; nutritionally, peas are simply wet beans without the poisons and with the bonus of vitamin C.

Nuts and seeds Nuts, like cereals and pulses, contain useful amounts of protein, dietary fibre, vitamins (especially B, E and folic acid) and minerals (including potassium, calcium, magnesium, iron and zinc). Seeds such as sesame, poppy and melon are similar but are eaten as garnishes rather than a main constituent of a meal.

The energy stored in nuts and seeds is in the form of fat instead of starch (as in cereals and pulses), so they should be eaten in moderation. As nuts are eaten dry, they appear – weight for weight – to contain more nutrients than pulses and cereals, but in practice we eat nuts in smaller helpings so the end result is similar.

Dried fruits and honey It seems curious that dried fruit, rather than fresh fruit, should find such favour as a health food. Dried fruit is only fresh fruit with much of the water and some of the nutrients lost in the drying process. Dried fruit makes a concentrated food package but is eaten in smaller helpings (by weight) than fresh fruit, so its nutritional contribution is about the same. Dried fruit is often used as a sweetener, and is to be preferred to sugar or Honey. Despite all the virtues attributed to honey, it is little more than sugar in another guise. Both provide kilojoules, but with only tiny amounts of other nutrients for maintaining the body.

Yoghurt and cottage cheese These both contain protein, vitamins (especially B) and minerals (including calcium and potassium) without an unhealthy excess of fat – provided you choose the right yoghurt. Yoghurt made with full-cream milk and sweetened fruit certainly cannot qualify as a health food.

Tonic supplements

What of pills? The massive increase in the sale of nutritional supplements indicates an upsurge of interest in personal health – an encouraging trend but one that is being satisfied by 'pill popping' rather than by sound dietary practices.

Should vitamin supplements be taken at all, or singly, or in combined 'multivit' forms? What is a health-promoting vitamin when supplied in tiny quantities by nature can, in overdose, become a dangerous poison. Vitamins A and D taken in excess can kill. Too much vitamin C can cause kidney stones. Minerals too carry dangers. Iron can inflame

Pulses, cereals, dried fruits and nuts are all part of a well-stocked 'health kitchen'. To get the most benefit from the food, they need careful weighing for a balanced diet.

the bowel and selenium is poisonous at quite modest overdose levels.

Even bran, source of the dietary fibre that Western-style eating lacks, has its dangers. It is widely available in health food shops as a concentrated, refined product that makes it easy to take in too much at one time – far more than you would eat in natural foods. Too much interferes with the absorption of iron, calcium, zinc and other essential minerals and nutrients.

Equally risky is taking every new fad substance that man's ingenuity brings onto the market. Individual amino acids have been offered as nutritional supplements in recent years. They are the basic building blocks of food and body proteins, but also serve as transmitter substances in the brain, passing information from one nerve cell to another. The body has sophisticated mechanisms to regulate the flow of the 22 different amino acids it needs and ensures that only those required are allowed to penetrate the brain, and even then only in suitable amounts. The amounts and balance of amino acids that you would take in from the proteins in foods are safe, but to load the body with individual amino acids can overwhelm its protective mechanisms and disrupt normal functioning of the brain.

A significant number of new fad substances are later withdrawn as useless, dangerous or both. The most recent is the mineral germanium, at first promoted as a wonder drug to stimulate the immune system and boost vitality. Now it has been withdrawn because it may cause kidney damage. In any

case, there is serious doubt that it ever did anything beneficial. An earlier example was Laetrile, the so-called vitamin B_{17}, that was supposed to cure cancer and produced cyanide in the body.

If you feel certain that you need supplements because your diet and lifestyle are so poorly managed, or because of illness, stick to safe and beneficial low-dose mixtures of minerals and vitamins from a reputable chemist or health shop. High-dose, high-potency single nutrients are quite likely to create more problems than they solve, by disturbing your metabolic balance. Megadosing, especially of individual nutrients, is nothing to do with nutrition. It is far better to use nature's supplements: milk, cheese or yoghurt for calcium, red meat for iron, carrots for vitamin A, greens for so many things.

Natural tonic supplements, such as ginseng, honey and GARLIC, have been used for thousands of years in the hope of improving strength and performance. Ginseng contains pharmacologically active substances that do something – but precisely what is not clear. There is no evidence that it does harm so long as the dosage is modest, and many people believe it has done them good. Honey is just a mixture of sugars with minute amounts of nutrients. There is no evidence that it does anything more than act as a fuel and taste nice. There is growing evidence, however, that garlic can reduce blood fats, blood pressure and blood clotting – all of which are helpful in the fight against coronary heart disease.

Another popular supplement, evening-primrose oil, has done well in some trials and may help PREMENSTRUAL TENSION, breast tenderness, ALCOHOLISM and ECZEMA. It contains the fatty acid GLA (gamma linolenic

acid) which the body converts into hormone-like substances. These appear to reduce inflammation, decrease cholesterol levels and regulate the female reproductive system. Side effects are rare, but epilepsy sufferers should not take the supplement.

In your search for a sound approach to health, observe three simple rules for nutritional sanity. Firstly, avoid extremes and overdoses. Just because a little is good, it does not mean that twice as much or a lot is better. Secondly, avoid single-nutrient supplements. In nature, micronutrients occur and work in complex groups, not individually. Thirdly, eat a well-balanced mixture of natural, fresh, nourishing foods – and put your trust in nature's delicate balance.

HEALTH HAZARDS

How to cope with some of the hazards – such as aerosols and lead pollution – which daily threaten our health? See IS THE ENVIRONMENT MAKING YOU ILL? p.172.

HEARTBURN

Despite its name, this discomfort or burning pain felt behind the breastbone is nothing to do with the heart. It is one of the symptoms of INDIGESTION or ACID STOMACH, and is avoided or treated in the same way.

HEART DISORDERS

The heart is one of the most efficient pumps ever evolved, beating approximately 2,5 billion times in a lifetime of 70 years. But like any other pump, if it becomes clogged it becomes less efficient – or even stops working altogether, threatening life itself.

In South Africa 31 people die of heart attacks every day (11 530 fatalities a year). This number represents just a quarter of the 124 people admitted to hospital daily for heart attacks.

From early adulthood onwards, plaques of the fatty substance cholesterol are deposited on the walls of blood vessels. Eventually this deposit may block the coronary ARTERIES that supply blood to the heart muscle itself and cause heart disease.

Partial blockage may result in ANGINA. More seriously, if a blood clot lodges suddenly in a coronary artery and blocks it completely, part of the heart is starved of oxygen, causing a 'heart attack' or even stopping it beating altogether.

Other complaints are associated with old age. Hearts become 'tired' and susceptible to both heart failure (weakening) and heart block, a condition which causes the heart to beat very slowly, sometimes only 30-40 times a minute. The rate does not increase on exertion, so the patient tires very easily. Heart valves may also become ineffective later in life, often as a result of rheumatic fever. Typical symptoms are breathlessness and WATER RETENTION, when the ankles swell towards evening.

Some babies are born with congenital heart disease in which the chambers or valves of the heart are not properly formed. Cardiomyopathy is general weakness and enlargement of the heart. There are many causes of this, and the condition can develop at any particular age.

Warning Anyone suspecting that they have a heart disorder should see their doctor before undertaking any alternative regimes or remedies.

What the therapists recommend

Autogenic Training This has been found helpful in reducing high BLOOD PRESSURE and cholesterol levels, and in steadying the heart rate and increasing blood flow to the body's extremities. All these things can help to increase the efficiency of the circulatory system and so help the heart to recover.

Naturopathy Practitioners will advise seeking orthodox treatment for heart disorders, but can advise on preventive measures. Reducing fats – especially animal fats – sugars and salt will be part of a dietary regime which includes increased intake of fresh fruit and vegetables, also whole grains. Regular EXERCISE is advised to maintain heart and lung fitness, and time should be set aside for relaxation and gentler exercises such as YOGA to combat STRESS.

An orthodox view

Doctors are concerned to try to prevent heart disorders by encouraging their patients to exercise regularly, eat sensibly and avoid SMOKING. Early detection and treatment of high blood pressure and raised blood cholesterol also helps some people who otherwise would be at risk.

Doctors can prescribe a variety of medicines to relieve angina. If these prescriptions are ineffective, bypass surgery to reroute the blood around the clogged coronary artery to the heart may help the condition. Modern medical treatment of a heart attack includes 'clot-busting' drugs such as streptokinase, which reduce the amount of damage to the heart muscle.

Increasingly ambulances, paramedics and doctors are equipped with defibrillators, which electrically shock the heart out of potentially fatal conditions. Heart block is usually treated successfully by inserting a battery-powered pacemaker under the skin of the chest wall. It produces tiny electric stimuli to keep the heart beating regularly and at the right rate – an average of 70-72 beats a minute for an adult male, awake but at rest, and 78-82 for a woman.

The risk of having a baby born with congenital heart disease is reduced if the mother has been immunised against German measles, and if she avoids smoking, drugs and medicines, particularly around the time of conception and during early pregnancy.

HEAT RASH

This harmless, but irritating, pimply skin rash most commonly affects babies and overweight people in hot weather. Also known as 'prickly heat', it appears around skin creases and where clothing is tight. The skin rapidly recovers on a return to cooler weather.

What the therapists recommend

Herbal Medicine You are advised to bathe the area with a cold infusion of marigold or lavender to reduce the inflammation. The leaves of many fleshy plants, such as the houseleek (*Sempervivum*, hen-and-chickens), may cool and soothe when applied to the affected area.

An orthodox view

There is no quick, conventional remedy. Doctors usually advise sufferers to wear loose clothing, avoid direct sunlight and take frequent baths or showers. Calamine lotion gives some relief. See also SUNBURN.

HELLERWORK

Realigning the balance of your body

The basis of this therapy is a series of 90-minute sessions of manipulation, movement and discussion designed to restore the body's balance, returning it to a more relaxed and youthful state and so releasing built-up TENSION and STRESS.

Hellerwork was founded in 1978 by a former American aerospace engineer, Joseph Heller. It does not set out to cure illness but to prevent it by freeing people from their set patterns of moving and thinking, thereby allowing them to adapt more easily to life's changes. The aim of the therapy is to release tension and rigidity, and to prevent it from occurring in the first place.

It concentrates on a form of connective body tissue called fascia, which wraps the individual fibres and bundles of fibres that become muscle. Fascia comes together at the end of the muscle and forms the tendon, which attaches the muscle to the bone.

Finding a practitioner Although there are no Hellerwork practitioners as such in South Africa, qualified physiotherapists (see entry on PHYSIOTHERAPY) learn similar therapeutic techniques as part of their massage training; and this enables them to relieve 'myo-fascial' pain – the pain that is associated with muscle fascia.

An orthodox view

Many physical therapies are similar in their approach, although they are known by different names. Hellerwork, ROLFING and the ALEXANDER TECHNIQUE, for example, all aim to bring about the harmonious integration of mind and body.

HERBAL MEDICINE

The popularity of medicinal herbs is booming as more and more people are turning to nature for their health's sake. See USING THE HEALING POWER OF HERBS, p.182.

HERPES

The term 'herpes' includes a variety of different skin diseases characterised by spreading clusters of tiny, painful blisters. (The word is derived from the Greek *herpein*, 'to creep'.)

Infection with the *herpes simplex* virus leads to, among other things, COLD SORES and MOUTH ULCERS, and to the sexually transmitted GENITAL HERPES.

Once this virus has invaded the body it remains there for the rest of life, dormant in the nerve ganglia. However, in about 40 per cent of affected persons there will be no recurrence of the complaint, and where attacks do recur they become gradually less severe and less frequent. Triggers to a recurrence are minor infections, stress of any kind, and exposure to the sun.

Herpes zoster is the medical term used for SHINGLES. The 'varicella-zoster' virus responsible for shingles is also the culprit responsible for CHICKENPOX. In both complaints the eyes may be affected.

Getting fit – away from it all

Modern health resorts follow the basic principles of naturopathy, with treatment centred mainly on diet and fasting (see NATURO- PATHY), and many people go there to lose weight, improve their health and change their lifestyle. A person may wish to stop smoking, improve poor eating habits, or embark on a comprehensive fitness and exercise programme. However, most health resorts – or hydros, as they are more often called – also offer a wide range of therapies such as AROMATHERAPY, SHIATSU, REFLEXOLOGY, HYDROTHERAPY, kneipp, sitz baths, YOGA, RELAXATION classes, PHYSIOTHERAPY or manipulation.

Their facilities include gymnasiums, saunas, steam rooms, swimming pools and hydrotherapy baths. Exercise facilities include such diverse pursuits as golf, snooker, tennis, water aerobics in heated pools, circuit training in a gymnasium, and the opportunity to go for scenic walks.

For both women and men there may be skin and body care salons.

Some health resorts insist that guests must be at least 16 – in some cases 18 – years of age; and if the guest has a medical problem, the health resort would insist on an appropriate letter from a doctor.

An initial consultation and physical examination by a doctor or registered nurse is normally held, and the weight and blood pressure of the visitor is checked daily. Many guests have chronic health problems such as ARTHRITIS, DIGESTIVE PROBLEMS, SKIN DISORDERS, high BLOOD PRESSURE or overweight.

Some people are suffering from stress-related symptoms, and others merely need to escape from the routine and pressure of business and domestic life. It is the clear-cut philosophy of many hydros to make sure that their guests unwind, and after a few days at a hydro, the stresses and strains of modern living tend to disappear.

Most hydros insist on a minimum stay of one week, during which time the guest will be prescribed a specific diet, have daily MASSAGE and hydrotherapy, and start a gradual exercise regimen.

The diet is usually vegetarian, and may start with a low-kilojoule fruit fast followed by salads, vegetables and whole grains. Drinking of water is encouraged, and coffee and tea are prohibited. Some health resorts may supply herb or rooibos tea. Guests are allowed to wander about the premises in dressing gowns or track suits, and to rest and relax as much as possible.

Some hydros offer educational lectures aimed at teaching guests about preventing illness and achieving optimum health. These lectures would cover all aspects of nutrition, exercise, positive thinking, relaxation and postural re-education.

The guest may be given information about his or her body composition, or may have a physical fitness assessment, or nutritional analysis.

The cost of staying at a health resort varies between R1 500 and R2 000 per week. This would include daily massage, hydrotherapy and other activities but excludes specialised beauty treatments.

Accommodation is invariably comfortable and at health resorts such as the High Rustenburg Hydro near Stellenbosch guests have the use of such luxuries as telephones, TVs, and air-conditioning or electric fans in their rooms.

The High Rustenburg Hydro near Stellenbosch, which lies among rolling hills, and is surrounded by breathtaking scenery, has an outdoor and indoor pool for the use of its visitors.

Treatment at a health resort involves several therapies for toning-up and stimulating the body. (Left) The visitor has her hands covered with hot paraffin wax to soothe them. (Centre) The visitor lies down comfortably on a couch while hot packs containing crystal gel are applied to her back and shoulders to relieve tension and draw out pain.

Hot packs, cold showers – and a puff in the 'Butt Hut'

The following is an hour-by-hour account of a young businesswoman's intensive day's toning-up at the popular High Rustenburg Hydro, Stellenbosch.

7:30 am The prescribed diet for breakfast is served in your bedroom.

9:00 am The guest is seen by a senior registered nurse and asked if she has ever had any serious illness, if she is currently taking any form of medication, and what – if anything – she feels is wrong with her.

In this, as in many cases, the nurse is told that the guest simply wishes to relax, be pampered, and leave feeling fitter and fresher than when she came.

The nurse takes her blood pressure to make sure it is not too high or low, and checks her weight and possibly her blood sugar.

A schedule of therapies is issued, and the guest changes into a swimsuit covered by a bathrobe, with slippers or soft shoes.

9:30 am The day starts with an invigorating session with a masseur. The guest spends 45 minutes having knots and nodules kneaded out of her shoulders and back.

10:15 am She goes from the massage room to the ladies' therapy rooms where she enters the sauna after showering. She may choose between having a sauna, which is dry heat, or the steam room, which is moist heat. The treatment is used to expel moisture from the body, get rid of waste products and poisons, to stimulate the circulation, and to help the person to relax. Following this she rests in a peaceful area and listens to music.

10:45 am The guest moves to the hydropools where she will relax in an individual heated bath with underwater massage for 20 minutes. Following this she will rest a while before her next appointment.

11:15 am Body composition is assessed on a device which measures body fat as well as lean body mass. This provides valuable information as to whether the visitor is overweight, correct weight or underweight.

11:30 am Physical exercise in the form of water aerobics is held in the spacious indoor heated swimming pool. The 30-minute workout is a combination of aerobic exercise, stretching and toning, and is led by a physical education instructor. Swimmers and nonswimmers are shown how to pedal or jog in the water, and do arm and leg exercises which benefit the whole body.

(Top right) Holding onto steel bars for support, the visitor stands naked – her back covered with salt – while she is sprayed with hot and cold water alternately. The so-called Scottish douche is for stimulating the circulation. (Right) The visitor relaxes in a warm bath which soothes the skin and the body.

12:15 pm Lunch is served in the dining-room overlooking sweeping lawns and gardens. High Rustenburg is famous for its salads, which are served from a lavish buffet decorated with imaginative vegetable garnishings. Afterwards the visitor is free to stroll in the grounds, or relax by the pool.

1:30 pm Time for reflexology, and some intensive foot massage.

2:00 pm Next stop is the skin care clinic where the visitor has a facial specially prescribed for her skin type and using natural herb products and essential oils.

3:00 pm The daily programme ends with a half hour relaxation class which concentrates on the importance of breathing properly, MEDITATION and VISUALISATION – all of which can help combat tiredness and stress.

3:30 pm Soup time at the hydro – a vegetable broth – is offered to all guests.

6:00 pm Dinner is served and everybody discusses their experiences during the day.

7:00 pm All guests are invited to attend a lecture on 'stress in our daily lives' by a guest speaker from the local university.

Is the environment making you ill?

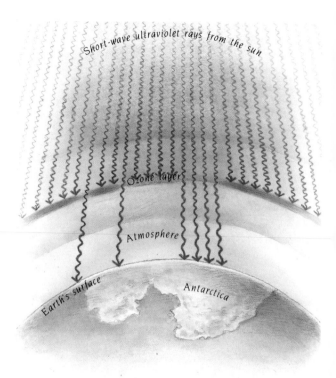

Daily life exposes us to all sorts of situations, substances, machines and gadgets that the human body was never designed to cope with. From aerosols to air conditioning and exhaust fumes to X-rays, hundreds of ordinary things in the immediate environment can damage our health.

Less direct but equally serious risks come from a multitude of industries, agriculture, power stations, mines and waste disposal, in the form of water and air pollution, noise, stress, exposure to dangerous chemicals, and even increased levels of radiation. There also exist longer-term perils, such as the much debated greenhouse effect, that may not pose an immediate threat but promise to affect the health, safety or comfort of future generations.

Although many of these hazards are beyond the power of individuals to control, there is still much that each person can do to make the environment healthier.

Air pollution

Poisons are continually being pumped into the air by industries, traffic, agricultural spraying, power stations, aircraft, aerosols, and wood, coal and garden rubbish fires.

Health risks include HEADACHES, EYE DISORDERS and irritation of the throat, lungs and respiratory tract, which can contribute to illnesses such as ALLERGY, ASTHMA, BRONCHITIS and EMPHYSEMA. Some chemicals may enter the blood from the lungs, eventually damaging the IMMUNE SYSTEM, causing CANCER, and contributing to defects in newborn babies.

Air pollution can have other serious consequences:

Lead from petrol   Three-quarters of the lead that poisons our air comes from vehicle exhausts. Lead can damage the brain and nervous system. It has also been associated with elevated blood pressure in adults and with HYPERACTIVITY and lower intelligence in children; and it may be particularly dangerous for pregnant women and their unborn babies.

What to do   Cut down car use if possible. Cycling, walking, public transport and car-sharing all help. Wrap a fine silk scarf over your mouth and nose or use a surgical mask when walking, cycling

The ozone layer lies 10 to 30 km above the earth, and protects us from cancer-causing short-wave ultraviolet radiation. Gases such as CFCs destroy ozone, and a large 'hole' in the layer – a thinning of the ozone – occurs each spring over Antarctica and a smaller one over the Arctic. However, by mid-1990, about 60 nations had agreed to phase out CFC production by the year 2000.

or jogging on roads with heavy traffic, but avoid such routes as much as possible.

Lead-free petrol cannot yet be bought at South African filling-stations. However, environmental groups and other concerned bodies have been campaigning for its introduction for some years; and it seems certain that eventually all South African cars will have been converted to run on unleaded fuel, which will be readily available.

Acid rain   A more correct name for this would be acid deposit or acid fallout, because the damage is done by pollutants in dry as well as wet form. Sulphur dioxide, nitrogen oxides and ozone are the main acid deposit gases. Sulphuric acid and nitric acid are chief among the wet deposits, which are formed when the pollutants are dissolved in rainwater. The burning of coal and oil in industry, and especially fumes from power stations and refineries, manufacturing (especially of chemicals), and vehicle exhausts are major sources of the pollution. Domestic users of fuels also play a part.

The pollutants may be carried for hundreds of kilometres by air currents before they are deposited. For example, large areas of the eastern Transvaal are gravely affected by sources of pollution in the industrialised Rand; as a result of complicated climatic factors, the pollution is highest in the dry (winter) season.

The earth is turning into a gigantic hothouse, for carbon dioxide, CFCs and other gases in its atmosphere act like the glass of a greenhouse. Short-wave heat rays from the sun pass through, but when the heat is re-radiated by the earth as long-wave radiation, the gases trap it. Significant global warming has begun; four years in the 1980s were the warmest since reliable records began.

Apart from the direct harm acid deposits do to health by causing respiratory diseases, they also alter the ecological balance of an area. They cause leaf loss and the eventual death of trees, increased acidity of soils, lakes and rivers, and the release of aluminium in soils where the underlying rock is granite. The aluminium runs into the rivers where it poisons fish, with a consequent increase in life-forms the fish would have eaten and a decrease in creatures that feed on fish.

What to do Individuals can reduce pollution by cutting their own consumption of coal and oil, and especially of petrol in cars. There is not much they can do about industrial pollution except to ask a local environmental officer to check the level of air pollution coming from factories in the area, and to monitor the acidity of rain and water in lakes and rivers.

To learn more about this problem, you should contact an environmental group such as Earthlife Africa, which has branches in many centres in South Africa, including Cape Town (P O Box 176, Observatory 7935), Durban (P O Box 38396, Point 4069), Pretoria (P O Box 40373, Arcadia 0007) and Johannesburg (P O Box 11383, Johannesburg 2000).

Carbon monoxide When carbon fuels are burnt with an inadequate supply of oxygen, carbon monoxide results. The colourless, odourless gas combines more readily with the haemoglobin in blood than oxygen does, and can cause suffocation. Most appliances produce some carbon monoxide, but motor vehicles are major producers.

What to do Catalytic converters convert the carbon monoxide, nitrogen oxides and hydrocarbons in a car's exhaust to less harmful carbon dioxide, water and nitrogen. The snag is that such converters are suitable only for cars that can use lead-free petrol.

CFCs Chlorofluorocarbons (CFCs) are nonflammable, virtually nontoxic gases widely released into the atmosphere. They are used mainly as propellants in aerosols, as coolants in refrigerators and air-conditioning plants, in the manufacture of plastic foam packaging, and as solvents in the electronics industry. They are very stable, and some last for more than 100 years. However, when they break down in the sunlight of the upper atmosphere they release chlorine, which persistently destroys ozone.

Although ozone is one of the acid deposit gases which are found in the lower atmosphere, it is essential in the upper atmosphere, where it forms a layer that shields us from too much ultraviolet light (see p.174 under RADIATION). The ozone layer has already been damaged by CFCs. If the damage continues, cases of skin cancer and of CATARACTS will increase in number and agriculture may eventually be harmed.

About 60 countries, including South Africa, have signed the Montreal Protocol, under which they have agreed to phase out use of CFCs by the end of the century. What is not certain, however, is whether the countries will be able to carry out their undertaking, or whether cutback by just these countries will be enough to prevent further damage to the ozone layer.

What to do Buy 'ozone-friendly' products instead of CFC aerosols and products in plastic foam packs. CFC-free refrigerators are becoming available.

Global warming As well as damaging the ozone layer, CFCs are among the gases that are causing the 'greenhouse effect' by trapping heat in the atmosphere. Carbon dioxide is another 'greenhouse gas'. The burning of wood and fossil fuels such as coal, natural gas and petroleum products – including oil, paraffin and petrol – produces carbon dioxide, and its output is increasing worldwide. Vehicle exhausts are a major source in the West.

At the same time, large-scale destruction of tropical forests in land-clearance schemes in the Amazon and other areas is worsening the situation. Trees and other green plants use up carbon dioxide and release oxygen as they manufacture their food, but now the earth's natural capacity to process carbon dioxide cannot keep pace with the increased emission.

The average global temperature has been rising very gradually over the last century. It is not clear how far this is part of natural fluctuation or how far it is due to the greenhouse effect. Rising sea levels from the expansion of water as it warms and from the melting of land ice are threatening to flood low-lying areas and submerge some islands. Many large cities and much prime farming land could be affected.

The food supply may be severely affected. A warmer climate may produce droughts in some areas, more rain in others. The distribution of plants and crops would change, and fish and animal populations would be different.

What to do Individuals can use less of the energy sources and goods that produce carbon dioxide in their generation, manufacture or use. Switch off lights and electrical appliances when they are not necessary; draught-proof and insulate the home; make garden rubbish into compost instead of burning it; cut out unnecessary driving and use a car with low fuel consumption; and stop using CFC aerosols.

Water pollution

Rivers, lakes, reservoirs, domestic water Some of the main pollutants are: the run-off from nitrate fertilisers, pesticides, silage and slurry used in agriculture; phosphates from detergent washing powders; and industrial wastes such as dioxin, which is a by-product from the manufacture of chemicals and from bleaching paper products. Nitrates convert to other substances in the body, where they reduce the amount of oxygen in the blood. Bottle-fed babies are at risk, even if the water used to make up their feeds is boiled before use. Some scientists believe they can also cause cancer of the oesophagus and stomach, but the evidence on this is not conclusive. Even small quantities of dioxin can result in SKIN DISORDERS such as chloracne, miscarriages, cancer and birth deformities; larger quantities can kill.

Chlorine is added to water to rid it of bacteria, but although the water may smell and sometimes taste of chlorine, the amount permitted is not usually a health hazard. However, some people may be allergic to it.

Aluminium is also added, in order to make the water clear. The amount permitted is extremely small – but there is controversy about how much is harmful. Some studies have suggested that ALZHEIMER'S DISEASE could be linked to aluminium. South Africa is free at any rate from the controversy associated with fluoridation. Fluoride is a compound that occurs naturally in some water (in particular in the northern Cape); and in a number of countries – but not South Africa – additional amounts are added to help prevent tooth decay. Large doses of fluoride can cause mottling of teeth, and it has been suggested that they may also be associated with genetic defects and even cancer.

What to do An efficient, properly maintained water filter can remove many chemicals from drinking water. Always take drinking water direct from a cold tap on the mains, not from a storage tank, and run the tap for a few moments first – hot water and water that has been standing in the pipes tend to contain more dissolved impurities.

To make sure you do not contribute to the pollution of your environment, you can avoid garden fertilisers and household goods that produce toxic wastes. Some supermarkets now sell unbleached paper towels, toilet paper and other items, as well as phosphate-free, biodegradable washing powders, shampoos and other liquids. You can also make your own non-polluting cleaners – see box on p.178.

Sea water The sea has a limited capacity to break down waste, and parts of South Africa's shoreline are badly polluted. Industrial and agricultural waste and oil spills are all problems. But by far the greatest threat to health is the discharge of raw or only partially treated sewage into the sea, leading to dangerously high levels of bacteria, algae and viruses, and contaminating shellfish. Stomach upsets are the most common danger faced by bathers but swallowing or bathing in badly polluted water, or eating contaminated shellfish, can also lead to ear and eye infections or hepatitis.

What to do Avoid swimming in the sea if you have doubts about the quality of the water. Look for sewage outlet pipes, and check with the tourist board before bathing.

Radiation

Nuclear radiation We are all exposed to nuclear radiation from many sources, some natural, some man-made. Particles from space, rocks (see Radon under Hazards in the home, p.175), soil, plants and other natural sources are responsible for 87 per cent of the radiation, and man-made items for only 13 per cent. Of the man-made radiation, 11,5 per cent comes from medical sources such as X-rays, and the rest from miscellaneous sources, including nuclear weapons tests, mining and processing radioactive matter, power-station discharges, high-altitude air travel (where there is less protection given by the atmosphere), and some household items such as luminous clock and watch dials and smoke detectors.

Radiation is measured in sieverts (Sv) or fractions of this unit. The Atomic Energy Corporation of South Africa regards a dose of 0,25 millisieverts per year as the acceptable maximum for members of the public in the vicinity of any discrete – that is, self-standing – nuclear installation, such as Koeberg power station in the south-western Cape. For workers at such an installation the figure is much higher, at 500 millisieverts. By comparison a chest X-ray is about 0,5 millisieverts.

High doses of nuclear radiation can kill. Lower doses can cause NAUSEA AND VOMITING, DIARRHOEA, bleeding, hair loss and eventual death. Radiation can also cause damage to human cells which makes them reproduce abnormally.

This can give rise to cancer and genetic defects that can affect future generations. The long-term effects of continual exposure to small amounts of nuclear radiation are not yet fully understood by researchers but some researchers believe that it can cause allergies, ASTHMA, high BLOOD PRESSURE and muscular or bone defects.

What to do Before having an X-ray, ask your doctor or dentist if it is essential, and make sure a protective bib or sheet shields the rest of your body. Avoid luminous-dial clocks and watches.

An extra precaution is to make sure you are getting enough iodine (see MINERALS) – it helps to eliminate any radioactive matter in the body.

Ultraviolet light Too much ultraviolet light, whether from natural sunlight or from a sunlamp, can cause eye disorders such as cataracts. It can also cause skin cancer; the greatest danger is to people with a fair complexion whose skin does not produce a protective tan but burns and freckles.

What to do Instead of baring yourself to strong sun, protect yourself with a broad-brimmed hat, a loose shirt, and trousers or a skirt. Use an effective sun-blocking cream on parts that are exposed to the sun for any length of time (see SUNBURN). Report to your doctor immediately any changes in moles or dark patches of skin, or skin sores that do not heal. They are easily treated in their early stages.

Electromagnetic fields A multitude of high and low-frequency electromagnetic waves emanate from man-made equipment – high-voltage cables, radar systems, microwave communications systems, domestic cables and appliances, computer and word processor terminals (see VDUs under Hazards at work, p.179). We are only beginning to recognise the effects that long-term exposure to these fields may have. The evidence is growing, but not conclusive, that they may cause head-aches, nausea, impaired concentration, STRESS, cataracts, disturbances of the nerv-ous system, and even cancer and genetic damage.

What to do It is difficult to avoid the effects of electromagnetic fields set up by power cables. However, you can reduce the fields in your home by remembering always to turn off unnecessary lights and appliances.

When watching TV, sit at least 2 m away from the screen, where the field is weaker. Some manufacturers are now producing computers with shielded parts, to reduce the electrical fields set up.

Hazards in the home

Lead in water Chlorine, aluminium and fluoride may be present in drinking water (see p.174 under Water pollution), but the greatest hazard is lead. It is very rare for lead piping to be used to transport water into a property from the local main; but if such piping does exist it should be re-placed without delay, for lead in drinking water is a serious health hazard. If you can-not afford to do so immediately, let the tap run for a time whenever you draw water, so that you do not use water that has been standing in the pipes.

Carbon monoxide See p.172 under Air pollution for the dangers of this gas. Paraffin heaters and gas appliances – including cookers, boilers, water heaters and fires – all produce it, along with small amounts of nitrogen dioxide, formaldehyde and sul-phur dioxide, which can aggravate bron-chitis, emphysema, asthma and ANGINA.

What to do Check that all appliances are properly adjusted – their flames should burn blue with no orange showing. If an item of gas equipment is not burning effi-ciently and you cannot adjust it, your local gas appliance centre should be able to

There is increasing evidence that the invisible electromagnetic fields around electrical appliances and power lines can be hazardous. The fields of 220-volt domestic power cables extend only a few centimetres. However, those around high-power lines such as those of the national grid, which operate at anything up to 800 000 kilovolts, can extend for hundreds of metres. The extremely low-frequency electromagnetic radiation from such lines has been linked speculatively with depression, insomnia, headaches and even with cancer. Our exposure to electromagnetic radiation from all sources – from the extremely low-frequency rays emitted by power lines and VDUs, through radio, microwaves, infrared (heat), light and ultraviolet rays to ultra-high-frequency, ionising X-rays and gamma rays – has increased nearly 10 000 times in the last 50 years.

help. Use all appliances only in well-ventilated rooms; if doors and windows are sealed for insulation, make sure there is an efficient ventilator. Have the flue cleaned regularly. Do not use a paraffin heater constantly. Have all appliances serviced regu-larly by professionals.

Fumes from open fires Carbon monoxide is also among the gases given off by burning wood and coal, and wood smoke also contains cancer-causing fumes. Burning plastic and rubber, on a garden fire for example, may give off the deadly gas dioxin.

The plastic foam filling which is com-monly used for furniture and mattresses will give off deadly cyanide fumes if it cat-ches fire. Latex is less hazardous, and a fire-retardant plastic foam has been developed in the last few years, but furniture already in the home or on sale secondhand may contain the more dangerous type of plastic foam filling.

What to do If you use an open fire in your home, make sure the chimney is swept regularly and is not letting smoke drift back into the room. Closed stoves are safer. En-sure that the room is well ventilated.

If you intend to buy foam-filled furni-ture you should bear in mind that a fire-retardant brand of foam can be ordered; it is considerably more expensive than other foam, however.

Install smoke detectors in your home. They will give occupants the crucial time necessary to get away from dangerous fumes, which kill more people – and kill them sooner – than are killed by flames.

Radon This colourless, odourless gas which is radioactive comes out of the ground, where it is produced by the decay of the element radium in rocks. Although radon is present in minute quantities everywhere, it comes mostly from granite rocks, which contain small amounts of radium. Radon can seep into homes through floors and walls, and in rare instan-ces remain trapped there until there is a dangerous build-up. It accumulates in people's lungs, and can eventually cause RESPIRATORY DISORDERS and lung cancer.

Houses which are built in granitic areas – for example, the Paarl Rock area of the western Cape – are considered to be at the greatest risk, especially if the structure is an old one in which the space beneath the wooden floor and the foundations lacks ventilation. Solid concrete floors provide greater protection. The concentration of gas is measured in becquerels (Bq) per cubic metre; if the count exceeds 200 Bq, the affected home may need to be treated.

What to do Ensure that ground-floor and under-floor ventilation are efficient. If the house is in a high-risk area, floors and pipe inlets should be well sealed.

For advice about radon contamination in your area, and how to prevent it, you can contact the Atomic Energy Corporation of South Africa, P O Box 582, Pretoria 0001. Your municipality's environmental health officer should also be able to help with any enquiries about radon contamination.

Formaldehyde Pressed timbers and plastic goods contain this chemical in the adhesives which are used to make them, and it is also used in some types of plastic foam, including some cavity-wall insulation. It gives off a vapour that can irritate the eyes, throat and skin, cause headaches and general fatigue, and is a suspected cause of cancer.

What to do Use as many solid and natural materials as you can to avoid an accumulation that causes discomfort. Make sure there is adequate ventilation in rooms where you detect the sharp smell of the vapour.

Air imbalance The natural balance of positive and negative electrically charged particles (ions) in the air is appreciably disturbed by electrical fields from nearby television sets and various other electronic appliances, by static from synthetic fabrics and by polluted or dry air. The negative ions are reduced from their normal fresh-air proportion of four parts for every five parts of positive ions. A similar reduction occurs before thunderstorms. A drop in negative ions may cause TENSION, irritability, MIGRAINE and HAY FEVER.

What to do Choose natural fibres such as wool and cotton rather than synthetics for clothes, home furnishings, carpets and curtains. Turn off television sets, computers and other electronic equipment when not in use. Good ventilation is another way of preventing positive ions from building up, as is a negative ionising machine (see IONISATION).

Cleaners Most commercial cleaners such as detergent washing powders, bleaches, scouring powders, window cleaners, polishes and air fresheners can cause health problems, including skin and eye irritations, and allergies. Many cleaners are poisonous if swallowed, and some give off fumes that can irritate the nose and throat – chlorine bleach and ammonia-based products are particularly dangerous.

What to do Use cleaners sparingly, following the instructions and ensuring the room is well ventilated. Wear gloves if you are going to touch them. Use hydrogen peroxide bleach rather than chlorine. Do not mix different products, especially chlorine and ammonia-based ones. For example, do not put bleach in the sink if you have been using scouring powder; the combination gives off chloramine vapour.

If sprays such as window cleaners irritate your eyes, nose or throat, look for alternative products that are used as solids or liquids. 'Green' cleaners are now available in most supermarkets, and cause fewer health problems, as well as less pollution. Alternatively, you can make your own simple cleaners by following the instructions in the box on p. 178.

Plenty of light at any workplace

Good insulation to conserve heat

Good light for reading in bed

Natural fibre bedding for warmth and air circulation at night

Fire-retardant mattress

Plenty of curtains, cushions and rugs for noise insulation

Television set at least 2 m from viewers

Natural fibre carpet to reduce positive ion build-up and reduce fire risk

Fire-retardant newer furniture, or older pieces covered with fireproof fabric

Lead-free paint on walls

Smoke detectors out of reach of children.

Half-hour fire door

Toiletries made without the use of CFC s and harsh chemical ingredients

House plants to contribute oxygen

Ozone-friendly fire extinguisher

Double glazing for warmth, preventing draughts and cutting down noise

Fire blanket for emergencies

Flue from gas stove

Good ventilation and natural light

Window boxes to provide noise insulation

Outlet duct

Radon-proof suspended floor

Radon-proof solid floor

'Green' cleaners stored out of children's reach

Gas cooker with flue for gases

Trench

Note Make sure that you store all household cleaners upright and out of reach of children.

Toiletries Cosmetics, perfumes, soaps and other toiletries can cause allergies, skin irritations and rashes in sensitive people; and if hairspray is used regularly it can collect in the lungs, causing breathing trouble. Frequent use of some hair dyes that contact the skin is suspected of causing cancer.

What to do Read the labels before you buy toiletries and choose those made from plant extracts rather than mineral oils. The plant extracts are less likely to have ill effects, especially if they are also free of added colours and scents. Many toiletries can be simply and cheaply made at home (see NATURAL AIDS TO BEAUTY). Use hair dyes that give paint-on highlights or treat selected areas only.

Insecticides Most household insecticides such as fly killers, mothballs and house plant sprays are poisonous if swallowed or inhaled. Many contain chlorine or hydrocarbons – naphthalene in mothballs is a hydrocarbon. Even when correctly used, they can cause irritating rashes, allergies, breathing problems, and eye, nose and throat irritations.

What to do Do not attract insects. Cover food, empty rubbish bins often and do not let washing up accumulate. See box for natural insect repellents.

You can often rid house plants – and garden plants – of pests by washing them with soapy water, taking care to treat both sides of the leaves. Or treat them with derris powder.

DIY products Many glues, paints, paint strippers, wood preservatives, varnishes, fillers and sealants, and other decorating and hobby products give off poisonous vapours until completely dry. If inhaled, these can cause sickness, dizziness, respiratory disorders and allergies. Flexible sealants which are not meant to harden completely continue to give off minute amounts of vapour. Glue or solvent sniffing can also become a dangerous ADDICTION.

Dust from timber, asbestos and cement sheets, bricks, and glass-fibre insulation material can irritate the lungs and cause chest disorders. Asbestos dust can also cause cancer.

What to do Follow the instructions carefully when using DIY products and wear gloves, safety goggles and a face mask whenever necessary. Do all possible jobs outside and make sure any indoor work area is well ventilated. Use glues that dry hard whenever

Greener cleaners

Some simple ingredients can be used to make safe and inexpensive household cleaners. Soap and water is the most useful and can replace many special-purpose cleaners. Stubborn dirt will often yield to soaking in soapy water – or you can wipe it at intervals over dirty surfaces until the dirt softens.

Washing-up liquid Put small slivers of hand soap in a warmed jam-jar, cover with boiling water and let them dissolve. Add 1-2 tablespoons of washing soda in hard-water areas. Use the mixture for washing up. Add a tablespoon of washing soda or vinegar to the washing-up water for greasy dishes.

Washing powder Use equal quantities of soap flakes and washing soda. A few tablespoons of washing soda also makes commercial biodegradable washing powders work a lot better.

Bleach Borax is a good bleach and disinfectant, although not as strong as a chlorine bleach. Keep borax out of children's reach.

Scouring powder Mix salt and sodium bicarbonate in equal quantities and rub on with a moist cloth.

Mirrors and tiles Use equal quantities of white vinegar and water. Mix and use for wiping off splash marks.

Fabric softener Combine one part bicarbonate of soda, one part white vinegar and two parts water. Use as you would a commercial softener.

Air freshener Good ventilation is best. For a pleasing scent use fresh flowers, herbs, potpourri or essential oils (see AROMATHERAPY).

possible. Do not work on any asbestos products or installations – it is a job for professionals only.

Food

Agricultural methods Unless they are labelled as organically grown, nearly all fruit and vegetables have been sprayed with chemicals, and grown with artificial fertilisers. Some of these substances are absorbed, and traces are found in most foods. Animals reared for meat are often given drugs such as antibiotics and artificial hormones to prevent disease and increase their weight. Some of these accumulate in the animal's body, along with chemicals that it absorbs by eating sprayed crops.

Intensive rearing methods often confine animals in unhygienic spaces and feed them the ground-up remains of other animals – sometimes of their own species – not thoroughly sterilised and even containing animal droppings. In these conditions salmonella, listeria and bovine spongiform encephalopathy (BSE) have passed down the generations and from one species to another.

Salmonella and listeria are commonly known to cause food poisoning; listeria also damages unborn babies. The effects of BSE are not yet known; there is no evidence so far that it is a hazard to humans, but some scientists fear that it might affect the human brain.

Many doctors and alternative therapists believe that allergies are often a reaction to small quantities of impurities and chemicals which may be found in some types of food. Other long-term effects of consuming these substances are not known, nor is it known how they may interact in the body with other chemical FOOD ADDITIVES.

What to do The best solution is to buy or grow as much organic produce as you can. It will also help to buy fruit and vegetables that are in season, since these need less spraying. Wash and peel non-organic produce, and trim fat from meat, since this is where most impurities accumulate.

Unless you have a butcher who sells organically produced meat, you should avoid liver and kidneys, as high concentrations of drugs and other chemicals can build up in these particular organs. Fish, game and free-range poultry are said to be safer than other types of meat.

Packaging, cooking and storage Many soft plastics, especially some types of thin, transparent film, contain minute traces of cancer-causing substances which may contaminate food. Traces of dioxin have been found in some cartons of fruit juice and milk. The aluminium linings to certain fruit-juice cartons may also pose a health hazard.

What to do At home, store or pack foods in lidded glass, china, glazed earthenware or stainless-steel containers. Wrap food for taking out as packed lunches or picnics in Cellophane or kitchen foil. Never use cling wrapping or plastic containers in a microwave oven. Avoid paper containers of milk and fruit juices. Buy your milk in bottles, and squeeze fresh fruit juice at home whenever possible.

Irradiation Treating food with radiation kills bacteria that would normally cause it to go bad after a certain time. It also eliminates insects in stored grain, fruit and spices. Irradiated foods can therefore be kept for longer 'on the shelf', and so producers and manufacturers save on the costs of spoilage.

The Department of National Health and Population Development has cleared certain foodstuffs for irradiation. Among these are processed spices, herbs, herbal teas, condiments and dehydrated vegetables; fresh fruits and vegetables such as strawberries, bananas, mangoes, pawpaws, tomatoes, potatoes, onions and mushrooms; and fresh poultry.

There is no way of telling for certain which foods have been treated, for while bulk packages are labelled, individual items are not. It is feared that irradiation may not only adversely affect the nutritional value of food, but mask bacterial contamination of rotting food. For although all bacteria are destroyed, some of them leave dangerous substances behind which can still cause FOOD POISONING.

What to do To avoid irradiated food, you should shop in stores that have guaranteed not to sell it; buy from small, local suppliers whose procedures you can question; buy organic foods; or grow your own food. Demand that your supermarket clearly marks all irradiated products.

Hazards at work

Offices and factories Various aspects of the indoor environment can affect the comfort and health of workers in offices and factories, causing the so-called sick building syndrome in serious cases. Possible causes include insulating materials, cigarette smoke, poor ventilation, artificial lighting, temperatures

---

Alternative ways to deal with insects

Some safe and simple insecticides can be made at home.

Ants Although they do not spread diseases, ants make for any food or food debris. To deter them, block up visible holes, then sprinkle dried mint, chilli powder and borax where they are coming in. Keep out of children's reach.

Cockroaches Food can be contaminated by the droppings of cockroaches. To deter them, put down a mixture of cocoa powder, borax and flour; icing sugar and sodium bicarbonate; or plaster of Paris and flour. Keep out of children's reach.

Flies Bacteria are spread by flies. If you do not want to use a fly swatter or sticky fly paper, make bunches of bay, mint, pennyroyal or eucalyptus leaves, or crush them and sew into cheesecloth bags with some cloves and a few drops of citrus or eucalyptus oil. Hang them in windows or doorways to deter flies.

Moths The destruction that moths cause to fabrics is not a health hazard but mothballs are. Put sachets of lavender, camphor, rosemary, peppercorns, conkers or cedar chips in drawers and wardrobes with woollen clothes. Before packing clothes away, wash and air well, then tumble in a drier or iron with a steam iron to kill moth eggs.

Weevils Stores of starchy foodstuffs are where weevils live and breed. Place a bay leaf in each container of rice, lentils or other dry goods – including flour, if the slight flavour of bay is acceptable.

---

that are either too high or too low, excessive dryness of the atmosphere, pollen, viruses, bacteria, moulds and other fungi, and chemical fumes from correcting fluids, glues, paints, industrial processes and even some photocopiers.

The most common symptoms caused are dizziness, headaches, EYESTRAIN, skin irritations, allergies, breathing problems, COLDS, stress and TIREDNESS. In and near air-conditioned buildings a type of PNEUMONIA known as legionnaires' disease can be spread if there is inadequate cleaning of the cooling system and its water.

What to do Employers have a statutory responsibility to provide a safe place of work, to control air pollution and noise, and to keep machinery and work practices safe. There are also strict rules about the amount of air space each worker should have.

The Machinery and Occupational Safety Act is the primary piece of legislation in this field. Guidance notes on various aspects of workplace legislation can be bought from the National Occupational Safety Association (NOSA), a quasi-government body which is represented by various branches throughout the country.

Tell your employer, personnel officer or head of department about anything you may feel is a health risk. If nothing is done about the problem, contact your environmental health department. Other organisations that could possibly help you are the University of Cape Town's Industrial Health Research Group; Natal University's Industrial Health Unit; the Workplace Information Centre, P O Box 5244, Johannesburg 2000; and the National Centre for Occupational Health, P O Box 4788, Johannesburg 2000.

Something you may be able to control is your own lighting. To reduce eyestrain, work in natural or non-fluorescent light as much as possible, or if fluorescent lighting is unavoidable do not use the ordinary tubes, whose flickering can cause headache, eyestrain and disturbance of vision. Instead, use a full-spectrum tube, in which the flickering is too rapid to be perceptible to the human eye.

It has been proved that passive smoking carries risks similar to SMOKING itself. Some of the smoke – if not all of it – that smokers exhale has not been 'filtered' by their lungs, and still contains tar and other cancer-causing substances.

If cigarette smoke is a problem, ask your employer to designate nonsmoking zones in the office. If separate zones are not possible, try to sit next to a window or use a desk fan to clear your immediate area of smoke.

VDUs The electromagnetic radiation from the visual display units (VDUs) of computers and word processors is still being studied, but it is known that pregnant women who work mainly at VDUs are more likely than others to miscarry. The World Health Organisation considers VDUs a health hazard, and the European Community is currently drawing up regulations for their use. The length of time spent at them is likely to be limited, and safe distances from terminals at which others can work safely will be designated.

Eyestrain, BACK PAIN and tendon strain in the arms and hands can also be caused by constant work at VDUs.

What to do Make sure that terminals near you emit only low-level electromagnetic radiation and that you are not within a metre of other people's terminals. Make sure the position and height of your chair and of the terminal are adjusted for you. Glare on a VDU screen can be reduced by using special shielded lights, attaching a clip-on protective filter, and placing the screen at right angles to a window – never facing it. Have a break of at least ten minutes in every hour you spend at the VDU.

Dangerous substances People who work with acids and other irritating chemicals can develop disorders ranging from ECZEMA to skin cancer. Asthma, allergies, lung cancer and other lung complaints can all be caused by breathing in chemical fumes or dust containing particles of asbestos, coal, sand or brick.

Leukaemia and other cancers can result from exposure to some products refined from petroleum (crude oil), dyes, X-rays, radioactive materials, and chemicals used in paints, glues and plastics. In other industries, heavy metals such as lead, cadmium and mercury are a danger. They accumulate in the body, causing damage to the brain and nervous system.

What to do The safest course is obviously to avoid or reduce contact with harmful substances. Follow the instructions for use issued with such substances, and make sure your employer observes the regulations and approved codes of practice for work systems and equipment. Wear protective clothing, including masks and gloves, where necessary, to reduce the risks.

People who work in or around substances likely to cause a risk to health should get regular medical checks, which should include blood tests. If you work with or near radioactive materials, make sure your personal dose recorder is checked frequently to ensure you are not receiving more than the permitted radiation. See p.174 under *Radiation* for permitted levels.

Noise

The environment in which we live is fast becoming noisier. People in the bigger cities suffer the effects of traffic in busy streets, suburban trains ferrying commuters to and from the workplace, aircraft overhead, and sirens (from ambulances, fire engines and home alarms); while motorways and farm machinery make even the countryside far from peaceful. Noise level is measured in decibels and the noise perceived by listeners is adjusted and recorded as dB(A). The noise of ordinary conversation heard one stride away is 60dB(A). Street traffic produces about 70dB(A).

The official safety level in South Africa is 85dB(A). Levels above that will cause damage, be it ringing in the ears, sound distortion or loss of hearing. The length of exposure to the noise plays a part in the severity and duration of damage. Permanent damage to hearing can result from four hours at 93dB(A), or from just a few seconds at 110dB(A).

The decibel scale does not rise evenly but multiplies: 90dB(A) is ten times louder than 80, and 100dB(A) is 100 times louder than 80. Caps in a toy pistol (up to 170), a screaming baby (up to 117), a pop concert (110) and a food blender (up to

A good working environment: it is well lit by natural light; the plant absorbs carbon dioxide from the air, and the worker's desk and chair are the right height for good posture.

100) are among the many noises above the danger limit. Many young people have experienced temporary deafness after an evening at a disco, and workers in heavy industry or construction suffer some permanent loss. Power tools used at home carry the same dangers but they usually operate for short periods.

Apart from the dangers to hearing, loud noises cause instinctive reactions which tense the muscles and increase the heart and breathing rate. If they are persistent or occur often, the re-sults can be tiredness, stress, high blood pressure, headaches, ULCERS, SLEEP DISORDERS and even HEART DISORDERS.

What to do Reduce noise at home by improving the insulation of floors, walls and lofts. Fit solid doors and double glazing; plant hedges and even trees, if possible, to block off noisy roads. Carpets, curtains, rugs and cushions also absorb sound. Wear earmuffs at home when you use noisy tools or machines, and at work if your job or workplace has dangerous noise levels.

Jet engine at 30 m: 110dB(A)

Thunder: 100dB(A)

Train on bridge: 110dB(A)

Gun shot 140-150dB(A)

Pop group at 1,2 m: 110dB(A)

Inside average factory: 90dB(A)

Telephone at 1 m: 80dB(A)

Moving traffic in the street: 68dB(A)

Talking at 1 m: 60dB(A)

Whispering at 1 m 30dB(A)

Rustling leaves: 10dB(A)

Quiet street: 50dB(A)

Noise is measured in decibels (dB), but the dB(A) scale includes the impact on our ears. The South African official safety level is 85dB(A), but anything more than 80dB(A) can damage hearing. The decibel scale rises by multiples – 40dB(A) is 10 times louder than 30dB(A).

Using the healing power of herbs

The medicinal use of herbs is said to be as old as mankind itself. Until the 18th century it was the usual form of medical treatment in the West. Today the World Health Organisation estimates that, worldwide, herbalism is three to four times more commonly practised than conventional medicine. And even conventional doctors rely heavily on plant-based medicines – in South Africa, an increasing number of GPs' prescriptions are plant-based.

Although many of the herbs and plants used medicinally in South Africa today were imported from Europe, there is a vast array of indigenous medicinal plants here too. For example, more than 400 species of indigenous plants are sold commercially as traditional medicines in Natal and KwaZulu. And it is commonly accepted that traditional medicine using herbs is widely practised throughout the rest of southern Africa. (Some plants are so popular that the demand for them is threatening their very survival on the subcontinent.) From the days of Jan van Riebeeck to the present, succeeding generations have passed on a wealth of knowledge about plants and their healing properties. During the 19th century, the Dutch Voortrekkers used plants such as wild ginger and *inkomfe* (*Hypoxis rooperi*) as herbal remedies.

In the early civilisations, food and medicine were inextricably linked, and many plants were eaten for their health-giving properties. For example, the armies of slave workers who laboured to build the Egyptian pyramids took a daily ration of GARLIC in order to ward off the pestilential fevers and infections that were rife at the time. And by this time, written records of herbs and their beneficial properties – the first 'herbals' – were being produced.

Most of our knowledge and use of herbs can be traced back to the ancient Egyptians, whose priests were also herbal practitioners. A papyrus from the city of Thebes, dating from 1500 BC, lists hundreds of medicinal herbs – including many that are still in use today, such as caraway seed and cinnamon.

As well as the Egyptians, the ancient Greeks and Romans were practitioners of herbal medicine. As their armies conquered the then known world, military doctors took the plants and their uses with them – and also gained new skills as they travelled. For example, the Roman conquerors of Britain brought with them many Mediterranean herbs, including lavender and rosemary.

Two more peoples who have always relied heavily on herbal medicine are the Chinese and the Indians. To this day in China herbs play a vital part in health care, and there are numerous schools of herbal medicine and herbal dispensaries in most hospitals. In India, the use of herbal drugs is part of the all-embracing system of AYURVEDIC MEDICINE.

From the Dark Ages well into medieval times, herbals were painstakingly hand-copied in British monasteries – each of which had its own physic garden for growing herbs to treat both monks and local people.

Setting up shop

The advent in the 15th century of the printing press encouraged the compilation and publication of herbals. John Parkinson of London, a herbalist-physician, listed 3 000 useful plants in a publication of about 1630. Such herbalists set up their own apothecary shops, and the most renowned of Britain's herbalists in the medieval tradition was Nicholas Culpeper (1616-54). He wrote several books, including his famous herbal, *The English Physician Enlarged* (1649), which have been in print ever since.

By the time Henry Potter established himself as a 'Supplier of Herbs and Dealer in Leeches' in London in 1812, a vast amount of traditional lore on the medicinal use of herbs was available from Britain, Europe and, in addition, the Middle East, Asia and the Americas.

The opening up of the world following the advances in navigation had made this possible. And by this time, too, preparations containing not just one herb, but a combination of several, were in use. Potter's firm continues today, and *Potter's Cyclopaedia of Botanical Drugs and Preparations* is still published.

Herbalism flourished in ancient Egypt. Queen Hatshepsut travelled to the Land of Punt around 1419 BC, and this wall painting in her temple at Deir el-Bahari shows her men returning with herbs.

However, soon after Potter founded his firm, the growth in popularity and power of scientifically inspired conventional medicine sent the profession of herbal medicine into a decline – although as the main element in folk medicine it continued to flourish in the countryside. Then, in 1864, a number of herbalists founded the National Association (later Institute) of Medical Herbalists, an organisation for training and maintaining standards of practice which remains in existence today.

In its early years – and until well into the present century – the institute resisted attempts by orthodox medical pressure groups to have herbal medicine banned.

Public opinion was with the herbalists, helping them to stay in business. Gradually interest in herbalism increased – especially over the last 20 years – as more and more people questioned the use of synthetic drugs and their prolonged and sometimes alarming side effects.

International research

Increasingly, the apparently safer approach of herbal medicine matched the growing support – throughout the world – for ecological matters and natural remedies. Today, in suburban and rural areas throughout South Africa herbal medicine is once again widespread and popular.

Countless people of diverse ethnic groups buy over-the-counter herbal remedies for various minor complaints and ailments. Health shops abound in the cities and many chemists have special herbal and health food sections. In addition, an ever-increasing number of professional herbalists treat patients for most illnesses.

However, while owing a large debt to traditional herbalism over the centuries, herbal medicine has not stood still. The incorporation of American herbs and practices in the 18th and 19th centuries has been followed by a continuing investigation of various other plants. International scientific research not only confirms the healing powers of herbs, but also enlarges herbalists' knowledge with new ones.

As medical herbalists have become more scientifically minded in their research, so a new word has been coined to describe their work: phytotherapy, from the Greek words *phyton*, meaning 'plant', and *therapeuein*, 'to take care of, to heal'. In Europe, most phytotherapists are conventional doctors who believe in the effectiveness and safety of herbs. Organisations such as The European Scientific Co-operative for Phytotherapy (ESCOP), in the Netherlands, promote the study of plants for healing purposes.

Because herbalists use only natural sources, they consider the pharmaceutical industry's search for 'active ingredients' in plants – which are then extracted or produced synthetically to make medicines – to be misguided. In many cases, they say, the whole plant offers a safer and more effective treatment than isolated ingredients which are artificially bound together.

Herbal therapy

Herbalism claims to treat the patient as an individual, with individual weaknesses and needs, and not as just another medical case history. So its treatment is tailored to specific and varying requirements – and there is no such thing as an 'automatic' repeat prescription.

Who it can help Herbalists state that their medicines may benefit most people suffering from most kinds of illnesses, including long-standing conditions such as ARTHRITIS, MIGRAINE and SKIN DISORDERS. In some cases, where plant medicines alone will not effect a cure, patients may be advised to undergo another therapy, such as CHIROPRACTIC or OSTEOPATHY.

Finding a herbalist There is no association of qualified herbalists in South Africa, nor can herbalists be registered with the Associated Health Service Professions Board (the Pretoria-based body that strictly controls the practice of 'alternative' therapies). However, in TRADITIONAL MEDICINE, there exists a large number of voluntary associations, none with official status, to which African herbalists belong.

Most Western-style herbalists have qualifications acquired overseas; and many combine herbalism with other therapies, such as HOMOEOPATHY or NATUROPATHY. Ask such a practitioner for the name and address of a herbalist in your area; or make inquiries at any health-food store.

A course in medicinal and therapeutic herbs is offered to interested parties by The Herbalism Training Centre, P O Box 15134, Impala Park 1472.

Consulting a herbalist At the initial consultation, a herbalist will ask the patient about his medical history, eating habits, how much EXERCISE he takes, if he feels under STRESS – as well as questions about his present state of health.

The patient's BLOOD PRESSURE will be taken and he will be given a thorough physical examination. Then he will receive detailed advice about improving his general health. Finally, the herbalist will prescribe a suitable treatment – which may take the form of a herbal tincture, lotion, cream or ointment. Individual prescriptions may be modified or changed to suit the patient after further consultations.

As a general rule, herbal medicines work more slowly than some conventional drugs, because they are less concentrated. This is particularly so when the patient has a long-standing ailment. However, as the herbs begin to enhance the body's natural healing powers, it is claimed that patients often soon feel better in themselves.

In addition to curing or relieving specific illnesses, herbalists aim to restore the patient's overall health and vitality. Herbal medicine has much in common with NATUROPATHY, sharing its concern for the importance of preventing and treating disease.

An orthodox view

Herbal medicine can be viewed as the precursor of modern pharmacology, and many powerful drugs are indeed derived from herbs. Like drugs, herbs are not always as safe as the practitioners suggest. In addition, the claim to be 'holistic' is somewhat spurious, as a glance through a herbal book will show – like orthodox medicine, herbalists will treat 'just the symptoms'. Nevertheless, there is much wisdom and know-how in the general approach of herbal medicine and there are undoubtedly fewer side effects.

For further information on the use of herbs, see pp. 184-7.

Making the most of herbs

The best way of using herbs as a means of keeping healthy – or for clearing up and avoiding minor ailments – is in your daily diet. They provide extra minerals and vitamins, as well as giving flavour to the food.

Medicinally, one of the most valuable herbs is GARLIC. It contains a variety of nutrients and is a potent protection against bacterial, fungal and viral infections.

However, it is not always practicable or pleasant to use herbs in food. For example, many people dislike the taste or smell of garlic. However, garlic's strong smell is neutralised by parsley, and as such it is usually available as a mixture in pill form. Some of the commoner herbs can be bought from a health shop in tea-bag form – and drunk as a refreshing beverage.

Alternatively, you can make your own drink, putting a heaped teaspoon of the herb in a cup of boiling water. Leave it to steep

To make a decoction: Put a dessertspoon of powdered dried herb into a stainless steel or enamel (not aluminium) saucepan. Add about 300 ml of boiling water. Bring to the boil and simmer for 10-15 minutes. Strain while hot, and drink.

To make a tincture: Put about 120 g of ground or chopped dried herb into a container. Pour on about 600 ml of 40 per cent alcohol such as gin or vodka, and seal the container. Leave in a warm, dry place for two weeks, shaking well twice a day. Then decant the liquid into a dark wine bottle. Seal, and use when required.

for two to three minutes and then drink it without milk or sugar, using a little honey to sweeten, if desired. Although decoctions and infusions (see below) are for home medical use, they should only be used for up to a week.

Herbal drinks   There are four main ways in which herbs can be taken as liquids:

Decoction   Suitable for preparations made from roots or bark, so that their soluble contents enter the water. To make a decoction put a heaped tablespoon of powdered dried herb into a stainless steel or enamel – not aluminium – saucepan. Add about 600 ml of boiling water. Bring to the boil and simmer for 10-15 minutes. Strain while the tea is hot, and drink.

Infusion   Popular in the home for drinks or gargles. Fresh or dried herbs can be used in loose or tea-bag form. To make an infusion, warm a teapot and put in 1 dessertspoon of herb for each cup required. Pour in a cup of boiling water for each cup of tea; allow to steep for 10-15 minutes.

Tincture   Herbalists prescribe more alcohol-based tinctures than any other form of medicine. They are long-lasting, highly concentrated and taken in small doses. They can be made at home with a 40 per cent spirit such as vodka or gin.

Put about 120 g of ground or chopped dried herbs into a container. Pour 600 ml of alcohol on the herbs and seal the container. Leave it in a warm, dry place for two weeks, shaking it well twice a day. Then decant the liquid, leaving the residue, into a dark wine bottle. Seal and leave until needed.

Tisane   Essentially a milder version of an infusion. It is sold in tea bags and is made with boiling water. It can be drunk straight away, without long steeping.

Herbal dressings   Herbs can be used in two ways to dress wounds, bruises, injuries and local infections:

Compress   To make a compress, soak a clean cloth, or piece of cotton wool, in a hot herbal decoction or infusion made from various anti-inflammatory herbs, such as borage, buchu, marjoram or mint. Place the cloth on the affected area and maintain the heat by holding a hot-water bottle against it. Helps cuts and bruises to heal more quickly.

Poultice   To make a poultice, soothing herbs such as comfrey root, camomile and mallow can be used. With fresh, untreated herbs, you can apply the leaves directly to the skin. Alternatively, put the leaves on a piece of gauze and place on the skin.

With dried herbs, make a paste with hot water and apply accordingly. Maintain heat by holding a hot-water bottle against the poultice. Used to draw out pus, promote healing and reduce inflammation.

Other herbal preparations   Herbal products are also sold by chemists and health food shops in a variety of other forms. Some of the best known include:

Creams, ointments   Used externally for helping wounds to heal and for relieving skin inflammations. Comfrey and marigold ointments, for example, can be bought in most health shops.

Essential oils   For external use only. They have many healing properties, from treating infected wounds (camomile, lavender) to clearing and concentrating the mind (basil, rosemary). For more details see AROMATHERAPY.

Creating your own herb garden

All the common herbs shown here – and more –
are available at nurseries and garden centres.
Planning and growing a herb garden can be a
rewarding experience in itself. Most herbs are
quite easy to grow, and some, such as garlic
and parsley, are often already part of an
average vegetable plot.
Most of the commoner herbs need a fairly

sunny aspect, and this should be borne in
mind when choosing a plot. In general, the
soil should be moderately fertile and well-
drained. Herbs are best grown organically
and should not be overfed. To obtain the
maximum aroma and flavour, a light mulch
of garden compost is all that is needed.

Herbs can be ornamental. A patch of golden
marjoram lies behind a border of box (left),
wild strawberry and germander.
Clockwise behind are purple-leaved sage,
sorrel, wormwood, lady's mantle, fennel (top
left), purple meadowsweet (top right), fennel.

A good spot for a herb bed is on the
sunny side of a wall or hedge. The
one shown here is roughly 2 m
long and 1 m wide, with
the groups of plants about
45 cm apart. (Use several
plants of smaller types.)
Make sure that tall
plants will not shade
shorter ones.

Most herbs can flourish in pots, as the wild
strawberry (left), and bay and parsley here.

Fennel

Comfrey

Lemon balm

Lavender   Chives

Borage

Camomile

Marigold

Garlic

Basil

185

Herbs for your health's sake

You do not have to be an expert gardener to grow health-giving herbs – which can be used for cooking, brewing herbal teas, or making poultices and compresses. The following list includes growing advice and recommended culinary and medicinal uses.

Basil Best treated as a half-hardy annual and planted in a warm, sunny situation; it can also be grown successfully in pots. Aids the digestion and eases stomach cramps.

Borage Will self-sow easily; simply pull out the excess seedlings. As a tisane it is used against rheumatism and respiratory infections. Its flowers can be eaten in salads.

Camomile Grow from seed. The flowers can be used fresh or dry to make a refreshing tea, which is good for digestive troubles. Apply as a poultice for inflammations.

Chives Buy a plant or grow from seed. Divide it each year or so to promote new growth. It stimulates appetite and helps digestion during convalescence. It is said to be effective against infections and anaemia.

Comfrey (or Knitbone) Unearth the roots each spring or autumn, split them down the middle and dry in a moderate temperature of about 50°C (122°F). Comfrey ointment is used to mend broken bones and tissue. The pounded sticky roots are wrapped around a fracture and, when dry, hold the bone in place.

Fennel Start with a plant, or obtain a seedling. Place at the back of a border or plot. Do not grow near dill, as cross-pollination will occur and seedlings will be hybrids. Both seeds and feathery leaves can be used against excessive wind, as well as indigestion, insomnia, nausea and vomiting.

Garlic Fairly heavy feeder needing plenty of organic matter. Divide a bulb into its cloves and plant in April or September. Harvest the following summer. Try using your own bulbs to repeat growth. See GARLIC.

Lavender Buy a plant or take cuttings. The flowers contain a very relaxing essential oil. Can be drunk as a tisane, or used as an infusion in the bath. Good for coughs, headaches, wind and rheumatism – and as an antiseptic for cuts.

Lemon balm Very easy to grow from seeds or cuttings. Makes a refreshing tea, good for anxiety and nervous exhaustion, as well as indigestion, headache, nausea and vomiting.

Marigold The old English variety, *Calendula officinalis*, is easily grown from seeds. It should be thinned out to about 23 cm apart. The flower heads are held to be ideal for treating local skin inflammations, as well as minor burns and scalds.

Marjoram Pot marjoram and wild marjoram (oregano) can be grown from seeds, cuttings or divisions of roots. Perennials, they prefer a dry, warm soil. They are good for relieving colds, indigestion and minor respiratory infections.

Mint Fast-spreading, it ideally needs its own border. Prefers moist, fairly rich soil. It greatly aids the digestion, and hot infusions can be helpful at the start of a cold. Black peppermint is used against headaches, stress, constipation, wind, insomnia, and nausea and vomiting.

Nasturtium Easy to raise from seed. Its peppery-tasting leaves are rich in vitamin C. Take for minor respiratory infections. Use in salads. The dried seeds can be ground in a pepper mill and used for seasoning.

Rosemary Needs plenty of sun and good drainage. It will thrive in a chalky, lime-rich soil; some ground-up chalk or a few eggshells should provide enough lime. A useful, space-saving variety is Miss Jessup's Upright. Good as a tisane for headaches, neuralgia, colds, and as an antiseptic gargle.

Sage A temperamental herb to grow; the drainage must be good, and the soil not too rich. Purple or red sage makes a useful gargle, or a lotion for wounds. Sage tea is recommended for indigestion, anxiety and depression, and excessive sweating.

Thyme Essential to any herb plot, taking up little space. Plant either in the garden or in pots and window boxes. It is propagated by cuttings or layered side shoots. A highly antiseptic gargle or expectorant for coughs and catarrh. Lemon thyme makes a pleasant tisane, with similar medicinal effect.

Mint

Comfrey

Lavender

Chives

Calendula

Garlic

Oregano

Fennel

Rosemary

Basil

Lemon balm

Nasturtium

Camomile

Borage

Sage

Thyme

HICCUPS

Hiccups are repeated sharp inhalations of breath caused by involuntary spasms of the diaphragm – the powerful muscle that separates the chest from the abdomen and which increases the volume of the chest when air is breathed in – accompanied by involuntary closing of the larynx (upper windpipe). They are caused by irritation of the diaphragm, for example by an overfull stomach or inflammation of the membrane around the heart.

If hiccups tend to recur frequently or an attack lasts longer than a day, you should consult your doctor.

What the therapists recommend

Traditional Medicine Traditional and folk remedies for hiccups are numerous. Here are some popular ones: Breathe in deeply and hold your breath while slowly counting to ten, or as long as possible. Gargle for a couple of minutes with hot or cold water. Sip several cups of cold water slowly. Drink a glass of water slowly, from the side of the glass farthest from you. Surprise the sufferer with, for example, a sudden slap on the back or by dropping something cold down the back of the neck – a door key or an ice cube often works.

Herbal Medicine Sipping peppermint or lemon balm tea may reduce the spasms.

An orthodox view

Doctors sometimes recommend inhalation of increased concentrations of carbon dioxide – an easy way is to cover nose and mouth with a paper bag (*never* a plastic one) and breathe in and out into it for a couple of minutes. Or a tranquilliser may be prescribed to control the symptoms.

What the therapists recommend
MASSAGE

Self help Massage is considered to be a valuable treatment for post-traumatic and post-operative conditions of the hip joint, in the relief of stress and strain around the joint, and as an aid to improving mobility in the stiffening, ageing joint.

Firm upward effleurage strokes (p. 225) are made over the front, outside and back of the thigh to improve general circulation and nourishment. This is followed by wringing and kneading of the same areas to improve muscle tone.

Lifting, squeezing and wringing over the buttocks should precede deep kneading and frictions over the hip joint. Once the muscles are softened and relaxed, intersperse the massage with passive mobilisation, moving the joint as far as possible both ways, providing the movement is pain-free.

Never force a movement and never massage an inflamed arthritic joint, but be content to persevere with treatment, daily if possible, and with just a little improvement at a time in cases where the joint has been stiff for some years.

ACUPUNCTURE

Consultation Hip joint pain is said to respond well to acupuncture. Points along the gall bladder, stomach and large intestine meridians may be treated. MOXIBUSTION may also be used.

An orthodox view

Doctors may prescribe non-steroidal anti-inflammatory drugs (NSAIDs) to relieve symptoms, but these can have side effects which include rashes or digestive upsets. If pain is persistent and severe, surgeons replace a damaged joint with a metal artificial one. Hip replacement operations have proved to be extremely successful.

into the skin. Often the cause is an ALLERGY to certain foods such as strawberries or fish, FOOD ADDITIVES, or drugs such as aspirin and codeine.

Sensitivity to cold, house dust, pollen or even sunlight can also trigger an attack of hives, but in many cases there is no identifiable cause.

What the therapists recommend

Herbal Medicine A cool infusion (see p.184) of camomile can help to alleviate itching. As well as treating the symptoms, a herbalist may use herbs such as yarrow, golden seal, gentian and camomile to improve the functioning of the liver and digestive system.

Naturopathy Relief may be gained by having cool baths or using a vitamin E cream. A naturopath may also recommend high levels of vitamin C, taken internally: 1 g or 2 g daily. In the longer term, exclusion diets (see DIETS AND DIETING) are advised to find and eliminate any food causes.

Homoeopathy If the sufferer is restless and full of anxiety, try A*rsen. alb.* If the rash is caused by stinging nettles, give U*rtica urens.* If there is burning and swelling, made worse by warmth, A*pis mel.* is recommended. When a rash burns and itches, there are blisters and the patient is restless, try R*hus tox.*

An orthodox view

The symptoms are usually treated with antihistamines, many of which are usually readily available from chemists without prescription. Doctors also try to help patients to pinpoint the cause of their hives. Sometimes this may be obvious, but in other cases careful experiments with diet and exposure to substances to which a patient may be allergic might be necessary.

In rare emergencies, where a swollen mouth, tongue or throat prevents breathing, an adrenaline injection can be lifesaving.

HIP COMPLAINTS

The head of the femur – the thigh bone – forms the ball of the ball-and-socket hip joint. It can be damaged by Perthé's disease (inflammation and softening of the top of the thigh bone) in children, or by a FRACTURE or ARTHRITIS in older people. The bone and joint surfaces become deformed so that movement is limited and painful.

Pain in the hip is also commonly caused by a back or knee complaint because of a common nerve supply to these areas.

Physical examination of the hip, sometimes aided by X-rays, helps to diagnose the cause of the pain.

HIVES

Itchy red weals on the skin are the major symptom of hives – also known as urticaria or nettlerash.

They can appear anywhere on the body and vary in size from small, pimple-like spots to raised patches several inches across. Sometimes the weals disappear after only a few minutes, but in other cases they can last for days or even weeks, and may move to different parts of the body.

Hives are the result of histamines and other substances being released by the body

HOMOEOPATHY

Boosting the body's healing powers

By using natural remedies to boost the body's own healing ability, homoeopathy aims to treat the whole person. Illness is seen as a sign of disharmony or inner imbalance, so homoeopaths try to resolve underlying problems rather than simply deal with particular symptoms.

To do this they use specially prepared homoeopathic remedies which are highly diluted forms of natural substances that, in a full-strength dose, would actually produce the symptoms of the illness in a healthy person. These applications are thought to help, since symptoms are seen by homoeopaths as the body's way of fighting illness.

Homoeopaths say that the more closely a remedy imitates a patient's symptoms, the better it promotes healing; and the more dilute the dose, the greater its effect, since the remedies are prepared in a special way that is said to strengthen them with each dilution (see box, p. 191).

Each remedy is carefully tested ('proven') on volunteers who take very dilute mixtures for up to a year, and record all their symptoms in detail. The relevant records taken include subjective impressions of sleeping and eating habits, moods and relationships, since homoeopaths believe that the body functions as a whole. Once the remedy has been proven it can be prescribed to patients, who usually receive only one high-potency dose. Remedies rarely cause any effects other than the symptoms already present, although occasionally these may worsen at first – known as a 'healing crisis' – but usually this does not last long, and is taken as a sign of imminent improvement.

Homoeopaths pay the most attention to symptoms that have the greatest effect on the patient's overall ability to function – particularly mental or emotional symptoms. Disorders of the heart, for example, are invariably regarded as more important than disorders of the skin.

The severity of symptoms within each bodily system is graded in order of importance, but unusual symptoms have greater significance. So a person's mental and emotional state, general problems such as INSOMNIA, and any additional 'peculiar' symptoms (such as a tingling sensation on the left side of the body only) may receive more attention than a symptom such as a rash, although this may have been the original reason for seeking help.

Who it can help Unlike conventional medicine, homoeopathy stresses the uniqueness of the individual, and holds that the individual's make-up determines which diseases he or she is most susceptible to and which symptoms are likely to occur. Homoeopathic remedies must be matched both to the symptoms and to the individual. So the same symptom, a cold for example, may be treated differently if the victim is a jovial, outgoing, overweight person, than in the case of a thin, nervous patient with few friends. Conversely, the same remedy may be used for different symptoms in different people.

Finding a therapist No homoeopath is allowed to set up a practice in South Africa unless he or she is registered with the government-appointed South African Associated Health Service Professions Board; and to do so, the homoeopath must be in possession of specialised qualifications recognised by the board.

There are no homoeopathic hospitals in this country (unlike in Britain, for example, where no less than five such hospitals, each staffed by medically qualified homoeopaths, exist). However, some doctors treat patients by means of homoeopathy as well as allopathic (conventional) medicine.

For names and addresses of homoeopaths, write to the Associated Health Service Professions Board, P O Box 17055, Groenkloof 0002; to the South African Homoeopathic Association, 20 Botanic Grove, Berea 4001; to the South African Complementary Medicine Association (SACOMA), 229A Main Road, Plumstead 7800; or to the Homoeopathic Society of South Africa, P O Box 9658, Johannesburg 2000. This last body is a lay society that promotes the use and understanding of homoeopathy; monthly evening meetings are held at a Johannesburg venue.

The Natal Technikon's Department of Homoeopathy (P O Box 953, Durban 4000) offers a five-year programme leading to a master's diploma in Technology: Homoeopathy. This must be followed by a one-year internship, required by the South African Associated Health Service Professions Board, before registration with the board as a homoeopath can take place.

Consulting a therapist The homoeopath will carefully assess not only your symptoms, but also your manner and appearance; your mood and state of mind; how worried or anxious you are; and your personal circumstances, emotional responses, fears and beliefs. This usually takes an hour or more.

In most cases, homoeopaths give only a single dose of one remedy, and wait to see what effect it has before offering further treatment. Any change is thought to show that the remedy has boosted the body's healing process, and that no other treatment should be necessary. For simple, temporary problems such as a HEADACHE, the remedy should be effective almost at once. Patients with more long-term conditions need to be monitored over many months, and extra doses or different remedies would be given if improvement stops or new symptoms develop.

Homoeopaths believe that in the course of a cure, symptoms change from more important to less important bodily systems, and from the inside of the body outwards – so, for example, heart symptoms may 'move' to the skin as healing occurs. Symptoms are thought to disappear in the opposite order to their appearance, the most recent being the first to go.

How homoeopathy began

The origins of homoeopathy go back to 1810 when a German physician, Samuel Hahnemann, first proposed a new system of medicine as an alternative to the orthodox practices of the day. These practices included blood letting and purging, which Hahnemann thought were too harsh, and often weakened patients more than did their illnesses. By contrast, the new system was to be based on gentle ways of helping the body to cure itself.

Hahnemann's ideas of how this could be done were inspired by the discovery that a herbal remedy for malaria, cinchona tree bark, actually *produced* symptoms of the disease, such as headache and FEVER, when taken by a healthy person. He concluded that symptoms were the body's way of fighting illness, and that medicines which produced the same symptoms as an illness could help recovery. (It was later discovered that cinchona bark contains quinine, the first drug used against malaria).

Hahnemann's ideas were in effect a rediscovery of an ancient principle first expressed by the Greek physician, Hippocrates, in the 5th century BC – 'like cures like'. Hahnemann called the new system homoeopathy (meaning 'like disease'), in contrast to conventional medicine, which he termed allopathy (meaning 'other disease') since it uses medicines to suppress or prevent symptoms (see ALLOPATHIC MEDICINE).

Hahnemann thought that small doses of homoeopathic remedies would be safer than large ones, while still being effective. He spent many years experimenting on himself and his family and friends with a wide range of natural substances in dilute forms. His approach was 'holistic', for it concentrated on the whole person, and his homoeopathic remedies aimed to restore the body's natural balance and to strengthen it to fight disease.

The first homoeopathic hospital in London opened in 1850. Although interest declined in the early 20th century, the popularity of homoeopathy has begun to increase, spurred on by concern about the side effects of conventional drugs and publicity about its use by the British royal family.

This is known as the 'law of direction of cure'. Sometimes symptoms get worse before they improve, or symptoms of old complaints may reappear briefly, this time to be healed permanently.

Homoeopathic remedies are sold in many health food and chemists' shops throughout South Africa.

An orthodox view

Homoeopathy is not taught in South African medical schools (see section on 'Finding a Therapist'), and it is often mentioned by doctors disparagingly.

Many doctors find it particularly difficult to accept the homoeopathic notion that the greater the dilution of a remedy, the greater its effectiveness, because this is contrary to orthodox medicine and orthodox medical thinking. They do not accept the homoeopathic theory that minute doses of a particular remedy will cure a patient because such doses are so dilute that they are likely to contain very few molecules, if any, of the original substance. Homoeopaths, however, maintain that the power comes from the dilution process itself, which leaves 'footprints' of the original extract in the solution even if none of the substance itself remains.

But since there is no scientific explanation of how this is possible, many doctors reject the theory. It is especially difficult to compare homoeopathy, which uses a variety of different remedies to treat the whole person, with orthodox medicine, which relies on specific remedies for particular diseases with established and accepted symptoms.

Many doctors attribute any benefits of homoeopathic treatment to the PLACEBO effect – the idea that some treatments are effective simply because the patient believes in them, rather than because they do any good themselves.

Nevertheless, a few scientific trials have shown that homoeopathy in general has benefits greater than can be accounted for simply by the placebo effect – although these findings have been hotly disputed by some practitioners of orthodox medicine.

Even if relatively few doctors believe in the effectiveness of homoeopathy, most say that the remedies are so dilute that they must be completely safe.

Common homoeopathic remedies and their uses

Aconite (wolfsbane, blue monkshood): for COLDS and COLDNESS, especially when there is dryness and thirst; CROUP; ANXIETY and anguish; also recommended for gastric complaints.

Allium (from red onions): symptoms of a cold, including sneezing, running nose and headache; also HAY FEVER.

Antimonium tart. (tartar emetic, potassium antimony tartrate): for STOMACH COMPLAINTS, especially if there is NAUSEA and VOMITING from sour food or drink.

Arnica (leopard's bane): BACK PAIN, SPRAINS, NOSEBLEEDS, BRUISING (as ointment), sore muscles and toothache.

Arsenicum (arsenic trioxide): this is used for DIARRHOEA or vomiting from FOOD POISONING; cold symptoms such as fever, sore throat, thirst, disturbed sleep; also used for general restlessness, anxiety, panic attacks and DEPRESSION.

Belladonna (deadly nightshade): throbbing headaches, especially when worsened by light; earache; fever; flushed or irritable teething baby.

Calcarea (calcium carbonate: a mineral which is extracted from oyster shells): this is said to be very effective for such widespread ailments as INDIGESTION, CONSTIPATION, OBESITY, ECZEMA, ARTHRITIS and heavy menstrual periods.

Chamomilla (German camomile): for teething babies, especially when they are irritable or will not sleep.

Drosera (common or round-leafed sundew): a remedy recommended for COUGHS which are accompanied by spasms and constrictions and are painful and frequently exhausting; usually a dry cough with tickling in the throat.

Dulcamara (bittersweet, woody night shade): said to help to clear up CATARRH, when there is also ulceration of the mucous membranes.

Eupatorium (boneset or thoroughwort): recommended for winter colds, when there is severe aching in the bones.

Euphrasia (common eyebright): for catarrh, especially when this is accompanied by a painful headache, and tired, light-sensitive eyes.

Gelsemium (yellow jasmine): FEAR and PHOBIAS may be successfully treated with this preparation, especially if there is trembling and a need to urinate; also, if there are overwhelming fears of falling, attending a dental surgery, or a sensation of the heart stopping.

It is also recommended for feelings of dullness and drowsiness – as well as for the opposite: excitement, inability to sleep and a feeling of inadequacy.

Physical complaints which may be treated include: headaches which lift after vomiting, sleeping or urinating, but which are aggravated by bright light; DIZZINESS, faintness, earache, double vision, summer colds, catarrh, sore throat, dry coughs and, in women, painful periods.

Glonoinum may be prescribed for a feeling of dizziness and headaches which are triggered by extreme heat or cold, hot flushes during the MENOPAUSE and the cessation of menstrual periods.

Hepar sulph. (calcium sulphide): a preparation used to treat sinusitis, CONJUNCTIVITIS, COLD SORES and mouth ULCERS, TONSILLITIS and INFLUENZA. It may also be prescribed for irritability caused by anxiety, for hypersensitivity to touch, and for restlessness beneath a calm exterior.

Hypericum (St John's wort): used as an ointment or tablets for burns and SUNBURN, small cuts and grazes, and bites.

Ipecac. (ipecacuanha): this is prescribed for fainting attacks , nosebleeds, general nausea, ASTHMA, back pain, a weak pulse, and copious bleeding, of blood that is slow in clotting.

Lachesis (bushmaster, sutucucu snake): sore throat; BOILS and abscesses; sinusitis; headaches; sore muscles; painful periods.

Ledum (marsh tea, wild rosemary): prescribed for anxiety, timidity and aloofness; also recommended for black eyes, stiffness of the joints and cold, purplish complexion during cold weather.

Lycopodium (wolfsclaw club moss): prescribed for ACNE; recurrent colds, lymphatic disorders (see IMMUNE SYSTEM), moodiness, premature ejaculation.

Nux vomica (poison nut tree): recommended for DIGESTIVE PROBLEMS, especially when caused by a poor diet or by overeating; constipation; PILES; influenza and colds with blocked nose and sore throat; MOTION SICKNESS; CYSTITIS; CRAMP; period pain; MIGRAINE.

Pulsatilla (Pasque flower): prescribed for colds that keep coming back, wheezy coughs, hay fever, obesity, depression, PAIN, swellings, headache.

Rhus tox. (poison ivy): recommended for arthritis, backache after physical exertion, SCIATICA, sprains, RINGING IN THE EARS, children's fevers. It is also prescribed for restlessness, nervousness, irritability, depression (especially for those who burst into tears for no apparent reason, or have thoughts of suicide).

How homoeopathic remedies are made

Plant, mineral and animal substances are used to make homoeopathic medicines. The substance is first soaked in alcohol to extract its active ingredients. This solution is diluted many times over in measures of tens or hundreds, with a vigorous shaking after each dilution.

The shaking is said to 'potentiate' the mixture and increase its powers by transferring energy to it. This means that homoeopathic remedies are held to become *more* powerful with each dilution, ending up with a very low concentration of the original substance, but with a very high energy level. Sugar is added to the diluted and energised solution for the purpose of making homoeopathic tablets.

Successive ten-fold (also called decimal or X potency) or hundred-fold (centesimal or C potency) dilutions are indicated on remedies as 1X, 2X, 6X or 3C, 12C, 30C and so on. Sometimes 1M is used instead of 1000C, and sometimes the X is omitted.

HOMOEOPATHIC POTENCIES
The decimal scale
$1X = 1/10^1 = 1/10$
$2X = 1/10^2 = 1/100$
$6X = 1/10^6 = 1/1\,000\,000$
and so on.
The centesimal scale
$1C = 1/100^1 = 1/100$
$2C = 1/100^2 = 1/10\,000$
$3C = 1/100^3 = 1/1\,000\,000$
up to:
$6C = 1/100^6 = 1/1\,000\,000\,000\,000$
and beyond.

A 3C dilution is a 1:100 dilution of the original mixture, further diluted in the same proportion and shaken twice more. A typical homoeopathic remedy for a mild condition might have a potency of 6C, while higher potencies of up to 200C or more are used for severe symptoms. As well as selecting a remedy suitable for the individual and his symptoms, the practitioner also has to decide which potency to prescribe.

HONEY

'Food of the gods'

Man has prized honey as a sweetener and food since the days of the Stone Age hunter-gatherers. The viscid liquid is produced by bees from the nectar they collect from flowers. The foraging bees carry the nectar, a mixture of sugars and water, together with pollen, back to the hive.

There, worker bees add enzymes that reduce the water content to less than 20 per cent and break down the larger sugar molecules. The honey is then sealed in the honeycomb, and later fed to the larvae or saved for winter food.

The smaller sugar molecules, including glucose and fructose, are readily absorbed by the human digestive tract, so honey soon gained a reputation as a high-energy food. The Egyptians, Persians and Chinese all knew its value. King Solomon recommended it, saying: 'My son, eat thou honey, because it is good; and the honeycomb, which is sweet . . .' (Proverbs 24, verse 13.)

The honey sugars break down into substances that inhibit the growth of bacteria, and the ancients used it to treat wounds, burns and skin problems – a practice that continued into the Middle Ages.

Besides sugars (about 75 per cent) and water, honey also contains small amounts of such valuable minerals as calcium, iron, magnesium, potassium, sodium, sulphur, phosphorus and protein.

Traditionally, honey has been used as a 'tonic' or 'pick-me-up', and in the treatment of ANAEMIA, KIDNEY COMPLAINTS and CIRCULATION PROBLEMS. Its soothing effects are universally well known.

Try a glass of hot milk with a teaspoon of honey for a sore throat, and the same with an added measure of brandy to relieve the symptoms of INFLUENZA.

A glass of hot water taken with 2 teaspoons of honey and the fresh juice of half a lemon is a soothing bedtime drink. You can use honey as a skin softener and conditioner: just spread it gently over the face and hands, leave for 15 minutes and then wipe off with a damp flannel.

Honey may also help HAY FEVER victims. But to be effective it must be gathered in the area where you live, so that you ingest the local mix of pollens.

An *orthodox view*

Doctors have long recognised honey as a high-energy foodstuff. A few of them think that its antibacterial properties are sufficient to warrant its use in the treatment of such problems as bedsores, BURNS and other ailments. Claims that honey tends to slow down the ageing process or has particular therapeutic effects for those who eat it are generally rejected. See also ROYAL JELLY.

HOOKWORM

The hookworm is a small round, bloodsucking worm some 3 mm long, with four sharp, curved, tooth-like structures with which it attaches itself to the small intestine. Infestation by hookworms is particularly associated with bad sanitation in tropical and semi-tropical countries.

Hookworm larvae hatch from eggs in the soil, and they enter the human body by penetrating the skin – usually that of the bare feet, which display an itchy rash – and entering the bloodstream. Should they migrate through the lungs in large numbers, symptoms include coughing and bronchitis. In the small intestine the adult worms develop; their consumption of blood leads to chronic ANAEMIA. Abdominal pain and diarrhoea are further symptoms.

What the therapists recommend

Herbal Medicine A strong infusion of fresh leaves of the wild geranium is among indigenous herbal remedies recommended for expelling worms. It should be drunk at the start of the day, for at least a week. The leaves of the wild parsley tree and of the small knobwood or wild cardamom may be used for the same purpose.

An *orthodox view*

A drug such as mebendazole is administered to kill the worms. To counter the anaemia the doctor will prescribe iron tablets or, in severe cases, arrange for a blood transfusion.

HOSPICES

In recent years, specialist care for the dying has increasingly been provided by hospices. Few nursing homes and hospitals are equipped to care for terminally ill patients for any length of time, and families may find it difficult to cope with a dying relative's needs. Patients, too, may prefer to spend their final days or weeks in a hospice where they are cared for in a positive spirit, and are less of a burden to others.

In addition, the hospice staff are skilled in dealing with the emotional and spiritual pain – along with any physical pain – that the dying may suffer. Patients, whether visited and cared for at home by hospice staff or in an actual hospice, are treated with respect and compassion, and their personal needs are attended to. Hospice staff also try to help relatives to cope with their own emotions.

To obtain a directory of hospices in South Africa write (enclosing a stamped, self-addressed envelope) to The Hospice Association of Southern Africa, P O Box 59, Kenilworth 7745.

See also TERMINAL ILLNESS.

HUMANISTIC PSYCHOLOGY

Taking responsibility for your life

Every living person is different from everyone else and must therefore accept final responsibility for his or her own actions and behaviour, regardless of influences exerted by genetic make-up, family, society and circumstances. This is the basic philosophy behind humanistic psychology – a reaction against what are seen as the dehumanising effects of today's technological society. Theories that behaviour results mainly from unconscious fears and desires, childhood experiences, social pressures and environmental forces are rejected.

The main driving force behind an individual's behaviour is held to be the need for personal growth – or 'self-actualisation' as it is called. Humanistic PSYCHOTHERAPY aims to help people to achieve this. While everyone is influenced by their genetic make-up, family background, society and environment, it asserts that the individual alone is responsible for choosing how he reacts to these, and what he makes of his life.

Unlike many other psychologists who study only certain types of behaviour – and those mainly in artificial laboratory settings – humanistic psychologists prefer to concentrate on the overall well-being and feelings of those who come to them – often called 'clients' rather than 'patients'. When they do try to analyse society, they usually do so in terms of its effects on individuals and their personal responses to social pressures.

Humanistic psychotherapies The different therapies within the humanistic movement concentrate on current problems and on individuals' own feelings about themselves and events. These therapies do not try to find objective explanations for various people's behaviour, and they prefer to avoid deep examination of childhood experiences or inner motives. Instead, they try to develop clients' self-knowledge and ability to communicate, and to help them to feel more positive about their lives.

Humanistic psychologists embrace different theories, but all are based on a belief in the individual's freedom to direct his own life. They reject psychoanalytic and behaviouris-

tic approaches as dehumanising, since they portray people as helpless victims of internal instincts or external circumstances.

The two most important spokesmen of humanistic psychology have been the American psychologists Carl Rogers and Abraham Maslow. Rogers pioneered a method of so-called 'client-centred' therapy – more often called COUNSELLING – in which the therapist tries to help the patient to make his own decisions without directing him – to assist him to develop his own view of a situation and how to handle it.

Rogers thought that problems arise when patients get out of touch with their true selves by being surrounded (especially in childhood) by others whose affection and approval are conditional – for example, a parent who implies: 'I will love you only if you are good.' He believed that trying to live up to such demands can leave people with a sense of failure, make them unable to admit their true feelings, and cause long-lasting psychological problems.

His methods became known as ROGERIAN THERAPY, and aim to decrease dependence on the judgment of others, restore the value of self, and help people to take charge of their lives. This is not a selfish attitude, say therapists, since self-reliant, fulfilled individuals can be more caring towards others and have better relationships with them.

Abraham Maslow became interested in finding which characteristics make some people more mature, fulfilled and successful. He drew up a list of human needs, from basic biological necessities such as food and warmth, through psychological needs such as love and security, and ending with the need for self-development and personal growth. Fulfilment, he decided, depends on meeting all these needs and keeping all aspects of the personality in harmony.

From a study of successful public figures, Maslow formed a general idea of the self-fulfilled personality, and defined the characteristics and ways of behaving associated with it. He took an optimistic view of human nature, viewing people as innately sociable and co-operative, and reasoning that destructive or antisocial behaviour occurs only when people cannot meet their basic needs.

The different types of humanistic therapy all aim to help people who are unhappy with the way they are leading their lives by encouraging them to make changes to improve matters. Therapists generally try to get some idea of the individual's view of himself – whether he is confident or fearful about his own abilities, for example. They try to match this self-image with what he would *like* to be and how he actually behaves in the real world. Discrepancies between how a person feels and

how he appears to others are discussed. For example, someone holding a good job may still lack confidence in himself; or a person may think himself helpful while others see him as interfering. The individual's ability to share his thoughts and feelings, and to portray himself honestly to others, is encouraged as characteristic of a healthy personality.

Who it can help Most clients helped by humanistic psychotherapists are people who have emotional problems that they want to talk about without delving into complex childhood experiences. People who feel that they tend to react inappropriately to circumstances, or who have problems in their day-to-day lives and relationships, may also benefit, as may those who just want to make more of their lives or who feel that they have simply lost sight of their goals.

Finding a therapist As with all forms of psychotherapy, there is no single recognised qualification for a humanistic psychotherapist. Some psychiatrists or other medically qualified doctors may offer this form of treatment, but usually the therapist does not have medical training – and such specialised training as he or she *has* received can vary greatly.

Therefore try, if possible, to contact a therapist by means of a personal recommendation from a doctor or friend. Or else write, enclosing a stamped, self-addressed envelope, to the Psychological Association of South Africa, P O Box 2729, Pretoria 0001. The Association has a directory of all practising psychologists, with their specialities.

Consulting a therapist Usually client and therapist sit in comfortable chairs facing each other, in an informal, relaxed atmosphere. Therapists tend to be flexible, seeing you as often as you wish. However, many require one or two meetings before letting you commit yourself – or them – to further therapy, and some will suggest a contract for a certain number of sessions.

At the first session, the therapist generally asks about your reasons for seeing him, and what your main problems are. He will usually stress that responsibility for change during therapy will be yours, but that he will be there to help and to act as a sounding board.

In further sessions he will try to build a relationship in which you can come to terms with the anxiety and confusion that can result from challenges to your view of yourself. A sense of personal value, openness to new experiences and feelings, trust in yourself, and freedom to develop in accordance with your true self should then grow.

An orthodox view

Doctors and conventional psychiatrists believe that the humanistic view of each person as responsible for his or her own life encourages a healthy, helpful self-reliance. Many clients report feeling more complete, fully alive, and better able to take charge of their lives after therapy.

Recently, psychotherapy as a whole has moved away from deep analysis of the childhood roots of unhappiness towards a more humanistic approach. However, some humanistic therapists may give the impression that people who feel trapped by circumstances are avoiding making choices, and that saying they feel unable to change things is just a way of not facing up to the truth. For some people this can create anxiety about choice and responsibility, or make them feel a failure if changes are not achieved.

HYDROTHERAPY

Water to stimulate the body into curing itself

We have all eased ourselves into a comforting bath of warm water to soak stiffness and pain from overworked limbs; or we have splashed on invigorating cold water to make ourselves alert. Hydrotherapy – water treatment – is much more specific in its use of water's properties to cure ailments.

At the root of hydrotherapy is the belief that water is the essence of life. It forms the major part of our bodies and is a constituent of most foods. We can live only a few days without it. In its various forms – liquid, solid ice, steam or gas – it can be used to induce relaxation, to stimulate blood flow, to remove impurities, drugs or alcohol, to ease pain and stiffness and to treat diseases.

Your body may benefit from water in several ways – in a compress, as a spray or from a bath – but the most significant point is its temperature. Hot water or steam dilates blood vessels, encourages sweating and relaxes muscles and joints. Cold applications constrict blood vessels, reduce inflammation and congestion on the surface and stimulate the flow of blood to internal organs.

The beneficial powers of water have been valued since ancient times, and used by physicians for specific ailments as well as for general well-being. Many of the ancient Greek temples built to honour the god of medicine, Asklepios, were at the sites of hot springs renowned for their healing properties. Steam baths were popular among the Romans and Turks, and both the ancient Chinese and the American Indians knew about the healing effects of water.

In Europe, the use of springs, and mineral springs called SPAS, to restore health led to the establishment of hydros and fashionable resorts. A hydro is a hotel that offers treatments with curative waters. Towns such as Spa in Belgium, Baden-Baden in West Germany, and Bath, Buxton and Tunbridge Wells in Britain attracted the smart set as well as cure seekers. At Lourdes, in France, seemingly miraculous cures have occurred at the spa's Christian shrine.

Sebastian Kneipp (1821-97), who founded Britain's first hydrotherapy centre at Champneys in Hertfordshire, was a Dominican monk from Bavaria who believed that the body had an inherent ability to regulate and cure itself. Kneipp firmly believed that water was the principal means of stimulating the body's own healing powers.

Hot and cold baths, vapour baths, hot and cold compresses, showers and foot baths were complemented by a strict regime of diet and exercise which Kneipp recommended to cleanse the body of impurities. Many of the treatments he popularised are now incorporated in NATUROPATHY, but others have been added – aerated whirlpools and underwater massage among them.

Who it can help People with BACK PAIN, JOINT PROBLEMS and RHEUMATISM may find their discomfort eased by water treatment as part of their physiotherapy. It is also beneficial to people with muscle injuries and paralysis after disease, injury or a stroke.

In naturopathy, hydrotherapy is used to treat a range of diseases from GALLSTONES to diphtheria. The cleansing effects of various types of steam baths may help HEADACHES, while hot and cold water sprays help those with PERIOD PROBLEMS, ANAEMIA, ARTHRITIS or ASTHMA. People with minor strains and SPRAINS find cold compresses effective.

Anyone who is feeling run down, anxious or exhausted should be relaxed and start improving after most forms of hydrotherapy. Women throughout the world are increasingly asking for water births when they have babies, because of the comfort and gentle support they get from being in water (see NATURAL CHILDBIRTH).

Finding a therapist Very few private physiotherapy practices have facilities for hydrotherapy, but these are available at larger hospitals. If you have painful joints or other conditions that your doctor feels might respond to hydrotherapy he can refer you to a suitable hospital or, if there is one available, to a recommended private physiotherapist.

Or write (enclosing a stamped, self-addressed envelope) for information to: The South African Society of Physiotherapy, P O Box 47238, Parklands 2121.

Hot springs are a feature of several South African health SPAS, where specialist therapeutic facilities are available.

Consulting a therapist There are many different forms of treatment, depending on the nature of your problem:

Physiotherapy For patients whose muscles have become weak or wasted by lack of use after an operation or injury, or through disease or a stroke, the physiotherapist is likely to include water therapy as part of the treatment. A patient immersed in warm water is supported by the water, so that muscles and joints can relax. The warmth also dilates the blood vessels, increasing blood flow and making more oxygen available to aid healing.

Patients generally have daily sessions lasting up to half an hour. They can exercise muscles and joints more easily in water to build up strength and improve mobility. When massaging in water, the therapist can apply greater pressure without causing discomfort and so speed progress.

Compresses To increase the blood flow to a diseased area or organ and to flush out impurities by opening the pores and promoting sweating, the therapist may apply hot compresses. You can use hot compresses at home to ease stiff muscles. Wring out a cloth in water that is hot, but not uncomfortably so. Wrap the cloth round the painful spot and leave it there until it has cooled.

To constrict the blood vessels and so reduce inflammation – at a sprained ankle or arthritic knee, for example – the therapist may use a cold compress. You can use one at home, wringing out a cloth in water running very cold from the tap and applying it to the inflamed area for several hours. Pin or bandage round the affected spot.

Iced water compresses or ice cubes wrapped in a cloth can be used – but only for severe inflammation and swelling.

Wrapping Cold wraps are used for SKIN DISORDERS, COLDS and feverishness, strained back muscles, chronic BACK PAIN and chronic BRONCHITIS. You can use one at home for minor ailments, but for chronic conditions a trained therapist should supervise the treatment. In such cases it may be necessary to apply wraps daily for several weeks.

A sheet wrung out in cold water is wrapped round the body. A dry sheet and a warm blanket are in turn wrapped over the wet sheet. The patient lies in the wrap until the wet sheet dries out. A hot-water bottle may be needed to keep the feet warm. When the wrap is removed, the body is sponged with tepid water, then rubbed with a dry towel.

A wrap applied from waist to hips only is said by therapists to help ease DIGESTIVE PROBLEMS and CONSTIPATION.

Baths A common treatment in hydrotherapy is 20 minutes in a hot bath with the water just above 38°C (100°F) and deep enough to cover the shoulders – it relaxes muscles, eases pain, and promotes sweating, which removes impurities from the body. Because BLOOD PRESSURE may fall, you should leave the bath slowly and lie down for about half an hour when you are dry. A bath at about body temperature will give many of the same benefits, but sweating will be much less.

Adding Epsom salts to a bath is believed to help drive off chills and colds; adding salt to help flesh injuries to heal. Oats or bran (tied in muslin or thin cotton) put in the bath is thought to help in clearing up ECZEMA and other skin complaints. Seaweed may also be added for soothing relaxation.

Cold baths with the water at about 16-20°C (60-68°F) are given to reduce inflammation and improve circulation, so that oxygen and nutrients are carried around the body more efficiently. You will not be immersed in cold water, but sit in a shallow bath for only a minute or two while the water is splashed over the upper part of the body. Vigorous towelling afterwards makes you glow. Cold baths are not suitable for children, elderly people or those with HEART DISORDERS.

Sitz baths For conditions such as CYSTITIS, CONSTIPATION, PILES, anal fissures and prob-

lems with the reproductive organs, a therapist will often recommend sitz baths. Two baths – each about the size of a baby's bath and having a ledge to sit on – are used. One is filled with hot water, the other with cold.

You sit in hot water covering the hips and abdomen for three minutes, with your feet in the cold bath, then sit in the cold bath for one minute with your feet in the hot one. The process may be repeated. You can improvise sitz baths at home.

Sprays A jet of water – hot, cold, or alternately hot and cold – sprayed on part or all of the body is used for a wide variety of conditions, from anaemia and arthritis to DIABETES, gallstones and headaches.

Water temperature is the most important ingredient of the treatment; its benefits are the same as those of baths, but the impact made by a spray increases the effects. Whirlpool and aerated baths also increase the effects, but not as much as sprays. Sea water and the mineral-rich waters at spas make particularly effective sprays.

Young children, old or frail people and anyone with blood-pressure problems should not have spray treatment – and no-

body should have it until at least two hours after eating a meal.

Although a hand-held shower at home can give some of the benefits of spray treatment, an experienced therapist should supervise a course of treatment for curing particular ailments, so that the best combinations of temperature and duration are used.

Steam bath TURKISH BATHS and SAUNA BATHS are recommended when problems arise from impurities in the body, such as drugs or anaesthetics. The profuse sweating caused helps to carry impurities out through the skin pores. The sweating can also be a short-term answer to water retention.

The atmosphere in a sauna is less humid than in a Turkish bath, so perspiration dries on the skin and the process may feel more comfortable. Sometimes an individual steam cabinet is used, so that the head is kept out of the steam and the steam is not breathed. The treatment finishes with a cool – not cold – dip or shower and a rub-down. Do not have any steam bath with a full stomach.

Inhalation Blocked nasal passages and catarrh on the chest may be treated by INHALATION THERAPY, especially with eucalyptus,

Techniques of hydrotherapy

Water is used to stimulate or soothe the body's self-healing properties. The procedures shown here are used by hydrotherapists for a wide range of conditions, and can be safely used at home for minor ailments.

Sitz bath *The patient sits with hot water covering the hips and abdomen and the feet in cold water for three minutes, and then vice versa for a further minute.*

Wrapping *The therapist wraps a sheet wrung out in cold water around the patient (above), and then a dry sheet and a blanket (right). The wraps are removed when the sheet is dry, and the body is then sponged with tepid water and towelled dry.*

Water that 'unfroze' a shoulder

Stewart H, a journalist in his early forties, was a keen sportsman and enjoyed a hard game of tennis and shot a golf score in the low 80s. He awoke one morning with a slight stiffness in his left shoulder, and as the days, then weeks and months, went by, it got worse.

Finally, he had to give up tennis, and his golf suffered because he was unable to raise his left arm above shoulder height. He had the distressing complaint known as FROZEN SHOULDER. Moving the shoulder beyond a restricted range was uncomfortable, sometimes painful.

After living with the condition for two years, Stewart decided to try hydrotherapy. 'The effect was instant and amazing,' he said. 'They played a fierce jet of very hot water on my shoulder, and suddenly it began to feel easier. Within a few months the pain had gone entirely, and I was able to play golf and tennis again, with complete freedom of movement in the arm.'

menthol or another pungent oil added to the water. CROUP in children and bouts of coughing during WHOOPING COUGH are also eased by breathing steamy air. Skin conditions such as ACNE are improved because the facial pores open and sweat out impurities.

An orthodox view

Except in physiotherapy or for childbirth, hydrotherapy is rarely recommended by conventional doctors. They are often sceptical about the benefits claimed for minerals in spa water, and for hot- or cold-water treatments. However, doctors do not doubt the benefit for body and mind of a warm bath, and fully accept that exercising in water is easier for those who find movement painful.

There are some dangers to avoid in hydrotherapy. Anyone allergic to iodine should avoid any treatment with seaweed or its extracts. Patients with heart disease or high blood pressure should see a doctor before having hydrotherapy. Take special care when choosing a hydrotherapist to find out about qualifications and experience. Hot- and cold-water treatments always need to be administered with caution to avoid dramatic changes in blood pressure, or fainting. There are similar hazards in taking too cold a shower or dip after a steam bath.

HYPERACTIVITY

Children who are always on the go

An abnormally active child can be anything from a 'bit of a handful' to one who is aggressive, violent and may, if not helped, come into serious conflict with school authority and eventually the law. The hyperactive child is constantly on the go, does not know its own mind, will not settle to anything for any length of time, cries and shouts a good deal, will not sleep, and has no or little fear and so can be a danger to itself and others.

The child also tends to experience problems of thirst and regulation of body temperature.

Rearing such a child can be highly stressful, especially if those doing the rearing get little sleep and little sympathy from friends, teachers and doctors.

Hyperactivity affects about 2-5 per cent of children, and ten times as many boys as girls. It is generally thought to be an allergic reaction (see ALLERGY) to certain foods and chemicals, and sufferers often have other problems, such as ASTHMA, HAY FEVER, ECZEMA and CATARRH.

Foods that have been implicated include dairy products; sugar; wheat products; citrus fruits, especially oranges, tangerines, clementines and satsumas; substances with a high content of salicylates – aspirin-like chemicals – such as most fruits (including apples and grapes), peas, dried fruits, almonds, vinegar and alcoholic drinks; and FOOD ADDITIVES, especially tartrazine.

Other substances suspected of causing hyperactivity include cadmium (from cigarette smoke), aluminium, copper, mercury (including amalgam tooth fillings), household chemicals, deodorants, perfumes, fluoride (see FLUORIDATION), vehicle exhaust fumes and chlorine (in treated water). Deficiencies of magnesium, manganese, zinc, vitamin B_6 and fatty acids may also play a part.

What the therapists recommend

Many therapists give nutritional therapy, with mineral, vitamin and other supplements, such as evening primrose oil, and exclusion diets to find allergens. The procedure can be lengthy, and may induce tantrums, but persevere. See DIETS AND DIETING, EATING FOR HEALTH, FOOD ADDITIVES.

Naturopathy Practitioners consider consultation essential. They see food intolerance as a major source of hyperactivity, with certain food additives posing significant problems. Careful thought is given before changing a child's diet, and non-food factors

are considered and eliminated before any diet restrictions are advised. Simply switching from high-additive foods to those with natural ingredients has been known to help.
Homoeopathy Individual treatment will include advice on avoiding food additives, and also toxic metals in the atmosphere.
Dance Therapy The child is given an opportunity to express himself without criticism. The therapist moves in harmony with him, and as their relationship develops the child is encouraged to explore new movement skills.

An orthodox view

This condition has been diagnosed more frequently in the last 20 years, and doctors feel that allergy to dyes in sweets may play a large part in it. Family medical problems may also be present. A doctor will advise a diet that cuts down on sugar, and may suggest seeing a child psychologist.

HYPERTENSION

This is the medical term for high BLOOD PRESSURE, which increases the risk of HEART DISORDERS, KIDNEY COMPLAINTS and stroke. About one middle-aged person in every ten is thought to suffer from hypertension.

HYPER-VENTILATION

It is not unusual at moments of great nervousness or ANXIETY for people to find that their heart starts thudding and their breathing becomes hard and rapid, as though they had been running for a bus. Hyperventilation, or overbreathing, is particularly common at moments of social tension – before making a speech in public, for instance, particularly if the speaker is not practised in the art. It happens because too much carbon dioxide is expelled from the bloodstream through the lungs.

Although the condition is basically harmless, it can result in DIZZINESS, FAINTING bouts, and feelings of light-headedness. In addition, sufferers feel pain or tightness in the chest, and tingling or numbness in their fingers, toes and sometimes lips. Excessive sighing and yawning is common.

Strangely enough, another symptom of hyperventilation is shortness of breath. To compensate for this, sufferers tend to breathe even faster and so make the condition worse. In extreme cases, they hyperventilate until they collapse. On some occasions, victims of hyperventilation are taken to hospital, mistakenly thought to be suffering from HEART DISORDERS such as ANGINA, in which chest pains are a symptom.

If public speaking is an ordeal, you can combat hyperventilation by taking several deep breaths beforehand – each time expelling as much air as possible from the lungs, then breathing in as deeply as possible.

What the therapists recommend

Yoga Therapists encourage patients to relax and to practise calm, rhythmical breathing, using the free movement of the lower ribs to activate the pumping action of the diaphragm. They should then aim to develop a slower breathing rhythm, relaxing in the pauses between inhaling and exhaling.

Biofeedback Practitioners believe that biofeedback instruments can literally show patients how to breathe properly, by providing the precise information needed to correct the mode of breathing, its rhythm and its gaseous composition. A tube around the abdomen, or one to breathe into, is connected to a computer which can display the extent of chest and diaphragmatic movement taking place, or show whether carbon dioxide levels in the breath are abnormal. The information provided can increase the patient's awareness of what is involved in his problem and help him to fight and overcome it.

An orthodox view

First of all, a doctor will examine the patient to make sure that there is nothing seriously wrong with him. He may then tell the patient to breathe into and out of a paper bag so that the exhaled carbon dioxide is returned to his bloodstream. (Never use a plastic bag, which could cause suffocation.) He may also send the patient to a physiotherapist to learn how to breathe correctly.

HYPNOTHERAPY

Seeking cures at a deeper level of consciousness

Somewhere between wakefulness and sleep is the state of consciousness that hypnotherapists use to try to improve a person's health. The trance-like state induced by therapists is similar to the one that occurs spontaneously in sleepwalking or daydreaming.

Someone in this condition can perform tasks efficiently, avoid hazards, obey instructions and speak lucidly. A sleepwalker, how-

ever, has not handed over control to another person, whereas someone in a hypnotic trance temporarily hands over a large measure of personal control to the therapist.

The therapist uses it to bring about physical or mental changes in the patient. Such changes can include healing physical illness, reducing pain, inducing relaxation, and gaining insight into present difficulties and past events that may have a bearing on them.

The word 'hypnosis' (based on the Greek hypnos, 'sleep') was coined for such induced trances in 1843 by James Braid (about 1795-1860), a Scottish surgeon working in Manchester, who revived the use of mesmerism (see box) for some of his operations. Other practitioners were, at about the same time, also using hypnotism as a painkiller. James Esdaile (1808-1859), a surgeon in Calcutta, performed many operations with hypnosis as the only anaesthetic. These surgeons were flouting established medical opinion, which had for some 60 years condemned Mesmer's theories and practices.

Although the effectiveness of hypnotism in deadening sensation was apparent from the surgeons' work, the technique once again fell into disfavour – ousted this time by the introduction of ether, chloroform and other such anaesthetics.

At the turn of the century, the British Medical Association looked into the subject of hypnotism and disapproved of it. Only in the last 50 years has it been used again. Practitioners now see the trance as a healing state that allows the mind and body to achieve a calmness and tranquillity in which changes can be created that are inaccessible in the fully conscious state.

There is no question of the hypnotherapist simply waving a magic wand and taking control of the patient. Instead, the therapist and the client work on a problem together.

Who it can help Hypnotherapy has successfully treated SKIN DISORDERS, MIGRAINE, peptic ULCERS, IRRITABLE BOWEL SYNDROME and other conditions caused by ANXIETY and STRESS, including hysterical illnesses (see HYSTERIA). ASTHMA, INSOMNIA and PHOBIAS (of heights, air travel, exams, for example) are commonly treated.

Patients gain self-confidence from reliving and coming to terms with past events. The confidence gained often eases difficulties in relationships. Hypnosis can help to control habits such as SMOKING, and give some help with drug and alcohol ADDICTIONS.

Finding a therapist The first requirements in a therapist are competence and adequate training, but almost as important are personality and character. You must trust and feel comfortable with a therapist with whom you may well discuss sensitive areas of your life.

In South Africa hypnotherapists are unable to register with the S A Associated Health Service Professions Board, nor can they be registered with the S A Medical and Dental Council unless they are additionally qualified (in, for example, psychology, psychiatry or – in certain circumstances – dentistry).

However, a number of trained, non-medical therapists do have practices here, many of them with specialist qualifications ob-

Mesmerised by magnets

Centuries ago, medicine men, shamans and the priests of ancient Greece seem to have used hypnotic powers to treat bodily and mental ills. Modern Western hypnosis, however, began its chequered history with an Austrian doctor, Franz Anton Mesmer (1734-1815).

His investigation of the natural phenomenon of magnetism led him to believe it existed as an invisible fluid flowing through and connecting everything in the universe, and that ill health occurred when the flow was distorted.

Mesmer believed that by using magnets he could restore a proper balance of fluid and cure illness. He became a celebrity in his fashionable Viennese practice by successful use of his 'animal magnetism', as he called it. But failures led to condemnation by Vienna University and in 1778 he moved to Paris.

Again he built up a circle of influential admirers who came just to be amused by his theatrical demonstrations. Patients clustered round a tub of water and iron filings, holding on to the tub while music and dim lighting relaxed them into a trance. Mesmer, holding an iron rod, would then practise his 'magnetism' on them. Modern investigators think that it was Mesmer's magnetic personality and powers of suggestion that brought about cures in patients who were in fact 'mesmerised'.

This time the French establishment was provoked by Mesmer's methods and notoriety. After scrutiny, they failed to find a scientific basis for his cures. Mesmer was eventually branded a charlatan and his treatments faded from the medical scene.

tained abroad. You can find some of their names in the advertising columns of alternative health magazines. Or write to the South African National Association of Hypnotherapists, 22 Ladbrook Street, Kenwyn 7764.

Generally five to ten sessions of therapy may be all that is required, but some conditions can take a great deal longer.

Consulting a therapist The procedures followed in hypnotherapy sessions vary widely from one therapist to another. At the first session the therapist will take a detailed history of your case, of past and current treatments and of any more general matters that may be relevant.

You will be given a full explanation of what will happen at sessions and should be ready to take part in discussions of what you are both trying to achieve. The therapist is unlikely to use hypnosis at the first session, but may test your susceptibility to it.

At following sessions, you will sit comfortably or lie down while the therapist puts you into a trance, usually by talking quietly and making repeated suggestions that you are tired and that your eyelids are gradually becoming heavy.

You may be asked to look at some particular thing – a pool of light or a slowly turning wheel, perhaps – which will increase your wish to close your eyes.

The feeling is similar to dozing off to sleep. While in this state, a patient can be led to recognise positive abilities, be guided by the therapist to view problems from a better perspective, and gain insight into past and future behaviour. The entire session usually lasts 30-60 minutes.

Very occasionally a client may pass from a trance into a natural sleep; this is only a sign of tiredness and the need for sleep. Clients should have no fear that they will remain in a trance or that they will be controlled by the therapist. Therapists have no wish to control their clients – and in fact work to return control to clients whose illness or condition demonstrate loss of control.

It is common for a hypnotherapist to teach a client to carry out self-hypnosis after an illness has been brought under control. This is particularly suitable for asthmatics, insomniacs and many others who may need frequent or on-the-spot help with their condition (see also AUTOSUGGESTION). With half an hour's practice a day between sessions, a client can reinforce and re-explore points reached during sessions. Some therapists supply a tape-recording to give the familiar lead-in to the trance state.

An orthodox view

Many doctors still have doubts about the scientific basis of hypnosis, but others are

Overcoming a fear of flying

Mrs C was a fine musician whose career had taken a distinct turn for the better. However, many of the invitations to perform came from abroad, and she had a phobia of flying. She had to turn them down, and it seemed she would not have an international career. In desperation she went to a hypnotherapist.

At the first consultation she was put into a trance and the therapist told her to imagine she was going on a trip to the airport. At the next session she was again hypnotised and told to visualise herself at the airport and getting onto a plane. At the third hypnotic session she saw herself boarding a plane and taking a short flight around the airfield. And at the fourth and fifth sessions, while again in a trance, she visualised herself making a flight to and from a foreign capital. In addition, the therapist made a short tape-recording of the sessions, which Mrs C afterwards played at home.

Soon after she flew to Vienna to give her first concert abroad. When she returned from her trip, she was overjoyed and said, 'The only thing that bothered me was the long delays at the airport!' Her career is now well established and she travels abroad extensively – her fear of flying a thing of the past.

themselves qualified hypnotherapists who use hypnosis as one of their techniques. It is best to find a hypnotherapist who is also a doctor. This avoids the danger of hypnosis being used for a wrongly diagnosed condition which needs different treatment.

Tests show that physiological signs during hypnosis match those that would be expected if events being recalled were actually happening; pulse rate and brain activity in a person reliving a traumatic accident, for example, will be the same as during the accident itself.

Patients who are taken back to earliest infancy will display one reaction that occurs only in small babies: if stroked under the foot, their toes curl upwards – a reaction that changes after the age of six months to curling the toes downwards.

Despite such evidence, some doctors dispute that anyone really goes into a hypnotic trance, although they do not suggest that

there is deliberate faking. It may be that the part of the consciousness that is geared to reality stops functioning and a part in which intuition and imagination flourish takes over.

Normally a self-critical aspect of full consciousness would reject ideas allowed to surface and develop under hypnosis. There is concern that pseudo-memories are woven into actual memories to produce what the therapist or the client thinks desirable.

Doubts about a hypnotic trance do not, however, prevent recognition of its effectiveness in giving drug-free release from pain, cures of many forms of PSYCHOSOMATIC ILLNESS and easing of a variety of conditions rooted in stress and anxiety.

HYPOGLYCAEMIA

The brain cannot store glucose, the energy source it uses for all its functions, so it must get it from the bloodstream. If it is starved of glucose because the bloodstream contains too little of this sugar the patient rapidly becomes sweaty and confused, and has a rapid pulse. Without treatment, unconsciousness and brain damage may follow.

Hypoglycaemia is most commonly caused by uncontrolled DIABETES, when there is an imbalance in the dose of insulin taken and the patient's carbohydrate intake. It can also be caused by ALCOHOLISM, and its symptoms are mimicked by excessive adrenaline production in ANXIETY. Rarely, non-diabetic people can suffer from hypoglycaemia, experiencing hunger, confusion, irritability, and sometimes sweating.

Self help If you are diabetic, always carry barley sugar or glucose tablets around with you in case of emergency. Eat a suitable snack or meal every two or three hours, especially if you are about to do something strenuous. Avoid becoming over-tired and try to get a full night's sleep.

What the therapists recommend

Naturopathy Avoid refined carbohydrates (sugary and starchy foods); instead eat whole grains that are digested slowly and thus maintain a more stable blood sugar level. Eat regularly to avoid wild swings in energy. Bitter salad vegetables, like chicory and endive, play a part in stimulating liver functions and digestive processes; the liver stores glucose in the form of glycogen, releasing it again as glucose when required.

An orthodox view

Doctors treat acute hypoglycaemia in diabetic patients by giving sugar, if necessary by intravenous injection, or by a glucagon injection. A glucose tolerance test, in which blood glucose levels are measured regularly for several hours after ingestion of 100 g of glucose meal, confirms the condition in non-diabetics. Doctors may then do further biochemical tests to exclude serious hormone or enzyme disturbances.

Minor symptoms can be relieved by regular, light meals. Symptoms in non-diabetics are more commonly caused by anxiety than by a disturbance of glucose metabolism.

HYPOTENSION

Some healthy people with a normal heart and blood vessels have blood pressure far below average for their age. Those with naturally low blood pressure – known medically as hypotension – tend to live longer than those with high blood pressure, but sometimes suffer from DIZZINESS and FAINTING. A drop in blood pressure during an illness or after an accident can be a serious sign of SHOCK.

The most common type of hypotension is known as postural hypotension in which the symptoms occur after abruptly standing up or sitting down.

HYPOTHERMIA

Elderly people and babies are the most vulnerable to hypothermia or abnormally low body temperature. However, mountaineers, sailors and anyone exposed to extreme cold can be affected.

Normally, body temperature is regulated at about 37°C (98.6°F) – by shivering, if necessary, to produce heat. But if someone stays cold or wet for long, his temperature may fall and hypothermia occur.

The situation becomes dangerous when the body temperature drops to about 35°C (95°F) and body metabolism starts to slow down. At about 33°C (91,4°F) shivering stops and the victim becomes totally confused.Unconsciousness invariably occurs at about 30°C (86°F), and then death if help is not urgently received.

What the therapists recommend

Naturopathy Maintaining adequate circulation becomes more difficult with advancing age. Naturopathic advice is aimed at preventing any deterioration reaching a critical level. EXERCISE is important at all ages, even when it is too cold to go outdoors. Hot drinks or soup give a boost to body heat.

How to prevent hypothermia

Always wear plenty of warm clothes when outdoors in severe weather and indoors when heating is inadequate – several thin layers are better than one thick one. Thermal underwear, long socks, scarves and gloves can help even indoors – or in bed, if necessary.

Wear a hat, for much heat is lost from the head. This is particularly so for children, whose heads have a proportionately larger surface area.

Keep the heat up to 21°C (70°F), even if this means using fewer rooms, or living and sleeping in one room.

Eat at least one good hot meal daily, and take hot drinks when needed.

Keep active – staying in one position for a long time makes you feel colder.

Check for draughts from doors and windows, and block up any gaps.

Use a hot-water bottle or an electric blanket – never both – in bed. Electric blankets are cheap to run, and an overblanket can be left on. A woollen or fleecy underblanket also helps.

People who move around little during the day may find electric heating pads and footwarmers cheaper and more effective than extra heaters.

Autogenic Training Although this can help to prevent the incidence of hypothermia in the elderly, it is certainly not a substitute for adequate food, clothing and heating.

An orthodox view

Anyone suffering from hypothermia needs urgent medical help – if you are on the spot, call an ambulance or a doctor without delay.

While you are waiting, wrap the victim's head and body in blankets, and place him in the recovery position if unconscious. Warming up too suddenly can be dangerous, so be sure to avoid direct heaters and hot-water bottles. If the victim is conscious and uninjured, offer a sweet, warm – not scalding – drink and comfort.

Never give alcohol to a hypothermia victim, or massage the body – these draw blood away from the vital organs to the skin.

HYSTERIA

Anxiety built up by conflicts during the formative years is the usual cause of hysteria – a medical term for a far more serious, deep-rooted disorder than is implied by its everyday meaning. Susceptible people under STRESS can become hysterical to avoid facing a difficult situation, or to divert attention from what they see as their inadequacy.

The symptoms are genuinely felt and not in any way faked. The subconscious mind has converted the individual's anxiety into physical symptoms. These take many forms, from uncontrolled screaming and thrashing about to loss of sight or memory, or apparent paralysis of a limb. Sufferers see themselves as gaining in some way, however crippling the symptoms may seem to others. The gain is the ability to opt out of a situation that is too difficult to deal with.

What the therapists recommend

Yoga Emphasis is on relaxation and natural breathing to calm the overactive, easily aroused nervous system. Restoring steady breathing is of primary importance, to reduce TENSION. Relaxation and MEDITATION can benefit longer-term conditions.

To those who study yoga, its philosophy can offer a new interest and motivation in life, which may help to free them from the conflicts at the root of their condition.

An orthodox view

No treatment will be effective for this condition unless the root of the anxiety is found and recognised by the patient. It is not enough to treat current symptoms. They may go, but the underlying cause will tend to produce new ones. And accurate diagnosis by a doctor is essential in case what are thought to be hysterical symptoms are those of a real physical ailment.

Tranquillisers will give relief for a time while PSYCHOTHERAPY tries to get to the root of the problem. HYPNOTHERAPY has proved a successful form of psychotherapy for many hysteria cases – but only when carried out by a qualified hypnotherapist who is also a doctor. Patients are taken back to the origin of the anxiety and allowed to vent feelings they suppressed at the time. Once the patient is freed from the unacknowledged anxiety, the symptoms go.

When faced with a fit of hysterics, be calm, firm and reassuring. Take practical steps to deal with whatever has triggered the attack. Get rid of any onlookers.

Warning Never slap a hysterical person – the shock can cause psychological damage. Get the victim to see a doctor.

IATROGENIC ILLNESS

When seeing the doctor brings its own problems

Illnesses that arise as a direct result of the application of medical treatment itself are called 'iatrogenic' – this comes from the Greek words *iatros* meaning 'physician' and *genesis* meaning 'origin'.

Since orthodox forms of treatment such as drugs and surgery involve interfering with the body's normal functioning in ways that may lead to iatrogenic conditions, doctors and patients have to carefully weigh the advantages and risks of treatment before they consider starting it.

In some cases, iatrogenic illness may be unavoidable – as, for example, when anti-CANCER medication causes hair to fall out. Unfortunately, iatrogenic disorders can occasionally be the result of accidents and errors during treatment or of rare and unexpected reactions to certain treatments.

Concern about the side effects of orthodox medical treatment is often an important part of a decision to consult an alternative practitioner such as a naturopath, herbalist or aromatherapist, rather than a doctor.

Not all alternative treatments are completely free of side effects – some herbs, for example, can be dangerous or even fatal if incorrectly used – but in general if you consult a suitably trained and qualified practitioner the chances of developing iatrogenic problems are less.

An orthodox view

Doctors say that as conventional medicine becomes increasingly sophisticated, the incidence of iatrogenic disorders will inevitably increase. However, by improving training and holding regular reviews – called 'medical audits' – they hope to reduce the risks considerably. In South Africa, doctors can report bad reactions to particular drugs to the Medicines Information Centre (Department of Pharmacology, UCT Medical School, Observatory 7925) which will then issue a warning if a new iatrogenic illness is suspected.

IMMUNE SYSTEM

The body has a system of organs, cells and antibodies to fight a constant attack of bacteria, viruses, fungi and parasites. It both resists first-time attackers and recognises previous ones. See THE SECRET SERVICE THAT DEFENDS OUR BODIES, p. 204.

IMPETIGO

This is a highly contagious bacterial skin infection, which is common among children, and minor epidemics sometimes occur in nurseries and schools. Red spots with yellow crusts usually affect the victim's face, hands or knees, but they may spread over other parts of the skin. Usually, the child does not feel ill; but without treatment the sores can linger for weeks.

If impetigo is suspected, consult a doctor immediately, because of the high risk of spreading the infection, particularly in a school environment.

What the therapists recommend

Herbal Medicine Local applications of antiseptic herbs, such as infusions (see p. 184) or tinctures of marigold, myrrh and thyme, are said to be effective. Most essential oils – especially eucalyptus, lavender, lemon and thyme – are also said to work. Put ten drops of an oil in a dessertspoon of water and dab onto the spots with cotton wool.

Herbalists may also prescribe internal treatment with tinctures of burdock or echinacea to cleanse the system.

Naturopathy Attention to hygiene is vital to prevent the spread of this infection. Use separate face cloths and towels, and even boil clothes. Natural antibiotic effects may be gained from GARLIC – three or four cloves or capsules a day might be needed. Extra vitamins A, B and C may help to boost healing and resistance.

Aromatherapy A mixture of essential oils is said to kill the bacteria that cause impetigo and so prevent the infection from spreading. Dilute three drops of thyme, three drops of savory, and six drops of tea-tree oils in three tablespoons of carrier lotion and apply to the affected area three times a day.

An orthodox view

A doctor will probably prescribe a course of antibiotics in tablet, medicinal, or ointment form, and advise that the child should be kept at home.

IMPOTENCE

A strong association exists between a man's ability to have and maintain an erection and his image of himself. Partly this is due to the common assumption – whether right or wrong, instinctive or conditioned – that the man should take the initiative in sexual intercourse. Partly it is because, unlike his female partner, he is not able to complete the sexual act without being fully aroused, with an erect penis.

Add to this the thought that normal reproduction is impossible unless the man can perform effectively through to ejaculation and it is not surprising that men are both proud of and fearful for their erections. There is so much that can go wrong . . .

In both sexes, sexual arousal or excitement is marked by increased blood flow to the genital and pelvic areas. In a man, blood pumps into the spongy tissues of the penis, causing them to swell and become stiff, making the penis erect.

The process depends on a complex arrangement of blood vessels in the penis and pelvic region, on the nerves controlling them and the central nervous system itself, on the correct balance and sequence of hormones triggered by the brain, and on an erotically focused mental state.

If any one of these should go wrong – whether for physical, neurological, chemical or psychological reasons – an erection may be impossible to achieve or may subside at a crucial moment. This is commonly called impotence but is medically termed *erectile insufficiency*. No wonder, then, that many causes of STRESS and disease, as well as more subtle psychological factors, can lead to impotence (see also SEXUAL PROBLEMS).

Many drugs such as tranquillisers, antihistamines, beta-blockers (prescribed for high BLOOD PRESSURE) and so on can also impair or prevent erections, yet doctors and pharmacists may not warn about such effects. The result can be very troubling to the man concerned, and may even create the kind of secondary anxiety about performance that makes the impotence worse.

Self help Many of the recommendations given under SEXUAL PROBLEMS will be beneficial. In addition, it is particularly important, in order for your body to re-establish sexual responsiveness, that when erections begin to return after a period of impotence, you allow them to subside without insertion, so that you have the experience of an erection coming and going in response to the flow of sexual stimulation.

What the therapists recommend

Autogenic Training This can help many kinds of sexual disorders, including impotence. Standard exercises are often enough, but sometimes the use of a personalised formula added to the exercise may be needed. Even better results occur when the training is used with orthodox techniques.

Behavioural Therapy With impotence, the important aim is to reduce any anxieties about sexual intercourse, and take away the pressures involved. Therapy usually focuses on physical contact – kissing, caressing, massage and foreplay – rather than intercourse itself, placing emphasis on the pleasant sensations. When an erection can be successfully produced and maintained, then sexual contact is made increasingly intimate until intercourse can take place.

An orthodox view

Effective diagnosis depends upon distinguishing between physical and psychological causes of impotence; or, if both are present, how they are interacting. Consequently treatment may involve both physical and psychological methods. As with all treatments for sexual problems, relaxed circumstances free from anxiety are crucial.

In recent years, surgical methods of treating erection failure have been developed – such as implants of permanent flexible splints; inflatable devices, and vacuum systems applied to the outside of the penis, to promote blood flow and cause an erection.

There are also drugs which, when injected into the penis, relax muscles and encourage blood flow. This technique is seen by doctors as best used as a way of breaking the cycle of anxiety and fear which persistent loss of erection can produce.

INCONTINENCE

The inability to control the passing of urine and/or faeces can be embarrassing to adults, teenagers and older children. It can be hard to cure and a doctor should be consulted.

Incontinence in children may result from certain insecurities (see also BEDWETTING). In women, urine incontinence may be caused by a PROLAPSE, or organ displacement, sometimes as a result of childbirth. In men, PROSTATE PROBLEMS may be the cause. Either sex can be made incontinent by a stroke that damages the nervous control of the bladder (see BLADDER PROBLEMS).

The most common cause of faecal incontinence is, oddly enough, CONSTIPATION, in which the bowel can become so obstructed by solid faeces that only liquid faeces can be discharged.

Looking after an incontinent person – particularly one who is elderly or bedridden – can be a trying and difficult chore. The unpleasant odours of wet or soiled clothes or bed linen can cause embarrassment and distress to both the sufferer and the carer.

A district nurse should be able to offer professional advice about home care. A wide range of aids is available, including incontinence pads. There are also special deodorants that can be used on affected items to get rid of the smell.

What the therapists recommend

Herbal Medicine To clear the bowels herbalists may prescribe a mild astringent such as marigold or meadowsweet, taken three times a day.

Naturopathy You are advised to see a doctor first. Naturopathic measures that may help are hot and cold sitz baths (see HYDROTHERAPY), or alternating hot and cold compresses over the lower abdomen and back to improve local circulation and muscle tone. Also, pelvic floor exercises (see PREGNANCY) may help the patient to regain considerable control.

An orthodox view

Bladder and bowel incontinence need careful examination, especially with the elderly, and expert treatment should be sought.

INDIAN MEDICINE

Traditional Indian medicine, AYURVEDIC MEDICINE, has developed over 4 000 years. It deals with all aspects of life – physical, mental and spiritual – and treats the whole person, not just diseases. Methods involve herbal remedies, diets, and practical aids such as MASSAGE, MEDITATION and YOGA.

INDIGESTION

Eating too quickly and too much is one of the main causes of indigestion, or discomfort in the upper abdomen or in the chest. It is often accompanied by belching WIND and the bringing up of acid through the gullet and into the mouth (see ACID STOMACH). Other causes include a diet of rich, fatty foods, smoking, and drinking too much alcohol and drinks containing caffeine.

Occasionally indigestion is the result of stomach CANCER, but this is unusual in anyone below the age of 40. Symptoms of indigestion can also be caused by a variety of other ailments, including GALLSTONES, hernia, OBESITY and ULCERS.

What the therapists recommend

Herbal Medicine For short-term indigestion, drink hot teas such as peppermint, camomile, fennel, lemon balm or cinnamon.

For recurrent, long-term indigestion, a herbalist should be consulted. He will treat each case individually, and may prescribe any one of a range of herbs, including dandelion, ginger, golden seal, marigold, marshmallow, meadowsweet and thyme.

Acupuncture An acupuncturist will usually treat the bladder, conception governor, spleen and stomach meridians.

Acupressure First treat a point on the lower leg, four fingers' width from the crown of the inner ankle bone, against the shin bone. Press inward beside the bone. Also, press inward from beneath the kneecap, three thumbs' width from beneath the kneecap, in the hollow on the outer edge of the shin.

Naturopathy For simple causes such as overeating or an excess of rich foods, fasting for 24 hours, taking only liquids such as apple juice or herb teas, may help the digestive tract to recover.

Longer spells of indigestion, however, require a consultation. In general, slippery elm powder in hot water may give some relief if the digestive tract is inflamed, while warm compresses over the abdomen will ease COLIC or stomach cramps.

An orthodox view

People who develop indigestion for the first time after the age of 40, or whose bowel movements change (see BOWEL DISORDERS), or if there is weight loss or frequent pain, should see a doctor. To reach a diagnosis a practitioner may send you to hospital for a barium meal and X-ray, or to have an endoscopy (an examination of the stomach and first part of the intestine by means of a flexible, lighted tube). He may also, as with other cases, prescribe an antacid or a drug to reduce the amount of stomach acid.

Indigestion may be aggravated by aspirin and most anti-ARTHRITIS medicines.

INFERTILITY

Difficulty in conceiving a baby, commonly called infertility, may be more properly termed 'subfertility', since most couples with this problem do eventually manage to have children. The condition is quite common, affecting about one in every ten couples in the West. Some women naturally take longer to conceive than others, so infertility is not diagnosed until a couple have been having regular sexual intercourse without using contraceptives for at least a year.

A variety of causes can reduce a couple's fertility: SMOKING, drinking too much alcohol, illness, and strenuous exercise by women may all play a part, as well as more specific physical disorders.

WORRY, STRESS and ANXIETY – especially about trying to have a baby – can also make things worse. In about a quarter of all cases, doctors can find no sure reason for infertility; for another quarter the problem lies with the woman; for another quarter with the man; and in the remaining quarter the problem lies with both partners.

The normal process of fertilisation

In most fertile women, one of the two ovaries produces an egg every month in about the middle of the menstrual cycle, although this varies greatly between individuals. The egg then travels down the uterine tube (Fallopian tube or oviduct) and into the womb.

For fertilisation to occur, the couple must have sexual intercourse shortly before or after ovulation, so that the man's sperm can pass from the vagina through the cervix – the muscle at the entrance to the womb – into the womb and the uterine tubes, where one of them must fertilise the egg. Since the egg survives for only about 36 hours after ovulation, and sperm for only about two or three days, fertilisation depends on timing.

The best chance of a woman becoming pregnant is to have intercourse 12 to 24 hours before ovulation, although this can be hard to estimate. Nevertheless, many women experience pain or discomfort when they ovu-

How good health can be a help

Good general health will make conception easier. Both partners should eat a balanced diet (see EATING FOR HEALTH), take a reasonable amount of EXERCISE – though very active women may need to cut down – get ample sleep, and make plenty of time for rest and relaxation (see RELAXATION and BREATHING).

Women can find out when their fertile days occur by taking their temperature every morning first thing before getting out of bed. When ovulation occurs, the temperature will rise by about 0,2 to 0,5°C (0,5 to 1°F). Conception is possible for about two or three days before and after the day of ovulation. Special kits are available from pharmacies which allow women to detect ovulation by testing urine samples. (See also CONTRACEPTION, for more information on telling when ovulation occurs.)

Men with a low sperm count are sometimes helped by splashing their testicles with cold water several times a day, since too high a temperature can interfere with sperm production.

late; sometimes they notice a little blood in the vagina, and a woman can identify fertile days by taking her temperature regularly, first thing every morning (see box). Once an egg has been fertilised it embeds itself in the womb lining as a foetus, and gradually develops into a baby.

Many physical problems – some of them quite small – can interfere with the process of fertilisation and pregnancy. Here are some of the most common ones:

Problems affecting women

Failure to ovulate About one-fifth of all infertility occurs because the woman ovulates very infrequently or not at all. The cause can be a hormonal imbalance, a problem affecting the ovaries, sudden weight loss, or even simply stress and anxiety. Usually the woman has irregular periods, or these may have stopped altogether.

Too little progesterone The hormone progesterone prepares the lining of the womb to receive the embryo. If too little is produced by the woman's body, the embryo cannot implant itself into the womb.

Blocked uterine tubes Usually an infection – either at the time or one which occurred in the past – is the cause. Conception is prevented as sperm are unable to reach the egg, and the egg to travel to the womb.

Endometriosis Pieces of the womb lining begin to grow around the ovaries or uterine tubes, reducing the woman's chances of becoming pregnant.

Problems with cervical mucus To prevent germs from reaching the reproductive organs, sticky mucus is secreted around the cervix at the entrance to the womb. Normally it becomes thinner during ovulation, to allow sperm to pass through, but if this does not happen infertility may be the result. In a few rare cases a woman's cervical mucus may contain antibodies which actually attack and destroy her partner's sperm.

Abnormalities of the womb Sometimes these can prevent the fertilised egg from implanting itself into the womb. The most common problems are fibroids (non-malignant tumours in the womb), adhesions (old scars in the womb lining, which are often the result of previous infections) or an abnormally shaped womb.

Problems affecting men

Sperm abnormalities Some men have a low sperm count or produce abnormal sperm which cannot fertilise an egg. Many factors can cause this, including illnesses such as MUMPS, VARICOSE VEINS near the testicles, OBESITY, tight clothing, and allowing the testicles to get hot – for example, by working in an overheated environment. In other cases, stress or hormone imbalances affect sperm

production. About one in ten infertile men produce antibodies which make their sperm clump together so that they cannot move freely; this can occur after a vasectomy operation has been reversed.

Difficulties with ejaculating sperm Infertility can result from blockages in the sperm ducts, premature ejaculation which occurs outside the vagina, and so-called 'retrograde ejaculation' when semen is passed into the bladder instead of out through the penis – a condition which affects some diabetics and men who have had prostate surgery.

What the therapists recommend

Acupuncture Treatment depends on the cause of the problem, and generally includes advice on diet and vitamin supplements as well as acupuncture or MOXIBUSTION treatment to the bladder, kidney, stomach and conception meridians.

Autogenic Training This may help when infertility is related to stress or TENSION.

Naturopathy The nutritional intake of the couple trying to conceive may need improving. A high-potency, multivitamin and mineral supplement is often very valuable. Hot and cold splashes of the genital area will stimulate local circulation (but hot baths should not be taken before intercourse). It should also help to avoid alcohol and tobacco; to take plenty of exercise; and to get adequate rest and sleep.

An orthodox view

Once a couple have been trying to have a baby for about a year without success, the doctor will begin tests to investigate the causes. Most of these can be treated by means of drugs, artificial hormones, surgery or special techniques such as in vitro ('test tube') fertilisation – where eggs are removed from the woman's body, fertilised with the man's sperm in the laboratory and then replaced in the womb.

If no cause can be found, couples are simply advised to improve their general health as much as possible, stop worrying, and keep trying – sooner or later many of them will manage to have a baby. If this does not happen, or the cause of infertility cannot be treated, the doctor may suggest that the couple consider adoption.

INFLUENZA

Winter epidemics of this virus infection are common. Many people incorrectly refer to COLDS as flu, but true influenza is more severe. It produces high FEVER with a sensation of feeling cold, sweating, HEADACHE,

Alternative remedies for influenza

HERBAL REMEDIES — EFFECTS

Remedy	Soothes sore throats	Eases muscle pain	Relieves headaches	Brings down fever	Fights infection	Decongestant	Cough suppressant	Expectorant	Sedative
Garlic	■			■	■			■	
Steam bath with olbas or eucalyptus oil				■		■			
Valerian or hop tablets			■						■
Camomile infusion			■	■					■
White willow bark	■	■	■	■					
Sage, nettle, eucalyptus or fenugreek infusion	■				■				
Meadowsweet	■	■		■					
Coltsfoot, white horebound, mullein, wild lettuce, wild cherry bark						■	■	■	
Yarrow, angelica				■	■				
Elecampane, elderflower	■			■	■	■			

VITAMINS AND MINERAL REMEDIES

Remedy	Soothes sore throats	Eases muscle pain	Relieves headaches	Brings down fever	Fights infection	Decongestant	Cough suppressant	Expectorant	Sedative
Calcium and magnesium	■	■	■	■	■				
Zinc	■	■	■	■	■	■	■	■	
Vitamin B complex (take in the morning or it may disturb sleep)	■	■	■	■	■	■	■	■	
Vitamin C	■	■	■	■	■	■	■	■	

BIOCHEMIC TISSUE SALTS REMEDIES

Remedy	Soothes sore throats	Eases muscle pain	Relieves headaches	Brings down fever	Fights infection	Decongestant	Cough suppressant	Expectorant	Sedative
Ferr. phos.				■					
Kali mur.							■		
Combination J							■		
Combination Q					■				

OTHER NATURAL REMEDIES

Remedy	Soothes sore throats	Eases muscle pain	Relieves headaches	Brings down fever	Fights infection	Decongestant	Cough suppressant	Expectorant	Sedative
Propolis	■				■			■	
Coltsfoot, pine and honey balsam					■			■	

If you stay at home and choose the right remedies, you can stave off the worst miseries of flu, from the shivers and soreness of the early days to the tiredness and cough that may linger. Wise treatment avoids spreading the virus and cuts the risk of complications.

The chart shown above gives a selection of alternative methods of treating influenza – and the specific effects that each particular remedy has. For example, taking garlic eases sore throats, reduces fever, combats infection and acts as an expectorant.

aching muscles, weakness, loss of appetite, COUGHS and pain behind the breastbone. It is caused by any of numerous influenza VIRUS INFECTIONS, which change with time to produce new strains so that long-term immunity is impossible.

Symptoms may last up to a week, and a period of depression is common afterwards.

What the therapists recommend

HOMOEOPATHY

Self help Medicines prescribed include: B*aptisia*, when there is severe prostration, gastric symptoms, stupor, and the patient has a red face and feels 'in pieces'; E*upatorium perf.* when the bones feel broken, the eyeballs are sore, and the patient dare not move; and *Gelsemium* when there is a bursting headache, great heaviness of head and eyeballs, absence of thirst, and hot and cold waves alternate down the back.

HERBAL MEDICINE

Self help In the early, shivery stages, hot ginger, cinnamon – or even cayenne pepper – teas are recommended to increase the circulation and warmth. When there is a fever, try infusions (see p. 184) of elderflower, yarrow and peppermint, to regulate the temperature; take a tablespoon of hot infusion every hour. Two or three cups of yarrow and lemon balm tea a day are said to improve the appetite during convalescence.

NATUROPATHY

Prevention would be ideal, although during epidemics this is not easy. Taking only fluids during the early stages may help. When aching and chilled, try a hot bath, perhaps with 2 tablespoons of Epsom salts, just before retiring. At the feverish stage, take elderflower tea and/or fruit juices, and apply a cold pack on the trunk. As always with cold packs and compresses, immediately cover with a thick towel or blanket to encourage warmth and sweating. Vitamins, especially vitamin A (about 5 000 iu) and vitamin C (3-4 g) may be prescribed.

BIOCHEMIC TISSUE SALTS

When there is feverishness, Nat. sulph. is recommended hourly, in alternation with Ferr. phos. during the early stages. Kali sulph. may be alternated with Ferr. phos. when there is a feeling of stuffiness, yellow discharge and a desire for cool air. It should help to reduce the temperature. Calc. phos. may be taken during convalescence.

An orthodox view

With rest, extra drinks and paracetamol or aspirin as required – up to two tablets every four hours, up to a maximum of eight in 24 hours – most healthy young people recover from influenza without medical treatment. Antibiotics are ineffective against viruses, but doctors prescribe them for secondary bacterial infections such as BRONCHITIS or PNEUMONIA, or to prevent complications in the elderly or infirm.

Flu sufferers should not struggle to work. They only spread the disease – by coughs and sneezes – and increase their risk of complications.

Every autumn, vaccines against the viruses that are expected the following winter are produced. Immunisation may be offered to high risk groups such as people over 65 and those who have DIABETES, lung disease or heart disease. However, the vaccines will give protection only against the particular viruses, not against other strains of flu – or against common colds.

INHALATION THERAPY

Many practitioners of HYDROTHERAPY as well as orthodox doctors recommend steam inhalations to clear CATARRH and to improve skin conditions such as ACNE.

Various kinds of aromatic oil or proprietary remedies, often with a eucalyptus or menthol base, are added to hot water to increase the effect of the vapour. You can use the treatment at home, breathing in the steam deeply over a bowl and holding a towel over your head and the bowl to keep the steam in. Take care not to have the water too hot, in case the steam scalds you, and be careful also not to upset the bowl.

INSOMNIA

Almost everyone experiences insomnia – or sleeplessness – at some time of their life or another. Noise, pain, coffee, irregular hours, unfamiliar surroundings and worry can all lead to restless nights. Because time drags when they are trying to sleep, most people overestimate their sleeplessness. There are no rules about how much sleep is necessary: everyone's needs are different. Babies – and some teenagers – may sleep for up to 18 hours each day, but elderly people may require only five or six hours.

There are two types of sleep: orthodox sleep and rapid-eye-movement (REM) sleep, during which dreaming occurs (see SLEEP DISORDERS). Both types of sleep are necessary if a person is to start the next morning feeling refreshed.

Lack of sleep causes irritability, inefficiency and inability to concentrate at school

---

Do's and don'ts of insomnia

Do note your sleep pattern in your diary; it will help you to find the causes of your insomnia.
Do persevere to find the alternative therapy that suits you.
Do take plenty of EXERCISE.
Do try to relax as often as possible during the day, and try to follow a regular routine.
Do keep regular sleeping hours.
Do ensure that your bedroom is well ventilated but warm, quiet and dark.
Do make sure that your bed is comfortable and gives your body proper support (see BEDS AND BEDDING).
Do allow yourself time to relax and unwind before trying to sleep.
Do listen to soft, 'easy' music while preparing for bed.
Do take a warm, not hot, relaxing bath.
Do put the bedside clock out of sight.
Do relax in bed. For example, imagine doing something peaceful, such as sunbathing on a beach.
Don't take alcohol or stimulants such as tea, coffee and cola drinks before going to bed.
Don't eat anything immediately before going to bed, or a heavy meal less than three hours before bedtime.
Don't over-stimulate your mind near bedtime – for example by smoking, taking a hot drink or watching a violent film on television.
Don't put off going to bed.
Don't lie awake for hours worrying; get up and do something relaxing for 20 minutes or until you feel tired again.

---

or work. However, the body can make up for sleep loss without catching up on every lost hour. People who have had several nights' broken sleep can recover after a single sleep of about 12 hours.

Some insomnia sufferers become so wound up that they cannot relax enough to sleep. A vicious circle of overtiredness and insomnia develops.

Insomnia, particularly early waking, may be a symptom of DEPRESSION. Sufferers also lack energy, finding everything an effort.

What the therapists recommend
HOMOEOPATHY
Self help Treatment of general health with homoeopathic remedies is said often to bring about an improvement in sleeping habits. In the meantime, one of the following may help: *Aconitum* when kept awake by a sense of fear and panic, possibly following a shock or fright; *Arnica* when overtired mentally and physically, and when the bed feels too hard and constant movement is necessary to get relief; *Coffea* when wide awake with an active mind.

HERBAL MEDICINE
Self help Infusions of camomile, lavender, lemon balm, lime blossom, marjoram or vervain are gently relaxing, so take 2 tablespoons at night.
Consultation Individual treatment and counselling may be needed for chronic insomnia due to STRESS and TENSION. In short-term (acute) cases, herbalists may prescribe 1 teaspoon (5 ml) of passion flower or cowslip tincture each night.

MASSAGE
Self help Provided the insomnia is not a result of indigestion or a medical condition, a soothing, relaxing, sedating massage can work wonders if applied at bedtime, or as near as possible before that.

The patient's head rests gently on the pillow during treatment, and the body is kept well covered and warm. The therapist uses mainly slow, rhythmic stroking movements, with fairly deep kneadings using the palms of the hands. Contact is maintained throughout, as removing the hands or even changing the stroke can be irritating or disturbing to the person.

A full massage of the legs and back is applied, taking extreme care to avoid hypersensitive areas and the abdomen.

Other alternative treatments
Traditional medicine A glass of warm milk with a teaspoon of honey helps induce sleep.

An orthodox view
Doctors can treat some forms of depression by prescribing antidepressant drugs, and so relieve insomnia. Other diseases that interfere with sleep, particularly painful ones, can also be diagnosed and treated.

Sleeping pills may be effective in breaking a vicious cycle of sleeplessness and overtiredness. However, users can become addicted within as little as three weeks of regular use, and the pills must therefore be used only for short periods. Caffeine-containing drinks such as coffee and tea, and certain soft drinks should be avoided.

The secret service that defends our bodies

A host of 'germs' – micro-organisms from the environment we live in – constantly attack and invade our bodies, where our immune system is ever at war with them.

The complex system acts as a secret army which begins preparing for war before we are brought into the world. When invaders strike our vulnerable human defence system, they immediately activate teams of chemical dispatch riders – messengers that carry the orders for deployment of the troops and their engagement with the enemy. And once an engagement has been fought, the troops remain in reserve against any future attacks by the same invader.

The unwanted 'germs' that invade the human body and live there as parasites include fungi such as *Candida albicans*, which causes THRUSH, and protozoa such as *Plasmodium*, the cause of malaria. However, by far the commonest invaders are bacteria and viruses which are responsible for a whole host of infectious diseases, ranging from COLDS and INFLUENZA to SHINGLES, PNEUMONIA and POLIOMYELITIS.

Our first line of defence consists of the skin itself (a physical, largely impenetrable barrier) and mucous membranes, which keep out many would-be invaders. However, close behind is a complex defensive system which allows us to remain immune to most infections, even when they do get into the body. That is why it is called the *immune system*. The discipline behind this system is known as immunology.

This system must be ready at all times to neutralise or destroy a vast array of micro-organisms and the poisons they make wherever they attack the body, and the extensive lymphatic system fills the bill.

The spleen, thymus gland, tonsils, bone marrow and other bodily organs are vital to it, and its network of capillaries and lymphatics, or lymph vessels, drain the clear body fluid known as lymph from the body's tissues and into the bloodstream (see diagram). And it is by special cells called *lymphocytes* – a type of white blood cell originating in bone marrow – and complex blood protein molecules called antibodies that the immune system mostly does its job.

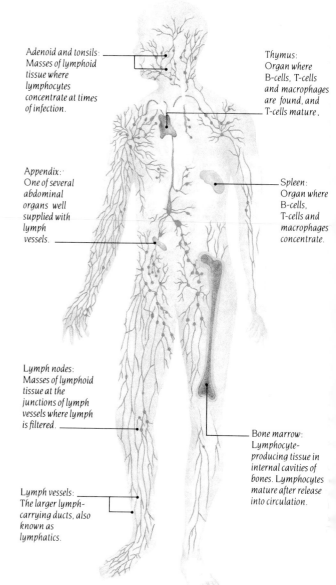

Adenoid and tonsils:
Masses of lymphoid tissue where lymphocytes concentrate at times of infection.

Thymus:
Organ where B-cells, T-cells and macrophages are found, and T-cells mature.

Appendix:
One of several abdominal organs well supplied with lymph vessels.

Spleen:
Organ where B-cells, T-cells and macrophages concentrate.

Lymph nodes:
Masses of lymphoid tissue at the junctions of lymph vessels where lymph is filtered.

Bone marrow:
Lymphocyte-producing tissue in internal cavities of bones. Lymphocytes mature after release into circulation.

Lymph vessels:
The larger lymph-carrying ducts, also known as lymphatics.

The lymphatic network – the body's one-way drainage system

The lymphatic system consists of a network of vessels extending to all parts of the body. The fluid in them is colourless lymph, containing white but no red blood cells, and valves ensure that it flows only one way, away from the body's extremities. (Lymph also bathes the body's tissues and is very similar to blood plasma.) Disease-fighting white blood cells called lymphocytes originate in bone marrow, and develop and mature in other parts of the lymphatic system, such as the thymus and spleen. The tonsils, adenoid and other organs are made of lymphatic tissue, but their exact role remains unclear.

Two types of immunity

We have two kinds of immunity. The first is a very general form of defence that we are born with or acquire through our mother's milk. This is called *passive* immunity, and it protects young babies while they are developing their own much more powerful system of adaptive, or *acquired* immunity. It is called 'acquired' because it develops in response to contact for the first time with some new virus or bacterium. The immune system adapts its response specifically to the particular enemy.

Having been acquired, this immunity remains with us, so that the next time we encounter the same organism we can mount a defence against it very quickly.

This is one of the immune system's key features: its ability to 'remember' attackers (or *pathogens*) encountered in the past, recognising them so that it can instantly switch on a set of ready-made defences. A second feature of the immune system is its diversity: its ability to develop a whole range of immune defences against different pathogens.

Immunity in the face of an attacker is not immediately acquired: it takes days or even weeks. The child, meanwhile, may grow seriously ill and be in danger of dying. Vaccination – artificial immunisation – forestalls this possibility. Immunising babies against, say, MEASLES or WHOOPING COUGH involves exposing them to a small amount of the dead or weakened pathogen. The body recognises this as a 'foreign' substance, or *antigen*, and creates a defence against it (see also ALLERGY).

In later life, if the child encounters live measles viruses, the defence system is ready and needs only to be activated and directed against those particular invading organisms. But the defences against measles give no protection against, say, polio. Whether by vaccination or direct contact with disease, the

How the antibodies, lymphocytes and macrophages act to destroy invaders

A B-*lymphocyte is shown in section above. The parallel red bands (right) are the system of membranes where antibodies are made.*

A computer graphic (right) shows an antibody-antigen complex. At the top is the antigen – the 'foreign' substance or bodily invader (red). The green is the part of the antigen that the antibody has recognised. The antibody itself is below (blue).

A *macrophage engulfs and digests a yeast cell (large oval), a type of fungus. Macrophages – similar to white blood cells – occur in connective tissue, liver and the central nervous system as well as in the lymphatic system.*
The *process by which they destroy invading cells is called phagocytosis.*

1 A B-cell detects invading bacteria, producing antibodies specially tailored to deal with the invaders.

2 Antibodies specific to the invading antigen (bacteria) are then released into the bloodstream.

3 Antibodies attach themselves to the invading bacteria, marking them for the macrophages.

4 Macrophages – scavenger white cells – engulf and digest the marked bacteria.

immune system has to develop a host of programmes, each defending the body against a particular invader.

In the front line

The actual defences of the immune system consist of two closely connected main parts – the lymphocytes, white blood cells which are found in lymph as well as the bloodstream, and antibodies, which are produced by certain types of lymphocytes and circulate in the blood.

Antibodies have a branching structure with special sites shaped to lock on to invading micro-organisms, or to the poisonous substances they are producing, and neutralise them. But the process goes further than that: scavenger cells called *macrophages* are constantly on the lookout for antibody-coated antigens. Any of these they encounter they engulf and destroy. In fact, antibodies act as 'markers' to ensure that invading material is destroyed by the macrophages.

Antibodies also act in other ways. When they stick to a foreign cell, the process mobilises groups of blood proteins known as *complement*, which have the ability to break up cells and so kill them. It may also be involved in the 'calling' of scavenging cells to the site of the ongoing conflict.

The body's production of antibodies depends on two types of lymphocytes. The B-*lymphocytes* (or B-*cells*), are the ones that first recognise the foreign antigens in the body and produce the first antibody reaction against them. During any subsequent attack by the same micro-organism, particular B-cells specialised for that antigen mature rapidly and produce the appropriate antibodies in large quantities.

A *cytotoxic* T-*lymphocyte attacks a virus-infected cell (the large cell at top). Such T-lymphocytes recognise antigenic components on the surface of invaders. They then bind directly to their outer cell membranes, and destroy the invader cells. In this process the invaders' outer membranes are broken, so allowing their cell contents to escape.*

However, they cannot do so on their own. They are controlled by a second group of lymphocytes known as the T-*lymphocytes* (or T-*cells*), so called because they develop and mature in the thymus in the upper chest. There are several types of T-cells. Helper T-cells 'switch on' B-cells, and suppressor T-cells switch them off again (see diagram, p. 207). So the balance of helper to suppressor cells is vital for controlling immunity. The Aids virus (HIV) attacks the immune system at this point, infecting and destroying the helper T-cells. The same mechanism is used to prevent the rejection of transplants.

Cytotoxic T-cells

Apart from the helper and suppressor cells, other types of T-cells play a direct part in destroying invading organisms or even the body's own cells once they have become infected – with a virus, for example. One type is the so-called *cytotoxic* ('cell-poisoning') T-cells, which learn to lock on to particular antigens on the surface of infected cells in much the same way as B-cells learn to make antibodies, which also lock on to antigens. The cytotoxic T-cells then break down the outer walls of the infected cells, thus causing their destruction. Other T-cells are known as *natural killers*. They do not need to be programmed, and can recognise and destroy any foreign materials even if they have not encountered them before.

Some CANCER cells are recognised as foreign by natural killer T-cells and are destroyed, but unfortunately not all. One of the great challenges of cancer research is to find out why, and to devise ways of boosting the immune system so that it can fight cancerous tumours.

An enemy cell is recognised, and a 'killer cell' locks on to it

1 A T-cell in the thymus is activated in response to the invading antigen – virus, fungus, parasite or cancer cell.

2 The activated killer (or cytotoxic) T-cell is released into the bloodstream to home in on the invader.

3 Now the alerted T-cell attacks the target antigen cell, or virus-infected body cell, binding itself on to it.

4 The invader's cell wall is then broken down by the T-cell and the disease-producing antigen is destroyed.

Why your 'glands' swell

The B- and T-cells and the macrophages, which together make up the body's system of cellular immunity, are found in high concentrations in the thymus (two soft, pinkish-grey lobes near the root of the neck) and the spleen. They constantly monitor the contents of body fluid as it flows through the lymphatic system, where lymph nodes (junctions in the network) filter it.

If foreign material is detected, mature lymphocytes concentrate in large numbers in the nodes and migrate to the bloodstream to deal with it. (This concentration causes the swollen 'glands' – in fact, lymph nodes – in the neck, armpits or groin during some illnesses.)

The way the body co-ordinates cellular immunity through chemical messages has only recently been discovered. Helper T-cells stimulate B-cells to produce antibodies by secreting a particular chemical substance called an *interleukin*. Other interleukins stimulate cytotoxic T-cells and natural killer cells into activity, and suppressor T-cells similarly exert their influence chemically.

So do macrophages, which produce similar substances when they encounter foreign cells in the body; the result is to boost the activity of T-cells nearby. And other chemical messengers act as 'help' signals. They make lymphocytes concentrate at the site of an infection.

Maintaining vital links

Chemical signals may also maintain links between the immune system and the brain. This traffic is apparently two-way, implying that the brain somehow monitors or responds to the condition of the immune system, and that state of mind can influence resistance to disease.

There is plenty of circumstantial evidence that this is true, and doctors have long known that a 'positive' attitude can help patients to overcome diseases ranging from common infections to cancer. But they have never been able to measure the effect or explain how it happens. The discovery of the chemical messengers involved may help us to both understand and influence this aspect of the body's defences.

Strengthening the defences

A number of alternative therapies suggest ways of boosting the immune system, to make the body better able to fight disease. Undernourishment is recognised as the primary cause of immuno-deficiency throughout the world, and most conventional doctors would endorse the need for a good, balanced diet. Alternative and orthodox practitioners recommend a diet based on unrefined and unprocessed foods, such as wholewheat bread, fresh fruit and vegetables, lean meat, fish and salads (see EATING FOR HEALTH, HEALTH FOODS and MACROBIOTICS). The high nutritional value of such foods can only serve to complement the immune system's natural defences. However, there is disagreement as to whether certain dietary supplements are beneficial, as many people claim. Vitamins A, B_6 and C are believed to play a vital role in enhancing the immune system. Adequate zinc and

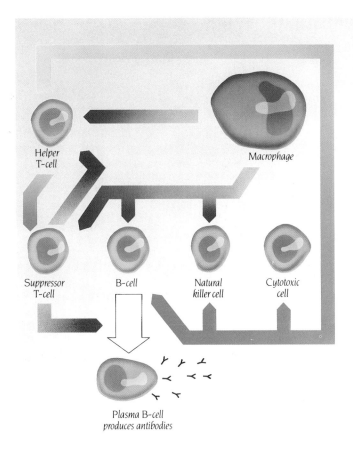

Plasma B-cell
produces antibodies

Chemical messengers

The various types of cells involved in the immune system – and, it now appears, the brain too – signal to and influence each other by a system of chemical messengers. Among the most important are the interleukins, by which helper T-lymphocytes (T-cells) stimulate other kinds of lymphocyte into action (green arrows), and the suppressor factors that suppressor T-cells use to keep helpers and B-lymphocytes (B-cells) under control (red arrows). Macrophages signal for help in a similar way (blue arrows).

iron levels (see MINERALS) are also nutritionally important. Conversely, excess consumption of sugar reduces the body's ability to fight disease – as does alcohol.

The immunity-boosting effect of EXERCISE may be difficult to prove or disprove, but there can be little doubt that a person in the peak of fitness has superior defences against illness and is therefore at an advantage when confronted with the threat of invasive micro-organisms. Obese people tend to have impaired immuno-deficiency, perhaps because of high blood levels of cholesterol and lipids.

The recent discoveries mentioned earlier – as well as commonplace experience – point to the importance of avoiding stress and adopting a consistently positive mental attitude to overcoming disease, whether it is the common cold or AIDS, influenza or cancer.

IONISATION

Mountain air from a machine

The well-known feeling of tension that builds up before a storm, and the sense of relief afterwards; headachy irritability after a day at work; or vigorous good health on a mountain holiday – these are some of the most common effects that different kinds of air seem to have on our well-being. One explanation – accepted by many doctors and scientists as well as by alternative practitioners – is that electrically charged particles in the air, called ions, are responsible.

Most air particles are electrically neutral, or contain no charge, but others can acquire a positive or negative charge. When there are too few negative ions or too many positive ones – before a storm, for example – many people experience HEADACHES, lethargy, DEPRESSION, irritability and a general feeling of being unwell. By contrast, a good supply of negative ions – as occurs after a storm – is associated with feeling alert and uplifted.

Charged ions are mainly the result of radiation from the sun and from space, but negative ions are also created by lightning, ocean waves and running water. Fresh mountain and seaside air is rich in negative particles, but most city air contains few or none. Pollution, air conditioning, central heating, dust, synthetic fibres and electrical appliances are all said to destroy negative charges, and may account for the oppressive atmosphere in many houses and offices.

Self help People in environments likely to be low in negative ions and those who are particularly sensitive to weather conditions – some ASTHMA sufferers, for example – often find ionising machines helpful. These are small electrical devices which use very little current but produce a constant stream of negative ions when turned on.

Small ionisers are available from some chemists and suppliers of medical equipment. They have a range of about 3-4 metres, so need to be plugged in at the bedside or placed on a desk where you work. Some manufacturers also make more powerful units for use in offices and larger areas.

Ionisers work best when doors and windows are closed, and should be no less than about 50 cm from walls and floors to allow a free flow of ions into the air. Wherever possible, avoid placing ionisers near windows or on polished surfaces, as static electrical charges on these can make the machines work less efficiently.

Keep ionisers and the surfaces around them clean, as they tend to attract dust particles – and sticky tar if you are a smoker – which may eventually interfere with their

Pure air for the home

The most effective ionisers are supplied by nature. For example, an electric storm fills the air with negative ions, making us feel refreshed and reinvigorated once the storm is over. Fresh running water – such as a mountain stream – is another highly successful way of providing the atmospheric ions that do us good. The balance of positive and negative ions in the home can be restored by installing an air ioniser in the living-room or bedroom. Bedroom ionisers should be placed no more than about 2 m from the head of the bed, and you can go to sleep in the reassuring knowledge that you are breathing in healthy, balanced-ion air that will help you have a good night's sleep. Home ionisers are believed particularly to help people suffering from chest and lung problems.

functioning. Ionisers are also more effective if air conditioning and central heating are used sparingly, and if electrical appliances are turned off when not in use.

Alternatively, taking a shower is a cheap and effective way of receiving negatively charged ions – which is one reason why most people feel refreshed and reinvigorated after a brisk shower.

Who it can help Regular night-time use of a bedside ioniser is said to benefit respiratory disorders such as asthma, BRONCHITIS, HAY FEVER and CATARRH. Depression, INSOMNIA, MIGRAINE and headaches have also been helped, and one study has even shown that burns may heal faster when there are more negative ions.

Ionisation is also thought to prevent illness by cleansing the air of bacteria and impurities such as cigarette smoke, pollen, dust and small fibres that can irritate the respiratory tract and cause ALLERGY. However, these impurities tend to collect on furniture and household surfaces, which then need to be cleaned more often.

An orthodox view

There are no known side effects or dangers associated with negative ionisation machines, and many conventional doctors and scientists accept the claims made for them. Studies in Britain have shown that many people with respiratory conditions, skin allergies and headaches were helped by ionisers at their places of work.

These studies suggest that air which is rich in negative ions has a stimulating effect, while too many positive ions have a depressing effect. The levels of the hormone serotonin in the blood, brain and other body tissues also seem to be reduced by the presence of negative ions, having a calming influence on the nervous system. This may explain why ionisers seem to help in cases of asthma, irritability and STRESS.

IRIDOLOGY

Diagnosing by eye

Studying the markings on the irises of the eyes and observing changes in them is the basis of iridology. It is a method of DIAGNOSIS and health monitoring used by iridologists and other alternative therapists. Iridology relates precise positions on the irises to parts of the body, and from changes at those positions, practitioners claim to locate and diagnose problems in the body – and mind.

Although early medical men sought clues in the eye for their patients' ailments, modern iridology began with the Hungarian doctor Ignatz von Peczely (1826-1911). As a boy he had cared for an owl with a broken leg. He noted a black line form in the owl's iris and gradually change to white marks around a black dot as the leg healed.

Later, as a doctor, Von Peczely became convinced that the same illness produced a telltale mark at the same point on the iris in patient after patient. After he published his findings in 1881, interest in them spread across Europe and, in the early 1900s, throughout the United States.

It was in America in the 1950s that Dr Bernard Jensen worked out a detailed chart of the irises, in which he carefully pinpointed the precise part of the body that each iris area is said to reflect.

The iris is divided into sections (like portions of a cake) linked to parts or functions of the body, and also into six rings or zones linked to bodily systems (see p. 210). The first and innermost zone relates to the stomach, the second to the intestines, the third to the blood and lymph systems, the fourth to glands and organs, the fifth to the muscles and skeleton, and the sixth and outermost to the skin and elimination.

The left iris corresponds to the left side of the body and the right iris to the right side. Many parts or functions are reflected in both irises. Generally, organs and functions in the upper body will reflect their condition in the top part of the iris and lower body organs and functions in the lower part.

White marks are thought to develop through inflammation, too much stimulation and STRESS; and dark ones when a part of the body does not work properly. A dark rim round the edge of the iris may indicate that poisons are accumulating in the skin because of inefficient elimination of waste.

Iridologists recognise ten different types of constitution with a different balance of strengths and weaknesses in their body systems, organs and glands.

Each type of constitution has a basic fibre pattern in the irises. A fine-grained pattern like woven silk indicates a strong constitution, an open hessian-like pattern indicates a weak one.

When the abnormal marks have been studied, the iridologist or other therapist may devise a suitable treatment to restore the correct balance for that particular patient's constitution. An experienced iridologist also looks for early warning of problems.

Who it can help People who do not like the more invasive techniques of conventional medicine – blood tests, swabs, X-rays, biopsies and the like – feel more at ease with an examination of the eye. Those who want early warning of a condition before it shows unpleasant symptoms or who want a regular check on what progress they are making with a more healthy life style, may also benefit from iridology.

Finding a therapist Iridology is not recognised as a therapy by either the South African Medical and Dental Council or the South African Associated Health Service Professions Board, and no register of practitioners is therefore available. Indeed, the strict rules by which alternative medical practitioners are governed in this country make it impossible for an iridologist officially to make a diagnosis, to cure, or take any form of remuneration. (To do so could be construed as a criminal offence.)

However, many alternative therapists, in particular naturopaths and homoeopaths, use iridology as one of their diagnostic methods, and some will use it as a matter of course when you consult them.

Consulting a therapist A practitioner who examines your irises as only one of several diagnostic techniques is likely to use a torch and a magnifying glass, and make a detailed record of your markings. A specialist iridologist may also use a camera with a closeup lens and side lighting to take slides of your irises for a permanent record.

When the slides are projected onto a screen, the iridologist will explain the significance of the markings and suggest a course of treatment, or recommend you consult a therapist. At follow-up consultations further slides can be compared with the originals to show progress.

If signs of degeneration, malignancy, or chronic disease are found, patients are advised to see their GP.

An orthodox view

Although doctors often find the general appearance of the eye – yellowing, inflammation, dullness or unnatural brilliance, for example – an indication of ill health, few of them accept the detailed links between parts of the body and areas of the iris that practising iridologists do. Most doctors tend to challenge the assumption that iridology is scientifically based; therefore they consider it of little or no use.

The colour of the iris, and variations in it, result from the distribution of pigment cells on the back of the iris. The white fibres in the iris are simply part of the layers of muscle that open and close the pupil, the hole at the centre of the iris. Neither they nor the flecks of colour have any more meaning than the texture or colouring of hair – except in a few instances. For example, minute pale lumps may develop on the iris of people with tuberculosis; and an inflamed iris may be an indication of an auto–immune disorder.

Conventional doctors do not generally consider iridology harmful. They feel that the

Right Iris

Cerebrum sensory
Physiological
brain

Cerebrum motor
Psychological
brain

Animation/life

12
11
1
10
2
9
3
8
4
7
5
6

Neck
Face
Lung
Throat
Thorax
Upper back
Liver
Lower back
Upper abdomen
Pelvic
Testes/ovary
Kidney
Vagina
Lower abdomen

Colon
Stomach
Ascending colon
Nervous system
Small intestine
Cecum
Back

Left Iris

Brain
Brain
Animation/life

12
11
1
10
2
9
3
8
4
7
5
6

Face
Neck
Throat
Lung
Thorax
Upper back
Spleen
Lower back
Upper abdomen
Pelvic
Vagina
Kidney
Testes/ovary
Lower abdomen

Colon
Stomach
Cardia
Small intestine
Nervous system
Back
Thyroid

When consulting an iridologist, a special camera is used to photograph the irises. It can move in three different directions: left-to-right, up-and-down and forwards-and-backwards.

The contours of the eyes are lit from the sides so that the therapist can capture all their aspects on film – and then assess the patient's strengths and weaknesses.

Seeing the body in the eyes

An American pioneer of iridology, Dr Bernard Jensen, drew up comprehensive iris charts showing, in sections, how the different parts of the body are related to the eyes. The left iris reflects the left side of the body and the right iris the right side.

Studying the eyes of this patient, the iridologist decided that she was disposed to weakness in the nervous system (shown by the fibres radiating from the pupil) – prone to headaches, swollen glands and ulcers as her nervous system was subjected to stress. The patch of white light at three o'clock is a camera light reflection.

chief danger may lie in failure to diagnose a condition that needs urgent surgery or control by a drug.

IRRITABLE BOWEL SYNDROME

A perplexing problem

Young and middle-aged adults are those most prone to this bowel disorder, commonly called IBS. It is more common in women of 20 to 45 years than in men of the same age, but children can also suffer. The symptoms come and go, and there may be many years of respite between bouts. However, in some cases IBS persists for months or years, even with treatment.

The condition has also been known by such names as spastic colon and mucous colitis, and the causes are still not firmly established, though it is thought that STRESS may play a significant role in many cases.

IBS restricts the contraction and relaxation of the rings of muscle in the walls of the gut, which push down through the intestines, into the colon and rectum, and finally out through the anus. When the sequence of muscle action is weak or disturbed, spasmodic pain with explosive, watery DIARRHOEA or CONSTIPATION results. Bouts of the two often alternate. Usually the diarrhoea is worse in the morning, and it may also contain slimy mucus.

Cramp-like pain in the lower abdomen is commonplace, but this is sometimes relieved by passing WIND or evacuating the bowel. Other symptoms may include BACK PAIN, a feeling of bloatedness, and general weakness and TIREDNESS.

The muscles of the bowel are controlled by the autonomic nervous system; they are not consciously directed. This means that IBS can be brought on and aggravated by ANXIETY, stress and certain NERVOUS DISORDERS. Scientific tests in which balloons and tubes were introduced into the colon have shown that sufferers have rapid, jerky contractions there, instead of a smooth sequence of muscle activity. Irritable bowel syndrome may also be the result of a severe infection affecting the intestines.

Warning If you have any bleeding from the bowel, see your doctor immediately. It may be the result of an unusually severe type of IBS, but it could also indicate something more serious. In any case, if you experience IBS symptoms together with a rapid loss of weight, especially if you are over 60, seek expert advice at once.

What the therapists recommend
NATUROPATHY
Consultation Naturopaths do not just regard irritable bowel syndrome as a matter of nervousness affecting the bowel. In fact, they often associate it with imbalanced diets and/or an intolerance towards certain foods. A wholefood diet (see EATING FOR HEALTH) is usually recommended to maintain regular bowel action. You will be asked to avoid stimulating laxatives, and instead rely on dietary FIBRE and bulk laxatives, such as linseed or psyllium seed, for restoring some degree of regularity.

A practitioner will also be concerned to rule out any food sensitivities. In any case, potential irritants such as alcohol, coffee and strong spices should be avoided.
Self help Abdominal massage can be helpful, and attention to ways of relaxing generally is considered vital (see RELAXATION AND BREATHING).

HERBAL MEDICINE
Self help Initial measures include hot infusions of peppermint or camomile, possibly with a little ginger added, two or three times a day. Use linseed as a soothing bulk laxative: put a dessertspoonful on a serving of cereal, and eat it with at least 200 ml water.

HOMOEOPATHY
Self help One of the following remedies may help ease the symptoms. Take a dose three to four times a day for 10-14 days. For griping pains, which are better when the sufferer is doubled up or pressing on his abdomen, and to give warmth, *Colocynthis* 6 or 30. This is also helpful if the condition is brought on by anger. When constipation alternates with diarrhoea, and there is flatulence, colicky pain and mucus in the faeces, *Argentum nit.* 6. If there are nausea, tearing pains and watery stools with jelly-like mucus, and an aversion to food, *Colchicum* 6.

An orthodox view

Doctors diagnose irritable bowel syndrome by testing samples of faeces, by X-raying the bowel after a barium enema (or meal), and/or by inserting an endoscope up into the rectum. These procedures eliminate any possibility of LACTOSE INTOLERANCE, diverticular disease – in which 'pockets' develop in the wall of the colon in which its contents become trapped – or CANCER of the bowel being the cause of the problem.

Treatment is aimed at controlling the abnormal activity of the bowel-wall muscles and relieving stress, if that is a factor. Doctors may tell the patient to eat more dietary fibre, and may prescribe antispasmodic and anti-diarrhoeal drugs.

ITCHING

Many skin disorders, including ECZEMA, HIVES and scabies, cause itching. Chronic itching and scratching of exposed areas can be symptoms of some psychological problems, and in jaundiced patients, some LIVER DISORDERS that cause excess bile in the blood can also give rise to itching. PILES, threadworms (see WORMS) and ANXIETY can cause itching around the anus – which is more common among men. This sometimes persists or recurs for months or years. In addition, lice and nits cause severe itching of the scalp.

What the therapists recommend
Herbal Medicine Full treatment depends on the cause of the itching. Well-proven rural remedies are the freshly squeezed juice of bulbinella ('cat's tail') or of a sour-fig leaf, applied to the itchy area. Or dab onto the itch a strong infusion of the leaves, flowers and stems of wild dagga ('minaret flower' or 'lion's ear'). Wild dagga twigs added to a hot bath are also soothing.

A dry skin aggravates an itch, and an oil such as sweet almond can help if gently massaged into the skin regularly.
Naturopathy The advice depends very much on the cause. In skin conditions such as eczema, the excessive dryness of the skin aggravates the itchiness and this may be relieved with oils such as sweet almond, avocado or wheat germ.

An orthodox view

Avoid heat and anxiety, both of which are apt to make any itching worse; and try not to scratch the skin severely, as sores will develop. If itching (medically known as 'pruritus') persists for more than two or three days, see a doctor, who may be able to diagnose and treat the cause.

Hydrocortisone cream or ointment, which is available without prescription, may relieve symptoms, but should be used only for conditions such as eczema that have already been diagnosed. Antihistamine tablets such as terfenadine or chlorpheniramine, which are also available without prescription, may provide some relief, but may also cause drowsiness.

Itching around the anus is embarrassing as well as distracting. Observe scrupulous hygiene in this area; avoid tight–fitting clothes; and if you are overweight, reduce your mass. If anal itching is caused by threadworms, or scalp itching is caused by lice and nits, all members of the household should be treated at the same time to prevent recurrence. A daily bath or shower and the use of soft wipes instead of toilet paper may relieve anal itching.

JAUNDICE

In cases of jaundice, the patient's skin – and the whites of the eyes – turn a sickly yellow. This is due to the presence in the bloodstream of a yellow pigment called bilirubin, which is produced in the spleen when old or damaged red blood cells are destroyed. Normally, the pigment is passed by the liver into the intestine, where it causes the stools to be coloured brown. There are various reasons why bilirubin may accumulate in the blood, causing jaundice.

The yellowing may be a symptom of a serious underlying disease – often of the liver – such as CANCER, cirrhosis or hepatitis. In addition, GALLSTONES in the bile duct can block the outflow of bile from the liver, preventing the excretion of bilirubin.

The most common type of jaundice in young, healthy people is a virus disease, infectious jaundice, or hepatitis A. Patients usually recover within three weeks without any specific treatment. Less common, but much more dangerous, is hepatitis B. See LIVER DISORDERS.

Otherwise healthy babies often suffer from jaundice during the first week of life, but in their case the condition is not very serious and quickly passes. It is a normal result of the destruction of excess red blood cells that are not needed once the baby is able to breathe on its own.

Warning Jaundice is often hard to recognise in its early stages, and may take anything from a few days to several weeks to develop. It can indicate serious (possibly fatal) disease so, as soon as it is suspected, medical advice should be sought.

What the therapists recommend

Herbal Medicine Medical herbalists have a range of remedies for helping the liver, including dandelion root, golden seal and milk thistle. They are usually prescribed as tinctures or decoctions.

Naturopathy Practitioners advise treating liver imbalance by avoiding fats and alcohol. Two or three glasses daily of fresh vegetable juices – celery or carrot, for example – may also be recommended.

Reflexology Massage is given to the reflex areas relating to the liver and gall bladder; and also to areas relating to the solar plexus, and the adrenal and pituitary glands.

An orthodox view

Once jaundice has been diagnosed, a general practitioner will try to determine precisely the root cause of the disease. Tests may include the taking of blood samples, X-rays, or a scan of the gall bladder or the liver. See LIVER DISORDERS.

JET LAG

Fatigue and feelings of sluggishness are normal after east-west or west-east air journeys that cross any of the world's 24 different time zones. The body's natural 24-hour cycle (known as the circadian rhythm) is disturbed. This causes sleepiness at the 'wrong' time of day. With north-south or south-north flights time changes do occur, according to how far east or west your destination is, but they are not as great as when travelling long distances from east to west or west to east.

One of the major problems in dealing with jet lag is that the condition varies from one person to another. However, some researchers have discovered that doses of melatonin, a hormone which is produced in the body during sleep, can help some people's systems to adjust to time changes on arrival in other countries.

Contributory causes that have been suggested include the body's overproduction of 'free radicals' – toxic chemicals. This is thought to be caused by factors such as low cabin pressurisation (generally equivalent to the air at about 3 000 m) and exposure to radiation through flying at heights where earth's protective atmosphere is thin. (It has been estimated that a trip across the Atlantic, for example, exposes a passenger to the equivalent of two X-rays.)

One way of getting rid of excess free radicals after a flight is EXERCISE, such as JOGGING or AEROBICS. This is thought to produce enzymes which help to counter unwanted chemicals in the body.

Other suggested ways to avoid the effects of jet lag include eating only light salads during a flight, sleeping as much as possible, and resting again on the first day after the flight. Supplementary VITAMINS are also believed to help: during a journey, try one 50-100 mg strength extra-stress B complex in the morning and another in the evening, along with 1 g of vitamin C with bioflavonoids, and 400 iu vitamin E.

It is also worth noting that both airline crews and passengers have attended courses in AUTOGENIC TRAINING, intended to help relax the traveller and to counter jet lag.

An orthodox view

Doctors say that jet lag can be greatly reduced by drinking plenty of non-alcoholic fluids during long air flights, and so avoiding dehydration. Do not drink alcohol, which not only dehydrates the body but has a stronger effect in low-pressure conditions. If possible, try to ensure that you will arrive at your new destination in the evening (local time). Then take a mild sedative or sleeping pill and go to bed early.

For a short visit – say a few days – try to eat and sleep according to your clock back home. For longer visits of a week or more, start to live according to local times as soon as possible. Set your watch to the new time as soon as you are seated in the aeroplane, and then go to bed at the same time as the residents at your destination. Recent research has suggested that exposure to bright lights can hasten the adaptive process.

JOGGING

Pacing yourself to fitness

Many people go jogging as their main form of EXERCISE, preferring its easy movement to that of running or more energetic sports and pastimes. Ideally, jogging should last for no more than 20-30 minutes at a gentle, comfortable pace. Run at a pace that allows you to have a conversation. If you cannot, then you are jogging too fast.

As your fitness improves you will find that you will be able to jog faster for the same rate of breathing.

Although jogging on grass or tarmac is generally regarded as a 'safe' activity, injuries such as SPRAINS and strains can occur – especially if you do not wear the right kind of shoes, socks and clothing.

Jogging, or sports, shoes should be flexible enough to promote a springing step and firm enough to give good support around the heel. Buy them from a specialist sports shop, where you can get expert guidance. A well-cushioned inner sole reduces impact shock and supports the arches. Make sure the shoes fit comfortably. There should be about a thumb's width of space between the big toe and the front of the shoe to allow the toes to move freely. Break in the shoes by wearing them at home or when out shopping or going for a walk.

The shoes, which can be expensive, are the most important investment. Remember, you get what you pay for; the higher the price, the better the quality and the more support they will give you. Good-quality shoes should last for many months, or even a year or two.

Sports socks should be made of cotton to absorb sweat – nylon socks do not do this. Again, make sure they fit comfortably and do not wrinkle up. A cotton (or cotton-mix) T-shirt and shorts are best for jogging in warm weather, and a well-fitting tracksuit when it is cold.

Before you start jogging, it is important to warm up for about five minutes with bending and stretching exercises (see illustrations, right). This prepares the heart and lungs for the effort to come, helps the muscles to work well, and cuts down the chance of injury.

When jogging, never ignore any pain or signs of breathlessness, discomfort, weakness or fatigue. If these feelings are experienced, slow down or stop. Carrying on regardless may lead to further distress, pulled muscles, stiff muscles and joint damage (see SPORTS INJURIES).

Jogging is a safe activity in terms of serious health risks such as heart attack. But if you are aged over 35, or suffer from bad health, do not take up jogging without first consulting a doctor.

Remember, vigorous activity never harmed a healthy body; it is inactivity that causes the damage. However, vigorous activity following years of inactivity may just bring unseen damage to the surface.

JOINT PROBLEMS

People with inflamed or worn joints find it increasingly difficult to move as the areas become stiffer and more swollen and painful. Most joint problems are caused by ARTHRITIS in one form or another.

Sometimes a joint may be damaged by injury, and the tough, fibrous ligaments that hold it together tend to become weak and painful. This may occur during strenuous games, for example (see SPORTS INJURIES; SPRAINS).

Usually, different diseases affect different joints. For example, OSTEOARTHRITIS affects mainly the hips, spine and knees of the elderly. RHEUMATOID ARTHRITIS tends to affect mainly the hands, knees, elbows and feet of middle-aged men and women. And GOUT, another common affliction throughout the world, affects mainly people's finger, leg and big toe joints.

What the therapists recommend

Chiropractic The aim is to remove abnormal stress from an injured joint, and improve overall mobility and muscle tone. But manipulation is not advised for acutely inflamed joints, as in rheumatoid arthritis.

Hydrotherapy For stiff and/or painful joints, therapists advise cold baths or packs for acute cases; and underwater douching, vortex baths, warm paraffin wax, Vichy massage and supervised exercises in the warm hydrotherapy pool for less serious cases.

Homoeopathy An experienced homoeopath will probably prescribe one or more medicines – for example, *Rhus tox.* for aching and stiffness which wears off as the patient gets moving, and which is worse after rest; *Colchicum* for pain and stiffness which is worse during the night; *Dulcamara* for pain which is worse in damp weather.

Acupuncture The practitioner will treat points on the abdomen, gall bladder, liver, spleen and stomach meridians. MOXIBUSTION may be applied to the abdomen, bladder, gall bladder and liver meridians.

Acupressure For knee pain, a therapist will treat the outer side of the knee, four fingers' width down from the kneecap in the hollow between the shin and smaller leg bone.

Massage A therapist will show the patient how to start the treatment with deep stroking of the limb and, if there is joint swelling, to concentrate on the part of the limb nearest to the trunk. Kneading and wringing follows to tone the muscles. Friction is then applied, gentle at first, then firmer, deeper movements around the affected joint.

Reflexology Massage is given to reflex areas related to the affected areas, and direct massage to the zone-related area – shoulder for hip, elbow for knee, wrist for ankle, hand for foot and so on. Areas relating to the solar plexus and the adrenal and pituitary glands are also treated. See chart, p. 295.

An orthodox view

If a joint is painful or swollen with fluid, a doctor will strap it with a crêpe bandage. He will then raise the limb – on cushions or a stool, for example – and apply an ice pack to reduce inflammation and swelling. In hospital a special hoist may be used.

If a FRACTURE is suspected, or if the symptoms are severe or last for more than a week, an X-ray or PHYSIOTHERAPY may be advised. If arthritis is suspected, blood samples may be taken to identify the cause.

See also BACK PAIN, CHIROPRACTIC and NECK PAIN.

Warming up for jogging

Ease into the stretches, and go only as far as is comfortable. Stretch in straight lines and breathe normally. Hold each breath for 10 seconds, and if comfortable, continue to time given.

Calf *Gently push through the hips, keeping heels on the floor. Hold for 30 seconds each leg.*

Hamstring *Pull knee towards the chest, hips on floor. Keep knee straight, as far as possible. Hold each leg for 20 seconds.*

Shoulder *Push arm gently back with hand. Don't arch the back; keep it rounded by bending the knees. Hold for 15 seconds each arm.*

Groin *Push knees down with elbows, feet together. Hold for 30 seconds.*

KIDNEY COMPLAINTS

Most people have two kidneys, although very occasionally a baby may be born with only one, or a kidney may be lost due to illness or an accident. Their job is to filter waste products from the blood into the urine, which then passes to the bladder and out of the system. They also play a vital role in controlling fluid balance in the body (see WATER RETENTION) and BLOOD PRESSURE.

Several disorders can affect the kidneys. The most common is kidney stones, small lumps of calcium and uric acid that crystallise in the kidneys or the ureters (the tubes that carry urine to the bladder). They result from urine that is too concentrated, or from an infection.

Usually the stones do not cause pain while in the kidney, but can do so when they become dislodged and start to travel down the urinary tract, or block it. When this occurs, there can be short bursts of severe BACK PAIN in the kidney region (see illustration below), sometimes spreading to the abdomen and genitals. This is also known as renal or ureteric colic. Other symptoms include pain on passing urine, and sometimes blood in the urine.

The kidneys may also become infected by bacteria, causing a disorder called pyelonephritis. This is usually the result of another condition, such as CYSTITIS or PROSTATE PROBLEMS. The sufferer experiences pain over the kidneys and in the sides, waist and sometimes the abdomen. There is usually a FEVER, and blood, protein and white blood cells are found on analysis of the urine. There may be a frequent need to urinate.

Nephritis is a rare but more serious kidney complaint. The cause is generally a disorder of the IMMUNE SYSTEM, in which antibodies produced by the body attack kidney tissue. The symptoms are red or smoky-coloured urine passed in small quantities, water retention, HEADACHE and backache, along with high blood pressure. A few cases eventually lead to kidney failure, making a transplant or regular treatment on a dialysis machine – a type of filter system – necessary. Other problems include CANCER of the kidney, in which there is blood in the urine, but no pain, and kidney failure brought on by DIABETES. Always consult a doctor about any kidney trouble, since it can become serious without attention.

Warning Untreated infections can cause permanent damage to the kidneys. It is vital to exclude them before seeking alternative treatments.

What the therapists recommend

Acupuncture Kidney problems are often thought to involve a deficiency of the yang element (see YIN and YANG). If the symptoms include burning heat, severe pain or FEVER, the disorder is usually regarded as an excess of heat disturbance of the bladder. If there is an infection, the patient will also be advised to seek orthodox medical treatment.

Acupuncture for kidney problems is given at points on the governor, conception, bladder, large intestine, kidney and spleen meridians (see chart, p.14). MOXIBUSTION may be applied at points on the gall bladder, bladder, kidney, liver and spleen meridians to strengthen the kidneys.

Herbal Medicine Responsible herbalists advise orthodox treatment for kidney complaints, although they may also recommend remedies such as parsley and wild carrot when there is inflammation or tiny kidney stones. These plants are said to have a soothing, diuretic effect and to help flush out the urinary system.

Waste-disposal system

Many times a day the blood passes through the kidneys, which adjust its content of water, salts and acids.

The X-rayed kidney on the left has a stone blocking the entry to the ureter. An inadequate flow through the ureter has allowed damaging deposits to form there.

Kidney
A mass of tubes in the kidneys processes the waste filtered from the blood and produces urine.

Ureter
A ureter from each kidney carries the urine to the bladder, where it can be stored before being expelled through the urethra.

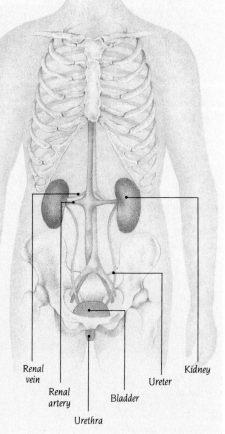

Renal vein
Renal artery
Urethra
Bladder
Ureter
Kidney

Caring for your kidneys

Drink up to 1,75 litres of liquid a day, especially when hot weather or activity increases perspiration. Dehydration makes the urine highly concentrated, increasing the risk of kidney stones and disorders such as cystitis.

Do not take diuretics – drugs that increase urination – unless they are essential. In that case, ask your doctor to prescribe those that do not increase uric acid levels in the blood.

Empty your bladder as soon as you feel the need. The longer urine remains in the body, the more likely minerals are to crystallise into stones, and the greater the chance for bacteria to breed.

If you suffer from kidney stones, avoid dairy foods, which are calcium-rich, and drink low-calcium bottled mineral water rather than tap water.

Acupressure can be helpful in countering incontinence – apply strong pressure upwards in the hollow between the inner ankle bone and the Achilles tendon.

Acupressure The therapist will apply firm pressure at appropriate points on the kidney, spleen, conception and bladder meridians.

T'ai-chi Ch'uan This is said to help by balancing the various energy flows of the body and mind, and generally improving the circulation of body fluids and the expulsion of waste. The gentle, co-ordinated movements of T'ai-chi Ch'uan, coupled with full abdominal breathing and good posture, are said to release TENSION and to have the effect of internally massaging the kidneys. A teacher would also be likely to advise the patient on a more suitable diet and about possible causes of tension.

Naturopathy Small stones and gravelly deposits are usually calcium based, and patients will be advised to reduce their intake of calcium-rich foods such as dairy products – and also foods high in oxalic acid, such as spinach, rhubarb and chocolate. Naturopaths may advise patients to take a little cider vinegar each day, or possibly a magnesium supplement. They will also be encouraged to drink plenty of fluids – in a hard-water area this may necessitate the use of a water filter to remove calcium.

Reflexology Manipulation would be applied to reflex areas that correspond to the kidneys, the bladder, and the pituitary and adrenal glands (see chart, p. 295), and to areas that relate to the lymphatic system.

An orthodox view

Kidney complaints can be serious if left untreated, so alternative therapies, although they may help to get rid of infections, should be used only alongside orthodox treatment. When consulting a doctor about kidney trouble, take a sample of urine along to help with the diagnosis. The doctor will probably also examine the abdomen to see if the kidneys are enlarged or tender, and may use blood tests, a kidney scan or X-rays to discover more. The urine will be analysed for evidence of blood, protein or cells. Sometimes it is also necessary to take a sample of kidney tissue for testing.

Treatment depends on the individual problem. Stones can be broken down with ULTRASONICS, while infections can usually be cleared up quickly by antibiotics. More serious disorders are treated in a variety of ways and, if all else fails, a kidney transplant can restore good health in certain cases.

Despite doctors' caution about alternative medicine, much of the advice from alternative therapists on diet and care of the kidneys is useful and appropriate. Naturopathy, herbal medicine and acupuncture, which help both to diminish toxin build-up and to increase the expulsion of toxins, can be useful on a long-term basis.

KINESIOLOGY

Balancing health by testing muscles

Most people are familiar with the 'knee-jerk' test, when your knee is tapped to test your reflexes. If they are working properly, your leg will involuntarily jerk upwards. A system of diagnosis and treatment based on this and similar reactions was developed in 1964 by an American doctor of chiropractic named George Goodheart. It became known as kinesiology from the Greek word *kinesis*, meaning 'motion'.

Practitioners believe that each group of muscles is related to other parts of the body – the organs, digestive system, glands, bones and circulation – and that when the muscles are in good working order, so is the body. How a muscle responds in tests to gentle, manual pressure reveals to the practitioner how the whole body is functioning.

Kinesiologists do not diagnose illness. They look for imbalances or deficiencies in nutrition and energy, or locate physical problems. Having pinpointed any trouble spots, practitioners try to revitalise them by giving a light, fingertip massage to 'pressure points'

on the body and scalp. Most of these points are some distance from the muscles they relate to. The pressure points for the main leg muscles between the hip and knee, for example, are along the border of the rib cage. The theory is that because muscles rely upon good supplies of blood and lymph (a body fluid which carries away poisons and drains the tissues), stimulating appropriate pressure points enhances the blood flow to the muscles concerned and balances the lymphatic system.

It is also believed that our bodies contain an invisible energy, like an electric current, running through 'computer circuits' that control bodily functions – a stomach circuit, a pancreas circuit and so on. The energy flow may be compared with the electrical impulses that make a washing machine run through a series of functions according to a programme. These circuits are said to 'blow a fuse' under stress or during illness, and you become weak if you use up more energy than they can generate.

Who it can help Practitioners believe that this therapy can help anyone, but it is perhaps best known for aiding people who have an ALLERGY or sensitivity to certain foods. The body is thought to recognise and react instantly to nutrients and chemicals, and these reactions affect (among other things) the way muscles work.

If certain foods cause instant muscle weakness, then the patient is said to be allergic to them (see box, p. 217). The allergy can result in many symptoms, such as CATARRH, COLDS, DEPRESSION, HEADACHES, TENSION, general TIREDNESS and a weakened IMMUNE SYSTEM.

Muscle tests are said to monitor the effect of foods on the body, and patients can use the techniques at home with the aid of a partner (see box, p. 216). Kinesiology also claims the ability to pinpoint deficiencies in VITAMINS and MINERALS and digestive problems.

Conditions such as lack of ENERGY, frequent minor illnesses, and being generally run down are believed to be made worse by internal stagnation of body fluids. Practitioners claim to treat the conditions by balancing the lymphatic system and improving blood flow. They treat BACK PAIN and NECK PAIN using muscle balancing techniques without the danger of stretching ligaments or loosening joints.

Patients can learn to use some of the techniques at home – for example, massage of the inner thigh, which is said to strengthen many weak muscles which cause or aggravate back pain.

Kinesiologists also claim that their methods can relieve or resolve PHOBIAS and FEAR. For example, gently tapping the bone under the eye in line with the pupil is said to help relieve fear.

How did kinesiology develop?

The chiropractor George Goodheart discovered kinesiology while trying to help a patient who had severe leg pains. As he was massaging along a muscle called the *fascia lata* – which runs down the outside of the leg, from the hip to just below the knee – the patient felt the pain easing.

Goodheart found that the muscle had been strengthened, but massaging the fibres of other muscles did not produce similar results. He then recalled research that had been done by an osteopath named Dr Frank Chapman at the turn of the century. Chapman had shown that massaging specific 'pressure points' could improve the flow of the lymph fluid in various parts of the body.

Goodheart patiently matched Chapman's pressure points to the sets of muscles to which they were related, and found that the pressure point for the *fascia lata* was the only one which lay over the muscle that is affected – nearly all the other pressure points were some distance away in various other parts of the body.

An American osteopath named Terrence J Bennett had claimed in the early 1930s that blood circulation to various organs could be improved by lightly touching certain pressure points on the skull. Bennett used a type of moving X-ray machine to monitor changes in the body after touching points on the head. Goodheart found that touching these points with his fingertips for a few seconds also strengthened specific muscles; eventually he mapped an association between 16 different pressure points on the skull, just above the breastbone and behind the knee, and all the major muscle groups.

Wondering how such a light touch could strengthen a muscle so quickly, Goodheart studied ACUPUNCTURE, which is also concerned with particular points on the body, located on invisible channels or 'meridians'. He concluded that these meridians are common energy channels for both organs and muscles. Kinesiology channels are identical to the meridians that are used in acupuncture.

Muscle tests to identify possible trouble spots

Weakness in major muscles can forewarn of health problems. A weak shoulder muscle, for example, may warn of a lung-related problem. When the muscle is tested (left) the person should be able to resist gentle, steady downward pressure on the elbow.

Weak abdominal muscles are a factor in most back pain. When these are tested (below), the patient should be able to hold up against pressure on the chest.

Finding a practitioner For information, names and addresses write to the South African representative of the International College of Applied Kinesiology: Dr Frans Kromhout, 12 Kloof Street, Sea Point 8001. Most practitioners have completed at least 200 hours of kinesiology, and some use it along with other professional skills.

There are some osteopaths, chiropractors, physiotherapists, naturopaths, homoeopaths and herbalists that use kinesiology. If the problem relates to bones, muscles or ligaments, an osteopath or chiropractor who uses the therapy may be able to help. For digestive problems a dietician-kinesiologist or a herbalist who uses muscle testing can be consulted. For mental or emotional disturbances, a psychotherapist or counsellor who uses kinesiology is the logical choice (see also TOUCH FOR HEALTH).

Consulting a practitioner The therapist starts by asking about your case history. Then your major muscle groups are systematically tested – a painless procedure. You are shown how to put an arm or leg into a particular position and hold it steady.

The kinesiologist presses gently for a few seconds to assess your ability to exert an equal and opposite pressure. If the muscle does not respond normally, the practitioner makes a series of touch tests to find out why it is not 'firing' properly.

More tests will determine which imbalance is most in need of correction, then the therapist works on the appropriate pressure points. Some points will be sore or tender when touched – due, it is believed, to poisons building up in the tissues and preventing proper nerve impulses from going to and fro between brain and muscle. This in turn affects the working of the muscle – tight shoulder muscles which cannot relax are a common example.

Soreness may persist for a day or two as poisons disperse, but an improvement of the main discomfort and in well-being should be felt almost immediately.

An orthodox view

An increasing number of doctors use kinesiology as an aid to diagnosis, but the therapy has not yet been the subject of much research that orthodox medicine would consider valid. Most conventional practitioners still take the view that the body's flow of electrical energies cannot be adjusted by mechanical means.

There are marked similarities in the approach used by kinesiologists and acupuncturists. Both parties subscribe to the point of view that the human body contains 'energy channels' which can become blocked for some reason or other, and which can be relieved by physical treatment.

Self-help test for food allergy

Kinesiology therapists often use a simple test made on a strong chest muscle (the pectoralis major clavicular muscle) to check whether a patient has an allergy or sensitivity to a particular food.

You can carry out the test at home with the aid of a partner – but note that this is not a trial of strength, and actions must remain firm but gentle. First, however, you must test the muscle itself.

The muscle test

1 Hold your body upright and stretch your left arm out in front of you with the elbow turned outwards and fingers and thumb hanging down.

2 Your partner faces you, resting two fingers of the right hand on your outstretched left wrist and placing the left hand on your right shoulder.

3 Now ask your partner to push your wrist downwards while you resist by exerting pressure upwards. Breathe normally (do not hold your breath) while your partner applies firm but gentle pressure for as long as it takes to say 'One thousand, two thousand and off'.

If you matched your partner's pressure and the muscle felt firmly locked, not 'spongy', go on to the allergy test. If, however, your arm moved downwards under pressure, the muscle is unsuitable for the allergy test. In this case, try the test on the other arm or test a different muscle. For example, hold your arm straight by your side with the palm turned outwards and resist your partner's pressure to pull the arm away from your side. If you cannot match the pressure again, you should contact a trained practitioner.

The allergy test

1 Take up the same position as before, with left arm extended, elbow outwards and fingers and thumb hanging down.

2 Place a sample of the suspect food – cheese, for example – under your tongue, or even just between your lips.

3 Your partner places the first two fingers of his or her left hand on a point in the soft tissue just under your right ear, while applying downward pressure on your left wrist. As before, you resist.

If you match the pressure and the muscle remains firm, it is believed that you are not allergic or sensitive to the suspect food; if your arm feels less strong, or moves, practitioners say you should avoid the food or eat it only occasionally – and never in excess.

If you are sensitive or allergic to a food, you may not be able to keep your arm raised against steady downward pressure when that food is held to your mouth.

KIRLIAN PHOTOGRAPHY

Capturing auras on film

The aim of Kirlian photography – named after a Russian engineer, Semyon Kirlian, and his wife Valentina – is to produce prints of the auras that reveal people's mental and physical disorders before they display any outward symptoms (see AURA THERAPY). Diagnosing from the photographs, practitioners may suggest appropriate treatments ranging from ACUPUNCTURE to YOGA.

For centuries, mystics, spiritual healers and psychics have been fascinated by the 'auras' – luminous, misty outlines – said to surround people, animals, plants and other animate or inanimate objects.

The auras are said to reflect the subjects' general well-being, and their colours and brightness to be open to medical interpretation. Kirlian high-voltage photography, or electrophotography, is a development of this; it claims to capture the interference pattern created when the high-frequency electrical sweep comes in contact with the subject's electromagnetic field, or aura.

Semyon Kirlian made his discovery in 1939 while repairing machinery in a laboratory. A spark flew off the machine, there was a vivid flash and he received a jolting electric shock. On recovering, he wondered what would happen if he put a sheet of light-sensitive paper between another electric spark and his bare hand – and had a photograph taken at the very instant of shock.

This was done and the developed film showed that his fingers were fringed with glowing streaks of light. The Kirlians then set up their own laboratory and spent the next 40 years taking their mysterious pictures.

To begin with, the Kirlians put two similar leaves, one from a diseased plant, the other from a healthy one, between photographic plates and high-voltage, high-frequency electrical charges. No light sources were used. When developed, the photographs showed a vivid aura around the leaf from the healthy plant. The other leaf had only a weak aura.

In another experiment, a leaf from which a section had been cut was photographed. This time the picture showed a faint outline of the missing section. The so-called 'phantom-leaf' phenomenon was compared with the experiences of many amputees who feel pain or tingling in the 'phantom limb'.

Semyon Kirlian also photographed his own hand at a meeting of scientists and doctors. His equipment consisted of an electric coil which sent a high-voltage charge to an aluminium plate, on top of which were a glass plate and a sheet of photosensitive film. The film was covered with a clear sheet of plastic to protect it from salt in the skin.

Kirlian placed his hand firmly on the plate for a few seconds – and the photograph was taken. To his alarm, however, his aura was shown to be vague and cloudy, with dull, blurred colours. His wife's hand was then photographed and her aura came out strong and clear. A few hours afterwards Semyon Kirlian went down with a bad case of INFLUENZA, while his wife remained well.

From this it was deduced that sickness in humans could be detected at an early stage, before symptoms became evident.

An orthodox view

Conventional doctors do not believe that Kirlian photography can accurately detect and record human auras. Nor can auras – providing they exist – be used as a reliable means of diagnosis. However, some doctors agree that dead and live objects give off 'energy emissions', which vary in intensity and degree. And that these emissions may indicate the presence or absence of disease.

KWASHIORKOR

Severe malnutrition accounts for kwashiorkor, a disease found predominantly in young children in poor rural areas.

The condition is characterised by a deficiency of proteins and often of vitamins, and the symptoms include stunted growth, a swollen abdomen, flaky skin, hair that loses its colour, diarrhoea, and general weakness and irritability.

The word 'kwashiorkor' is Ghanaian and means 'displaced child'. It was so-named because it was seen as a disease syndrome affecting babies displaced from their mother's breast – and a protein-rich supply of milk – by another pregnancy and, in due course, a younger sibling.

What the therapists recommend

Naturopathy Spacing the birth of children allows the mother to breastfeed her young. Breast-milk provides a more natural sustenance than artificial feeds.

An orthodox view

The victim must be supplied with frequent small amounts of milk (or powdered milk), supplemented with vitamin and mineral tablets. Zinc can prevent the skin from flaking any further. In the longer term a protein-rich diet is necessary; however, even despite this diet, the growth of very young children may be permanently stunted.

Kirlian photographs of the menstrual cycle

Day 3

Day 7

Day 12

Day 21

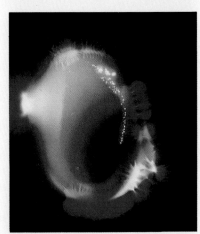

Day 3

These Kirlian images show finger-pad auras which are claimed to reflect the hormonal changes that occur during a woman's monthly cycle. The colours all have a meaning. Red-yellow within a dotted halo represents follicle-stimulating hormone (FSH), which stimulates the follicles in the ovaries to ripen into ova (or eggs). Blue denotes luteinising hormone, which stimulates ovulation (release of an ovum from an ovary). White represents the level in the blood of oestrogen, one of the steroid hormones that promote the functioning of the female sex organs.

On day 3, menstruation is in progress. Day 7 shows increasing hormonal activity. By day 12, hormonal activity has reached its peak before ovulation (about day 14). The activity has subsided by day 21, and by day 3 a new cycle has begun.

LACTOSE INTOLERANCE

This condition – the inability to absorb lactose, or milk sugar – results in watery DIARRHOEA. The sugar is a baby's main source of energy. Normally, more than 99 per cent of the lactose in a baby's feed is digested and absorbed into its bloodstream. As a result, there is virtually no sugar in the baby's normally solid faeces. However, if not enough is absorbed, lactose and water remain in the faeces, causing diarrhoea.

Lactose intolerance is usually a temporary problem, and most commonly occurs in babies and children after they have had an attack of gastroenteritis (diarrhoea and vomiting). Taking milk only makes it worse. In rare cases, the condition is present at birth and lasts for life.

What the therapists recommend

Naturopathy As with any food intolerance, the practitioner will make sure that this really is the problem before advising a restricted diet, particularly if the patient is a child. You will be asked for details of everything that is eaten, and changes will be suggested to improve digestion generally. If lactose is found to be the cause of the upset, foods containing it will be excluded from the diet.

An orthodox view

A doctor will determine if lactose intolerance is present by testing a baby's faeces for sugar. As the condition is intensified by taking milk and other dairy products such as cheese, he will advise avoiding them until the digestion of lactose is back to normal. In the meantime, the baby can be fed on soya milk substitute, which contains no lactose.

Short-term lactose intolerance following gastroenteritis usually lasts two to three weeks. Milk can then be safely reintroduced into the diet. Adults with lactose intolerance should avoid many pharmaceuticals, confectionery and bakery products, which also contain lactose, as well as dairy products.

LARYNGITIS

Loss of voice and hoarseness are the two main effects of laryngitis, or inflammation of the larynx (voice box). There are two main types of laryngitis: acute, which is infectious, short-lived and usually accompanied by pain or discomfort in the throat; and chronic, which is longer-lasting or keeps recurring, and affects only adults.

Acute laryngitis is usually caused by a VIRUS INFECTION. Chronic laryngitis is frequently the result of emotional STRESS and strain. It can also be brought on by irritating the vocal cords through singing or shouting – as well as by smoke, fumes or dust.

What the therapists recommend

Herbal Medicine For immediate relief, gargle with marigold, myrrh, raspberry leaf, sage or thyme. These are most effective in tincture form. Or use as a gargle a decoction of camomile, comfrey, fennel seeds, lavender, rosemary and thyme, diluted in warm water.

To boost resistance to laryngitis infection, take two to four garlic capsules a day for a few days. Herbalists may also prescribe herbs such as echinacea or wild indigo to fight infection, and may also advise you to take extra vitamin C.

Acupressure The points to be treated are the bottom corner of the nail on the outer side of the thumb, press upwards and inwards; and at the end of the crease in the web between the forefinger and thumb, press towards the finger bone.

Homoeopathy For a harsh cough and dry, ticklish throat try *Drosera*. For a dry, hard cough and loss of voice, try *Phosphorus*.

An orthodox view

In cases of acute laryngitis doctors advise patients to rest their voice, drink plenty of fluids, and, if needed, take painkillers such as aspirin or paracetamol. Antibiotics are not normally prescribed unless the infection has spread to the lungs (see BRONCHITIS).

With chronic laryngitis, patients are advised to avoid smoke, dust and irritants – and not to shout or sing until the voice returns to normal.

If hoarseness lasts for more than three weeks, you should consult a doctor in case there is a more serious underlying cause. He may send you to an ear, nose and throat specialist, who will examine your throat for a non-cancerous polyp or nodule on the vocal cords and remove it if necessary.

LAUGHTER

How it does us good . . .

We share our ability to laugh with our fellow primates – for example, chimpanzees 'laugh' when tickled – and this behaviour goes back to earliest times. Primitive man bared his teeth as a sign of aggression or warning. But by screwing up his face at the same time – and making strange, inarticulate, rhythmic noises – he turned aggression into friendliness, and warning into welcome. 'Do you want to fight?' became 'Do you want to play?'

Laughing together is a way of strengthening social bonds between people, for laughter brings us out of ourselves and provides the human contact we need in order to survive. But it has other benefits – both physical and psychological.

When we laugh we draw air in and out of our lungs more than during normal breathing. So laughing may push more oxygen into the bloodstream, stimulating the circulation. Our heart rate often goes up at the same time, helping the process. And studies of blood samples taken from people while they were laughing show higher levels of the 'arousal' hormones, adrenaline and noradrenaline. During a bout of laughter we become physically more aroused and, as a result, afterwards we may be mentally sharper.

Finally, when we laugh we experience a burst of activity followed by a period of relaxation, when our muscles are less tense than they were before. These alternating cycles of tension and calm stop us getting physically keyed-up about daily problems.

The mental benefits relate more to our underlying sense of humour than to the act of laughing. Seeing a problem as funny breaks the overwhelming sense of TENSION that often goes with it, and an intimidating difficulty suddenly becomes manageable.

Psychologists regard humour as a vital way of dealing with day-to-day problems. It helps promote and sustain mental good health, for people with a well-developed sense of fun usually have few emotional problems.

People who laugh together – such as husbands and wives – have a better chance of staying together, and being happy together. And laughter on the surface is a sign of something deeper and more significant – it reflects a particular way of looking at the world which makes us feel better, and may even help us to live longer.

LAYING ON OF HANDS

Since earliest times, some people have believed that they have the ability to bring about cures for physical and mental illness by placing their hands on or near the affected person or part, so transferring some sort of power. The early Christians developed such a 'laying on of hands' using God's power through the Holy Ghost (or Spirit), and it is still practised by Christian healers, especially those of the charismatic churches (see CHARISMATIC HEALING). A similar 'hands on' technique, sometimes called 'hand healing', 'contact healing' or 'touch healing', is an integral part of SPIRITUAL HEALING.

LEPROSY

Leprosy has uniquely unpleasant connotations – the very word 'leper' is synonymous in the English language with 'outcast' – and yet this infectious disease is by no means highly contagious. What is more, it can be cured, if the prescribed drugs are taken over a period of years. Early diagnosis is essential, however, if disfigurement is to be avoided; and any damage that has taken place before treatment is permanent.

Leprosy is a chronic bacterial infection that initially affects the nerves of the limbs and face. Colourless blotches form on the skin, accompanied by reduced sensation. Muscle paralysis leads eventually to deformity. Other longer-term effects include blindness, and the destruction of bone tissue in the nose and other areas.

What the therapists recommend

Herbal medicine A rural remedy is to apply an infusion of wild dagga twigs to the affected area. Some indigenous peoples of South Africa treat leprosy with a decoction of the bark of the raasblaar (large-fruited bushwillow); taken orally, this is said to purify the blood. Another indigenous remedy – which can either be drunk or applied to the skin – is a strong tea made from the Christmas berry plant (wild gentian).

An orthodox view

The diagnosis is made by biopsy, when a fragment of skin tissue is examined microscopically. The drug dapsone, which is taken orally, destroys most of the leprosy bacteria within days; but this treatment must be continued for at least three years in order to prevent a recurrence. No leprosy vaccine is available.

LEUKAEMIA

This uncommon form of CANCER affects the blood cells. If not treated, most cases are fatal, but with appropriate treatment many patients are cured. There are two forms, depending on the type of blood cells affected: *lymphoblastic* and *myeloid*. Either of these can be acute (rapidly developing) or chronic (slow-developing and long-lasting).

The most common childhood leukaemia – which starts between the ages of three and six – is acute lymphoblastic leukaemia, in which major advances in treatment have been made. Symptoms develop rapidly and include FEVER, ANAEMIA, HEADACHES and excessive NOSEBLEED. In adults, symptoms include fever, loss of energy, loss of appetite,

Herbalists collect liquorice in this Italian illustration of about 1385. It has been used in Mediterranean lands for centuries.

weight loss and weakness. Women may menstruate excessively (see PERIOD PROBLEMS). Chronic leukaemia, especially in the elderly, can be relatively harmless.

If leukaemia is suspected, you should consult a doctor without delay.

LIQUORICE

For more than 3 000 years, Chinese physicians have been using liquorice to treat LIVER DISORDERS, and it is still their popular remedy for hepatitis, JAUNDICE, a distended abdomen and NAUSEA AND VOMITING.

The liquorice root and stolon – creeping underground stem – are dark reddish-brown and wrinkled, with a yellow, fibrous interior. They are usually sold cut into sticks some 15 cm long and 13 mm in diameter, and may be chewed raw. The hard, though pliable, black solid used in medicine and confectionery is prepared by crushing and boiling the roots, then reducing (evaporating down) the resulting juice. Medicinal extracts are then prepared from this solid, and sold in liquid, powder and lozenge form.

Modern research has confirmed many of the medicinal properties claimed for liquorice. It is a demulcent (soothing agent) and spasmolytic (countering muscle spasms such as those that cause COLIC and some bronchial disorders). It is an expectorant (increasing the production of sputum so that it may be coughed up more easily), an anti-

tussive (suppressing coughing), and an anti-inflammatory and antiallergic substance, making it particularly useful in the treatment of ASTHMA. It is generally 'hepato protective' (protecting the liver), and may be used in the short term to relieve stomach ULCERS.

The other ingredients of liquorice may give it antidepressive properties, inhibit histamine release and act as muscle relaxants. It is a mild laxative, and may have detoxifying effects on poisons such as strychnine.

Liquorice root, either from your garden or bought from a chemist's or herbalist shop, may be prepared as a decoction. Put ½ -1 teaspoon of the root in a saucepan. Add a cup of water, boil, and allow to simmer for 10-15 minutes. Drink when cool.

LIVER DISORDERS

The liver is the largest gland in the body. Situated in the upper right part of the abdomen, it weighs 1,1-1,6 kg in adults. It performs more than 500 different functions, ranging from storing VITAMINS and carbohydrates to excreting waste products from the bloodstream.

The liver produces bile, which aids food digestion and makes the faeces brown. It metabolises proteins and carbohydrates, and helps to regulate the amount of sugar in the bloodstream. It stores and metabolises fats, producing cholesterol.

It also produces blood-clotting chemicals and heparin, an anticoagulant. It synthesises vitamin A, and stores it together with vitamins B_{12}, D and K. One of the liver's most important roles is the removal of drugs, poisons and worn-out red blood cells from the bloodstream.

Because the liver is such a complex organ, it has a vast number of possible disorders. Inflammation of the liver is called hepatitis. 'Infectious hepatitis' (hepatitis A) is caused by a virus and is transmitted by food and drink. It causes FEVER, sickness and the yellowing of the skin known as JAUNDICE, which may last up to three weeks. It is rarely serious, but is frequently followed by a period of post-viral DEPRESSION, and your doctor should be informed.

The much more serious 'serum hepatitis' (hepatitis B), also a virus infection, is spread by sexual intercourse and by infected blood and blood products, syringes or needles, and drug addicts who share syringes are particularly vulnerable. Health care workers are also vulnerable. Its symptoms – HEADACHES, fever, chills, general debility and jaundice – appear suddenly after an incubation period of one to six months. Even with treatment, recovery may be slow or incomplete – and in about one case in ten the disease is fatal. Cirrhosis, in which scar tissue replaces dead or injured liver cells, has several causes, including ALCOHOLISM, hepatitis, blockage of the common bile duct by GALLSTONES or other obstructions, disorders of the IMMUNE SYSTEM and chronic heart failure.

Or it may occur for no known reason. Because of the organ's importance, CANCER of the liver is extremely serious.

Warning If you suspect any liver disorder, consult your doctor before embarking on a course of alternative treatment.

What the therapists recommend

Herbal Medicine To cleanse the liver, drink a weak tea made by boiling in water the shoots of the wild asparagus ('haakdoring').

Acupuncture Practitioners will usually give treatment at a combination of points on the patient's liver, gall bladder, stomach and spleen meridians.

Homoeopathy Treatment of chronic (persistent) hepatitis is constitutional and must be carried out by an experienced homoeopath. For acute (brief but severe) hepatitis, *Phosphorus* 30 is indicated. *Chelidonium* 30 is indicated for jaundice when the abdomen feels distended and there is right-sided pain extending to the shoulder.

Naturopathy You are advised to avoid fatty foods and alcohol, and take two or three glasses of fresh vegetable juice every day. Cold packs on the abdomen and exercises such as YOGA can help to stimulate the liver, and in some cases supplements such as multivitamin and mineral tablets or lecithin to counteract cholesterol may also help.

Reflexology Massage is applied to the reflex areas relating to the liver, gall bladder, small and large intestine, spleen and lymphatic system, and also to the areas related to the solar plexus and adrenal and pituitary glands. See chart, p. 295.

An orthodox view

Patients with hepatitis A are advised to rest, eat little or nothing – or a fat-free diet (see LOW-FAT DIETS) – and to take plenty of fluids. Since the condition can be spread by faeces, people should avoid water that could be contaminated by sewage.

Pay careful attention to hygiene – especially when travelling to places where the disease is prevalent, such as poorly developed tropical and subtropical countries. An injection of gamma globulin before going to high-risk areas gives some protection against hepatitis A.

Corticosteroids may reduce inflammation in hepatitis B. The disease can be prevented by immunisation, by avoiding contaminated needles, and by the use of condoms.

There is no cure for cirrhosis, but it can be halted by removal of the cause – alcohol, hepatitis, blockage of the common bile duct (removed by surgery), or heart failure (see HEART DISORDERS).

LOW-FAT DIETS

Helping to keep arteries clear

Small quantities of fats and oils are essential for a balanced diet, but in large amounts they are thought to contribute to ailments such as heart disease (see HEART DISORDERS). Between 35-38 per cent of the kilojoules – or energy value – of the average westernised South African diet comes from fat. Doctors and alternative practitioners agree that this is far too high, and a figure more like 30 per cent is generally recommended.

Reducing fat intake to about this level is particularly important for patients with conditions such as hardening of the arteries (see ARTERIES [HARDENING]), heart disorders or ANGINA. This is because excess fat in the bloodstream can build up on the inner walls of the arteries, obstructing the flow of blood and straining the heart and circulation.

Low-fat diets may also be recommended for OBESITY, or for people who just wish to lose weight. Weight for weight, fat is the most concentrated form of food energy, containing about 38 kilojoules per gram, while proteins, starches and sugars – the other main energy-giving food components – contain only about 17. This means that fat helps to keep us warm and gives us energy for activities (though it is digested much more slowly than sugars). But it also makes it easy for us to put on weight if we eat a lot of it.

Nevertheless, a certain amount of fat is necessary. It contains essential substances known as fatty acids, some of which the body cannot make and must get from food. In addition, fat-containing foods are sources of vitamins A, D, E and K, and fats can make food tastier and more satisfying. Most people can easily cut down on fat in their diets and still meet their needs, but if in doubt, ask a doctor, nutritionist or naturopath for advice.

Different kinds of fat Whether or not you need a low-fat diet, you can benefit a lot from careful choice of the type of fats you consume. Depending on their chemical structure, the fatty acids in food oils and fats can belong to three groups: saturated, monounsaturated or polyunsaturated (see EATING FOR HEALTH). Most fats contain a mixture, usually with more of one than the others.

Nutritionists advise eating mainly monounsaturates such as olive oil and the oils in

fish, and polyunsaturates such as sunflower oil. In moderate quantities unsaturated oil is safe even for people who are on low-fat diets, and monounsaturates are believed even to reduce the risk of artery disease.

Saturated fats can cause damage to the circulatory system and are generally reduced

Cutting down on fats

If you begin to apply some simple changes to your ordinary, everyday diet, you will reduce your intake of fat considerably:

Butter, margarine, low-fat spreads Reduce or stop using spreads altogether. Although most soft margarines and low-fat spreads are made from mainly unsaturated oils – be sure to check the labels – they also tend to contain additives and preservatives, and have been highly processed.

Meat, chicken Although the flesh of red meat contains fat, the overall amount can be reduced if you choose lean cuts, trim off any visible fat and remove the skin from chicken. Skim fat from soups, stews and curries before serving, and look out for low-fat products such as special sausages. Eat meat sparingly, substituting with fish or occasional vegetable dishes.

Milk, cream Skimmed milk and buttermilk are low-fat alternatives, as are some soya milks and plain yoghurts, but you will need to check the labels to make sure.

Hard, full-fat cheeses such as cheddar Cottage cheese or even medium-fat types such as Brie, Camembert and Edam are better.

Mayonnaise, salad dressings Home-made dressings containing low-fat yoghurt or cottage cheese are less oily than bought products. Flavour them with herbs, garlic, mustard, lemon juice or other seasonings.

Cooking oils and fats Reduce your intake by frying, sautéing and roasting food only occasionally. Baking, boiling, grilling, poaching, steaming and stir-frying all use less or no oil or fat.

Snacks Avoid nuts, crisps, chocolates, biscuits and cakes, all of which are high in fat. Instead try eating fresh or dried fruit, carrot or celery sticks, or eat a wholewheat sandwich.

The fat content of foods

This table gives the amount of fatty acids – saturated and unsaturated (including both poly- and monounsaturates) – and total fat (including glycerol) per 100 g of food. No one is likely to eat 100 g of butter at a time, but for foods such as meat and chicken 100 g is about the size of an ordinary portion. In some prepared foods, the saturated and unsaturated content depends on the fat or oil used.*

FOOD		SATURATED FATTY ACIDS (g)	UNSATURATED FATTY ACIDS (g)	TOTAL FAT (g)
Cheese	Camembert	13,9	8,0	23,2
	Cheddar	20,0	11,6	33,5
	cottage	2,4	1,4	4,0
	processed	14,9	8,7	25,0
Cream	double	28,8	16,7	48,2
Milk	whole	2,3	1,3	3,8
	skimmed	0,04	0,03	0,1
Yoghurt	low-fat	0,6	0,3	1,0
Butter		49,0	28,3	82,0
Chocolate		17,7	10,8	30,3
Lard		41,8	50,6	99,0
Margarine	soft, vegetable oil	25,6	51,7	81,0
Oil	olive	14,0	80,9	99,9
	sunflower	13,1	81,8	99,9
Bacon	grilled	13,6	17,6	33,8
Beef	lean grilled steak	2,5	3,1	6,0
	roast (lean only)	3,8	4,7	9,1
Chicken	roast with skin	4,6	8,4	14,0
	roast, no skin	1,8	3,3	5,4
Egg		3,4	5,4	10,9
Lamb	roast (lean only)	4,0	3,5	8,1
	grilled chops	14,1	12,3	29,0
	kidney	0,9	1,0	2,7
	liver	3,2	4,2	10,3
Pork	roast (lean only)	2,7	3,6	6,9
	grilled sausage	9,7	13,6	24,6
Mackerel	smoked	4,0	10,4	16,3
Prawns		0,2	1,0	1,8
Sardines	tinned	2,7	10,1	13,6
Almonds		4,2	46,7	53,5
Hazelnuts		2,6	31,7	36,0
Peanut butter		10,6	40,7	53,7
Peanuts		9,2	37,4	49,0
Bread	wholewheat	0,5	1,6	2,7
Muesli		1,3	5,8	7,5
Oatmeal porridge		0,1	0,7	0,9
Biscuits	plain	7,9	7,7	16,6
Fruit cake		3,9	6,3	11,0
Most fruits (e.g. apples, pears)				Traces only
Avocado		2,6	18,6	22,2
Most vegetables (e.g. carrots, beans, peas)				Traces only
Potatoes	boiled, baked	0	0,1	0,1
	roast*	-	-	4,8
	chips*	-	-	10,9

to a minimum on a low-fat diet. They come mainly from animals, and include butter, lard, suet, cheese and the fat on meat, all of which are highly saturated. Coconut and palm oil, which are used in hard margarines, though vegetable oils, also fall into this category (see table, left).

LUMBAGO

The pain of lumbago in the lower back, or lumbar region, can be so severe that the back 'locks' – and the patient is stuck in a bent position. Symptoms may be caused by strained back muscles or ligaments, a SLIPPED DISC or displacement of a vertebra. The pain is often triggered by stooping, sitting or lifting, and may also accompany SCIATICA.

What the therapists recommend

Herbal medicine A soothing remedy is a poultice made from the baked and powdered roots of the buffalo-thorn (or 'blinkblaar') tree. Camomile tea also provides relief.

Acupuncture In addition to points that are painful, other channels treated are gall bladder, bladder and large intestine. MOXIBUSTION may also be used.

Acupressure The pressure point in the centre of the back of the knee-crease should be used – but *not* if the patient has VARICOSE VEINS. Press inwards at this point.

Massage Before the pain becomes acute, deep effleurage and frictions should be given to the lumbar region, extending the movements upwards, to improve general circulation. This should be followed by petrissage, concentrating on kneading and rolling movements over the muscles at the sides of the waist and upper buttocks. Next, friction is applied along each side of the spine.

Hydrotherapy Ice packs are recommended for severe pain. Other treatments offered include hot packs, needle sprays and underwater douches.

Chiropractic Treatment is aimed at reducing spasm in the small muscles of the back and increasing flexibility in the joints of the spine. Exercises to ease the pain may also be suggested.

An orthodox view

Doctors often advise rest in bed – with a board under the mattress for extra firmness. They may prescribe painkillers or occasionally, for short-term use, muscle relaxants such as diazepam. EXERCISE to maintain muscle strength and the natural curvature of the spine can help, as does traction, physiotherapy, and advice about lifting and sitting properly (see BACK PAIN).

MACROBIOTICS

The aim of a macrobiotic diet is to help you get the most out of life in terms of health and enjoyment. It is based on a regime of vegetables and whole grains. See EATING YOUR WAY TO INNER HARMONY AND HEALTH, p. 228.

MALARIA

As many as 300-million people are affected each year by malaria, a widespread, parasitic infectious disease found in tropical and subtropical countries. The malaria parasites are transmitted by bites of infected female anopheles mosquitoes, when they pierce the skin to drink blood. The incubation period ranges from 10 days to six weeks, and symptoms include bouts of fever (sometimes with shivering attacks), severe headache, vomiting and muscle pain.

Once in the bloodstream the parasites invade the liver, multiply, invade the red blood cells and multiply further. The destruction of these blood cells is in itself a serious matter; but in addition the cells may block blood vessels in vital organs such as the liver, kidneys or even brain.

One form of this unpleasant disease in particular – malignant tertian or falciparum malaria – demands prompt treatment and probably hospitalisation at the first signs of any symptoms; a doctor should in any case be consulted as soon as malaria is suspected.

What the therapists recommend

Acupuncture Two points high up on the spine are stimulated, and seeds of the tropical pili tree may be inserted into the hole made by the acupuncture needle.

Naturopathy Suggested treatment includes a very hot bath followed by bed, with hot-water bottles and blankets to encourage perspiration. Perspiration can be further promoted if the patient drinks water flavoured with lemon-juice or orange-juice. A fast, as in the case of other fevers, is recommended for several days. Substances such as quinine are regarded as poisonous to the system. All-round fitness and a good, balanced diet are thought to be the best preventive measures against malaria.

Herbal medicine An assortment of plant remedies has been used as a cure for malaria by the indigenous peoples of southern Africa. The remedies include the bitter-tasting gum exuded from the bark of the baobab tree; an infusion of the leaves of the Cape willow; and similar infusions of leaves of either the crinum lily or the ginger bush. Sipped at regular intervals, tea infused from the leaves of the lemon bush ('fever tree') is said to be an excellent treatment for malarial fever; while another herbal infusion uses the leaves of the 'nastergal' or nightshade.

An orthodox view

Chloroquine is the standard drug administered to rid the system of the malaria parasite. Subsequent treatment makes use of primaquine.

Those travelling to infected regions must take anti-malarial drugs for several days prior to the visit, as well as during it and for up to a month afterwards.

MANIC DEPRESSIVE DISORDERS

Everyone has changes of mood – feeling 'high' sometimes and 'low' at others – but those who suffer from manic depressive illness experience excessive mood swings, ranging from extreme elation (mania) to profound DEPRESSION.

Symptoms of mania may include over-confidence, talkativeness, extravagance, HYPERACTIVITY, and the ability to remain extremely lively with little or no sleep. Such sufferers may make grandiose plans and be interfering and difficult. Although tolerable for short periods, relatives and friends eventually find manic behaviour exhausting.

When they are depressed, sufferers may be withdrawn and introverted, lacking in confidence and self-reproachful. They may even contemplate suicide. Swings from mania to depression may be sudden or gradual, and are usually unpredictable.

Some sufferers' mood may swing to only one extreme: at one end of the swing they behave normally, but at the other they are either manic or depressed. So some cases of depression are caused by manic depressive disorder, despite the fact that the sufferer is never manic.

Symptoms of manic depressive disorders may resemble those of SCHIZOPHRENIA.

What the therapists recommend

Aromatherapy A drop of thyme and two of clary sage in a teaspoon of carrier lotion, applied to the back of the hands every two hours and inhaled, is said to be helpful in balancing extreme emotions. A total of six to eight drops of basil and bergamot with sandalwood or patchouli in the bath or inhaled from a tissue may also be beneficial.

Bach Remedies For treatment of the manic state: Scleranthus for general instability, and for being introverted and out of touch with one's feelings. Vervain for overenthusiasm, fanaticism (especially if religious mania is apparent) and overextension of oneself. If there is impatience with others' slowness, try Impatiens. Give Chestnut bud for haste and an inability to control the repeating cycle of moods. Walnut may also help to regulate the cycle. Try Gorse for a feeling of despair that things may never change. For treatment of the depressive state, see DEPRESSION.

Homoeopathy Practitioners regard the condition as too serious for self help, and advise consultation with a qualified homoeopath. Remedies are available for both the manic and depressive stages and treatment is prescribed according to individual needs.

Biochemic Tissue Salts *Kali phos.* is believed to help sufferers to cope with the nervous STRESS that may accompany the manic depressive condition.

Naturopathy Since depression and other psychological imbalances may have a physical basis in part, naturopaths will encourage changes to provide more energy for the central nervous system. Cutting out alcohol, strong tea, coffee and sugar, and increasing protein as part of a wholefood diet may help. FOOD ADDITIVES should be excluded as far as possible.

An orthodox view

Without treatment, a manic patient's behaviour may be so bizarre and antisocial that he finds himself in trouble with the law, or being detained involuntarily in a psychiatric hospital. Doctors treat attacks of mania with tranquillisers such as haloperidol or chlorpromazine, and depression with anti-depressant drugs.

The mainstay of medical treatment is lithium carbonate which, taken daily, is a mood regulator and prevents dramatic swings from mania to depression and vice versa.

MANTRAS

Among the early Hindus, mantras were sacred words (or groups of words) used in prayers and incantations to invoke the gods. Later, similar formulas were repeated, either aloud or silently, in order to clear the mind for MEDITATION. They are now also used in YOGA, and were an integral part of COUÉISM. It was Emile Coué who coined the famous mantra: 'Every day, in every way, I am getting better and better.'

Sitting cross-legged in the Lotus position is an ideal way in which to say your daily mantra, either aloud or silently to yourself.

MASSAGE

Perhaps the oldest way of healing

As probably the oldest therapy known to man, massage has been practised in the Middle and Far East since at least 3000 BC. Physicians in ancient Greece were skilled in massaging stiff and painful joints – and Hippocrates, known as the 'Father of Medicine', wrote in the 5th century BC: 'The way to health is to have a scented bath and an oiled massage each day.'

Oil is still used for all forms of massage, which became increasingly popular in Europe from the 19th century onwards, when the Swedish gymnast Per Henrik Ling devised the aesthetic and scientific principles of what is now called Swedish massage. Based on various ancient massage practices, it combines therapeutic massage with exercises for muscles and joints.

The next major step forward came in the early 1970s, when the American massage therapist George Downing published his trend-setting work, *The Massage Book*. In it he formulated the idea of massage as a therapy taking into account a person's whole being – his physical, mental and emotional make-up. Downing also incorporated into his comprehensive system the beliefs and techniques of two other well-known massage therapies, REFLEXOLOGY and SHIATSU.

Since then, the art of therapeutic massage has grown into a way of creating and maintaining the best possible health for its devotees. It aims to do this by, in turn, relaxing, stimulating and invigorating mind and body.

Who it can help The most common – and most effective – use of massage is to relax the body and mind and so relieve the strains and TENSION of daily life. It is also used to treat people with some CIRCULATION PROBLEMS and HEART DISORDERS – as well as those suffering from high BLOOD PRESSURE, HEADACHES, HYPERACTIVITY, INSOMNIA and sinusitis (see SINUS PROBLEMS).

Physically, its therapies are aimed at improving the blood, muscular and nervous systems, and also helping the body to assimilate food and get rid of waste products.

On the simplest level, massage can ease the kind of BACK PAIN and NECK PAIN people frequently suffer from at the end of the working day – especially if they have been hunched over a desk, or sitting awkwardly behind the wheel of a car.

Athletes, sportsmen and dancers can also benefit greatly from massage – which eases the stiffness they often experience when their work is over. It does this by 'milking', or draining, the muscles of toxic chemical waste products which accumulate in them following strenuous activity.

Mentally, on a psychological and emotional level, its calm and soothing effects have helped people plagued by ANXIETY or DEPRESSION, allowing them to deal more constructively with everyday worries and problems – and to regain self-confidence.

Finding a practitioner In South Africa there is no professional board of masseurs and masseuses. Contact is therefore best made through personal recommendation, or at the suggestion of your GP. Alternatively, trained and qualified practitioners can often be contacted through a health hydro (if there is one in your area) or a health and fitness gymnasium. The South African Medical and Dental Council, P O Box 205, Pretoria 0001, keeps a list of all masseurs and masseuses registered with the council.

Do not simply pick a name at random from the *Yellow Pages*, and certainly not from advertisements in a local shop window. Treatment by an unqualified practitioner could do more harm than good.

Consulting a practitioner These days more and more practitioners are incorporating methods from other therapies into their work. These include ACUPUNCTURE and ROLFING (tissue massage), as well as AROMATHERAPY, reflexology and shiatsu.

Basically, however, massage takes four main forms: effleurage (or stroking), friction (or pressure), percussion (or drumming), and petrissage (or kneading). See illustrations.

Used individually or in combination, these techniques – and variations of them – aim to help people through the use of 'caring touch'. Practitioners stress that massage is fundamentally a two-way process, in which the therapist – by using his or her hands with skill and sympathy – benefits in terms of wellbeing just as much as the patient.

In most cases, people visit a masseur at his work place, or else attend a massage clinic. However, some private practitioners will visit clients at their homes. Whichever it is, the same basic procedure is followed. The client strips to undershorts or briefs and lies – usually face down – on a massage table or the floor. A thorough massage is then given, lasting for some 20-60 minutes.

An orthodox view

This form of therapy – one of the oldest and most humane in the world – has wide applications for many conditions. However, it should not be seen as a treatment for a specific disease – or as a substitute for conventional medical treatment. Its effect has more to do with its soothing, relaxing qualities and the close and sympathetic contact with another human being. A danger arises if its practitioners believe it can actually cure.

MASTITIS

Many women suffer from nodular mastitis, or fibroadenosis – tender, lumpy breasts, particularly in the week before a period (see PERIOD PROBLEMS). This is an uncomfortable and often worrying condition – but harmless. It is caused by the effect of female hormones on breast tissue.

Another form of mastitis is a breast abscess, which sometimes occurs in a nursing mother. Bacterial infection enters the breast through the nipple, which may be cracked. Any woman who discovers a lump in her breast should seek medical advice immediately – see BREAST PROBLEMS.

The four main forms of massage

Give massage in a warm, quiet room with the recipient lying on a firm, comfortable surface. Place a pillow under the torso as shown to protect the chest and stomach from uncomfortable pressure, and a small cushion or rolled-up towel under the ankles to take unnecessary strain off the feet.

Effleurage

This consists of slow, rhythmic strokes usually performed with the hands close together and the thumbs about 25 mm apart. For light massage, only the fingertips or palms are used. For deeper massage, the thumbs or knuckles are employed.

Percussion

These short, fast rhythmic movements are also known as tapotement, from the French word 'tapot', meaning 'to drum' (on a table). The percussive strokes are usually performed with the sides of the hands on the back or any broad, fleshy part of the body – such as the thighs, waist, buttocks and shoulders. The karate-like chops are delivered briskly but lightly so as not to cause pain; they are also meant to stimulate and tone-up the skin.

Petrissage

This form of massage involves grasping and squeezing sections of muscle, such as those at the waist and across the stomach. The flesh is kneaded like dough as it is picked up, 'rolled', and then released – with the masseur's hands moving steadily across the area. It stimulates circulation, and helps sportsmen to stretch and relax hard, contracted muscles. It also helps to 'milk', or drain the lactic acid that builds up in their muscles during periods of heavy exertion. It is the build-up of lactic acid that is often the cause of cramp.

Friction

Here a series of small, circular movements are made by one or more fingers, the heel of the hand, or the pads of the thumbs. The pressure stimulates circulation and enables joints to move more freely. It is particularly helpful to sportsmen and dancers, who tend to strain or damage tendons and ligaments. However, without a doctor's approval, it should not be applied at all to bruises, injuries, or sore areas of the body.

A complete body massage

Choose a quiet, warm room, with relaxing music and soft lighting – candles, for example. A futon mattress is ideal if you work on the floor, but a thick blanket will do. Support the head with a soft cushion, and have a large towel handy to cover your partner. Use a pleasantly scented massage oil, and confine yourselves to a face and/or back massage if time is short.

Starting with the face and head

A face massage is a deeply relaxing way to start a complete body massage. Use a couple of drops of massage oil – there are many available especially for the face. Alternatively use a luxury face cream.

4 Support your partner's head on one side. At the same time, glide your hand down the side of the neck towards the shoulder, gently squeezing the neck muscles.

5 While leaning in, glide the heels of your hands from the breastbone across the upper chest, working the pectoral (chest) muscles.

6 Stroke up and across your partner's abdominal area, using both hands.
7 Continue until your hands are under your partner's body in the waist area. Then lift your hands slowly, so giving the body a lift and stretch.

8 Work your hands gently over your partner's stomach area. Use the 'wringing' action, moving one hand gently in one direction while at the same time moving the other in the opposite direction.

1 Rest your thumbs on your partner's forehead, then gently but firmly stroke them towards the temples. Use the same gliding stroke across the cheeks.
2 Squeeze all along the jawline between your thumbs and index fingers, making small circles with the thumbs.
3 Massage fairly deeply, using all your fingers and small circular movements.

9 Support an arm at the wrist; stroke it up and down between thumb and fingers.
10 Gently squeeze and stretch each finger.

13 At this point, have your partner turn over, and lie with the cushion under the chest. Then effleurage stroke the back of a leg (using flat hands in a gliding movement; right), keeping the pressure firm but gentle.

11 Effleurage stroke the leg (with hands flat and gliding). Stop the inside hand before the groin area, but take the outside hand up to the hip.

15 Knead your partner's buttocks by using the 'wringing' action – moving one hand one way and the other in the opposite direction – and squeezing the muscles (below).

14 Make the stroke flow up the leg to the thigh and then down again (above). Keep using gentle but firm pressure except over the back of the knee. Repeat the procedure on the other leg.

12 Massage the foot with the thumb, using firm, circular strokes.

Especially for the back

A back massage is a good way to help relieve tiredness and tension after a busy and stressful day, and especially when there is insufficient time for a full body massage. Have your partner lie face down, with the cushion under the chest.

16 Place your hands on your partner's back, with the fingers together as shown. Make long, firm strokes all the way along the back, from the sacrum (back of the pelvis) right up to your partner's shoulders.
17 Continue the strokes across the shoulders, maintaining the pressure.
18 Take the strokes on down the back, but release the pressure so that the strokes flow in one direction only – up the back. Repeat these strokes several times so that you cover the whole of your partner's back.

19 Use the thumbs to make small circular movements along the back, on either side of the spine. Vary the pressure to suit your partner, and never press on the spine itself.

20 With both palms, use a 'wringing' action – moving one hand forwards and the other backwards – on the upper shoulder area. Have your partner's face away from the side you are working.

227

Eating your way to inner harmony and health

In the 1880s a Japanese doctor, Sagen Ishizuka, found that he could treat many common health problems with a diet based on wholegrain cereals and vegetables, and without white rice and refined sugar products. He kept case histories and published his ideas in two books. Early in this century the Japanese writer George Ohsawa put these ideas into practice and claimed that the diet had cured his tuberculosis.

Ohsawa went on to develop a whole dietary system based on Ishizuka's methods, which he named macrobiotics – from Greek words meaning 'long' and 'life', as he believed that it could make everyone healthy enough to enjoy life to the full.

Macrobiotics is based on the Chinese philosophy of YIN AND YANG, two qualities which complement and balance each other, and which are held to be part of every natural object. Yin represents the flexible, fluid and cooler side of nature, and yang the strong, dynamic and hotter side. Everyone has both yin and yang elements in combination – as does each type of food – and macrobiotics is aimed at balancing the two complementary principles in the right way for each individual.

People who are more yin than yang are thought to be calm, relaxed, peaceful, creative and social; those who are more yang are active, alert, energetic and precise. A balance between the two is said to be needed for good health, and an excess of either to result in illness. Too much yin is supposed to bring lethargy, DEPRESSION and difficulty in concentrating; too much yang to induce TENSION, irritability and inability to relax.

To overcome these problems – as well as more serious illnesses – the macrobiotic diet recommends foods with yin and yang qualities that complement the person's condition. For example, someone who needs to be alert at work but who lacks energy would be advised to eat more yang foods such as fish or bean stews, whole oat porridge and root vegetables. Someone who needs to relax and stay calm under STRESS should eat more yin foods such as salads, nuts, seeds, steamed vegetables and fresh fruit (see chart, p. 231).

Temperature and climate are also said to play a part – yang foods are warming and strengthening during a cold, wet winter;

yin foods are cooling and refreshing in hot summers. Even so, extremely yin and yang foods are not recommended: these include sugar, spices and alcohol (very yin), and meat, eggs and cheese (yang). Such foods are believed to have too strong an effect on the system, and may eventually cause illness.

The macrobiotic way of life involves other factors such as EXERCISE and environment as well as diet. For example, YOGA and T'AI-CHI CH'UAN are considered yin in effect, and 'aerobic' exercise, such as JOGGING or skipping, yang.

Followed consistently, macrobiotics is said to help in preventing or treating nearly all illnesses, and there are many case histories which claim cures for CANCER, ARTHRITIS, DIGESTIVE PROBLEMS and other serious disorders. But macrobiotics is not only for those who are ill, and it should certainly not be regarded as a last-ditch attempt at cure where all else has failed. Practitioners regard it as a way of life – everyone may benefit from the increased energy, healthy appearance and greater resistance to illness that it is said to bring.

Anyone wishing to try this way of eating is advised to attend a cooking course. Pregnant women, breastfeeding mothers, children, people who are ill, and anyone with special requirements should see a doctor before visiting a macrobiotic counsellor, who can draw up an individual diet and health plan. Health-food stores should be able to direct you to a counsellor resident in your area.

Two of South Africa's leading experts in this important field are Mrs Shirley Horwitz (nutritional guidance counsellor), 39 Eastwood Road, Dunkeld 2196; and Mrs Barbara Cohen (teacher of macrobiotic cooking), who you can contact at Amberley, Bishopscourt Road, Claremont 7700.

Warning During the 1960s and 1970s an extreme form of macrobiotics was widely followed. It involved eating almost nothing but brown rice. This dangerously narrow diet gave macrobiotics a bad name. However, the version of the diet that is given here is much more moderate, and meets the requirements of normal, good nutrition.

The macrobiotic larder

Most macrobiotic foods are everyday ingredients found in supermarkets and grocers' shops, but some special oriental products are also used – buy them from a health food shop or oriental grocers. Here are some of the most important ingredients to keep in stock:

Wholegrain cereals These include brown rice, barley, oats, wheat, buckwheat, maize (mealies), millet, rye and products made from these such as wholewheat flour, bread and pasta; whole oat porridge; couscous.

Vegetables Fresh, seasonal vegetables are used, preferably those that grow in the local soil and climate. A mixture of root, ground and leafy green ones is recommended.

Fruit Like vegetables, these should be bought often, to ensure absolute freshness. Choose seasonal and local varieties of both fresh and dried fruit.

Pulses Some of the best include lentils, chickpeas and adzuki beans (a type of kidney bean).

Nuts and seeds Peanuts, almonds, hazelnuts, walnuts, dried chestnuts, and sesame, sunflower and pumpkin seeds are all used in the macrobiotic diet.

Oils Polyunsaturated or monounsaturated, cold-pressed vegetable oils such as sesame, sunflower, maize (mealies) and olive oil are used (see EATING FOR HEALTH).

Seasonings Sea salt, gomashio (sesame salt), ginger, mustard, tahina (sesame seed paste), cider vinegar, garlic, lemon juice and apple juice are recommended in moderation.

Spreads Natural, sugar-free jams, tahina, barley malt, peanut butter and other nut butters can be used.

Snacks Always useful to have around for occasional eating are rice cakes, roasted nuts and seeds, and raisins.

Sweeteners Use barley malt or maize and barley malt, rice syrup – buy it at a health food shop – or fruit juice.

Beverages Natural drinks such as apple or carrot juice, real ale, organic wine, spring water and herbal TISANES are all allowed.

Special oriental ingredients

Bancha twig tea This is made from the twigs of the bancha bush. It contains virtually no caffeine or tannin, and is slightly alkaline – useful in counteracting the effects of stress.

This tea has a mild, soothing taste and does not need milk or sugar. Rooibos tea is an indigenous alternative, with many of the same properties.

Brown rice vinegar A tasty seasoning for vegetable dishes.

Kuzu This vegetable powder can be used to thicken sauces and desserts, and is said to settle the digestive system.

Miso A rich, salty seasoning for soups and sauces, made from fermented soya beans. It is said to fortify the blood and improve digestion.

Seaweed Use this to enhance the flavour and nutritional value of just about any savoury dish. Try wakame in soups or salads, kombu with beans, and arame or hiziki with vegetables. All of them are rich in calcium and iron.

Shoyu This dark, naturally fermented soya sauce is a good seasoning for bean and vegetable dishes.

Tofu A soft, white soya-bean curd, which is high in calcium and protein. It is quick and easy to prepare, and can be fried, steamed, boiled or grilled.

Umeboshi plums Salty, sour pickled plums which can be added to grain or vegetable dishes, or stirred into bancha tea. Umeboshi plums are also recommended for HEADACHES, INDIGESTION, upset stomachs and HEARTBURN.

A doctor's road to recovery

In January 1987 a retired English doctor living in Italy, Hugh Faulkner, was told after tests in London that he had cancer of the pancreas. The tumour was already the size of a cricket ball and could not be operated on, but a bypass operation was performed to prevent it blocking the passage of food from the stomach. Dr Faulkner knew that drugs and radiation treatment would be unlikely to help, and that he would probably die within a few months.

However, while recovering from the bypass operation, Dr Faulkner began to receive SHIATSU massage treatment, which he found greatly relieved his pain and stiffness. The shiatsu therapist mentioned that she thought a macrobiotic diet could help his condition further. After discussing it with friends and family, the doctor decided to try it, since orthodox medicine had nothing more to offer. He contacted Britain's Community Health Foundation, which provided advice, books, cookery lessons and food supplies.

When the doctor and his wife Marian got back to Italy, they began to follow the macrobiotic diet as carefully as they could. They grew many of their own vegetables and drank water from a well on their land. In addition, they practised self MASSAGE and took lessons in shiatsu and the ALEXANDER TECHNIQUE.

Three years after the operation, at the age of 77, the doctor was not only still alive, but fitter and more energetic than for many years. He was engaged part-time in local health work and was also doing research, writing, and learning woodcarving and the jazz harmonica.

He has admitted that there is no scientific proof that macrobiotics cured him. However, a scan showed that the tumour on his pancreas was shrinking and that its centre was being destroyed – and spontaneous regression is rare in pancreatic cancer.

Utensils in the macrobiotic kitchen

Using the correct tools is just as important in macrobiotics as having the right mix of ingredients to start with. Pots, pans and other utensils are chosen with care and treated with respect. Most kitchens already contain many of the essential items, but you may find that you need to buy one or two. Basic equipment includes:

Pots and pans Cast-iron utensils are generally preferred because they distribute heat evenly, but they are also very heavy and can be hard to lift when full. Stainless-steel pots – particularly those with a heavy, reinforced base – are a good alternative, but need to be used on a lower heat or food may burn. Enamel pots can also be used – treat them gently to avoid chipping, and do not use harsh scouring pads which can scratch the surface.

Copper and aluminium kitchenware is not advised, as traces of the metals may contaminate food and affect its vitamin content.

Ovenware In addition to stainless steel, enamel and cast iron, ceramic and Pyrex are suitable for baking utensils and oven dishes. These materials are more fragile, however, so avoid exposing them to strong direct heat. Sudden changes of temperature such as transferring dishes straight from refrigerator to oven or pouring cold water on a hot dish can also cause breakage. Treat ovenware with care.

Knives A good knife – or several if you like to use different sizes – is an indispensable part of macrobiotic cookery. Carbon steel blades are best, followed by stainless steel, which cuts well but chips more easily. Sharpen knives regularly on a whetstone or butcher's steel.

Vegetable chopping board Choose a wooden board of the biggest size that you can handle comfortably. If possible, avoid scrubbing or washing with soap and hot water – instead, wipe down with a damp cloth before and after use, and between chopping different vegetables. Rubbing in a little sesame oil occasionally will help to keep the wood in good condition.

Steamer Few methods of cooking vegetables are better for retaining taste, texture and vitamins than light steaming. Special steamer pot sets are available, but a folding steamer rack that fits inside an ordinary pot works just as well. Whichever method you use, stainless steel is recommended.

Vegetable brush Brushes of natural bristle are available from many health food shops and stores that sell kitchen equipment. Use them gently to remove sand and grit from root vegetables.

Containers and jars Airtight containers made of natural materials such as glass, ceramic or even wood are recommended for storing dry goods such as nuts, seeds, pulses, rice, other grains and flour.

Pestle and mortar Use these for all mixing, crushing and grinding jobs, such as pulverising nuts and seeds, making sauces and salad dressings, and blending herbs.

Spoons, spatulas and ladles Wooden or bamboo ones are preferred as they do not scratch pans or taint food.

Cooking and preparation methods

Macrobiotic cooks believe that the way food is prepared affects both its nutritional value and its yin and yang qualities. In general, raw foods are considered more yin than cooked foods, and the more heat and the longer the cooking time the more yang food is thought to become. Different kinds of food respond best to different methods of preparation and cooking:

Vegetables The freshness of vegetables is of great importance in macrobiotic cookery. Buy small quantities regularly rather than occasionally stocking up with large supplies. Store vegetables carefully, removing plastic bags so that they are able to breathe, and keep them in a cool, dry place such as a refrigerator vegetable box.

To preserve their vitamin content do not remove soil or wash vegetables in advance. Treat vegetables gently when preparing them and, if possible, scrub off soil with a vegetable brush rather than peel them. Avoid lengthy soaking which will leach nutrients into the water. When cutting, use a sharp knife that slices cleanly rather than a blade that has to be drawn back and forth.

Because the upper parts of plants are considered more yin than the lower parts, vegetables are usually cut from top to bottom or diagonally to get a cross-section of yin and yang in each piece. Make the pieces quite small and use different shapes such as triangles, matchsticks, rolled strips, semicircles and cubes to add variety to your meal.

Vegetables are often eaten raw in a macrobiotic meal, usually with a sauce or savoury dip to accompany them. When cooked, they are generally steamed, boiled or stir-fried. Leafy green ve-

getables need only a minute or two, while root vegetables will take a little longer, but no vegetable should be cooked so long that it loses its crunchiness and texture. Save the water from boiled or steamed vegetables to use in soups, stews and sauces, and when stir-frying use just enough oil to coat the pan, never heating it so much that the oil smokes.

Grains In their whole form grains can be kept for a year or even longer, but as soon as they are ground into flour or pressed into flakes they begin to lose some of their freshness and nutritional value, and will last only a few months. Many macrobiotic cooks dislike buying ready-milled flour for this reason and prefer to use a small hand mill with which to grind fresh flour.

Grains and grain products are best stored in airtight containers and kept in a cool, dark place. Whole grains should be cooked slowly, using just enough water so that the pot is left dry at the end of cooking – about four measures of water to every one of grain. Remember that the unpolished grains used in macrobiotic cooking take longer to cook than polished ones – about 40-60 minutes for brown rice, for example, compared with 15-20 for white (which also needs less water).

To add variety, sprinkle rice or other grains with roasted nuts or seeds before serving, or you could serve them with a sauce made from miso, fried onion and a little water or stock.

Pulses Beans, peas and lentils are a rich and inexpensive source of protein. Stored in airtight containers away from heat and moisture, they can last for several years, but careful preparation is necessary to avoid indigestibility.

Begin by spreading dry pulses on a clean tea towel and picking out any stones, husks or broken pieces. Then rinse thoroughly and leave to soak for 4-8 hours or overnight in plenty of water. Before cooking, throw out the soaking water, rinse the beans and bring them to the boil in a saucepan with four measures of fresh water to every measure of beans. Sometimes a strip of kombu or wakame seaweed is added to improve digestibility. Reduce the heat and simmer gently until soft, about 40-60 minutes or even longer in some cases. When soft add soya sauce or sea salt to taste and cook uncovered until the remaining water has evaporated. Adding salt any sooner will harden the skins of the pulses and increase cooking time.

Beans and other pulses can also be baked. Soak as above and boil for 20 minutes. Place a strip of kombu seaweed in the bottom of a baking dish, pour in the beans and cooking water, cover and cook in a medium oven (180°C or 350°F) for 3-4 hours. Top up the water in the baking dish halfway if necessary, and add diced vegetables such as onion and carrot if wished, or miso, salt or soya sauce to season.

Legumes
Lentils
Beans
Peas
Tofu

Fruit

Soups

Seafood

Wholegrains
Wholewheat bread
Oatmeal porridge
Wholewheat pastry
Brown rice
Couscous
Wholewheat pasta

Vegetables
Green vegetables
Salads
Seeds
Seaweed

Balancing your diet
This diagram indicates approximately the proportions of different types of foods that should be eaten in a balanced macrobiotic diet. However, they do not need to be followed rigidly.

Fish and shellfish Many people who follow a macrobiotic diet are strict vegetarians, but for those who are not, a little fish and shellfish can be included. They should make up no more than 5 per cent of a macrobiotic diet – only a couple of small portions every week – and their yang qualities should be balanced by helpings of vegetables, grains or pulses in the same meal. Buy only the freshest seafood, if possible on the day you are going to eat it. Pay attention to details such as the firmness of the flesh, the brightness of the fish's eyes, and the pinkness or redness of its gills. Seafood should really be cooked within a few hours of its being caught; if you have to store it, make sure that you wrap it tightly in air-proof and moisture-free wrapping.

Fish can be baked or roasted whole, or skinned, filleted and sautéed in a little hot oil, with stock, vegetables, seasonings or fruit added to make a sauce. It can also be chopped into smaller pieces and used in dishes such as paella, or stir-fried with vegetables – also good ways to use prawns or other shellfish.

Another tasty way to prepare seafood is in a casserole, with seasonings such as herbs, spices or miso, vegetables, and a little liquid such as stock or wine. Cook covered at 150°C (300°F) for about an hour, or until tender.

A *macrobiotic meal to try*

The three recipes below have been chosen to give an idea of the different tastes and textures which everyday macrobiotic dishes can provide. Together with rice or other grains they make up a light, well-balanced meal, with a good mixture of yin and yang ingredients. The quantities given should be sufficient for four average servings.

Corresponding yin and yang foods

MODERATELY YIN	MODERATELY YANG
Fruit	Wholegrain cereals such as brown rice, wholewheat bread and flour, whole oat porridge
Leafy green vegetables	Root vegetables such as carrots, potatoes, parsnips
Nuts and seeds	Fish and shellfish, cottage cheese
Tofu	Beans, peas and lentils
Fruit and vegetable juices	Salt
Jams (made without sugar)	Miso
Barley malt	Shoyu soya sauce

Extremely yin and yang foods to avoid

YIN	YANG
Sugar, sweets, cakes	Meat, poultry
Strong spices	Hard, salty cheeses
Alcohol, tea, coffee	Eggs

Miso Soup

1,1 litres water
7,5-10 cm strip wakame seaweed, plus a little water for soaking
225 g sliced vegetables (try combinations of carrot, onion, celery, leek, broccoli, cauliflower or others)
1½ tablespoons miso
Lemon juice or crushed ginger to season (optional)
Chopped spring onion or parsley to garnish

Soak the wakame in water for a few minutes, then remove and slice, retaining the soaking water. Bring the 1,1 litres of fresh water to the boil, add onion if used and simmer for 10 minutes. Then add the other vegetables, wakame and soaking water, and simmer for another 5 minutes.

Turn the heat right down, mix the miso into a little of the soup liquid and add. Simmer gently for 3-4 minutes without boiling, add seasoning, pour into bowls, garnish with the spring onion or parsley, and serve.

Chickpea and Vegetable Stew

175 g chickpeas (dry measure), soaked overnight
15 cm piece of kombu seaweed
900 ml water
1 chopped onion and 2 chopped carrots
¼ teaspoon sea salt or 1-2 teaspoons shoyu soya sauce
Parsley sprigs and lemon slices to garnish

Boil or bake the chickpeas and seaweed in the water as described in *Cooking and preparation methods* for pulses. When nearly done, add the chopped vegetables and seasonings, and cook until the water has evaporated and everything is soft. Garnish the stew with the parsley sprigs and lemon slices. Serve with rice, couscous, pasta or other wholegrains, and a dish of steamed, blanched or raw vegetables, or a salad.

Fruit Compote

Fresh or soaked dried fruit – use the equivalent of 2-3 whole fruits per person, or more if using small fruit such as berries, apricots or prunes
Water or apple juice to cover fruit
3-4 tablespoons raisins
Pinch sea salt
Pinch ground cinnamon or ginger
1 teaspoon arrowroot
Roasted almonds and lemon slices to garnish

Peel the fresh fruit if not organically grown, core and chop. Place fruit, including raisins, into a pan with the water or the apple juice and salt.

Simmer gently until the mixture is soft – 5-10 minutes for fresh fruit, but slightly longer for dried fruit, depending on the time that was spent soaking. Stir in the arrowroot to thicken, remove from heat, add the cinnamon or ginger, and scoop into individual bowls. Serve the compote cool, decorated with the roasted almonds and the lemon slices.

Yin

Wholewheat
pasta

Wholewheat
flour

Balancing yin and yang

*A good variety of natural, unprocessed
foods make up the healthy macrobiotic
diet, with cereals and vegetables
making up the largest part,
and pulses, soya products,
fruit, fish, nuts and seeds
used more sparingly.*

Wholemeal
bread

Rye flour

Jumbo
oats

Rice cakes

Brown rice

Root
vegetables

Barley

Wholegrain
cereals

Buckwheat

Turnips

Couscous

Carrots

Potatoes

Fish

Seasonings

Shoyu
soya sauce

Umeboshi plums

Pulses

Varieties of lentils – re
brown, green and blac

Flageolet beans

Miso

Butter beans

Blackeye
beans

Aduki
beans

Yang

Sweeteners

Barley malt

Brown rice vinegar

Fruit

Lime

Tomato

Kumquat

Orange

Apple

Lychees

Grapes

Nuts

Chestnuts

Walnuts

Peanuts

Hazelnuts

Vegetables

Watercress

Spinach

Soya products

Tempeh

Tofu

Seeds

Sesame seeds

Hiziki seaweed

Melon seeds

Mustard and cress

Sunflower seeds

Cabbage

Lettuce

MEASLES

One of the most common infectious diseases in the world is rubeola, or measles – a major cause of death in less-developed countries. The virus is spread by direct or close contact and, after an incubation period of eight to 15 days, causes FEVER, a dry cough and sore eyes, followed by a characteristic brownish-pink rash over the entire body.

White spots, known as Koplik's spots, on the insides of the cheeks, may be visible a day or two before the skin rash appears.

Recovery is usually complete within about ten days, although adults who catch the disease may take up to four weeks. Complications arising from measles, which are more common in adults, include ear infections, PNEUMONIA and, rarely, brain inflammation. **Warning** Measles is a notifiable disease, and you must report any suspected case to your doctor whether or not you also seek complementary remedies.

What the therapists recommend
HERBAL MEDICINE
Self help   To relieve the feverish symptoms, make infusions (see p. 184) of yarrow, elderflower or boneset; drink a cupful hot every three to four hours. For restlessness and aching, add camomile to the mixture.

To relieve itching, sponge the skin with a cool infusion of lavender, or a teaspoon of distilled witch hazel added to 300 ml of water.

NATUROPATHY
Consultation   You will be advised to avoid dairy produce and take plenty of fruit and vegetable juices both to replace fluids and provide nutrients. A practitioner may prescribe 1-2 g of vitamin C per day to improve resistance to the viral infection.

HOMOEOPATHY
Self help   The aim is to aid recovery, relieve distress and reduce the risk of complications. A*pis mel.* is prescribed for a high temperature, when the patient is hot but wants to be uncovered, has sore eyes and/or ears, and is tearful and irritable. *Euphrasia* is for streaming, sore eyes and sensitivity to light. *Gelsemium* is given for high fever and extreme prostration – even delirium. If a child is restless and irritable, needs to be comforted, has a troublesome cough, try *Pulsatilla*.

An orthodox view
There is no cure for measles, although secondary ear infections or pneumonia respond to antibiotics. Measles vaccine, given along with MUMPS and German measles (rubella) immunisation, to two-year-olds, is 95 per cent effective as a preventive. The side effects of the vaccine are the same as those of measles, but the risk is less after vaccination than after infection.

Conventional advice to measles patients is to rest, drink extra fluids, and take paracetamol to reduce fever and ease discomfort. To ensure that there are no complications, consult your doctor.

MEDITATION

Finding your way to the still, calm centre
When life heaps upon us problems that must be solved, decisions that cannot wait and changes that disrupt settled ways, we sometimes feel unable to manage, lose confidence in ourselves and become plagued by TENSION and ANXIETY. These may persist beyond immediate crises, robbing us of energy, setting a pattern for INSOMNIA, raising BLOOD PRESSURE, and causing many other physical ailments. To gain relief, millions of people go to their doctors for help and are given tranquillisers, sleeping pills and anti-depressants; such drugs are by far the commonest prescribed for patients.

Meditation is seen as a way of shedding your cares and strains – reaching, without drugs, a tranquil state that refreshes the mind and relaxes the body. Such a respite, which you can take as frequently as you wish, is aimed at restoring both the will and the ability to manage your life. A little time spent simply staring into space and pleasantly daydreaming may give an inkling of the feeling and benefits.

In India and much of the rest of Asia, meditation has been practised for thousands of years as a way of achieving spiritual enlightenment. YOGA developed from it. There have long been small numbers of people in the West who practised it, mostly people who were interested in Buddhism. But meditation was thrust into the limelight in the 1960s, when Eastern music and culture attracted pop musicians, among them the Beatles, and masses of young people looking for new approaches to life's problems.

Maharishi Mahesh Yogi was the best known of their teachers, and his MANTRAS for transcendental meditation attracted devoted followers – an unusual occurrence because the association of meditation with Oriental or eccentric religions, and descriptions such as 'transcendental', which wrongly imply that unearthly powers are involved, tended to put off most Westerners.

However, forms of meditation have been, and are, practised by members of various Christian religious orders – the retreats of Jesuits, and the spiritual exercises of their founder, St Ignatius Loyola, for example, may be considered to involve elements of meditational techniques.

Meditation is regarded by its practitioners as a supreme self-help method. Using nothing more than your own powers of concentration, you control your thoughts and calm and slow your body. This is not to say it is easy. Switching off racing thoughts and keeping worry at bay may at first prove difficult, but practitioners offer simple procedures which they say help most people to reach the utterly relaxed and at the same time self-controlled meditative state.

Who it can help   Meditation requires concentration, persistence and time – anything from ten to 20 minutes a day. Most people can learn to meditate without too much difficulty. Although some benefits – such as lowering of the pulse and blood pressure – may occur immediately, long-term benefits require regular practice. For some people, this can be difficult.

A large group among those who benefit are people with high blood pressure: many are able to cut down or even cut out the drugs prescribed for them. The exaggerated reactions which their bodies have to everyday stresses diminish and their blood pressure remains lower as long as they continue with meditation, especially if they also practise RELAXATION AND BREATHING.

Machines that record the electrical impulses sent out by muscles show that muscular tension drops almost to nil during meditation. As a result, chronic pain and discomfort from injury are relieved – for tension causes, or at least worsens, many pains.

Circulation has been shown to improve during meditation, so conditions as comparatively minor as CHILBLAINS or as serious as RAYNAUD'S DISEASE may be helped by meditating. It can also relieve tension HEADACHES, where the blood supply to the scalp is affected.

The slower, deeper breathing and the reduced rate of consuming oxygen that occur during meditation are beneficial to people with chest complaints. Combined with the relaxation of muscles, this is particularly good for asthma sufferers.

Pain, breathing difficulties, tension and a mind racing uncontrollably are all common causes of insomnia. Monitoring the brain's pattern of electrical activity with an EEG (electroencephalograph) machine shows that a person's brain activity during meditation becomes similar to that during sleep.

Meditation makes people sufficiently relaxed to go off to sleep. It breaks the pattern of sleeplessness which is particularly difficult to alter. Insomniacs who meditate will not necessarily sleep longer, because their need to switch off is partially satisfied by the meditative state itself. They will, however, be able to get to sleep and feel properly rested by the sleep they have.

Finding a teacher Traditional meditation techniques intended to empty the mind with the aim of allowing consciousness to expand and reach a higher reality require formal programmes of teaching. A special posture and a mantra (a phrase or sound chanted over and over) are used in transcendental meditation, with a teacher to lead and supervise. People rooted in Western cultures often find this difficult to accept, and simpler methods may suit them far better.

Some people find it impossible to start meditating on their own and welcome joining a group where they can seek advice and practise suggested techniques. Your neighbourhood library may include such groups in its list of local societies. You will also find meditation groups listed in the advertising columns of alternative lifestyle publications. Various YOGA schools are good points of contact. The South African Association for the Age of Enlightenment (SAAAE), P O Box 4738, Cape Town 8000, specialises in transcendental meditation.

How to meditate Whether you choose to meditate on your own or in a group, the procedure will be similar. Details may vary, but the basic rules are common.

It is best not to eat or drink in the half hour before meditating. Choose a quiet room where you will not be interrupted. Some people lie down and close their eyes, but many teachers say that you should sit comfortably but upright, with eyes open and hands resting in your lap. In this way you can relax but remain alert and controlled; lying with eyes closed, your mind may simply wander or you may fall asleep.

What you are aiming to do is stop troublesome or stimulating thoughts from entering your mind. This is most easily done by filling up your mind with one neutral or calmly pleasing thought. Breathing is made the focus in some methods, by feeling the air entering your nostrils, moving it down to fill your lungs completely and then slowly expelling it. Concentrate on making your diaphragm move down and your abdomen (not chest) swell out as you breathe in. Count as you breathe in and out, taking as long to expel the air as you did drawing it in – and making sure it is all expelled.

When this breathing pattern becomes automatic you may find unwanted thoughts creeping in. You can shift your concentration from breathing to relaxing your body. All your muscles should be completely relaxed. With one breath, check that your forehead is not tight, with the next that you are not clenching your teeth, then that your shoulders, elbows, knees, calves and feet are loose.

If thoughts keep intruding, do not follow them up. Merely acknowledge that they have come and then resume concentration on your chosen focus. When you can easily follow the breathing and relaxation pattern, you may prefer to focus on an object – a favourite ornament perhaps, or a photograph of a tranquil place whose smell, sounds and air you can feel surrounding you.

You may find that playing a soothing tape-recording helps you into the meditative state. Special meditation tapes can be bought at health food shops or specialist book shops, or you could compile your own.

Maintain your meditation for ten minutes or more. As you become practised you will be able to fall into it almost anywhere – on a train going to work, between chores, or at your desk during your lunch break. At the end of your meditation, shuffle about and exercise your muscles gently for a minute or two before you stand up, otherwise you may feel giddy because of lowered blood pressure.

Obviously you must not practise meditation at all while driving or using tools of any kind. But otherwise it holds no dangers and is a useful way of improving well-being, whether or not you are receiving any other form of treatment.

An orthodox view

The key to meditation probably lies in managing to concentrate on just one thing at a time instead of on a welter of things as we normally tend to do. Reducing the flow of information and sensations we are trying to accept reduces the mental responses we have to make. This respite from any thought also diminishes stress.

Research shows that breathing, brain activity, blood pressure, and heart and pulse rate are all affected by meditation. The calm and rested feeling it produces should not only ease disorders of the moment, but also improve your ability to cope physically and mentally with forthcoming activities or future problems.

MEGAVITAMIN THERAPY

Treatment based on large doses of vitamins

The American biochemist Linus Pauling (1901-) first attracted popular attention to the use of huge doses of VITAMINS to improve health. His book *Vitamin C and the Common Cold* (published in 1970) described for ordinary readers what he discovered.

It was research into the way MEMORY works that led Pauling to investigate the role of vitamins. His findings during studies of vitamin C led to his claim that large doses of the vitamin could ward off the common cold. The medical establishment rejected his claim – but many people tried the vitamin remedy and have found it effective.

Pauling's researches went much wider into other vitamins and MINERALS. He gave the name ORTHOMOLECULAR MEDICINE (*ortho* means 'correct') to a new approach to health which came out of his work. It was based on preserving and restoring good health by finding the right level of vitamins and minerals to suit each individual.

He claimed that orthomolecular medicine could add 20 years of good health to people's lives. He also claimed benefits for large doses of vitamin C that went far beyond fighting the common cold – chiefly in helping people with CANCER. He said that it could improve healing and strengthen the IMMUNE SYSTEM – especially the resistance of tissue around a cancer, so that malignant cells cannot spread.

Although Pauling's fertile mind and communication skills drew attention to the potential of vitamin megadoses, he was not the first in the field. From the early 1950s his compatriots, Dr Abraham Hoffer and Dr Humphry Osmond, had been using high doses of vitamin B3 to treat SCHIZOPHRENIA, and claimed success rates of more than 75 per cent in some 2 000 cases. A whole field of 'orthomolecular psychiatry' has grown since, to treat mental illnesses.

At the core of all these treatments for physical and mental ills – now generally referred to as megavitamin therapy – is the belief that the daily intakes at present recommended by orthodox practitioners for vitamins and minerals are only a very rough guide. Individual needs can vary enormously – many people are said to need quantities ten times greater than the recommended amount, and some are thought to need doses 100 or more times greater.

Taking vitamins as remedies is now common practice. Vitamin C supplements which are aimed at preventing VIRUS INFECTIONS are available from chemists and some health shops abroad without prescription; the amounts taken are much smaller than megavitamin doses.

Vitamins and minerals are also prescribed as part of standard medical practice – for example, for ACNE, ANAEMIA, DIABETES, high blood cholesterol, ALCOHOLISM and PREMENSTRUAL TENSION (PMT) – but again the doses do not reach megavitamin proportions.

Who it can help Megavitamin therapists take the view that most people's illnesses will be relieved by their therapy because a principal cause of illness, they say, is metabolic abnormality resulting from an incorrect intake of vitamins.

The therapy also helps those people who are unable to absorb enough vitamins and minerals even from a diet that would normally be adequate. Megadoses are prescribed so that the tiny proportion absorbed by their faulty system will approach their required level.

Some illnesses and medical treatments are believed to alter the ability to absorb vitamins and minerals, and very large doses are prescribed in such cases; conventional chemotherapy and radiotherapy, for example, are said to triple the needs of cancer patients for vitamins B and C.

Megavitamin therapists have worked out complex combinations of vitamins to treat cancer patients, especially after they have had orthodox treatments.

Vitamin C and the B vitamins are also claimed to restore the biochemical balance in the brain of people with mental illnesses including schizophrenia and DEPRESSION. Hyperactivity and drug dependency (see ADDICTION) have also been found to respond to megavitamin treatment.

Finding a therapist   For further information about megavitamin therapy, and details of where it is available, contact the Vitamin Information Centre, P O Box 182, Isando 1600. Enclose a stamped, self-addressed envelope with your letter.

Another source of information on this subject is the Association for Dietetics in Southern Africa, P O Box 13904, Northmead 1511.

Consulting a therapist   Large doses of vitamins and minerals should never be taken without the advice and supervision of a qualified dietician. Vitamins and minerals interact in complex ways which it is the dietician's job to know. Indeed the most important part of a series of consultations will be devoted to drawing up an accurate profile of your particular needs.

This process will take time and may involve skin tests and hair analysis. Only then can a suitable course of high-dose supplements be decided upon. The therapist will want to keep a close check on your progress because vitamins can cause uncomfortable, even dangerous, side effects from quantities that can easily be eaten.

An orthodox view

Despite the many individual cases where megavitamin treatment has been successful, orthodox practitioners view the therapy with suspicion. This is largely because it works in the dark. Very few controlled trials have been done on matched groups of people to pinpoint the effects of vitamins and minerals,

alone or in combination, compared with other treatments.

Trials which have been carried out, mainly in the United States, have produced poor or confusing results. There are so many variables in the biochemistry of individuals, whether in normal or in ill health, that it may never be possible to get enough answers to predict the effects of treatment.

Meanwhile, the possible harm done by megadoses is causing concern. If vitamin D, for example, is taken in excessive amounts it can quickly cause muscle weakness, bone pain, hypertension, irregular heartbeat and kidney deterioration. If vitamin A is taken in excessive quantities for a long period it can cause painful joints, cracked skin, anaemia and amnesia in adults; in children it can cause severe visual disturbance and painful swellings over bones; and in unborn children it is suspected of causing deformities.

There are also doubts about the skill of those who prescribe, and fears that big business interests are misleading the public in order to make profits.

At present it would be better to educate the public on what the daily requirements of vitamins and minerals are, what common foods contain them, and how to avoid destroying them during cooking or storage.

MEMORY

Ways of giving it a jog …

The brain may be likened to a computer, for in both a 'good memory' involves the successful input, storage and retrieval of information. Barring some forms of mental problems, we learn throughout our lives, receiving and storing information and experiences. This is thought to involve changes in the way nerve impulses are routed through the brain.

There are two kinds of memory, based on two kinds of changes. Short-term memory is thought to involve reverberatory activity in groups of nerve cells – a kind of 'echo' or 'bouncing back' effect. Long-term memory probably involves a more permanent 'trace' in the brain, in the way the nerve cells are connected to each other at the so-called synaptic junctions (relay stations between the nerve cells).

The two types of memory have different properties. For example, at any one time only about seven items can be retained in the short-term memory. Most people can read and remember a seven-digit telephone number, provided they keep rehearsing or repeating it. Larger numbers are not so easily

remembered, for the items become jumbled or lost. And without repetition, short-term memory lasts for only about 30 seconds.

Another difference is that specific items or detailed content tend to be stored in the short-term memory while usually only the general idea or meaning is retained in the long-term memory. For instance, most people will remember for about a day the actual words of a sentence that some friend or acquaintance said. After that, they will be able to recall only the gist or the meaning of the particular sentence.

Generally, the more easily recalled items fit into an existing framework, the more successfully they are stored in the long-term memory. All adults have built up a framework of the human face, and when confronted with a new one, need only to remember its distinguishing features to recognise it again.

Generally, too, recognition – or storage – is easier than recall or retrieval. We have all had someone's name 'on the tip of the tongue'; we feel we know the name, yet cannot recall it. Then as soon as the name is said, we instantly recognise it.

On the whole, the more easily a new item can be associated with earlier items, the more easily it is learned or stored. And this association works for new material too, for items are more readily learned if associated in groups. However, association with earlier information may confuse what we store. We may have preconceived ideas about a situation and these may affect what we remember about it.

Normally, the more interesting we find an experience, the better it will be remembered. This is probably because we concentrate on it and rehearse it more, so that a more permanent 'trace' is made in the brain.

Several factors can impair the memory. Head injuries often result in a total or partial loss of memory – a condition known as AMNESIA. Alcohol, nicotine, and the side effects of certain drugs, such as the tranquillisers prescribed for INSOMNIA and medications for BLOOD PRESSURE problems, adversely affect the memory. So do STRESS, DEPRESSION, ANXIETY, SHOCK and fatigue, which affect concentration. AMNESIA may also be a symptom of HYSTERIA.

We all experience deterioration of our mental faculties – including memory – to a greater or lesser degree in old age (see GROWING OLD). In its more drastic form, this is called senile dementia and is associated with loss of brain cells and synaptic junctions. Elderly people more readily recall things experienced in the distant past than recent happenings. However, in some people, severe dementia develops in middle age, and this condition is known as ALZHEIMER'S DISEASE for which no cure has been discovered.

Self help There are several ways in which you can improve your memory. Some people find that MEDITATION or the SILVA METHOD are a great help.

Dietary supplements of choline have been proved beneficial in tests carried out at the National Institute of Mental Health in Bethesda, Maryland, USA. Subjects given 10 g of choline were able to memorise a list of unrelated words more quickly than they could before. Choline is a substance that the body produces and converts into acetylcholine, which is essential for the smooth flow of nerve impulses.

Victims of Alzheimer's disease are deficient in the enzyme that produces acetylcholine, so the evidence for a link between choline and memory seems strong.

Lecithin, a fat sometimes included in the vitamin B complex, is the main dietary source of choline. It is found in soya beans, maize, egg yolks and liver. It is best to try an unsaturated type, such as that made from soya beans, available in granule or capsule form. Take as directed by the manufacturer. Alternatively, take 1 or 2 tablespoons of the granules each day, sprinkled on food or mixed in drinks. (Lecithin also has the property of dissolving cholesterol deposits, so it may also be helpful for HEART DISORDERS and GALLSTONES.)

Do not smoke, and cut out alcohol and any drugs that are not absolutely essential to your well-being (see ADDICTION, ALCOHOLISM and SMOKING).

Use 'tricks' of association. For example, conjure up a pleasing image for each of the numbers 0 to 9. You should find it easier to remember the images than the numerals, and through them, recall the digits more easily. When introduced to someone, imagine something connected with them, their name or their occupation, for example – a gigantic pen for a writer, or a green light for someone named Green.

Try to associate things to be remembered in groups. For example, you may find it easier to remember the shopping list if you group the items according to their location in the supermarket – and you will save time, too. Try to imagine things in a setting that you already have imprinted in your memory. Associate them with happy events or some pleasing scene.

These images need not necessarily be visual; they can be sounds, feelings, moods or postures. You will remember happy events better if you put yourself into a happy mood. Conversely, unhappy episodes will come to mind more readily if you are sad. Whatever you do, the more outrageous and unusual your images and associations are, the more effective they will be. The more you practise, the better your memory will become.

Mnemonics – devices such as formulas or rhymes – also aid memory by association. In music the notes of the treble clef can be remembered by the formula 'Every Good Boy Deserves Favour'. An example of a mnemonic rhyme lists the sovereigns of England from the Norman conquest: 'Willi, Willi, Harry, Ste; Harry, Richard, John, Henry' and so on.

Finally, arrange your 'memory training' according to the time of day. Short-term memory gets worse as the day wears on, possibly because of increasing tiredness. On the other hand, long-term memory actually improves as the day progresses.

MENOPAUSE

Technically the term menopause refers to the permanent ending of monthly periods, but in general use it often embraces the wide range of accompanying symptoms which make up the climacteric, or 'change of life'. This phase of a woman's life, when her ovaries stop producing eggs and her fertility declines and eventually ceases, may begin anywhere from the early forties to the mid-fifties and usually takes two or three years.

Bound up with this physical process are several psychological factors – fear about losing attractiveness, uncertainty about a purpose in life for middle-aged women, perhaps sadness that the fertile prime of life is over. These strong feelings are added to, and may outweigh, any physical discomforts or disturbances caused by complex changes in the hormone balance.

In a few women, menstruation may stop suddenly with no previous change in the cycle, but in most women the menstrual cycle becomes irregular. Often, periods become less heavy and occur farther apart. But they may also occur more often, or follow the usual timing but with some missing altogether. Bleeding or spotting which occurs between 'normal' periods, or after sexual intercourse, should always be discussed with your general practitioner promptly – as should any bleeding which occurs a year or more after the last period.

During the menopause, the ovaries reduce and finally cease production not only of eggs but also of oestrogen, the hormone that maintains the female reproductive function. Some oestrogen is still made elsewhere in the body, particularly in the layers of fat beneath the skin, so plumper women generally experience fewer effects.

Loss of oestrogen brings symptoms such as hot flushes, sweating at night, uncomfortable lack of lubricating fluid in the vagina, and a more frequent need to pass urine. About

seven in every ten women suffer these effects in varying degrees.

One result of the menopause in all women initially goes unnoticed – a gradual but progressive loss of bone mass, or OSTEOPOROSIS. This leads to a greater risk of FRACTURES, particularly of the hip, in later life. After the menopause, women also lose the greater protection against heart attacks, compared with men, which their higher oestrogen level may have given them previously.

During the menopause, many women suffer from ANXIETY, irritability, lack of concentration, INSOMNIA, swings of mood, or even DEPRESSION. As it often coincides with children growing up and leaving home, women who have had families may feel an acute loss of identity. Women who go out to work generally tend to have fewer menopausal problems than those whose life revolves around the family home.

Symptoms may be made worse by the STRESS, lack of zest for life and curtailment of activity and exercise which can result from the psychological hurdles.

For many women, however, the problems are few and the compensations welcome. They feel fit, vigorous, and glad to be rid of the slight (or considerable) nuisance of monthly periods (see PERIOD PROBLEMS). They find their sex life enhanced by knowing they will not become pregnant and being free at last of the need for contraception.

Vaginal dryness and shrinkage are greatly lessened by a regular sex life. And as lifespans have increased, the process of GROWING OLD has been slowed. Where once both men and women were considered elderly at 55, a postmenopausal woman can now expect many years of active life. There are many natural and medical ways of enhancing wellbeing during this time.

What the therapists recommend
NATUROPATHY
Self help A healthy diet, regular exercise and sufficient sleep will ease many menopausal symptoms.

Consultation Naturopaths may suggest a short period of supervised semi-fasting, taking only fresh vegetable juice or fruit juice, to cleanse the body of impurities. This is followed by a diet with a high proportion of raw foods, and a planned programme of EXERCISE and relaxation.

Some naturopaths also recommend vitamin and mineral supplements, particularly vitamins B, C and E and calcium.

ACUPUNCTURE
Consultation Although treatment varies according to the individual and her symptoms, menopausal disorders are generally treated at points on the bladder, conception, sto-

mach, kidney and liver meridians. MOXIBUS-TION to the governor, stomach and bladder meridians may also be suggested.

The practitioner may also be able to treat digestive disorders, peptic ulcers and gall-stones, to which older women are more prone, in addition to OBESITY, raised BLOOD PRESSURE, SMOKING and ALCOHOLISM, which can sometimes affect them.

HERBAL MEDICINE

Self help Regular drinks of camomile tea and lime-blossom tea act as general relaxants. Passiflora tablets may also reduce accumulated tension and anxiety. Oats included in the diet should provide a gentle tonic. Hot flushes may be relieved by taking liquid sarsaparilla, ginseng tea, life root or St John's wort. Hormonal disturbances can be effectively treated with herbs such as chaste tea, wild yam and false unicorn root. A bed-time drink of honey and hot water, with three drops of essential oil of sage added, is used to relieve night sweating.

Other alternative treatments

Homoeopathy Treatment is individually tailored for the woman's personality, circumstances and overall symptoms.

Pulsatilla may be recommended to stabilise the menstrual cycle of women with fair complexions, but *Sepia* for those women who are dark-skinned brunettes. *Glonoine* and *Lachesis* are believed to be most useful for reducing severe hot flushes.

Aromatherapy Essential oils of sage, cypress and geranium are said to ease physical symptoms – carry a mixture of the oils with you for inhaling if symptoms start while you are out. At home, put six or eight drops of the oils in your bath. For massage, add a total of 15 drops of the oils to 5 dessertspoons of carrier oil.

An orthodox view

Regular exercise and a balanced diet help to minimise menopausal symptoms, and reduce to some extent the risk of osteoporosis. Drugs such as clonidine can alleviate hot flushes and oestrogen cream eases vaginal dryness. Orthodox medicine also offers hormone replacement (HRT; see box).

MERIDIANS

Followers of Chinese medicine believe that Qi – the body's life-activating internal energy – flows through 12 channels known as meri-

---

Replacing lost hormones through HRT – panacea or meddling with nature?

An increasingly popular, but somewhat controversial, conventional treatment for menopausal problems is hormone replacement therapy (HRT).

Women using HRT are usually given oestrogen tablets which they take for three weeks out of every four-week cycle, or continuously for the whole four weeks if, for example, menopausal symptoms appear in the week in between. If the tablets cause nausea or DIARRHOEA, oestrogen implants, pessaries, creams or stick-on skin patches may be used instead.

Most women are also given a second hormone, progesterone, as protection against the major side effect of HRT: over-stimulation of the womb lining and a possible increased risk of developing CANCER. This does not affect women who have had a hysterectomy, and they are given oestrogen only.

HRT can make a dramatic difference to those women who find that coping with the menopause is a really uncomfortable struggle, but not all doctors unreservedly approve of its use.

They agree that it does relieve hot flushes and vaginal dryness, and may improve skin tone, lift depression and increase energy. But against this are slightly increased risks of some cancers and the possible inconvenience of continued monthly bleeding – similar to a period but without an egg being produced.

The greatest benefit of HRT is that it reduces OSTEOPOROSIS and the risk of hip, wrist and spine fractures of brittle bones that are common among post-menopausal women. Since hip fractures in particular are a major cause of disability and death in women over 65, HRT can literally save lives.

There is also some evidence that HRT brings down the risk of heart disease and strokes to pre-menopausal levels, because of the protective effects of oestrogen. However, other studies show an increased risk – possibly due to progesterone – so that HRT is not given to women who have had heart attacks, strokes or blood-clotting problems.

It is also unsuitable for anyone with a history of cancer of the breast or uterus, a family history of breast cancer, or undiagnosed vaginal bleeding. Here are the contrasting views of two women who have had HRT:

FOR …
Mrs Theresa Gorman developed unpleasant menopausal symptoms in her late 40s. She suffered hot flushes, MIGRAINE and pains in her wrists, ankles and back; she became forgetful, felt tired and lost interest in life.

As soon as she began HRT – now more than 10 years ago – all the symptoms disappeared and have never returned. She regained her confidence, energy and sense of well-being, and says she now feels just as she did in her 20s.

Mrs Gorman believes that ignorance about HRT condemns many women to unnecessary suffering, and she campaigns to publicise its benefits. A biologist by training, she views HRT as restoring something which nature takes away too soon.

The most valuable benefits, she says, are that it stops women from worrying about their physical state and get on with living, and that it can prevent the pain and suffering which are caused by osteoporotic bone fractures.

She believes also that the zest for life that HRT gives is important, especially for the number of elderly women to whom it might offer new hope – and prevent them from being placed in homes.

AGAINST…
Dr Margaret White, a retired general practitioner with a special interest in women's health, had a natural, trouble-free menopause at 48, without any unpleasant symptoms such as hot flushes. Two years later she was persuaded by a drug company representative to try HRT. Dr White took the lowest dose for a year and still felt well, but then visited an American medical professor who strongly advised her to stop, since not enough was known about long-term effects, including cancer.

Dr White gradually reduced her doses until she eventually stopped altogether. But she immediately began to suffer from menopausal symptoms – hot flushes, sudden sweats, giddiness and depression. The symptoms slowly subsided and it was another year before she felt completely normal again, bitterly regretting ever having started HRT.

Dr White believes that HRT should only be used for a short time to help women with symptoms to get over the worst of the menopause. She advises healthy women to wait until more research has been done before taking the treatment.

dians. These link related organs and body parts, and when they become blocked, energy imbalances result; it is these that cause disease. In order to restore the flow, practitioners of ACUPUNCTURE insert needles at points along the meridians, while practitioners of ACUPRESSURE and SHIATSU apply finger pressure. REFLEXOLOGY has ten similar meridians, which link the massage points of the feet with their related body parts.

METAMORPHIC TECHNIQUE

Manipulation as a means to health

A relationship between the foot and the body's development during the first nine months of life in the womb forms the basis of the metamorphic technique. Its practitioners believe that gentle manipulation of the feet, hands and head can help recipients to come to terms with an assortment of long-standing problems.

They do not claim an ability to heal or cure, but many of their clients say that they experience physical and emotional benefits, and are helped to develop a more positive and creative outlook.

In particular, people who feel trapped in a rut, or are aware of a need for change but cannot see what to do, may find that the technique opens up their lives.

The metamorphic technique began in the 1960s as a result of the work of a British naturopath, Robert St John (1912-). He was disappointed that many people who had been helped by treatment later fell back into their old ways of behaving and their former illnesses recurred.

Seeking a way to help these people to gain permanent benefits, St John turned to RE-FLEXOLOGY – a method of massaging areas of the feet thought to correspond to particular bodily systems and organs.

In addition to the normal reflex areas, however, St John came to feel that parts of the foot – particularly the reflex areas relating to the spine (see chart, p. 295) – also reflect the individual's development before birth. He attached great importance to this period, and thought that many of our physical and psychological characteristics develop during the nine-month gestation period.

He decided that for people to receive lasting benefits, treatment should go right back to these early patterns, removing and correcting problems that had their origin in the first stages of life.

Who it can help Generally metamorphic technique is designed to help anyone who feels mentally blocked, stuck or unable to make a necessary change. People who cannot shake off long-standing health problems, children and the handicapped are said to derive particular benefits – even those with such severe conditions as Down's syndrome and AUTISM.

Finding a practitioner There is no national association in South Africa, and only a limited number of practitioners. For further information write to 'Metamorphic Technique', P O Box 91863, Auckland Park 2006; P O Box 454, Honeydew 2040; or 15 Seaforth Court, Simon's Town 7995. Or make enquiries from a practitioner of REFLEXOLOGY, a closely related therapy.

To find out more information about the subject, you can read *The Metamorphic Technique: the principles and practice* by Gaston St Pierre (head of Britain's Metamorphic Association) and Debby Boater.

Consulting a practitioner No attempt is made to diagnose or treat problems directly. Instead, practitioners of the metamorphic

technique call themselves catalysts – agents of change and healing who remain personally detached from the processes which they spark off in the client.

Sessions begin with the client sitting comfortably, with legs raised and well supported. The practitioner sits at right angles and gently manipulates first the right and then the left foot. Using a light circular or vibrating finger movement, he strokes or touches the bony ridge on the inside of each foot, then moves on to the big toe and ankle areas. Later, the thumbs, wrists and top of the head are worked on.

The feet are considered to represent movement and energy; the hands and head, respectively, to express action and thought. As each is touched, old patterns of behaving, feeling and thinking are said to be loosened, allowing new and better ones to develop.

Throughout the process, the practitioner remains detached, allowing the client simply to express whatever he feels. Acceptance is offered, but not approval, disapproval or advice, since practitioners do not see themselves as therapists. Instead, their attitude

A practitioner of the metamorphic technique begins a session with the right foot, using light circular or vibrating movements to stroke or touch the bony ridge on the inside of the foot. The practitioner then moves on to the big toe and ankle as shown, before working on the left foot, hands and head. At the same time, the client may talk or fall asleep. Sessions are said to help people come to terms with, or sometimes permanently overcome, both physical and mental problems – especially those determined before birth.

encourages the client to take responsibility for his or her own health, and they believe that their work simply helps to activate clients' own inner healing powers.

Sessions usually last for about an hour and take place weekly until the client feels ready to stop. However, daily sessions may be arranged in certain cases where the clients are, for example, children, mentally or physically handicapped people, or patients confined to a hospital.

Family self help Practitioners encourage their clients to learn a simple form of the technique and to practise it on family members. Although you can use the technique on yourself, there is a drawback since this creates what practitioners call a 'closed circuit' of energy, and you lose the sense of 'sharing' with another person. At least two members of each family should learn and take part.

An orthodox view

There is no scientific evidence to support practitioners' claims that areas of the feet correspond to particular body systems and organs. However, massaging the feet is a harmless activity that seems to reduce anxiety and encourage relaxation.

MIASM THEORY

Treating the roots of disease

The belief that illness can signify an underlying disease that is not directly apparent was initially proposed by the founder of Homoeopathy, Samuel Hahnemann (1755-1843), of Meissen, Germany. He noted that many patients would recover only to become ill again later, and reasoned that some deep-seated condition was creating within them a predisposition to develop certain diseases.

He used the word 'miasm' – from the Greek *miainein*, meaning 'to pollute' – to describe the condition. He felt that various diseases, including SKIN DISORDERS and TUBERCULOSIS, were 'miasmatic' in character. Accordingly, he sought to get to the roots of his patients' illnesses, and to treat them with appropriate homoeopathic remedies.

Hahnemann also tried to improve their ways of life. For example, he told them not to smoke or drink too much, not to eat rich food, or to waste their energies on such pursuits as gambling and horse-riding.

Some homoeopaths believe that miasms are the underlying causes of ANXIETY, DEPRESSION, CANCER, MIGRAINE and STOMACH COMPLAINTS. However, other homoeopaths reject the theory that diseases have an essentially miasmatic character.

MIGRAINE

A common problem that goes straight to the head

One of the most common ailments of the nervous system, migraine causes recurrent HEADACHES and sometimes other neurological symptoms, such as numbness, tingling or weakness on one side of the body.

The first sign of a migraine may be an 'aura', or a premonition that an attack is imminent. There may be visual disturbance, such as bright spots or zigzag lines before both eyes. An aura is caused by temporary narrowing of the blood vessels supplying part of the brain. Minutes later, when the blood vessels, which had been tightly constricted, suddenly open up to allow a gush of blood to the brain, a severe, one-sided, throbbing headache follows, often with an aversion to light, and vomiting. Symptoms may last from a few hours to several days.

However, not all migraines follow the same pattern – and in some cases only the headache occurs.

Typically, migraine occurs after, rather than during, times of STRESS – for example, after an examination or important interview. It may also be related to sensitivity to certain foods (see ALLERGY and FOOD ADDITIVES). Women are prone to migraine during menstrual periods. The oral contraceptive pill can also cause migraine, particularly during the pill-free week.

What the therapists recommend

ACUPUNCTURE

Consultation Practitioners ascribe migraine to a blockage of Qi energy in the yang channels of the head. Individual treatment depends upon the location of the pain, but the stomach and the large and small intestine meridians would probably be treated. MOXIBUSTION is also said to be effective.

ACUPRESSURE

Self help There are three points to be treated for migraine: on the hand, press at the end of the crease between finger and thumb towards the first finger bone; press in and upwards at the top of the neck beneath the skull and close to the sides of the spine; on the feet, press the web between the big and second toe inwards and up towards the centre of the foot.

BIOFEEDBACK

Consultation By visualising comfortable surroundings (see VISUALISATION THERAPY), such as being on the beach, in the bath, or in front of the fire, patients can relax – and, in doing so, restore normal blood circulation.

This technique, it is claimed, can be learned by using a biofeedback instrument that measures the temperature of the fingers – and informs the user when warmth is restored. With practice, sufferers are said to be able to ward off a migraine attack when they feel one coming on.

HOMOEOPATHY

Consultation Advice is given according to individual diagnosis, but one of the following remedies may be prescribed: *Iris vers.* for blurring of vision before the onset of headache, vomiting and/or when the scalp feels tight; *Nat. mur.* for throbbing, burning headache, or when tingling or numbness in the face signals an attack; *Sanguinaria* for a right-side headache which starts at the back of the head and extends to the right shoulder; and *Spigelia* for a left-side headache made worse by bending or movement, and when pain pulses in time with heartbeats.

IONISATION

Whether related to stress or sensitivity to some foods, a migraine attack is thought to release a substance called 5-hydroxytryptamine (serotonin) from blood platelets. Negative ions are believed to reduce the amount of serotonin carried by the platelets, so that when something triggers an attack, less of the substance is released and both the chances of an attack or the severity of it are reduced.

One of the three acupressure points for treating migraine is the area at the top of the neck. To gain relief, the sufferer should press inwards and upwards below the skull and near to the sides of the spine.

Other alternative treatments

Reflexology Massage is given to the reflex areas relating to the head, and to the spine, eyes, sinuses, pituitary, thyroid and reproductive glands, the digestive system, liver and solar plexus (see chart, p. 295).

Massage The treatment is the same as that recommended for HEADACHES.

An orthodox view

Anyone who suffers severe, recurrent headache should consult a doctor, who can make a diagnosis and check the patient's BLOOD PRESSURE. If migraine attacks are preceded by an aura, the doctor may prescribe ergotamine tablets. Ergotamine can be dangerous if taken in excess or during pregnancy, but if it is taken early, during the blood-vessel-narrowing stage of migraine, before headache develops, it can prevent the development of a full-blown attack. Newer drugs, such as sumatriptan, can bring relief even after attacks have started. For frequent sufferers, a doctor may also prescribe a drug to be taken every day to reduce the frequency of attacks.

If it is not possible to prevent or avert an attack in the early stages, doctors advise rest in a darkened room, painkillers and, if necessary, medicines to control vomiting.

A woman who has ever experienced numbness, tingling or weakness of part of the body during a migraine attack should tell her doctor, because some oral contraceptive pills may be inadvisable.

MIND AND BODY

Ways of keeping them in harmony

Most of us know only too well that illness and DEPRESSION often go hand in hand. We also know that when we feel at our best physically, we tend to be brighter, more optimistic and to have more mental energy.

Everyday language is full of phrases that link feeling with physical states. We speak of having 'butterflies in the stomach', 'shouldering a burden' or 'having a lump in the throat'. Similarly, physical factors both inside and outside the body (muscle tension, TIREDNESS, light and WEATHER, for example) can influence our thoughts and feelings.

Despite this, orthodox Western medicine generally makes a sharp distinction between mind and body. Doctors tend to confine their care to bodily illnesses and psychiatrists confine theirs to the mind.

Alternative therapies, however, are nearly always directed at the interaction of the two.

From ACUPUNCTURE and BIOFEEDBACK to YOGA and ZEN, they tend to view the person as a whole, needing harmony between body, mind and feelings before complete health can be achieved.

Most alternative therapies use one – or more – of four basic approaches to influence body and mind: food and drink, breathing, EXERCISE, and mental activity.

Of these, the food and drink approach is probably the most familiar. In alternative medicine, herbal extracts, vitamin supplements or HEALTH FOODS are likely to be recommended. Fasting for 24 hours is known to lower the adrenaline level in the blood and so reduce STRESS.

In AYURVEDIC MEDICINE, particular foods and drinks are used to produce mental and emotional changes, and many spiritual traditions believe that certain diets can enhance spiritual well-being.

Like food and drink, breathing is essential for life. Again, language reflects the link between breath and state of mind. We speak of being inspired (from Latin *inspirare*, to breathe in), we sigh when depressed, or talk of someone being a 'breath of fresh air'. In alternative medicine, rhythmic diaphragmatic breathing forms the basis of most relaxation techniques today, from NATURAL CHILDBIRTH exercises to HYPNOTHERAPY.

Exercise is a less common form of mind-body therapy in the West, where it is generally used simply to tone the muscles or to improve stamina. However, exercise can be very effective in relieving unpleasant moods and altering our state of mind.

Try going for a long walk next time you feel low or depressed – and notice how much better you feel. Or try a brisk run or some other form of demanding exercise to forget anger and frustration.

The process also works in reverse – changing the way we think can bring about changes in the body. MEDITATION is one of the most effective of these thought therapies, but it can be difficult to learn and keep up regularly. Easier, and more convenient to practise, is positive thinking – focusing on thoughts such as 'Every day, in every way, I am getting better and better'.

Images may be used as well as words, for example, in VISUALISATION THERAPY where a CANCER patient creates a mental picture of the body's defences attacking invading cancer cells.

Since alternative medicine is based on the idea of promoting well-being as a way of warding off (though often also curing) diseases, each of the four approaches is seen not just as a therapeutic measure, but as a vital part of daily life. Good health and a harmony of body and mind require the right balance of all four.

MINERALS

Getting enough of the essential traces

Your body contains about 25 essential minerals – chemical elements found mostly in inorganic (non-living) matter, but which are present in small proportions in living things. They are needed in small amounts for your body's chemistry to work properly. A diet which contains too little of any vital mineral, or anything that prevents it being absorbed into the body, can lead to deficiency disease and eventually to death.

Certain minerals, such as phosphorus and calcium, are present in the body in larger quantities than others. Phosphorus makes up about 1,5 per cent – just over 1 kg – of an average 70 kg healthy adult, mostly in bones and teeth, and the total body content of the mineral is replaced every three years. Calcium accounts for about 2 per cent of body weight, and again it is present mostly in bones and teeth.

Iron forms only some 0,006 per cent of body weight, the average adult body containing only 4,2 g. Yet it is critical for life. About half of it is contained in the haemoglobin of the red blood cells. The iron is part of the pigment haem, which gives the cells their colour. Combined with the protein globin this forms the haemoglobin molecule, which has the unique ability to combine reversibly with oxygen, and is the means by which the gas is carried from the lungs to the body tissues. There it combines with glucose and other 'fuels' to produce energy for essential metabolic processes.

Some elements present are needed in even smaller quantities. These minerals are known as 'trace elements'. See the tables of the most important minerals and trace elements on pp. 242 and 243.

The amount of a mineral needed by the body varies with age and circumstances. Generally children require less than adults, but growing children – those under 17 years – need more calcium than adults. Women need more iron than men, and pregnant women and nursing mothers need more iron and calcium again.

Some minerals, notably sodium, can create problems because people tend to consume too much of them. Many doctors believe that too much sodium can be a cause of high BLOOD PRESSURE in some people. Excess sodium is usually taken as too much salt (sodium chloride). You can easily cut down the amount of salt that you add to your diet, but beware of manufactured foods. Salt is added to many of them, so read the labels and go for those items whose labels state that

Major minerals: what they do and how we obtain them

MINERAL AND NATURAL SOURCES	RECOMMENDED DAILY AMOUNT (RDA) AND BENEFICIAL EFFECTS	EFFECTS OF DEFICIENCY
Calcium Dairy products; hard tap water; fish, and especially sardines, pilchards and other fish whose bones are eaten; watercress; fortified cereals, white flour and its products.	RDA: 500 mg; 1 200 mg for pregnant women and nursing mothers. Growth and maintenance of healthy bones and teeth. Several essential processes, including nerve function, muscle contraction and blood clotting.	Deficiency of calcium is very rare. Its uptake is facilitated by vitamin D, and deficiency of the vitamin may cause rickets in children and osteomalacia (equivalent of rickets in adults).
Iron Red meat, kidney, liver; pulses; dried apricots and figs; cocoa; fortified white flour and products; fortified breakfast cereals; nuts, especially almonds.	RDA: 10 mg for men, 12 mg women, 13 mg pregnant women, 15 mg nursing mothers. Healthy blood function: distribution of oxygen to and removal of carbon dioxide and other waste products from body tissues by haemoglobin.	ANAEMIA. Extreme cases: depression of IMMUNE SYSTEM.
Magnesium Most foods, but especially green vegetables; wholewheat flour, cereals and products; milk; eggs; meat; nuts, especially peanuts; pulses; shellfish.	RDA: 300 mg; 450 mg for pregnant women and nursing mothers. Healthy bones and teeth. Proper functioning of muscles, nerves, metabolic enzymes, and vitamins B_1 and B_{12}.	Loss of appetite; nausea; weakness; ANXIETY; muscle cramps and tremors; INSOMNIA; rapid or irregular beating of the heart; HYPOGLYCAEMIA. Also PREMENSTRUAL TENSION.
Phosphorus Nearly all foods, but especially high-protein foods such as meat, dairy products, pulses.	RDA: 800 mg; 1 200 mg for pregnant women and nursing mothers. Healthy bones. Conversion and storage of energy in all cells. Muscle function. Function of some enzymes. The intestinal absorption of some foods.	Loss of appetite; weakness; bone pain; stiff joints; central NERVE DISORDERS; respiratory failure. **Excess** can prevent intestinal absorption of calcium, iron, magnesium and zinc.
Potassium Most foods, but especially fresh fruit; vegetables, including potatoes; meat; wholewheat flour, cereals and products; milk; coffee; tea. Salt substitutes.	RDA: 1 875-5 625 mg. Maintenance of body's balance of fluids, especially water. Maintenance of body's acid-alkali balance. Functioning of nerves and muscles.	Vomiting; abdominal distension; muscular weakness, paralysis; 'pins and needles'; loss of appetite; low BLOOD PRESSURE; thirst. Extreme cases, drowsiness, coma. **Excess** may be dangerous for people with some heart conditions – consult doctor.
Sodium Common salt (sodium chloride); baking powder; most foods, but especially cured meats, smoked fish, milk; tinned meats and vegetables; bakery products.	RDA: 2 000 mg (5 g common salt). As potassium.	May accompany dehydration, which causes low blood pressure. **Excess** causes oedema; hypertension (high blood pressure); HEART DISORDERS; some KIDNEY COMPLAINTS. In babies, DIARRHOEA and dehydration.

none has been added. Avoid also foods containing monosodium glutamate (MSG). This flavour enhancer and seasoning has a meat-like taste, and is widely used in soups and similar products.

On the whole, if you follow a healthy, well-balanced diet every day, you will undoubtedly get all the essential minerals that your body requires. The only possible exception is the mineral selenium.

It is estimated that many adults get only 20 per cent of the recommended daily amount (RDA) of selenium.

Several things affect the amount of food minerals that the body absorbs. One factor is the form that the minerals take. For instance, you will absorb far more of the iron present in meat than the iron which is contained in green vegetables.

Another factor is the combination of mineral sources at a single meal. For example, vitamin C from fresh fruit and vegetables will enhance the uptake of iron, but the tannin in tea will reduce it. Too much bran (see FIBRE) reduces the absorption of several minerals, including calcium and zinc. In addition,

anyone lacking vitamin D cannot absorb calcium properly.

Generally, refined foods have lost many of their minerals, including potassium, chromium and selenium. Refined flours and cereals have a greatly reduced calcium and iron content, so if you do eat these and their products, go for the fortified varieties to which calcium and iron have been added.

See also BIOCHEMIC TISSUE SALTS, HERBAL MEDICINE, HOMOEOPATHY, MEGAVITAMIN THERAPY, NATUROPATHY, EATING FOR HEALTH and FOOD ADDITIVES.

Trace elements: the minerals we need in minute amounts

TRACE ELEMENT AND NATURAL SOURCES	RECOMMENDED DAILY AMOUNT (RDA) AND BENEFICIAL EFFECTS	EFFECTS OF DEFICIENCY
Chromium Unrefined and unprocessed foods, but especially wholegrain flour, cereals and products; fresh fruits; nuts; liver; kidney; beef; brewer's yeast.	RDA: 0,05-0,2 mg. Metabolism and storage of fats and sugars; functioning of skeletal muscles; partial control of body's IMMUNE SYSTEM.	Very rare, but may cause irritability, confusion, weakness, DEPRESSION.
Cobalt Meat, liver, kidney; eggs.	RDA: none laid down. Essential component of vitamin B_{12}.	Lack of vitamin B_{12} leads to pernicious ANAEMIA, weak muscles, BOWEL DISORDERS, NERVE DISORDERS.
Copper Most foods, but especially shellfish (particularly oysters), nuts (brazils), cocoa, liver, kidney; brewer's yeast; tap water supplied through copper pipes.	RDA: 0,05-0,2 mg. Functioning of many enzymes; red blood cell formation; bone growth.	Very rare, but may cause low white blood cell count, changes in hair colour and texture (not normal greying), DIARRHOEA.
Fluorine Fluoridated toothpastes and the like; tea, especially China tea; fish such as sardines and pilchards whose bones are eaten; cereals; meat.	RDA: 1 mg Probably for healthy bones and teeth.	Dental caries (decay); OSTEOPOROSIS. **Excess** causes fluorosis – mottling and discoloration of teeth; calcification of ligaments; increased density of bones in spine, pelvis and limbs.
Iodine Iodised table salt; seafood, including seaweed (kelp); meat, fruit and vegetables produced where soils contain iodine.	RDA: 0,14-0,15 mg. Production in the thyroid gland of hormones that control metabolism, and therefore healthy growth and development.	GOITRE; drop in metabolic rate, leading to drowsiness, lethargy, fatigue, increased weight. In pregnancy and from birth can lead to cretinism.
Manganese Many foods, but especially wholegrain cereals, nuts, tea, pulses, avocados.	RDA: 2,5 mg. Control of growth; the functioning of many enzymes, nerves and muscles; strong, healthy bones.	Decreased growth rate; bone deformities. **Excess** may cause brain damage.
Molybdenum Many foods, but especially buckwheat, barley, oats, liver, pulses.	RDA: 0,15-0,5 mg. Prevention of dental caries; iron metabolism; male sexual function.	Increased dental caries; IMPOTENCE; in extreme cases, irregular heartbeat, coma.
Selenium Unrefined foods, especially wholegrain flour, cereals and products; seafood; egg yolk; liver; kidney; brewer's yeast; GARLIC.	RDA: 0,05-0,2 mg. Healthy liver function; with vitamin E selenium is an antioxidant, and detoxifies elements such as cadmium, lead and mercury; the proper functioning of red and white blood cells.	Cardiovascular disease; possibly infant cot death and some types of ANAEMIA.
Sulphur Animal and vegetable proteins (meat, dairy products, pulses).	RDA: none laid down. Normal protein synthesis; strong hair, nails and skin.	
Zinc Most foods, but especially liver and red meat; egg yolk; dairy produce; wholegrain flour, cereals and products; seafood, particularly oysters.	RDA: 15 mg; 20 mg for pregnant women; 25 mg for nursing mothers. Functioning of many enzymes, and thus normal growth and development; the release of insulin (see DIABETES) and of vitamin A; healthy reproduction; the healing of cuts and wounds.	Slow physical, mental and sexual development; INFERTILITY; and the slow healing of wounds.

MINERAL WATER

Better from bottles than your tap?

Drinking spring water for therapeutic reasons is mentioned in early Chinese writings, and in Britain the Celts and Romans practised a form of what is now called HYDROTHERAPY, notably at Aquae Sulis (Bath). However, it was on the Continent that 'taking the waters' or 'cure' became really popular, and by the 18th century it was the fashionable thing for the rich to do. Numerous medicinal properties were claimed for rival waters, especially as cures for RHEUMATISM and similar ills. In the 19th century South Africa, too, acquired its popular spas at places where spring waters with special health-giving properties were discovered. One of the best patronised of these resorts was on the outskirts of Caledon (where the chalybeate, or iron-containing, baths had been used since the days of the Dutch East India Company).

Another popular watering place in the Cape was Montagu, while in the Transvaal there were such well-established resorts as Warmbaths, whose curative mineral waters are rich in sodium chloride, calcium carbonate and other salts.

The bottling and sale of spring – or natural – mineral water soon followed, and today the industry is 'big business' both in Europe and South Africa. One of the world's largest firms is Source Perrier near Nîmes in southern France, which normally sells more than 2 000 million bottles a year. However, sales were affected early in 1990, when the company withdrew its entire stock of 160 million bottles from the market. This followed the discovery that the water was contaminated with the petroleum-derivative benzene, which is thought to induce CANCER. The company blamed the problem on inefficient filtration at its spring at Vergèze, but resumed normal production once the filters had been cleaned.

Natural mineral water is not healthier than good, clean tap water – you may simply prefer the taste of bottled water, and with ice and a slice of lemon or lime it makes a refreshing alternative to alcoholic drinks.

The most common MINERALS found in bottled waters are bicarbonates, sulphates, ni-

Visitors to Karlsbad (now Karlovy Vary in Czechoslovakia) in about 1895 drink from the Vridlo (der Sprudel), the best known of the spa's 17 active springs. Its alkaline, sulphurous water issues at 72°C (160°F).

Do's and don'ts of mineral water

Do use a brand of bottled water that you know if you doubt the purity of local tap water.

Do boil bottled water and allow it to cool before making up babies' feeds with it.

Do remember that mineral waters, like all water, have a mild diuretic effect – they increase your flow of urine – and the greater the mineral content, the greater the effect.

Don't drink natural mineral water if you are on a SALT-FREE DIET, for sodium chloride is one of the most common minerals in bottled waters. If you are on such a diet, you should read the label carefully and seek professional advice on what you can and ought not to drink.

Don't drink waters with more than 20 mg sodium/litre if you are on a low salt diet.

Don't regularly give water with more than 1,5 mg fluoride/litre to babies or children, as it can cause mottling and weakening of the teeth.

Don't assume that bottled water will necessarily help those people who are allergic to tap water – mineral water may also contain chloride and other substances that are implicated in the allergy. Seek professional advice.

Don't drink bottled waters instead of milk as a substitute source of calcium – even the most calcium-rich mineral waters contain only about 12 per cent of milk's calcium.

trates, chlorides, calcium, magnesium, potassium and sodium. Of these, calcium and bicarbonate are by far the most common. A few mineral waters contain iron and/or iodine.

While the European Community (EC) has strict laws governing 'natural mineral water', in South Africa the same legislation applies to bottled mineral waters as to any other bottled 'soft drinks'. On labels the word 'natural' has to be used with great caution: nothing must either have been added to or removed from the water. Any health-giving properties claimed for the drink must have been scientifically substantiated. And it is illegal to state that the drink has been recommended by doctors.

MORNING SICKNESS

Feelings of nausea and sickness which are common in early PREGNANCY are caused by increased hormone production, triggered by the woman's condition. This so-called morning sickness can actually strike at any time of the day or night. It usually comes during the first three months of pregnancy, but can happen even before the woman has missed a period – and it very occasionally persists right into late pregnancy.

In severe cases – known as *Hyperemesis gravidarum* – the mother vomits so much that she risks becoming dehydrated and must receive medical attention.

What the therapists recommend

Herbal Medicine Make an infusion (see p. 184) of fresh ginger and sip frequently. Since morning sickness may be associated with lowered blood sugar levels, ginger biscuits may give relief. Also held to be beneficial are peppermint or camomile teas.

Homoeopathy These remedies are believed to be particularly appropriate because their great dilutions mean they pose no risk to mother or child. *Ipecacuanha* is recommended for constant NAUSEA and VOMITING and lack of thirst; *Argentum nitricum* for nervousness and panic, and a craving for sweet foods. *Sepia* may help if the vomit is pale and full of mucus, but the appetite is good and the mother feels sad and indifferent. Try *Pulsatilla* when fatty foods aggravate the condition, symptoms are worse late in the day and the mother is tearful but better for fresh air.

Naturopathy Eating small, frequent meals and avoiding fried, fatty foods may be helpful. Wholewheat toast or a dry biscuit in the morning can often relieve the problem, and

the woman should take plenty of fluid – but not milk – to counteract dehydration if she is actually being sick.

An orthodox view

Conventional doctors are extremely reluctant to prescribe medicines in early pregnancy because of potential adverse effects on the developing baby. Practitioners can, however, examine the mother-to-be to ensure that the pregnancy is progressing normally, offer reassurance and give advice about the importance of small, regular meals.

In severe cases it is sometimes necessary to admit the patient to hospital and give her fluids through an intravenous drip to prevent dehydration.

MOSQUITO BITES

Mosquitoes are found all over the world, especially in association with stagnant water (in which the insect's eggs are laid and hatched). To man, mosquito bites are usually more of a nuisance than a danger, producing pain and skin irritation. However, in some tropical and subtropical countries mosquitoes transmit parasites that cause serious diseases, including MALARIA.

Only the female mosquito is potentially harmful. When it bites, it injects its saliva into its victim's skin, causing a local irritation that draws blood to the surface. If the mosquito takes blood from an infected person, it will carry the disease, which will be spread each time the insect bites and injects infected saliva into another victim.

Of the many diseases spread by mosquitoes worldwide, malaria is the most serious. Carried by certain mosquitoes of the *Anopheles* genus, it is endemic in large areas of Asia, South and Central America, and Africa – including parts of the Transvaal, Natal and northern Cape. Attempts at global eradication have so far failed.

Dengue fever (breakbone fever), YELLOW FEVER and some forms of encephalitis, including St Louis encephalitis, are all spread by mosquitoes. However, it seems the AIDS virus is not transmitted by them, probably because the virus is killed by mosquito saliva.

What the therapists recommend

HERBAL MEDICINE

Self help Dab the affected areas with distilled witch hazel, or with a drop of essential oil of lavender, to reduce the irritation and inflammation. If susceptible to insect bites, sponge exposed areas of skin with camomile infusion, which will help deter the insects. To prepare the infusion, put 2 teaspoons of dried

Do's and don'ts if mosquitoes are troublesome

Do sleep in properly screened rooms and use a knockdown flyspray to kill mosquitoes that may have entered the room during the day.

Do use mosquito nets around the bed at night, checking that there are no holes, and tucking the edges under the mattress before nightfall. Protection may be enhanced by impregnating the material with permethrin. Use 0,2 g per square metre every six months.

Do use mosquito coils or an electric mat to vaporise synthetic pyrethroids in the bedroom overnight.

Do wear long-sleeved clothing and long trousers, and avoid wearing dark coloured clothes when out of doors after sunset, as such garments can attract mosquitoes.

Do use adequate insect repellants, such as diethyl toluamide, on exposed skin.

Don't rely only on electronic buzzers to ward off or kill mosquitoes because they are inadequate.

leaves in a cup and fill it with boiling water. Allow it to infuse for five to ten minutes, strain and use when cold.

An orthodox view

Visitors to affected areas of Africa and South America should be immunised against yellow fever at least ten days before they travel. One dose gives protection for ten years.

If you are visiting malaria-infested areas, your doctor will prescribe daily or weekly tablets and will select them carefully, for some strains of the disease parasite have become resistant to certain drugs. It is vital that the antimalaria treatment starts a week before travel and continues for four weeks after you leave the malaria zone.

If you are bitten, calamine lotion and antihistamine creams or tablets will relieve the symptoms. After returning from an area where malaria or other serious diseases are endemic, seek medical advice without delay if you develop a feverish, sweating illness, particularly if accompanied by headache. Some malaria parasites have an incubation period of ten months, so the symptoms may develop up to ten months after your return from a malarial region.

MOTION SICKNESS

Seasickness can be the most uncomfortable manifestation of this all-too-common problem, and many sailors remain affected by it throughout their careers – Nelson, Britain's greatest naval hero, was believed to be a lifelong sufferer. However, as many know to their cost, motion sickness can also affect travellers by road, rail or air.

The cause is an imbalance between what the eyes see and what the delicate inner ear balance mechanisms feel during movement. The eyes adjust to motion, but the inner ear does not, and the resulting signals to the brain from eye and inner ear do not tally. Symptoms are usually less severe if the eyes can see dry land or the horizon, or if the eyes are kept closed.

The symptoms cease quickly at the end of a journey, but may last up to 72 hours during long journeys. Children are more vulnerable than adults. However, some people adapt to regular travel, and the sickness diminishes on subsequent journeys.

What the therapists recommend

Acupressure A widely used remedy is to press a point three fingers' width above the wrist crease on the inner wrist, centrally, in line with the middle finger (Pericardium 6; see p. 13). Apply the pressure towards the centre of the wrist.

In some countries abroad, wristbands are available from certain chemists and at seaports, airports and railway stations, which perform the same function and have proved effective.

Homoeopathy If sickness is worse for the smell of food, try taking *Cocculus*. Use *Tabacum* for giddiness, weakness, nausea, sweating, the feeling of a tight band round the head, and if the smell of cigarette smoke is particularly nauseating.

Petroleum is recommended for nausea, vomiting and increased salivation by a patient who feels better when eating or lying down and worse in bright light. *Borax* is advised for a fear of sudden downward motion – such as is experienced when travelling by air and there is turbulence.

Aromatherapy Two drops each of peppermint and ginger essential oils on a tissue, inhaled regularly on a journey, are said to ease the discomfort.

Naturopathy Ginger is said to be one of the best remedies: chew a few pieces of fresh or crystallised ginger root during a journey. Some practitioners also recommend taking vitamin B_6 – 25 mg every two hours for adults, 10 mg for children.

An orthodox view

Do not talk about being sick in the presence of someone who is susceptible to motion sickness. Anticipation makes sickness more probable, whereas regular breaks and fresh air make the condition less likely. Try to ensure that susceptible children can see out of a window and stay warm.

At the same time (if you are travelling by car) keep at least one window slightly open. Don't allow queasy passengers to read; and stop once every hour, or more often if necessary, to let passengers out. If you are travelling by boat, go up on deck (provided the weather permits it).

There are several antisickness medicines which help if taken before symptoms begin. Some contain atropine or related substances and may, as well as preventing sickness, cause a dry mouth and constipation. Others such as cinnarizine are antihistamines and may result in drowsiness, particularly if taken with alcohol.

If sickness does occur, lie down if at all possible and take small amounts of fluid regularly to prevent dehydration. Vomiting may in fact give some relief.

MOUTH ULCERS

Painful, small, shallow, round or oval ulcers, often with a grey base and yellowish edge, occur inside the lips or cheeks, on the tongue or elsewhere in the mouth. Sometimes known as 'aphthous ulcers', they can appear suddenly for no apparent reason, but may indicate that you are run down, or they may be STRESS-related.

Other causes can be dentures that are ill-fitting, or over-vigorous brushing of the teeth, which produces tiny abrasions that can then turn ulcerous. You may also inadvertently have bitten your tongue or the soft flesh inside the cheek.

A more serious cause is the herpes virus (see COLD SORES). The first attack can be severe, with sore throat and several unpleasant-looking ulcers inside the mouth. Subsequent attacks are less severe, with fewer, smaller ulcers. So-called hand, foot and mouth disease (which is nothing to do with foot and mouth disease in cattle) is a common infectious disease of childhood in which there are small blisters on the hands and feet, as well as in the mouth. More rarely, mouth ulcers occur in association with drug allergy and in ANAEMIA and TUBERCULOSIS, among other complaints.

Self help If the ulcers coincide with feeling run down, check that your diet is a well balanced one (see EATING FOR HEALTH), and take more rest, with a general vitamin and mineral supplement. The ulcers may possibly be due to GLUTEN INTOLERANCE, so try a gluten-free diet for a week or two.

Use a soothing mouthwash several times a day: add two to three drops of essential oil of lemon, tea tree, camomile, sage or fennel to a cup of warm water.

What the therapists recommend

Herbal Medicine As herbalists generally see mouth ulcers as a sign of being run down, treatment looks at the underlying health as well as the ulcers themselves. A mouthwash of tincture of myrrh, available from herbalist stores and chemists, should clear up the ulcers in 48 hours if used every two hours or so. Chewing a piece of LIQUORICE root is both soothing and healing.

Homoeopathy If there is bad breath and increased salivation, try *Merc. sol. 6*. When the ulcers feel like sharp splinters, try *Nitric acid 6*. When the ulcers are on the soft palate and bleed when touched or during eating, and the mouth feels tender and hot, *Borax 6* is the recommended treatment.

Naturopathy Practitioners consider that mouth ulcers are often caused by lowered vitality, stress and inadequate nourishment. Fresh vegetables and fruit are recommended to cleanse the system, although some foods may add to the acidity in the mouth. Occasionally, the problem may be related to vitamin B_2 deficiency; in this case wheatgerm or brewer's yeast, together with extra vegetables, are recommended in the diet. Practitioners may in addition recommend taking vitamin C with zinc.

An orthodox view

Most mouth ulcers disappear in a few days. Mouthwashes or local anaesthetic lozenges such as benzocaine (available without prescription) help to keep the mouth clean and relieve pain. However, take care that you do not numb the mouth before a meal as this might lead to choking.

Glycerine is a well-tried remedy to soothe the soreness of mouth ulcers: apply it with the fingertip. Repeat at regular intervals.

If the symptoms are persistent or severe, you should see a doctor to exclude any underlying cause. The doctor may prescribe local preparations which tend to encourage the healing process.

If you find a hard lump in your mouth and it persists for more than two weeks, consult your doctor or dentist to check that it is not a malignant growth. It could well be an abscess, or a non-cancerous cyst.

An old lump that ulcerates or changes in some other way should likewise be shown to a doctor immediately.

MOXIBUSTION

Toning the body's flow of vital energy

Practitioners use this technique as well as the insertion and manipulation (or electrical stimulation) of needles in ACUPUNCTURE. It is a way of applying heat locally to regulate, tone and supplement the body's flow of Qi (vital energy).

The practice is particularly popular in China and Japan, and has been found especially useful for relieving post-operative pain and for helping chronic conditions such as ARTHRITIS.

The word moxa is derived from the Japanese term 'mogusa' signifying 'burning herb'. Two methods of moxibustion exist, and they both employ moxa wool – prepared either by drying and shredding leaves of the common mugwort (Artemisia vulgaris, Chinese wormwood) or by drying the hairy white down from its leaves. Certain other plant materials are sometimes used instead.

In the heated needle method, the practitioner inserts acupuncture needles, then places small cones of moxa on the needle heads and ignites them. (The needles are sometimes inserted through discs of cardboard or similar material to prevent any ash falling onto the patient's skin.) The gentle heat so generated passes down the needles into the body.

Where moxibustion is used to relieve internal pain it is thought to act as a mild counter-irritant: by irritating nerve endings in

Roll of paper method
The practitioner fills a roll of paper with moxa wool and then lights it. She holds the lighted tip above the appropriate acupuncture point. The practitioner withdraws the tip when the heat becomes too hot for the patient's comfort.

Heated needle method
First of all, the practitioner inserts an acupuncture needle – or needles – in the selected acupuncture point. She then puts a small cone of moxa wool on the the head of the needle and sets it alight. As a gentle heat is generated, it travels down the needle and into the patient's body. Sometimes the needle is inserted through material so that hot ash does not fall onto the patient's skin. Both methods attempt to cure or relieve specific ailments and allow the unimpeded flow of good health.

the skin it alleviates deep-seated pain found in the same area.

In the other method, the therapist fills a roll of paper some 15 cm long with moxa, lights it, holds the glowing tip safely above the acupuncture point until it becomes too hot and then withdraws it. The number of times this is repeated varies according to the condition of the individual patient and the nature of the complaint.

Moxibustion has been compared to the Western medical practice of cauterisation – not accurately, however, for cauterisation entails burning or destruction of body tissue, for example in order to stop bleeding during a surgical operation. Moxibustion is an altogether gentler form of treatment.

MUD THERAPY

Putting dissolved minerals to work – on the body

The ancient Greeks discovered the therapeutic value of certain muds which are rich in dissolved minerals and plant substances, and mud baths are still available at certain SPAS and HEALTH FARMS. On the Continent, Black Sea resort spas in particular have long specialised in this form of treatment. See HYDROTHERAPY.

The benefits that are derived from the many different sorts of mud used are said to come from health-giving substances in decayed plant matter and soil that accumulate in them at certain sites over hundreds of years. The composition of each differs, according to the minerals and plants found in the area.

Mud at one of the most famous mud spas, Neydharting in Austria, has been shown to contain natural antibiotics, VITAMINS in large quantities, as well as MINERALS, trace elements and other organic matter.

Apart from taking mud baths, mud packs can be applied to the skin. Packaged mud products – including shampoos and cosmetics – from well-known spas such as Neydharting can also be bought from health shops for use in the home.

No one knows exactly how mud therapy works, but most theories assume that the beneficial substances in it penetrate the skin, possibly entering the bloodstream and circulating throughout the body. In addition, tiny nerve fibres in the outer layers of skin may be stimulated, so that the whole nervous system benefits.

Quite apart from the other properties of mud, its heat alone is of therapeutic value, toning and energising the bather's nervous

Patients of both sexes wallow in a therapeutic mud bath in the south American republic of Colombia. Such baths are recommended treatment for arthritis and rheumatism.

system. And mud can be tolerated at a higher temperature than hot water.

The drying, abrasive action of mud on the skin is thought to augment the cleansing and invigorating effects of mud baths which have been compared to taking vigorous exercise – increasing the heart rate, speeding up circulation and encouraging sweating, helping to rid the body of impurities.

The mud treatment can be used not only for toning the system generally, but for easing particular complaints – RHEUMATISM, ARTHRITIS, SKIN DISORDERS, INFERTILITY and other disorders of the female reproductive system. Some mud extracts can even be drunk and are claimed to relieve stomach ULCERS and other DIGESTIVE PROBLEMS.

MUESLI

Making your own good-health food

The German-Swiss doctor Max Bircher-Benner (1867-1939) initiated muesli's present popularity. He discovered that a staple part of the diet of the exceptionally fit and long-lived inhabitants of certain country areas of Switzerland was muesli. This was made from various combinations of wheat, oats or barley with nuts, fresh fruit and berries, honey and milk. The doctor's discovery confirmed his own faith in a RAW FOOD DIET, and he introduced at his small clinic in Zürich his own

recipe – a simple mixture of oatmeal, grated apples or berries and milk.

Today there are many brand versions of Dr Bircher-Benner's original low-fat, protein and fibre-rich muesli on sale. 'Swiss-style' mueslis are soft and usually have added salt, milk powder and sugar – up to about 20 per cent. So-called 'natural' mueslis contain no added salt and sugar. 'De luxe' brands have higher proportions of fruit and nuts, while the 'crunchy' mueslis generally include toasted or cooked ingredients, frequently coated with honey or sugar.

A bowl of your favourite muesli at breakfast makes a good start to the day, and making your own is both easy and much cheaper than relying on brand varieties. It allows you to use fresh fruits and berries in season, and to include different ingredients to ring the changes and suit your preferences. It also allows you to control the amount of sugar or salt – if any – that you add.

A useful basic recipe contains: 360 g mixed cereals – rolled oats or oatmeal; rye, barley or wheat flakes; millet; 240 g dried fruit – sultanas, raisins, chopped dates or figs, apple, banana, apricot, pineapple; 60 g seeds – sunflower, sesame, pumpkin; and 30 g chopped nuts – almonds, brazils, hazelnuts, walnuts, coconut. These quantities will be sufficient for about eight to ten average portions.

Mix the ingredients and store in an airtight container. Then serve as required, adding fresh fruit and/or berries and milk, preferably semiskimmed milk for adults. When buying the cereals, make sure that they contain no added sugar or salt. Additional

oat bran flakes or wheatbran will provide extra dietary FIBRE if needed, while wheat germ will boost the muesli's content of vitamins B and E.

See also EATING FOR HEALTH.

MULTIPLE SCLEROSIS

A disease that affects one in 2 000

Known for short as MS, multiple sclerosis results from damage to the sheaths surrounding the nerve fibres of the central nervous system. Like electric wire without insulation, affected nerves are unable to function properly. The cause of multiple sclerosis is unknown and subject to much research. About one person in 2 000 is affected, women more often than men. The average age of onset is about 30.

Symptoms usually develop over a period of hours or days. The disease may attack only once, but usually runs a course of relapses (attacks) and remissions (periods of recovery) over many years.

Some 40 per cent of cases begin with blurred, dimmed or double vision. Sufferers may develop weakness, numbness or lack of co-ordination. They may also become clumsy, develop slurred speech or lose full control over their bladder and bowels (see INCONTINENCE).

Self help MS sufferers should make sure that their diet is low in fats and high in FIBRE. Avoid sugar and all sugar-containing items such as chocolate. Do not drink stimulants such as coffee, tea and cola drinks; use fructose (fruit sugar), weak lemon tea, decaffeinated coffee, herb teas and fresh fruit and vegetable juices. Be sure to avoid pulses (beans, peas, lentils), white bread and pasta, peanuts, salted nuts, hot spices and other such flavourings.

Stop SMOKING and avoid other people's smoke. Cut out all alcohol, especially if your balance is impaired.

What the therapists recommend
YOGA
Self help Effective breathing, in which the diaphragm is the body's pump, is said to enhance the electrical charge running through the nervous system and stimulate activity. Where muscles are constricted, relaxation and relaxed breathing may ease the tension.

The stress factor in MS is severe, and yoga provides a force to counter this. The postures, linked with calm mental processes and improved breathing, are said to provide an important stimulus to the patient's use of the affected limbs.

MASSAGE

Consultation General massage of the entire body is applied, if possible using slow, rhythmic and fairly deep movements of effleurage and kneading. Massage of the legs is most beneficial in maintaining some degree of muscle tone and, equally important, abdominal massage helps avoid constipation, which is often suffered by those unable to take normal exercise.

In the early stages, regular treatment – on a daily basis if possible – helps the nourishment and tone of the muscles, and encourages patients to persevere with light trunk exercises.

In later stages, when the sufferer is confined to bed, massage of the legs and abdomen continues as long as the patient derives benefit from it.

NATUROPATHY

Consultation This is not a complaint for which self help can be advised, but there may be scope for individual advice on nutrition, to support the nervous system. In recent years, some benefit has been claimed with evening primrose oil capsules – but see a qualified practitioner first.

ANTHROPOSOPHICAL MEDICINE

The actual nature of the treatment by this holistic school of medicine depends on the therapists' diagnosis of the MS sufferer, and on the particular imbalances which exist in his or her system.

Rhythmic massage, dietary measures, herbal medicines (for example, arnica or belladonna), and a course of injections are some of the options.

An orthodox view

The first task of a conventional doctor is to diagnose the disease. As well as performing a thorough neurological examination, including testing skin sensation, muscle power, co-ordination and reflexes, the doctor may recommend a lumbar puncture. A local anaesthetic is given, and fluid is withdrawn for testing from around the spinal cord through a needle inserted into the small of the back.

Treatment includes prescribed courses of steroid injections such as prednisolone or ACTH (adrenocorticotrophic hormone), physiotherapy to maintain bodily function, and occupational therapy to help the patient cope with disabilities. He should be given encouragement to strengthen his muscles, so far as this is possible, and to keep them mobile; suitable exercises can be recommended by a doctor or therapist. Given the

determination, an MS sufferer can lead a long and relatively active life.

Although doctors, nurses, therapists and counsellors can help sufferers, there is no orthodox medical cure for MS. The South African National Multiple Sclerosis Society is a valuable source of support and advice for affected people and their families.

For more information write (enclosing a stamped, self-addressed envelope) to the national secretary, Mrs I Henderson, 295 Villiers Road, Walmer, Port Elizabeth 6070; or to the national chairman, Mr Norman Abbott, 52 Captain Proctor Street, Brandwag (Bloemfontein) 9301.

MUMPS

The most common recognisable sign of mumps is swelling in front of the ear and over the angle of the jaw as one of the saliva-producing (parotid) glands becomes enlarged. The corresponding gland on the other side may also swell a day or two later.

Mumps is an infectious disease which occurs in epidemics and mainly affects children over the age of two. Along with the swollen glands, there may be earache, particularly when eating. Other saliva-producing glands situated under the tongue and jaw may also become swollen.

Since the incubation period is 15 to 21 days before the visible symptoms appear, it is impossible to stop the infection from spreading. The virus, which is similar to that of INFLUENZA, is carried through the air, so the disease can be caught simply by being close to an infected person.

Adult men who catch mumps can suffer painful complications – swelling and inflammation of one (or rarely, both) of the testicles. In girls, inflammation of the ovaries or pancreas can cause abdominal pain. In some rare cases, encephalitis or meningitis – inflammation of the brain or its surrounding membranes, or meninges – can result.

What the therapists recommend

Herbal Medicine If there is an increase in temperature, infusions (see p. 184) of yarrow or elderflower are advised, to induce sweating; try a cupful, hot, every few hours. Marigold added to the infusion is said to relieve the swollen glands. Medical herbalists may use more potent remedies, such as poke root, which requires careful dosage.

Naturopathy Because of the difficulty in eating that can arise due to the swollen glands, it is sensible to increase liquids, such as soup, in the diet. However, it may not be advisable to drink too many fruit juices that are

acidic. Supplements to boost the IMMUNE SYSTEM may be prescribed, and a cold compress will reduce swelling.

Homoeopathy For the early, acute stages, when there is pain, fever, restlessness and thirst, *Aconitum* 30 is suggested; if the testicles are affected, *Pulsatilla* 6. Try *Belladonna* 3 when fever is accompanied by throbbing pain, worse on the right side. When worse on the left side, and in cold, damp weather, *Rhus tox.* 6 is indicated.

Biochemic Tissue Salts Try *Ferr. phos.* alternating with *Kali mur.* hourly while the fever lasts, *Kali mur.* alone for glandular swelling and pain when swallowing, and *Calc. phos.* during convalescence.

An orthodox view

Doctors recommend immunisation with MMR vaccine against MEASLES, rubella (German measles) and mumps, for all babies during their first year. As mumps becomes less common through immunisation, so too should serious complications, such as meningitis and inflamed testicles, which in adult males occasionally causes sterility.

There is no specific cure for the disease, but a few days of rest and, if necessary, paracetamol or children's aspirin to reduce fever and ease discomfort are all that is required. Consult a doctor if earache or HEADACHES are severe, if the neck becomes stiff, or if the testicles in adult males become painful or swollen.

MUSCULAR DYSTROPHY

Alternative therapists can offer both practical help and psychological support to victims of this progressive, muscle-wasting disease; but like conventional doctors, they cannot promise a cure. For the disease – commonly called simply MD – is hereditary and cannot be reversed. It usually appears in one of three distinct forms:

The Duchenne-type begins in childhood and affects only boys between four and ten years old. It starts with weakness in the legs. The child tends to waddle, cannot climb stairs properly, and can rise to his feet only by using his hands to 'climb up' his legs. In facio-scapular-humeral MD, the face, shoulders and arms are mostly affected. The disease tends to strike during the teens or young adult life of both sexes. Limb girdle MD affects the shoulders or hips during the twenties or thirties in both sexes. This type runs a slower, less-severe course than other forms of the disease.

In certain cases of MD, there is *pseudohypertrophy* of the muscles, meaning that they are enlarged, but weak. Generally, the best outlook is for those who develop the disease late in life.

What the therapists recommend

MASSAGE
Consultation A brisk, but very brief, full body massage is probably of most benefit. Otherwise, the massage should be confined to only a few minutes' treatment of the affected limbs: effleurage stroking and kneading movements should be given, with the aim of toning up the muscles and improving blood supply, and delaying atrophy and contraction for as long as possible.

Physical therapy is extremely important in the treatment of muscular dystrophy and massage can be valuable. However, on a long-term basis, its value is largely in making the condition seem less severe, rather than in bringing about actual improvement.

HYDROTHERAPY
Consultation Needle spray or vortex baths would be advised, to promote or improve circulation in the affected limbs. This would be followed by specific exercise programmes, suited to each patient's particular condition, in a HYDROTHERAPY pool.

An orthodox view

Despite intense medical research, there is still no cure for muscular dystrophy, or any sure means of determining whether affected potential parents will pass it on to their offspring. Doctors confirm their diagnoses by finding raised levels of muscle enzymes, or ferments, in blood samples, and by surgical removal and examination of a small sample of muscle. Sufferers may benefit from advice from specialist therapists, such as occupational therapists, and from the support and advice of a family contact group, of which there are a number throughout South Africa. For the address of a group in your area write to the Muscular Dystrophy Research Foundation, P O Box 81306, Parkhurst 2120.

MUSIC THERAPY

The rhythm of life as a healing force

The need for self-expression is satisfied not only by speaking but also by music. Its rhythms and harmonies, the pattern of its sounds and silences make a powerful impact on our senses, often touching feelings too deep or difficult to express in words. Continually bottling up such emotions can cause distressing mental – even physical – problems. See also PSYCHOTHERAPY and HUMANISTIC PSYCHOLOGY.

Since ancient times music has been closely connected with healing – an association that declined as a scientific basis for treatments became the test of acceptability. Only recently has the use of music in therapy been researched and found valuable. Individual responses may vary, but many of us are deeply affected by music. And actually making music – however crudely – allows us to express a range of emotions, from anger and frustration to tranquillity and joy.

It is these expressions and responses that music therapists, who are trained musicians, can observe and work with. Therapists believe that clients can be helped in the widest possible way – physically, mentally, emotionally and spiritually. The therapy depends, however, on a satisfactory reaction between therapist and client, as shared music-making frees the client to reveal deep – sometimes totally submerged – feelings and problems.

The improvised music that they play or sing together is ideally chosen or initiated by the client (who may, through disability, be unable to ask directly), no matter how simple the music or the means of making it may be. This improvised music, composed for that particular moment in the therapy, is considered an essential factor in the treatment.

It is not only in the psychotherapeutic approach that music is valuable. Physically handicapped people who may need to improve their movement or breath control, for example, are often more enthusiastic about playing even a simple instrument or singing than about doing pure exercises.

Who it can help South African practitioners of music therapy consider that it can be of help in a very broad range of situations, from childbirth to hospice work. The mentally handicapped, the mentally ill and the physically handicapped can also benefit.

Children who are referred by education authorities to child development and assessment centres, or who are being given special education, are treated.

Elderly people – whether they are attending care units or day centres – can also benefit, as can people attending community health centres, and those who need help in coping with STRESS. Even prison inmates have responded very well to this form of treatment.

The client does not need to have any musical experience. Striking results have been obtained from people claiming not to be musical and those who have never learned to play an instrument.

Finding a therapist For information about practitioners in your particular area write, en-

How music can help an autistic child

Geoffrey is a seven-year-old child suffering from AUTISM. He can't talk, although he can make a wide range of vocal sounds. Like all autistic children, he finds it extremely difficult to establish relationships with other people; he prefers to relate to objects. He loves music and for the past three years has been receiving music therapy at home – with his mother taking an active part in the sessions.

Each week the therapist fosters a special bond between the two, by encouraging Geoffrey's mother to respond to him on his own level, singing to him and imitating and developing his vocal sounds. Through sharing a musical experience, Geoffrey feels that someone is showing an interest in him and that he can participate in a family activity.

'These sessions,' says Geoffrey's mother, 'have been an opportunity not to be missed. With the aid of the therapist, I have been able to help Geoffrey to open out and have developed a brand-new relationship with him. It is the one time in a busy week when he and I can share an experience which means a great deal to both of us.'

closing a stamped, self-addressed envelope, to the Music Therapy Society of Southern Africa, P O Box 44482, Linden 2104. The *South African Journal of Music Therapy*, published by the society, appears three times a year and is available in libraries.

Another body that will be able to help you is the Professional Board for Occupational Therapy, c/o South African Medical and Dental Council, P O Box 205, Pretoria 0001.

Music therapists must have ability both in music and psychology. At present no specialised training is available in South Africa, and many local practitioners have qualifications acquired abroad. However, the College of Music at the University of Cape Town – which until a few years ago offered a postgraduate course in remedial music – is planning soon to introduce a four-year Bachelor of Music (Musical Therapy) degree.

Consulting a therapist What happens at a session varies according to individual needs, but the broad approach is the same no matter what your age or problem. The therapist first observes the client's musical responses, asks questions aimed at discovering his needs, and assesses what music therapy programme could be arranged to best serve those particular needs.

This is an important time for therapist and client to get to know one another and feel comfortable together. A variety of instruments, such as piano, xylophone, glockenspiel, keyboards, guitar and drums will be available, and the therapist will also have an instrument.

For those with physical problems, the music is used to motivate movement. With someone whose problems are emotional or physical rather than intellectual, the therapist may discuss music, to find out what the client enjoys and to agree on a starting point for the therapy.

For a client who has difficulty speaking and understanding speech, the relationship has to begin with the music-making. This may be as simple as sharing an instrument and playing together, or beating 'messages' to one another on drums.

The client's responses are carefully observed so that the therapist can follow them up, so it becomes important that the client is brought to realise that the therapist is communicating through the music. But always the therapist aims to let the client choose and control what happens in the music, and realise that he can express what cannot, perhaps, be put into words.

The music is seen not as an end in itself, but as a means of building confidence and self-esteem and facing inner conflicts.

An orthodox view

Music therapy with a qualified therapist is a completely safe and very effective form of treatment. Research has shown that it is beneficial for people with mental disorders that prevent communication through speech, and also for people with physical disabilities.

MYALGIC ENCEPHALO-MYELITIS

ME – a mysterious, exhausting illness

Extreme exhaustion is the most characteristic symptom of myalgic encephalomyelitis – usually referred to simply as ME. But a number of other symptoms may afflict sufferers: muscle pains, especially after exercise; a persistent itchy skin rash; twitching of the muscles and limbs; chest pains; localised sweating; FEVER and shivering fits; HEADACHES; visual disturbances and RINGING IN

THE EARS; nausea and STOMACH COMPLAINTS; INSOMNIA; swollen glands; frequent need to pass urine; and a strong body odour.

Patients feel generally unwell and often experience worrying mental symptoms such as loss of memory and inability to concentrate, or psychological effects such as mood swings and DEPRESSION.

The symptoms develop following a failure to recover fully from VIRUS INFECTIONS. The initial infection, such as INFLUENZA or gastroenteritis, may be fairly trivial, and sometimes passes unnoticed by the patient. After virus infections people are often tired and lethargic for some weeks. In ME, however, the symptoms are more severe: even the slightest exertion may make the sufferer's muscles so weak that they need several days' rest to recover.

Medical researchers have found a number of abnormalities in ME sufferers, particularly changes in the IMMUNE SYSTEM and in the composition of muscle cells; but they have not yet been able to pinpoint the cause. A genetic defect in the immune system or an unusual reaction to one particular virus may be what triggers off the condition. The virus that causes GLANDULAR FEVER has been found in some ME sufferers, and many ME symptoms resemble the prolonged debilitation which often occurs after glandular fever. Other viruses implicated include enteroviruses (which enter the body and multiply in the bowels) and the CHICKENPOX virus.

These viruses, however, may only be triggers for certain people. Another factor frequently shared by ME sufferers is recent physical or emotional STRESS. Whatever symptoms affect individual ME sufferers, they usually follow a fluctuating course, with some easing between severe bouts.

The condition often strikes active, successful people, and those in their late twenties and early thirties are the most frequent victims. When ME was first recognised it was often dismissed as over-dramatised debility or as psychological in origin, a result of high-pressure modern lifestyles. The media rather scathingly dubbed it 'yuppie flu', but as more cases were reported to doctors, and scientists began to take it seriously, it was more often called postviral fatigue syndrome. In many cases this was more appropriate than its current cumbersome full name, which literally means inflammation of the brain and the spinal cord with associated muscular pain, and is quite erroneous.

The wide range of symptoms added to the difficulty of recognising the condition. The sufferers seemed to be affected by totally different ailments. In fact, most patients suffer many of the same symptoms but in numerous permutations of severity.

However, although some doctors remain sceptical, ME is now generally recognised as

an illness in its own right, and sufferers are entitled to treatment in the same way as people who have other recognised, if not more straightforward, ailments.

The ME Association of South Africa supports a network of self-help groups for sufferers. For information about a group near you, or for other advice, write to MEASA, P O Box 461, Hillcrest 3650.

What the therapists recommend

Naturopathy Poor functioning of the immune system is seen as an underlying cause, and a proliferation of yeasts – especially *Candida albicans* – in the intestines has often been found in ME patients. A radical, long-term change in eating habits and lifestyle may be recommended to help sufferers.

A wholefood diet based on unprocessed, additive-free, raw foods is usually suggested. You will be asked to keep a note of what you have eaten, to identify foods that provoke symptoms or worsen them, so that you know what to avoid. Fresh air is generally thought to be helpful, but exercise should be avoided. Some practitioners prescribe supplements of MINERALS and VITAMINS to boost the body's defence system.

Do's and don'ts for ME patients

Do get an accurate diagnosis before following any programme of treatment.
Do take plenty of rest and avoid stresses, both mental and physical.
Do avoid alcohol, and any foods that make the symptoms worse.
Don't have an anaesthetic or a vaccination unless it is essential.
Do keep notes about your diet, activities and symptoms. You are the best person to pinpoint what improves or worsens your condition.
Don't take supplements of the trace element germanium, which some claim boosts the immune system. Tests suggest it can cause severe kidney damage. And no thorough clinical tests have yet been made of claims that vitamin B_{12} injections, capsules of evening primrose oil, or antifungal drugs are safe for treating ME sufferers.
Do find an activity to occupy you in your weakest periods to stave off loneliness and depression – simple card games, jigsaw puzzles or keeping a scrapbook, for example.

Acupuncture A practitioner will advise treatment according to individual needs. Generally this is aimed at stimulating the immune system, ensuring that breathing and digestive problems do not develop, relieving pain and increasing strength and energy. Stimulation is given to the points diagnosed as appropriate on the spleen, governor, liver, conception, heart and kidney meridians.

Aromatherapy Try oil of lavender, which relaxes and soothes, to alleviate tiredness, weakness, pain and shiveriness. Oil of lemon is said to calm the mind and, combined with oil of lavender, to promote refreshing sleep. You can put drops of any of these oils on a tissue to inhale, or take a ten-minute warm bath with six or eight drops of oil added. For a drink, put two drops of geranium, thyme, lemon or sage oil on a tea bag, put the bag in a jug or teapot, then pour onto it 600 ml of boiling water. Drink this infusion without milk, keeping any that is left over in the refrigerator, to reheat as and when required.

Hydrotherapy Russian, Turkish or sauna baths, or ordinary hot baths at home, are used to stimulate circulation and promote relaxation. They are seen as particularly helpful for ME patients who feel shivery at night or have difficulty in getting to sleep. Hot and cold sitz baths may bring relief where muscular pains are troublesome.

Herbal Medicine Gentle relaxants and tonics such as wild oats, skullcap, vervain and St John's wort are recommended to aid rest and increase vitality.

Homoeopathy ME patients are said to have gained considerable relief of symptoms through the care of an experienced homoeopath, but no general remedies are prescribed, as the condition is so complicated. The practitioner starts by making a detailed assessment of the patient's constitution and the symptoms causing most trouble, and seeking information about the illness which triggered the onset of ME.

Bach Remedies Wild rose is recommended to combat exhaustion and Crab apple to purify the system. Feelings of confusion and low vitality may be helped by Clematis, while Heather may help to alleviate depressive symptoms. Walnut and Willow are suggested to overcome feelings of resentment and help acceptance of the newly restricted lifestyle while the illness lasts.

An orthodox view

Because neither physical examinations nor laboratory tests produce findings specifically related to ME, some doctors are still sceptical about the illness. Many have in the past dismissed it as malingering, or seen it as a psychiatric condition, but it is now generally recognised as a distinct clinical condition. There is increasing evidence that it is associated with the Epstein-Barr virus, which also causes glandular fever. Diagnosis is not easy, for tests must be made for other causes of muscle weakness and possible stress disorders, in order to rule them out.

General practitioners have reported that among ME sufferers are schoolchildren, whose complaints of feeling unwell may have been disregarded as unwillingness to go to school, or put down to many other causes before their true condition is recognised. Delay in diagnosis and unsympathetic treatment can have particularly severe consequences for children. They may fall far behind their classmates and even have to take an extra year at school – by which time the disease has taken hold.

Although there is no proven remedy, many patients do benefit from a course of antidepressant drugs. Some people are reluctant to take antidepressants because they naturally do not wish their problems to be seen by others as psychological.

But where frequent mood swings, disturbed sleep and poor concentration are occurring, this treatment may help, whether ME has a physical or a psychological cause.

MYOPIA

Myopia or shortsightedness is among the commonest of all EYESIGHT PROBLEMS, and it has been estimated that as many as 60 per cent of the population suffers from it to some extent. Those who are handicapped by this defect of vision can see near objects clearly, but distant objects are blurred.

The cause is an error of refraction, the process by which light is normally focused on the retina or screen of nerve-cells at the back of the eye. A myopic person's eyeball is too long in relation to the combined focusing power of his cornea and lens; as a result the image of a distant object is focused in front of the retina, not on it.

Sometimes this is an inherited condition. It may start in early childhood, though it is often not detected until the child first goes to school and is unable to read what has been written on the blackboard.

Conventionally, a shortsighted person has his eyesight tested by an ophthalmic optician (optometrist) and is then prescribed corrective spectacles with concave lenses. Alternative therapies offer the hope that the myopic condition of the eyes can itself be improved – by, for example, a sensible diet, loosening-up exercises for strained neck muscles, special exercises designed to improve the eye muscles, and techniques to cultivate memory and imagination.

Trial and error for a schoolgirl sufferer

It was in the autumn of 1987 that schoolgirl Flavia Boyd's mother began to suspect that her daughter had ME. By Friday each week, 13-year-old Flavia would be exhausted and ashen-faced, and sleep all weekend to recover. At first Mrs Boyd thought overwork could be the trouble. Flavia – able, conscientious, and very keen to do well at her schoolwork – would stick at her books until 10pm.

Then a bout of flu and severe gastroenteritis struck Flavia. Once she was back at school the gastroenteritis recurred and she became very depressed. Mrs Boyd had seen similar symptoms in her own sister, who was suffering from ME, and so was alert to the danger. Both the school and the family doctor were sympathetic to the problem, but the doctor knew little of how to treat ME – a new and little understood disease.

Low point By December, Flavia was too ill to go to school and it was six months before she returned. She was constantly fatigued and her muscles ached; she was bewildered by her condition and resentful about the time lost at school. Her tiredness and depression were made worse by poor nights, when frightening, technicolour nightmares disturbed her sleep.

In the absence of firm medical guidelines for treatment, the Boyds tried whatever they could – vitamin and mineral supplements in case there was some deficiency, and a diet made up of wholefoods, avoiding any items that might foster an abundance of yeasts in the bowel. Treatment for a suspected liver condition only made her worse. Flavia had made no improvement by March of the following year, when she had colonic irrigation to wash out the bowel.

On the mend This proved to be the turning point for her. During the early summer she made such progress that in June she went back to school part-time. The school, still co-operative, kept her workload down when Flavia pushed herself too hard to catch up on the work she had missed.

Eventually Flavia recovered completely. Today she is not afraid to be active at her many interests – but she has learned not to overtax herself.

NAIL PROBLEMS

Nails serve a protective purpose and, like the skin and hair, their condition reflects your overall state of health, as well as the treatment they receive.

To keep your nails strong and healthy, wear rubber gloves for household chores, avoid soaking your hands in water for long periods, eat a balanced diet (see EATING FOR HEALTH) and follow the instructions for HAND CARE on p. 162. Particular problems can be dealt with as follows:

Deformed nails Hollow, spoon-shaped nails may show iron deficiency (see ANAEMIA) while with RESPIRATORY DISORDERS or HEART DISORDERS nails can become clubbed or grow around the fingertips. Pitted nails can be a result of PSORIASIS. Treatment can prove difficult and, like the skin rash in psoriasis, the problem can recur.

Flaking, splitting or chipping Rough treatment or lengthy immersion in water is usually to blame, or sometimes a shortage of unsaturated fats in the diet.

These problems can generally be overcome by massaging a moisturising cream into the nails every day, and wearing work or rubber gloves for gardening and indoor tasks as necessary. Keep nails fairly short and file them in one direction only, never to a point. Always use an oil-based polish remover if you paint your nails.

Practitioners of HERBAL MEDICINE regard nail problems largely as a sign of nutrient deficiency – such as calcium or silica – in the diet. But a consultation and full treatment is advisable to investigate the underlying cause of the problem.

Naturopaths also regard such conditions as split or brittle nails often to be the result of inadequate nourishment. Calcium and vitamins A, B and D are recommended and a multivitamin and mineral supplement might be suggested.

Hangnails Frequent soakings in water can make the outer layer of skin pull away from the cuticle, causing painful splits called hangnails. Prevent them becoming infected by snipping dead skin off with sharp nail scissors, and always keeping the hands clean.

Be sure to wear rubber gloves for washing up and other domestic chores, and moisturise the skin with hand cream and cuticle cream every night.

Loose nails Regular use of commercial nail hardeners containing formaldehyde can separate nails from the skin underneath, opening the way to germs. Psoriasis and ECZEMA may cause a similar condition. The problem takes time to heal, but is helped by trimming the nails short and avoiding the use of hardeners containing formaldehyde.

Nail biting This is a common habit of both adults and children, and often stems from ANXIETY, TENSION or insecurity. It weakens the nails and may damage sensitive skin underneath. Painting the nails with one of the bitter-tasting products sold by chemists and keeping the hands occupied when idle – by knitting, for example – may help to break the habit.

PSYCHOTHERAPY and HYPNOTHERAPY have been used to help nail-biters come to terms with any insecurity or anxiety at the root of the problem. In some cases, however, the best remedy is to appeal to the individual's vanity or self-respect.

Nails turn black or purple Dark discoloration under a nail is a sign of bleeding due to prolonged pressure or to a blow. Usually such spots just grow out, but if bleeding is extensive the nail may loosen and fall off. Pain caused by pressure can be relieved by having a doctor lance the nail. A new one should grow in due course – the actual rate of growth varies between individuals.

Pale nails Anaemia may be responsible. Whitish nails may show a liver condition which should disappear when the underlying cause has been treated.

Red, inflamed cuticles A bacterial or yeast infection at the base of the nail is usually to blame (see FUNGAL INFECTIONS). The cuticles become swollen and sometimes small blisters develop. Eventually nails may become discoloured or deformed.

Self-help measures include taking supplements of zinc, vitamin C and vitamin B-complex, but it is usually necessary to see a doctor, who will probably prescribe an antibiotic or another drug or ointment to clear the infection.

Belladonna 30C is used by homoeopaths when skin at the nail base is red, painful and throbbing; the biochemic tissue salt H*epar sulph.* 6C is advised if the tenderness is acute and there is pus.

Ridges Crosswise ridges are the result of a calcium or zinc shortage, illness or injury to the nail – for example, from pushing cuticles back too hard. The ridges grow out with time, and may be prevented by protecting nails from further damage and taking a multimineral supplement. Women can use a commercial ridge-filler to smooth the surface before applying varnish.

Lengthwise ridges sometimes develop in old age or illness, possibly because of vitamin and mineral shortages, and supplements may be of help.

White flecks These are usually a sign of too little zinc or vitamin A in the diet. Eating more spinach, whole grains and sunflower seeds may help, or taking vitamins and minerals.

White, soft and crumbly nails Fungal infections are the cause. Eventually nails may thicken or grow ridges. Orthodox treatment with antifungal drugs and ointments is usually necessary.

Homoeopaths will generally recommend treating brittle nails that are red, swollen at the base, and sore with *Thuja* 6, three times daily for ten days. For slow-growing, white-spotted nails you should take *Silica* 6 twice a day for a month.

Yellow nails Staining can result from SMOKING, dyes in nail polish, or too much chlorine in swimming pools. Rub gently with a nail buffer and soak nails in lemon juice (or paint it on) to lighten the stain. Women should be sure to use a base coat before they start to apply nail polish.

Four common kinds of nail disorder

Deformed, spoon-shaped nails may indicate an iron deficiency in the diet. It may help to eat iron-rich foods such as broccoli, watercress, raisins and parsley.

Painful splits called hangnails may occur if the hands are frequently immersed in water. To prevent this, rubber gloves should be worn when doing washing up.

Loose nails are often caused by using nail hardeners containing formaldehyde. This can separate the nails from the underlying skin, allowing germs to enter.

White-flecked nails are mostly the result of a diet containing insufficient vitamin A or zinc. They may be remedied by eating spinach and sunflower seeds.

NATURAL AIDS TO BEAUTY

Creams, lotions, face packs and shampoos to make at home

Nothing you put on your skin or do to your hair can take the place of good health when it comes to looking your best. But with a balanced diet (see EATING FOR HEALTH), regular EXERCISE, a good night's sleep and satisfying work and relationships, cosmetics and toiletries made from natural ingredients can help a woman make the most of her looks.

The recipes given here are easy and inexpensive to follow. Many of the ingredients may even be found in your kitchen; the rest can be bought from a chemist or health shop. They do not include any of the chemical dyes, perfumes and preservatives that can cause ALLERGY when used in certain commercial products. You will also have the satisfaction of knowing that none of the preparations has been tested on animals.

A double boiler is useful for some of the recipes, but a heatproof bowl placed over a pan of boiling water will work just as well. Otherwise you need only ordinary kitchen utensils, storage jars and bottles. Wash and dry all utensils and containers thoroughly before using.

When buying the recommended essential oils, make sure that they are pure, and not synthetic or adulterated (see AROMATHERAPY). Always count out the stipulated number of drops.

Note Allergies to these preparations are rare, and a simple test will soon show sensitivity. Dab a little of each cream or lotion on the inside of the forearm and leave for 24 hours. If there is no reaction, it is safe to use. All these preparations are intended for external use only, and should not be swallowed.

Caution Remember that, because no preservatives are used in the homemade preparations given here, the creams and lotions will not last as long as commercial products. Always store your preparations in a cool, dry place, and use a spatula to extract and apply them, since putting your fingers into jars can promote the development of bacteria.

Moisturiser Suitable for face and hands, a simple mixture using equal quantities of glycerine and rose water has been a favourite moisturiser for many years. Reduce the proportion of glycerine to make a less greasy cream for oily skins, or increase it if your skin is dry.

To make a moisturising gel, dissolve a teaspoon of gelatine in 150 ml of hot water, then mix in a teaspoon of rose essential oil and 3 tablespoons of glycerine. If you prefer, use lavender, orange or another flower water in place of rose.

Facial cleansing cream Finely pare about 8 tablespoons of beeswax – bought from a health shop – with a sharp kitchen knife or grater. Heat gently with 450 ml of liquid paraffin in the top of a double boiler until melted. Allow to cool to 50°C (120°F), while separately heating 300 ml of water to the same temperature. When both are hot, slowly add the water to the wax and oil mixture, stirring continuously. Leave the mixture to cool until it begins to solidify, then pour it into storage jars.

Cold cream Pure aloe vera gel is available from most health shops and gives a pleasant texture to this cleansing and moisturising lotion – make it as shown in the illustration on the next page.

Facial toning lotion This contains sage to tighten the skin, close the pores and soothe any spots of inflammation. Use the lotion after cleansing the skin and before applying any moisturiser.

To make the lotion, place 4 tablespoons of dried sage – or 8 of the fresh herb – into a clean jar, and pour on it 150 ml of vodka. Tightly screw on the lid and leave it to stand. After a week strain off and discard the sage, replacing it with a similar new measure of the herb and leaving it for another week.

The liquid should now have a strong herbal smell, but for an even stronger lotion, repeat the procedure once more. Finally, strain the liquid into a clean bottle, using a fine sieve or a coffee filter. Add four or five drops of tincture of benzoin – available from chemists – screw on the lid and shake well.

To make a milder lotion, dilute with distilled water or use a less astringent herb such as camomile instead of sage. Stronger herbs such as yarrow, or the addition of 2-4 tablespoons of witch hazel, will strengthen the mixture.

Skin refresher Pawpaw fruit contains various enzymes that help to remove dead skin, leaving the face fresh and clean. Apply pulped fruit all over the face, leave for a few minutes and then wipe off. Splash with cool water and apply moisturiser, as pawpaw tends to dry the skin.

Facial masks These will cleanse and tone the skin, drawing out impurities and soothing sore or inflamed spots. Make them as shown in the illustration on the next page, mixing dry and liquid ingredients chosen to suit your skin.

Oatmeal and ground almonds are good all-purpose dry bases, suitable for any skin type; wheatgerm and brewer's yeast are said to nourish the skin; and kaolin clay to draw impurities to the surface, heal spots and improve circulation.

Other clays may also be used: bentonite to soothe and heal, and fuller's earth to absorb excess oil and stimulate the skin. Sulphur is sometimes used to treat ACNE and oily skins, but it can cause allergies so use with caution and test on a small area first.

Liquids to use for a greasy skin include witch hazel, beaten egg white, yoghurt, lemon juice or an infusion of yarrow, agri-

A wide selection of natural aids to beauty is available at health shops and pharmacies in South Africa. These include skin moisturisers, cleansing lotions, herbal shampoos and hair conditioners.

mony, raspberry leaf or lady's mantle. Dry skin can benefit from an application of egg yolk, honey, sour cream, pulped bananas or avocado, rose water, almond oil, or melon or carrot juice.

To invigorate the skin and improve circulation, try using rosemary, peppermint, nettle, elderflower or eucalyptus infusions in the mixture; to soften rough, dry skin, use aloe vera gel or 1-2 tablespoons of linseed or kelp gently heated in 150 ml of water until it thickens.

Herbal shampoo Choose the right herbs for your hair type when making this gentle shampoo: sage to condition and enhance dark hair, camomile to lighten and soften fair hair, mullein to intensify blonde highlights, parsley to thicken hair and enrich its colour, southernwood to stimulate hair growth, burdock root and nettle to control dandruff, and kelp or yarrow to encourage growth and check hair loss.

Into a heatproof jar place 1½ tablespoons of your chosen herbs, a teaspoon of pure-grade borax and 3 tablespoons of dried soapwort leaves or 2 tablespoons of dried root. Pour on 450 ml of boiling water and stir well, cover loosely and leave to cool. Allow the mixture to stand for a day or two, shaking regularly; then strain and use.

In this recipe, soapwort takes the place of the soap or detergent used in most shampoos. It has a good cleaning effect, but you will need to use a little more of the shampoo than of most proprietary types.

Soap shampoo A gentle, effective shampoo which rinses out better than commercial ones can be made with Castile soap, which is made from olive oil.

For fair hair, place 8 tablespoons of dried camomile flowers into a saucepan with 1 tablespoon of dried peppermint, 2 tablespoons of dried rosemary and 600 ml of distilled water.

For dark hair, substitute dried sage for the camomile flowers. Bring the mixture to a boil, reduce the heat and simmer for ten minutes. Turn off the heat, cover, and allow it to soak for half an hour.

Strain the liquid into a mixing bowl, squeezing out as much as possible from the herbs before discarding them. Put 60 g of flaked or grated Castile soap into the saucepan and pour the herbal water back in. Heat gently until all the soap has dissolved, stirring with a wooden spoon. Leave and allow to cool.

Stir three drops of peppermint or eucalyptus essential oil into 2 tablespoons of vodka. Add this mixture to the soap solution. Pour into a jar and leave for three to four days in a warm place before using.

Herbal hair oil Place 12 tablespoons of suitable herbs (see herbal shampoo recipe

Making cold cream

Using a blender or whisk, thoroughly mix together a tablespoon of aloe vera gel and 150 ml olive or other vegetable oil. Then, in the top of a double boiler, melt a tablespoon of white beeswax and 2 tablespoons of anhydrous (water-free) lanolin. Slowly stir in the oil and aloe mix, remove from heat and add 2 tablespoons of rose, lavender or other flower water, and two or three drops of any essential oil you like. Stir until the mixture cools and thickens, then pour into storage jars.

Homemade face packs

To make these, combine 2 tablespoons of a suitable dry base with enough liquid to make a thick paste, choosing ingredients to suit your skin type – see text.
Before applying, wash your face and either steam it (see p. 194) or cover with a warm, wet facecloth for a few minutes to open the pores. Then spread the paste all over the face, not neglecting, as some women do, the neck and décolleté area; but avoid eyes and lips. Allow to dry completely – about 15-30 minutes – before washing off with warm water and a soft cloth.

on the previous page) in the top of a double boiler and add 300 ml of safflower, soya, peanut or sunflower oil. Olive oil may also be used if you do not mind the smell. Heat for half an hour, then pour the mixture into a wide-necked jar. Cover with a few layers of cheesecloth or muslin held by a rubber band. Leave in a warm place for about a week, stirring every day. Then strain and store in a clean container.

To use, pour out 5 tablespoons of the oil – 8 if your hair is very long or thick – and warm it gently for a few minutes. Wet your hair with warm water, squeeze out, then spread the oil evenly through the hair using your fingers. Cover the hair with a shower cap, and wrap around your head a wrung-out towel that has been soaked in hot water. When the towel cools down, remove and wet it with hot water again, wring it out thoroughly and replace around the head.

Make sure you leave the oil on your hair for about half an hour, then shampoo it out twice and rinse well.

Egg and oil conditioner You can use this mix like the oil above, or else just warm it slightly and apply 15 minutes before washing your hair.

Beat together an egg, 2 teaspoons of lemon juice and 1 teaspoon of honey. Pour into the top of a double boiler and heat until creamy, stirring continuously.

Remove this mixture from the heat, and when it has cooled down slowly whisk in 4 tablespoons of safflower or other vegetable oil – or the herbal hair oil above – into which you have stirred two or three drops of rosemary essential oil.

Green clay body treatment Mixed to a paste with water and two or three drops of an essential oil of your choice, green clay can be applied liberally to the whole body to cleanse and tone the skin, draw out unwanted impurities and invigorate your circulation. It removes dead cells, leaving the skin smooth and soft, and will not irritate even a sensitive skin.

A course of regular applications can be used to treat spots on the back and help dry out excessively oily patches. Leave the treatment on for at least five minutes, and up to a maximum of 15 minutes, depending on the sensitivity of your skin.

Pre-bath body rub To remove dead skin cells and improve your general circulation considerably, rub your body all over – excluding your face and neck – with fine sea salt. It is best to use it by the handful and apply it with a circular motion. Rinse off with cool water, then bathe.

Beauty baths Almost any herb can be used in the bath – choose according to the list on p. 186. To prepare, steep 60 g of herbs in 600 ml of boiling water for 20-30 minutes, strain

Natural hair colours from herbs and flowers

Test these tints on a strand of hair to check the colour before using. The infusions need to be used as regular rinses to keep up the effect, but a single 15-30 minute application of the paste colourings is usually enough, with retouching every four to six weeks to colour new growth at the hair roots.

COLOURING AGENT	EFFECT ON HAIR COLOUR
Henna mixed to paste with hot water.	Comes in different colours, but red is most popular.
Henna mixed to paste with hot camomile infusion, red wine or lemon juice.	Enhanced red tints.
Henna mixed to paste with hot black coffee.	Deeper colour.
Strong camomile infusion.	Lightens fair hair.
Camomile mixed to paste with kaolin powder.	Highlights mid-brown hair.
Infusion of marigold flowers, or saffron roots or flowers.	Gives reddish-yellow tint to white hair.
Infusion of powdered walnut bark or shells.	Darkens hair slightly (good for grey hair).
Rhubarb root infusion.	Lightens any hair slightly.
Sage infusion.	Gives brown tint to grey hair.
Sage infusion mixed with tea.	Deeper brown colour.

and add to your bath water. Alternatively, tie the herbs in a muslin bag and hang it from the hot tap so that water runs through it. One bag will do about three or four baths.

Half a pint of cider vinegar added to a bath, with one or two drops of peppermint essential oil added, may help to relieve irritating, dry and itchy skin.

The combination of cider vinegar and sea salt in a 3 per cent dilution in your bath is said to be very helpful in guarding against THRUSH or other irritating yeast infections. Alternatively, you can try four or five drops of tea-tree oil.

Oatmeal and bran baths are prepared in the same way as herbal baths and have a cleansing, soothing and whitening effect on the skin.

For a rich, nourishing bath, try adding about 60 g of powdered milk to the water or, for a fragrant treat, a few drops of aromatherapy oil.

Natural deodorant If chemical sprays and roll-ons irritate your skin, try using an alunite crystal moistened with a little water and rubbed under the arms for a few seconds.

You may also find that you have less need for deodorant if you eat plenty of foods that contain chlorophyll, such as green, leafy vegetables and salads. You should also make sure that your diet is balanced by adequate supplements of zinc, aluminium and manganese (see MINERALS).

NATURAL CHILDBIRTH

More and more women are choosing to have their children delivered without artificial aids. In South Africa, a significant number of women are opting for natural childbirth because they feel it will be less traumatic for the baby, and give them more control in the birth process. Many doctors endorse this attitude, and some hospitals now provide suitable facilities for natural childbirth. See A GENTLER WAY INTO THE WORLD, p. 260.

NATUROPATHY

Helping your body to heal itself

The first man to bathe his sprained ankle in a cool stream was practising naturopathy – as was the first woman to stop eating food to rest an upset stomach, and the first person to sit tight and sweat out a fever.

The term 'naturopathy' dates from only the late 19th century, but the philosophy on which this system is based is age-old. Since its earliest days, when it was known as 'nature cure', naturopathy has concentrated on helping the body to cure itself. One of the main pioneers of the movement, the Ameri-

The natural birth of naturopathy

The Knee-jet.   Fig. 2. The Head-affusion.

Walking barefoot in wet grass.

The origins of naturopathy go back more than 2 000 years to the Greek physician Hippocrates, known as the 'Father of Medicine'. He laid down the principle of 'first do no harm' – implying that cures should work with the body and be as natural as possible – and maintained that good health is based upon eating and exercising with moderation.

Modern naturopathy was pioneered in Germany in the early 19th century by therapists such as Vincent Preissnitz (1799-1851), who believed in the 'miraculous' healing power of water and founded hydrotherapy as it is now called. Towards the end of the century a Bavarian monk, Father Sebastian Kneipp, successfully treated an ailing American named Benedict Lust. After studying with Kneipp at his clinic, Lust returned to the USA and founded his own particular form of therapy – naturopathy.

Lust believed that, as far as health is concerned, man is his own worst enemy – hampered by 'narrow thinking' and beset by 'criminal eating, foolish drinking, sagged standing [and] congested sitting'.

The Kneipp water cure was recommended to people of all ages suffering from muscular aches and pains. Hosing, sprinkling with water and walking barefoot in wet grass were all part of the therapy.

can Benedict Lust, envisaged a three-part cure. First, 'evil habits' such as overindulgence in food and drink, meat-eating, late hours and aberrant social behaviour had to be eliminated. They were to be replaced by 'corrective habits' such as correct breathing and exercise, the right mental attitude, and moderation in one's lifestyle. The third part of Lust's cure entailed 'new principles of living' such as proper fasting and the correct selection of food; hydrotherapy, mud baths and Turkish baths; and various forms of massage and manipulation (mechanotherapy). There was only one real healing force in existence, he said, and that was Nature itself.

The therapies used by naturopathy today include CHIROPRACTIC, DIETS AND DIETING, EXERCISE, HYDROTHERAPY, MASSAGE, OSTEOPATHY, RELAXATION AND BREATHING and YOGA. It also encourages people to think positively in terms of good health, rather than of pain and illness – and to live as naturally as possible amid the pressures of our modern, everyday world.

When, for whatever apparent reason, our health breaks down, naturopathy sets out to identify the underlying cause of illness – and to treat this, rather than trying to suppress or merely alleviate the symptoms.

Basically, disease is thought by naturopaths to have one major cause – the breakdown of the body's normal balance. The particular type of illness a person suffers may be the result of various bacteria, viruses, ALLERGY, or other outside factors. But these are held to be of secondary importance to the patient's weakness and lack of resistance.

By treating each case as unique, and each person as an individual, naturopaths take into account the patient's entire physical, emotional, biochemical and social circumstances. They seek to complement and support conventional doctors – providing help and comfort whenever severe illness requires surgery or drastic orthodox treatment.

Who it can help Naturopaths believe that their holistic approach can help all kinds of people with all kinds of medical problems. Age is no barrier, and patients range from infants to the elderly.

Naturopathy is said to be particularly effective against degenerative diseases such as ARTHRITIS and EMPHYSEMA (damaged, inefficient lungs). It has reportedly been used to powerful effect on patients with ULCERS and various forms of inflammation. In addition, it aims to speed up recovery in cases of COLDS, INFLUENZA, DIARRHOEA and rashes (see SKIN DISORDERS).

It is often used in dealing with cases for which no clear medical diagnosis can be made – such as ANXIETY and TIREDNESS. And naturopathy is believed to be highly successful in helping to prevent disease in bodily tissues and organs such as the lungs, kidneys and heart.

As naturopaths concentrate on the person, rather than the disease, they emphasise that their success depends upon their patients' ability to heal themselves, as well as the amount of physical damage already done. For example, a young person full of vitality should respond well to treatment for, say, BRONCHITIS. On the other hand, a frail, elderly person with the same complaint may not get better as completely or as soon. Even so, naturopaths believe, old people should be able to cope with the illness effectively without the need for drugs.

Finding a therapist The best way to find a qualified naturopath is by recommendation from a friend. If this is not possible, study the advertising columns of alternative health publications; or write, asking for a list of names in your area, to the South African Homoeopathic Association, 20 Botanic Grove, Berea 4001. Be sure to enclose a stamped, self-addressed envelope with your letter.

Legally, naturopaths cannot be registered with the South African Associated Health Service Professions Board unless they also practise a therapy – such as homoeopathy – that the board recognises. Naturopaths work in private practice and will see patients only by appointment. Some therapists attend health farms and clinics.

Consulting a therapist Since naturopathy deals with you as a whole, a therapist will first take your complete case history, possibly by means of a questionnaire. He will want to know how you – and your symptoms – are affected by such things as changes in the weather, different times of day, the areas in which you live and work, the various events that make up your daily routine, your eating habits and sleeping patterns, and physical factors such as menstrual cycles and bowel activity.

This will be followed by a routine medical examination of the pulse, heart, lungs and BLOOD PRESSURE. The practitioner may also check the spinal joints and other parts of your musculoskeletal system to make sure that they are working freely.

Many naturopaths also use various special diagnostic techniques – such as IRIDOLOGY

Naturopathy in the home

The advice given by a naturopath will be directed at you as a person, rather than at a specific disease you may have. And most of what the practitioner recommends can be carried out in your own home.

For example, you may be told to make changes to your diet – such as eating more salads and fresh fruit, and avoiding caffeine in coffee and tea. In some cases of allergy you may be told to avoid dairy products and wheat. And people with arthritis and skin disorders may be prescribed dietary supplements of anti-inflammatory fatty acids (see EATING FOR HEALTH).

You may even be put on a short, water or juice-only fast designed to cleanse your system and give your organs a chance to rest. You may also be advised, if necessary, to stop SMOKING and give up alcohol.

Simple advice on hydrotherapy may also be given – such as taking hot and cold foot baths to help control high blood pressure, or applying cold compresses to the throat and waist to try to relieve TONSILLITIS. Other measures may include the use of herbal medicine and HOMOEOPATHY.

During the first few weeks of home treatment you will need to see your naturopath regularly so that the effect of any dietary changes can be checked, and for special muscle reflex treatments, counselling, or instruction in relaxation and breathing. But after that fewer consultations should be needed.

(examining the irises of your eyes for signs of illness) and HAIR DIAGNOSIS. Samples of your blood and urine may also be taken for laboratory analysis.

Naturopathic diagnosis is more concerned with establishing the exact reasons why your health has broken down than with putting a name to the illness. For the practitioner, the diagnostic findings are only part of the general assessment he makes. He will also take into consideration your own particular physical, emotional and environmental circumstances.

Many people are frightened of illness, feeling it is something over which they have no control. Naturopaths try to dispel this fear by explaining what the body is telling us when it is unwell.

For example, sudden or severe symptoms are indications that it is dealing with a particular illness and therefore the symptoms must not be suppressed – unless, of course, the patient's life is at risk. Sometimes during treatment of long-standing conditions such as bronchitis or skin disorders, there may be a short return of phlegm or irritation for a few days. These aggravations of old symptoms are known as the 'healing crisis', and are regarded as a good sign.

Measures may include changes in diet or herbal treatment (see HERBAL MEDICINE). In all cases, care is taken to ensure that the symptoms do not overcome the patient's reserves of energy or hinder his ability to make a satisfactory recovery. If necessary, therapists may arrange for patients to have emotional and spiritual COUNSELLING.

An orthodox view

Many of the treatments offered by naturopaths form the basis of good health care, both preventive and curative. Several are now advocated in health education programmes. Treatment of complex medical problems will respond well to a combination of orthodox approaches as well as naturopathy.

NAUSEA AND VOMITING

Nausea originally meant sea-sickness; these days it refers to any sensation of needing to be sick, and this unpleasant state is often accompanied by pallor, sweating and a reduction in the heart rate. Vomiting is simply the physical outcome. It is usually an involuntary process, although it can also be induced by medicines known as 'emetics'; ipecac is a common example.

Nausea and vomiting may be symptoms of many conditions, including overeating, MORNING SICKNESS, MOTION SICKNESS, MIGRAINE, VERTIGO and uncontrolled DIABETES. Often a patient is nauseous and sick after a general anaesthetic. Sometimes the trigger is psychological or emotional, for example an overwhelming disgust with food (of the kind associated with ANOREXIA). One of the most common causes is FOOD POISONING, or gastroenteritis, in which bacteria from contaminated food inflame the lining of the stomach and intestine – often resulting in DIARRHOEA, too. By ridding the body of the harmful agents, vomiting can make you feel much better.

But prolonged or excessive vomiting (with or without diarrhoea) can result in dehydration – the loss of too much body fluid.

What the therapists recommend

Acupressure Press towards the centre of the wrist, three fingers' width above the inner wrist crease, centrally, in line with the middle finger (Pericardium 6). Alternatively, press firmly inwards, centrally, on the midpoint on the stomach, between the breastbone and navel (Ren 12).

Herbal Medicine Sipping an infusion of ginger, peppermint, camomile or sage, or taking a combination of any of these, can bring some relief.

A fragrant tea which is made from the scented leaves of the pelargonium is a very popular indigenous remedy; a teaspoon of buchu brandy, taken twice daily, is another. A herbalist may also prescribe black horehound to give relief, while simultaneously treating the cause.

Naturopathy Once the cause is discovered and the vomiting controlled, some foods can be reintroduced, starting with clear vegetable soups, followed by wholewheat toast or boiled rice and vegetables, before gradually resuming a normal diet.

Homoeopathy For constant nausea and vomiting after meals, with a clean tongue, griping pains, headache and perspiration, homoeopaths recommend Ipecac. 6. If it follows rich fatty food and afflicts a weepy person who tends to feel better outdoors, try Pulsatilla 6.

If the vomit is very acidic and occurs soon after a meal, with burning pains, chilliness and exhaustion, Arsen. alb. 6 is recommended. Dosage in each case is every half hour until improvement is felt.

An orthodox view

Nausea and vomiting are symptoms – not diseases. The most important role of a conventional doctor is to diagnose and treat the cause of these symptoms. For example, it would be dangerous – and could even be fatal – to treat the vomiting of a patient with uncontrolled diabetes without giving insulin.

If a person vomits blood, bleeding somewhere in the digestive tract is usually indicated, and this is an emergency situation that calls for immediate medical attention. Blood vomited as a result of nosebleed is, of course, less serious.

If vomiting fails to relieve severe abdominal pain this must be treated as an emergency; a perforated ulcer or appendicitis are possible causes. Pending professional advice, take little or no solid foods and plenty of fluids, such as water or barley water.

Medicines such as metoclopramide or prochloperazine, taken in tablet form, suppository or injection, may control vomiting, once the cause is known. But medicines should be avoided during pregnancy.

NECK PAIN

Most people have neck pain and stiffness at some time in their lives. The cause can be trivial or serious – and it can be difficult to tell which.

The neck is the most mobile part of the spine, with seven bones separated by discs of cartilage and joined by ligaments. Wear-and-tear changes in the bones and joints, known as cervical spondylosis, begin at the age of about 25 and may result in pain and stiffness from bony fringes, called osteophytes, growing around the joints. ARTHRITIS can also develop in the joints between the vertebrae (spinal bones).

Ligament SPRAINS may occur after 'whiplash' injuries to the neck caused, for example, when a car is shunted by another from behind – an event that happens all too frequently in South Africa.

Neck pain is frequently accompanied by pain in the shoulder or arm caused by trapped nerves (see NERVE DISORDERS). It is also often aggravated by reflex muscle spasm in the neck, with increased stiffness and restricted movement.

Tension HEADACHES – the result of stressful living conditions – may also cause neck pain. If it occurs suddenly and the patient shows signs of general illness, it can also be a symptom of meningitis – infection of the membranes surrounding the brain – or a brain haemorrhage.

What the therapists recommend

Acupuncture Treatment can be given for most types of neck pain and stiffness. Points treated are on the small intestine, gall bladder, lung, bladder and large intestine meridians (see chart, p. 14). MOXIBUSTION may also be beneficial.

Massage If the pain stems from the neck muscles or joints – but is not glandular or disease-related – apply firm, stroking effleurage movements down the back of the neck and over the shoulder area. Also give deep frictions with the pads of the fingers along the band of muscle at each side of the vertebrae of the neck. But avoid the front of the neck and throat regions.

Reflexology Massage is given to the reflex areas relating to the neck, with rotation of the toe joints, plus massage to areas relating to the upper spine, the side of the head, the shoulders, the arms and the adrenal glands (see chart, p. 295).

Osteopathy Poor posture – particularly if it has been maintained for several years – can often lead to recurring pain and stiffness in the neck. Gentle manual traction and mobilisation may bring about rapid relief. Some simple exercises are recommended to help

Exercises to avoid neck pain

Maintaining flexibility is the key to keeping your neck free of tension and pain. To achieve this, try the following daily exercises. Make sure to move only your neck and head.

Neck rolls are performed by slowly rotating your head in a clockwise direction. Breathe slowly in and out and gently stretch the muscles at the front and back of the neck.

(Left) Inhale as you bend your head back. Then exhale and bring your head forward. (Right) Exhale as you bring your left ear to your left shoulder. Then repeat with your right ear and shoulder.

you to maintain mobility of the neck. First, when sitting, drop the chin to the chest and then slowly stretch the head up and backwards. Second, with the head upright, turn round as far as possible to the left and then to the right.

Third, again with the head upright, bring the left ear slowly down as far as possible to the left shoulder, then the right ear to the right shoulder. Repeat all three exercises five times.

Herbal medicine The Cape willow or river willow (*Salix mucronata*) provides a remedy to relieve neck stiffness and also headaches. Infuse the bark and soft twigs (stripped of leaves) in boiling water for ten minutes, and sweeten the bitter tea with honey to make it more palatable.

An orthodox view

X-rays are not particularly helpful in diagnosing the cause of various kinds of neck pain, because they frequently tend to reveal cervical spondylosis in patients who are over the age of 25 even when there are no symptoms of stiffness and pain.

On the other hand, severe symptoms sometimes occur in people whose X-rays appear to be fairly normal.

After taking a patient's history and physically examining the neck, a doctor may recommend a course of physiotherapy, heat treatment, traction or a cervical collar. Painkilling medicines such as aspirin, paracetamol or ibuprofen sometimes help, but they do not relieve muscle spasm.

A gentler way into the world

Nothing in this world is more natural than having a baby, yet through the ages few natural events have been more interfered with. The natural childbirth movement upholds the right of women to follow their instincts in the matter of childbirth, and since the pioneering work of this movement in the 1980s, women have increasingly opted for natural deliveries. Many doctors are sympathetic to the idea, and some hospitals, in particular private ones, now make special provision for women who want a minimum of medical interference while still ensuring the safety of their babies.

All births were natural until the 17th century, when King Louis XIV of France made his mistresses lie on their back during labour so that he could witness the birth of his children. Although childbirth is difficult and painful in this position, it soon became so fashionable that French doctors had to develop forceps to overcome some of the problems it caused. Soon so many special instruments were introduced that doctors came to regard childbirth as an emergency requiring medical intervention for the best results.

Women may give birth squatting, sitting or even standing up; there is no general rule. But even in the most primitive societies, first-time mothers usually get the advice of other women who have been through the experience of childbirth.

In Britain, natural childbirth was pioneered by Dr Grantly Dick-Read (1890-1959), after he assisted at a delivery in a Whitechapel slum. The woman refused to have chloroform. Later, when asked why, she replied: 'It didn't hurt. It wasn't meant to, was it doctor?' From this and other deliveries,

Dr Dick-Read came to believe that women who stayed calm and had faith in the natural process of birth tended to have a relatively painless experience.

He developed relaxation techniques to help women overcome their fears and these, with advice on posture, EXERCISE and diet, became basic principles of the National Childbirth Trust (NCT) in Britain.

A French obstetrician, Dr Michel Odent (1930-), went a step further. Instead of teaching women what to do, he encouraged them to believe that if they trusted their instincts they could all be natural experts at giving birth. He gave his patients the freedom and privacy to act as they wished during labour, including the chance to sit in a tub of warm water to ease painful contractions – and so the idea of water births was introduced to the West (see below).

Another recent development is the 'Leboyer method', named after Dr Frederick Leboyer (1918-), who considered birth from the point of view of the baby. He believed that instead of emerging into a world of bright lights and raised voices – and even being held upside down and slapped – a baby should enter the world as gently as possible.

In South Africa, the delivery unit at Goodwood's Libertas Hospital set a precedent some 12 years ago by agreeing to conform to the wishes of the mother-to-be and her husband in the matter

In many overseas countries water births are growing in popularity, and some hospitals even have pools big enough for both partners to enter, as shown here. The baby does not breathe until its head is out of the water.

of childbirth. The husband could even live on the hospital premises during his wife's confinement. Soon afterwards, in 1982, Professor Justus Hofmeyr established a Midwives' Natural Childbirth Unit at Johannesburg's General Hospital.

Today, a significant number of South African women opt for natural childbirth because they feel it will be less traumatic for the baby, and give them more control over the birth.

Preparing for natural birth

Start immediately – even before you are pregnant – to take regular exercise and eat a well-balanced diet rich in proteins, VITAMINS and MINERALS (see EATING FOR HEALTH). During PREGNANCY, choose gentler types of exercise such as swimming and walking, which tone the muscles and improve fitness without strain. Some simple YOGA exercises can help to increase your overall suppleness and flexibility.

Choosing where to have the baby is the next step – the most 'natural' place is wherever you feel most comfortable. For some mothers – particularly if it is their first baby or there are any problems – this is in hospital, where modern technology is available. Some women prefer the familiar surroundings of home, with the midwife present as a guest. Another option is to be looked after at home by a midwife during the first stages of labour, and then to be taken to a (private) hospital for the delivery, with one's own doctor in attendance.

Natural childbirth advisers generally recommend that every mother-to-be should draw up a 'birth plan' well in advance, setting out what she would prefer. You can easily make your own birth plan (see box, p. 263).

Natural labour and birth

Birth positions If squatting appeals to you it may be a good idea to practise during pregnancy (see illustrations, p. 262). Your partner can help by holding you up. You may also find that a kidney-shaped birth stool or birth chair helps you to stay in position, but ask the advice of your midwife or doctor, as some modern birthing chairs can restrict movement and may increase bleeding and tearing.

Alternatively, you could adopt a South American Indian method and stand up just as the baby's head is about to emerge – half the women who do this have no tears at all.

Traditionally African women give birth in a kneeling position, with the knees held apart and the heels together, supporting the perineal area. It is ironic that, with the adoption of Western customs, this natural position is replaced in the hospital setting by supine delivery.

Water births The first recorded underwater birth was mentioned in a medical report of 1805, but it was not until the 1960s that the idea started becoming popular. Now some modern hospitals abroad provide receptacles for women who want to try this method.

The tub or pool is filled with about 38 cm of body-temperature water – enough to reach the armpits when sitting. When contractions become painful, the mother-to-be eases herself into the water. Some receptacles are even big enough for her partner

Louis XIV of France began a fashion that became popular throughout the world when he insisted that his mistresses give birth lying down in spite of the problems it caused.

Childbirth can now be a happy, relaxed experience in which partners increasingly play an active, supporting role. In natural childbirth, the mother-to-be usually chooses where and how she will be delivered.
The old days when women were expected to give birth to their offspring on their back are over.

to get in with her and give support. The water's warmth tends to soothe away pain, and its buoyancy supports her weight. The water also provides a gentle and comfortable transition from the womb for the baby.

Although water births are still rare in South Africa, the Active Childbirth Unit at Johannesburg's General Hospital has a jacuzzi in which a mother-to-be may, if she wishes, spend her labour, either emerging from it for the actual delivery or else remaining in the water. Some labour wards are equipped with ordinary domestic baths, in which labour pains may likewise be relieved.

Coping with pain The first choice during a natural birth is to rely on RELAXATION AND BREATHING exercises to control pain. Simply concentrating on your breathing can have a soothing effect

261

Preparing for the birth

Two positions which can help women prepare for childbirth are the squatting pose (right) and the so-called 'frog position' (below). The first increases flexibility and gives a good stretch to thigh, groin and back muscles, while the second is said to enhance suppleness and aid relaxation, especially when combined with labour breathing exercises.

Gently lower yourself from a standing position into the squat, keeping your back straight and your feet flat on the ground if possible. Rest elbows on thighs and clasp hands together. Remain in the position as long as is comfortable.

Kneel on a soft carpet, rug or mat with your toes touching and knees a little apart. Keep your back straight and arms, neck and shoulders relaxed.

Place hands on the floor, palms down, and lower your bottom as far as possible. Slowly 'walk' hands forward, stretching out the spine and lowering the body towards the ground.

When you are stretched out as far as you can go, rest your forehead on a cushion. Hold for a minute or two, taking slow, rhythmic breaths with the emphasis on the out-breath.

Two simple ways of helping to make labour more comfortable for you

A gentle massage from a nurse, therapist or partner can soothe away pain and help women in labour to relax. It is said to work best for women who have had massage before, and who find the touch of human hands reassuring.

Pillows, cushions or a beanbag moulded into shape can help women to find the best positions for giving birth. These simple aids, which can be brought to the hospital if necessary, provide a useful combination of comfort and support.

(Right) A mother-to-be tries out the V-shaped birth cushion developed at Britain's Milton Keynes General Hospital by Dr Jason Gardosi in 1987.

(Left) The mother lies on her side or sits if she prefers, while the therapist or nurse massages her back and buttocks, relieving muscle tension and labour pains.

A birth plan for you and your baby

Prepare your plan well in advance with your partner, and try to include every aspect of the birth. Discuss the details of it with a midwife or your general practitioner, and prepare to be flexible.

Include the following information:

Other people Many women enjoy having a partner, relative or friend with them during labour. Your midwife or doctor can tell you if this is possible. If you would rather be alone, note this instead.

Induction This is not used in natural childbirth, as once contractions are artificially induced they become faster and more painful, increasing the need for painkillers. If induction is unavoidable – for example, if the baby is two or three weeks late, or if mother or baby shows signs of distress – you can still say that you want to try alternative methods first. Acupressure, acupuncture or homoeopathy may be able to balance your system so that your labour begins naturally.

Lovemaking, nipple stimulation, a long walk or a drink of castor oil and orange juice may all increase production of the hormone prostaglandin, sometimes causing labour to start.

If artificial induction is necessary, you can ask for it to be done by the gentler method of prostaglandin vaginal pessaries, rather than by having the waters broken or being given the hormone oxytocin by injection or through a drip.

Shaving and enemas Neither the shaving of a woman's pubic hair nor the administration of an enema is obligatory prior to having a baby, although both procedures are still usual in South African hospitals. If you do not want either of them, say so in your plan.

Moving around Freedom to move around and change position at will can relieve pain and assist labour, so put that in your plan. Electronic monitoring of the baby can restrict movement, and you can choose to have it done only intermittently, or with an instrument called a Pinard stethoscope, which allows you to move most of the time.

Pain control Painkillers are often administered without asking the mother, so say in writing if you want them only on request. However, in case natural methods such as relaxation and breathing prove inadequate, you should say which of the alternatives you would prefer.

The usual options are gas and oxygen (a mixture of laughing gas – nitrous oxide – and oxygen); injections of pethidine; or an epidural injection of an anaesthetic which goes into the outer lining of the spinal cord. This numbs the lower half of the body while leaving you conscious.

Cut or tear Neither may happen, but your plan should allow for all possibilities. In natural childbirth, natural tearing of the vagina is usually preferred to an episiotomy – a deliberate cut at the entrance of the vagina to help the baby out. Natural tears

are said to heal faster, but episiotomies are common in some hospitals, so say if you don't want to have one. They are avoidable unless forceps are used.

Giving birth Say what equipment you want available – a birthing stool or cushions, for example. Indicate also what sort of conditions you would like for the birth – with lights dimmed and the room quiet, or perhaps with a piece of music on a tape recorder. Talk it over with the midwife or doctor. In private care it should be possible to have all of these needs satisfied.

Delivering the placenta In a natural birth the placenta – often known as the afterbirth – is left to be delivered naturally after the baby's birth. However, most hospitals inject a drug called syntometrine to speed the process. Should you not want this, say so in your birth plan. If syntometrine is not given, then there is no immediate necessity to cut the umbilical cord, and you can wait until it stops pulsing or even until the placenta appears, if you wish.

After delivery You can choose to hold and breastfeed your baby immediately, and to have some time in private with your partner and the baby. You may also want to bath the baby yourself soon after birth. If both mother and baby are well, you can leave hospital after just a few hours, though it would be wise to have a private midwife pay visits to you for some days. Or you can choose to stay in the hospital for two or three days.

and is a well-known MEDITATION technique. During contractions, breathe rhythmically in to a count of four and then breathe out to a count of four.

Once labour begins in earnest, your breathing pattern will change naturally, as you breathe more deeply in through the nose and out through the mouth. Practising during pregnancy will help to make this pattern familiar and natural.

Gentle MASSAGE can also be tried to ease labour pain, especially in the region of the lower back. Downward strokes are particularly calming and soothing to some expectant mothers, but not everyone enjoys being touched during the time of labour. For anyone who is continually anxious or worried about being unable to relax, HYPNOTHERAPY can be used to teach simple calming techniques.

Many alternative therapists are happy to attend births and, if labour is tiring, painful or slow, ACUPUNCTURE, HOMOEOPATHY or ACUPRESSURE can often help. However, the practitioners of such alternative therapies are unlikely to be welcome in the labour wards of South African general hospitals.

Some hospitals abroad can provide transcutaneous electrical nerve stimulation (TENS) instruments for ELECTROTHERAPY. These

instruments use electrical impulses to block the body's pain signals and stimulate the production of natural painkillers called endomorphins in the brain.

Welcoming baby

A great advantage of natural childbirth is that it leaves mother and baby free from the after-effects of drugs, and feeling well – which makes bonding more successful.

Fathers are encouraged to participate – for example, by washing and cuddling the baby soon after birth.

The baby is generally put to its mother's breast as soon as possible after it is born. The sucking stimulates contractions of the womb so that the placenta is then expelled naturally. It also stimulates the production of milk containing colostrum, a substance rich in antibodies that give the newcomer substantial protection from disease.

To find out more about facilities for natural childbirth, write (enclosing a stamped, self-addressed envelope) to the National Childbirth Education and Parenting Association, P O Box 95050, Grant Park 2051. The association can put you in touch with midwives working in your area.

NERVE DISORDERS

When problems hit the body's intelligence network

Messages to and from the brain and around the body are conducted by nerves. The messages consist of electrical impulses that travel from one end of a nerve to the other and are then chemically transmitted to other nerves or to muscles. Sensory nerves carry messages to the brain or spinal cord about sensations such as PAIN, ITCHING and COLDNESS. Motor nerves deliver orders from the brain to the muscles.

Any interference with the operation of nerves can cause such symptoms as pain, numbness or paralysis. Neuralgia is pain arising from an irritated or damaged nerve and is felt in the part of the body served by the nerve – not necessarily at the site of the problem. NEURALGIA felt in an arm or leg that has been amputated is caused by the severed nerves and is known as 'phantom pain'.

Trapped nerves can also produce pain, numbness and tingling sensations in the part of the body supplied by the particular nerve. Compression of the median nerve at the wrist causes symptoms in the fingers, sometimes spreading up the arm, particularly at night (see CARPEL TUNNEL SYNDROME). Spinal problems may irritate nerve roots, causing pain in the shoulder or arm or down the back of the leg (see NECK PAIN; SCIATICA; SLIPPED DISC; LUMBAGO).

SHINGLES, caused by the CHICKENPOX virus infecting a nerve to part of the skin, produces a painful, blistering rash, especially on the chest of the victim.

Neuritis is inflammation of a nerve. Optic neuritis, for example – inflammation of the optic nerve which carries visual signals from the eye to the brain – results in temporary deterioration of sight. It can be a sign of MULTIPLE SCLEROSIS. Other types of neuritis may produce neuralgia.

Myasthenia gravis is a rare condition in which antibodies – part of the body's defensive IMMUNE SYSTEM against infection – interfere with the chemical connections between nerves and muscles. The muscles feel weak and tire easily. The eyelids droop towards the end of the day, and chewing and swallowing may be difficult.

What the therapists recommend

Herbal Medicine Infusions of rosemary or peppermint make gentle tonics. However, in individual cases herbalists may use stronger restoratives such as vervain, wild oats or St John's wort.

Naturopathy A naturopath will probably advise the patient to follow established relaxation methods, such as those employed in YOGA and MEDITATION, as long-term self help to maintain a calm and balanced attitude. MASSAGE may also be recommended to reduce TENSION and fatigue.

Many herbal teas – for example, lemon balm or rosemary – are held to be of great value in calming and restoring nerve function, and patients may be referred to a herbal practitioner. Vitamin B taken as a supplement is said to be particularly effective for nervous exhaustion.

Biochemic Tissue Salts For nervous debility, *Kali phos.* is suggested as a nerve nutrient. *Mag. phos.* is prescribed when motor nerves are involved and there are cramps, nerve pains and twitching.

An orthodox view

To diagnose nerve disorders, a doctor may carry out nerve conduction studies by placing electrodes at different points along a nerve and measuring the passage of impulses along it. Treatment depends upon the cause.

Trapped nerves can sometimes be released by steroid injections, by surgery or, in the spine, by traction.

Prescribed early enough, antiviral drugs may reduce the pain of shingles. So-called anticholinergic medicines – which enhance the effect of chemical transmitters between nerves and muscles – generally help myasthenia gravis sufferers.

Sometimes an operation to remove the thymus gland at the base of the neck (which influences metabolism in muscles) also provides relief.

NERVOUS DISORDERS

The distress and anguish of the disturbed mind

The distressing complaints known as nervous or psychiatric disorders are mental problems that are serious enough to be called illnesses – as opposed to the minor psychological problems that still permit the sufferer to lead a more or less normal life. They fall into two main groups.

The first group, known as neuroses, are generally less severe, and sufferers to a large extent recognise their problem. Their responses to situations – sometimes including physical symptoms – may seem exaggerated or inappropriate to outsiders, but they remain in touch with reality.

In the second and more severe group, the psychoses, patients are cut off to a greater or lesser extent from the reality of the world around them. Not only is their behaviour irrational, but they themselves cannot see that it makes no sense.

Neuroses When normal thoughts and feelings of vulnerable individuals are exaggerated to such a degree that they interfere with daily life, the result is known as a neurosis. The most common form is an ANXIETY state. Everyone feels anxious at times, and the increased circulation of the hormone adrenaline around the body and the heightened awareness and responsiveness that it causes are a useful reaction to STRESS. A neurosis occurs when the anxiety is aroused without adequate cause, or when it is excessively severe or persistent.

Anxiety neurosis may lead to panic attacks with PALPITATIONS, shortness of breath and a sensation of imminent disaster. Other sufferers develop PHOBIAS – unreasonable fears of going outdoors (see AGORAPHOBIA), of confined spaces (CLAUSTROPHOBIA), of heights and so on.

Neurotic DEPRESSION is another excessive response to stress. Unlike psychotic depression (see below), which can occur with no apparent cause, there is usually a reason for neurotic depression – although it may not be obvious. Sufferers find everything an effort, cannot get to sleep, feel worse as the day goes on, and may have either an increased or decreased appetite.

OBSESSIVE-COMPULSIVE BEHAVIOUR is also a neurosis. As a response to stress, a sufferer's mind is preoccupied, or is unable to shake off certain thoughts or impulses. Sufferers may feel extremely anxious if, for example, ornaments are out of their usual places. Or they may feel compelled to perform rituals, such as washing their hands many times a day.

HYSTERIA is another neurotic condition, in which a person subconsciously develops symptoms of physical disease – such as paralysis of an arm or leg – or displays unusual behaviour in order to attract attention or to avoid an unpleasant situation. Unlike a malingerer, the hysteric is unaware of the true psychological cause of his or her physical symptoms.

Psychoses Unlike neuroses, psychotic illnesses often occur for no apparent reason, although they do tend to run in families. The two most common psychoses are SCHIZOPHRENIA and MANIC DEPRESSIVE DISORDER.

Psychotic people experience life in a distorted way. Schizophrenics may suffer various delusions or hallucinations and can be unreasonably suspicious. Manic depressive illness produces uncontrollable mood swings, varying from profound depression to mania – a state of excessive cheerfulness and overconfidence accompanied by overactive (and often extravagant) behaviour. Most people regarded as 'mad' are actually suffering from some form of psychotic illness. Unfortunately, some psychotics do not realise that they are ill and tend to strongly decline all treatment.

What the therapists recommend

A number of alternative therapies offer help for sufferers of nervous disorders, particularly the less severe neuroses. For specific recommendations, refer to the main entries on individual neuroses and psychoses.

MASSAGE
Depending on how the neurosis shows itself, such therapy – whether rhythmic and relaxing, or rapid and tonic – may have some sedative, soothing, stimulating or other psychological effect. If the neurosis is accompanied by physical symptoms, such as PAIN, the massage will aim at generally improving circulation and mobility, relieving spasms and so on.

MUSIC THERAPY
The sharing of music-making between the therapist and client can encourage the expression of deep and sometimes previously unrecognised emotions. Music therapy may reduce anxiety and build up self-esteem. The cathartic ('cleansing' or 'purgative') effect of the music may make it much easier for patients to express their pent-up feelings.

ART THERAPY
The process of creating an image can be a valuable first step in sharing the distress of a neurotic condition. Art therapy often provides a means of uprooting buried feelings, in a process which may be described as 'dreaming on paper'. The art work can be kept and discussed either at the time of making it or later. It gives a tangible record of progress which can be useful for both the patient and therapist.

Other alternative treatments

Hypnotherapy Psychoanalysis originally made great use of hypnosis in analysing the deep causes of neurotic disorders, and, properly used, it is still held to be of great value. The therapist can use posthypnotic suggestion to instruct the patient in self-help measures that are undetectable after coming out of the trance.
Dance Movement Therapy The aim of therapists in this field is to help clients to regain contact with their deep feelings, to discover the personal resources that are needed to cope with their emotional problems and (when done in a group) to develop

the ability to make positive, satisfying and lasting relationships.
Herbal Medicine Therapies vary according to the exact condition, but an infusion of camomile, lemon balm, lavender or thyme is held to aid relaxation. In some cases, herbalists may suggest stronger relaxants such as valerian, passion flower, skullcap or cowslip.

An orthodox view

As with physical illnesses, the treatment of nervous disorders depends largely on DIAGNOSIS, and this usually needs the skills of a qualified psychiatrist (a doctor specialising in mental problems) and possibly a psychologist (a person who studies people's minds and behaviour).

Psychiatric treatment may include PSYCHOTHERAPY, drug treatment, or both. The behavioural approach, which aims to teach patients to understand and cope with their problems, involves skilled psychologists, psychiatric nurses and counsellors in individual or group therapy sessions.

At one time, tranquillisers and sleeping pills were widely prescribed for neuroses and lesser psychological problems, but they are losing favour because of the risk of ADDICTION. However, there are non-addictive antidepressant drugs, such as amitriptyline and imipramine, which may help in the treatment of depression.

A sufferer from schizophrenia or manic depressive disorder requires skilled psychiatric help – sometimes in hospital. If the illness is a potential danger to the sufferer's life, or to that of someone else, it may be necessary to detain him in hospital against his will. Treatment with antipsychotic drugs, such as chlorpromazine, haloperidol or lithium, may allow the sufferer to lead a reasonably normal life, although medical supervision and treatment may always be needed.

NEURALGIA
Pain signals that spell trouble

When pain signals reach your brain along a nerve, you sense the pain as coming from whatever part of your body is served by that nerve. If the real cause is irritation or damage to the nerve itself, anywhere along its route, the pain still seems to come from that part of your body.

For example, inflammation of the trigeminal nerve, which is a carrier of sensations and which enters the skull near the ear, produces spasmodic pain in one side of the face. This kind of pain is called neuralgia.

See also NERVE DISORDERS.

What the therapists recommend
Acupressure For trigeminal neuralgia, press inwards at the inner eyebrow, or press downwards towards the jaw at the points near the corners of the mouth.
Acupuncture When pain is acute, treat neuralgia every day. The points manipulated are on the governor, gall bladder, bladder, large intestine, stomach and liver meridians.

Acupressure can relieve the pain of neuralgia. Try pressing inwards with an index finger at the inner end of the eyebrow on the affected side of the face for trigeminal neuralgia.

Alternatively, press downwards with the index fingers at the points close to the corners of the mouth. For both treatments press lightly for 5-10 minutes, and repeat half-hourly.

Aromatherapy Facial pain may be helped by applying, when required, a mixture of two drops of clove oil, one of basil and one of eucalyptus in a tablespoon of carrier lotion.

Biochemic Tissue Salts The principal remedy recommended is *Mag. phos.* taken every half hour until the pain subsides. *Kali phos.* is prescribed when it is accompanied by irritability or sleeplessness.

Herbal medicine Relief may be obtained by drinking an infusion of camomile, lemon balm, mint, rosemary or vervain. Placed on the site of the neuralgic pain, a warmed leaf of the 'wilde als' (wild wormwood) makes a soothing poultice.

An orthodox view

Having diagnosed the cause, a doctor may then prescribe painkillers. Alternatively he may apply transcutaneous nerve stimulation – electrical impulses passed through the skin from a portable instrument which anaesthetise the nerve (see ELECTROTHERAPY). Another method of providing relief is a 'nerve block' – an injection of phenol into the nerve to destroy the hypersensitive fibres. Drugs normally used to treat epilepsy may reduce the pain of trigeminal neuralgia.

Some hospitals in this country now have special 'pain clinics' which provide professional advice and treatment for sufferers from neuralgia and the wide assortment of other chronic types of pain.

NOISE POLLUTION

Increasing noise levels are a fact of modern life, so much so that even our homes are often far from peaceful. Yet noise is not just a nuisance – doctors now know that at high levels or over long periods of time noise can be a major cause of STRESS and related problems, as well as a danger to hearing.

See HEALTH HAZARDS.

NOSE AND THROAT AILMENTS

The symptoms of a sore throat and a blocked nose have many different causes. Viral and bacterial infections are responsible for COLDS, LARYNGITIS, TONSILLITIS, ADENOIDS and QUINSY. HAY FEVER, on the other hand, is a seasonal allergy to grass and other pollens. Laryngitis often results in temporary hoarseness, but if prolonged it may be caused by

polyps or 'singer's nodes' on the vocal cords, particularly if the voice is abused.

A NOSEBLEED can be caused by injury or infection, but most commonly it just happens for no clear reason.

Cleft palate – a readily seen gap in the roof of the mouth – may be associated with a hare lip, and is present from birth. The baby has difficulty sucking from the breast or bottle, and will go on to develop a characteristic speech impediment.

What the therapists recommend
AROMATHERAPY

Self help For CATARRH and a blocked-up nose, mix four drops of eucalyptus oil with the same amount of cajeput and half the amount of peppermint, and inhale either from a kitchen tissue or a basin of warm water (see p. 37) – provided you are not asthmatic. Diluted in a carrier oil or lotion, this mixture can be applied to the outside of the nose.

For a runny nose, mix three drops of eucalyptus with equal quantities of cypress and lemon oil, and inhale from a kitchen tissue. To relieve a sore throat, try three drops of eucalyptus, one of tea tree and two of sandalwood oil, either gargled in a glass of water or mixed in a tablespoon of carrier oil or lotion and rubbed around the throat and behind the ears. Do it three times during the day and before retiring at night.

The same techniques can be used with various oils from eucalyptus, aniseed, camphor, hyssop, cedarwood and cinnamon to ease a cough. Two drops each of thyme, sage and geranium oil can usually soothe swollen glands.

Other alternative treatments

Naturopathy For many problems such as nasal congestion and catarrh, or recurrent throat infections, you are advised to avoid dairy produce and sugars and eat more fresh fruit and vegetables. Vitamin C can be helpful – a gram a day for a short period, then half that amount in the long term – for chronic catarrh or infection.

Herbal Medicine Gargles of tincture of sage, thyme or myrrh can ease sore throats. Catarrh is relieved by steam inhalations (see p. 37), using one or two drops of the essential oils of eucalyptus, pine, cypress and lavender. Infusions (see p. 184) of catmint can help to clear a blocked-up nose.

An orthodox view

Most nose and throat ailments eventually clear up by themselves, so although antibiotics are sometimes given to speed recovery from a bacterial infection, most doctors recommend just rest and simple home remedies, such as inhalants, camphor oil and nasal sprays.

Serious or continual problems, however, require other medical treatment. For recurrent tonsillitis or swollen adenoids, and also nasal polyps, surgery may be the answer. And through plastic surgery most babies with a cleft palate can now develop normally.

NOSEBLEED
Isolating the causes of a common complaint

Many people, especially the young and middle-aged, occasionally suffer from bleeding from one or both nostrils. The bleeding usually comes from the superficial blood vessels just inside the nostril, on the septum, which divides the nose in two.

Nosebleeds have a variety of common causes, including COLDS, HYPERTENSION, SINUS PROBLEMS, blood disorders, injury, nose-picking, or SNEEZING, but sometimes occur without obvious cause. In most cases, they stop within an hour.

What the therapists recommend
TRADITIONAL MEDICINE

Self help Most nosebleeds can be stopped by the sufferer sitting upright in a chair with the head tilted slightly forward and firmly pinching the soft part of the nose for at least 15 minutes. Any blood that goes down the back of the nose should be swallowed or spat out. Breathe through the mouth. If the bleeding restarts, squeeze the nose for a further 15 minutes. An ice-pack applied to the bridge of the nose may help to reduce bleeding.

NATUROPATHY

For persistent nosebleeds, a general investigation of health, including BLOOD PRESSURE, may be required.

If there is swelling over the nose, an ice-cold compress may help. Causes such as severe CATARRH or sinus congestion will call for treatment through diet, supplements and, perhaps, inhalations, although excessive heat is not desirable in recurrent nosebleeds, so seek advice.

An orthodox view

If a nosebleed does not stop, the sufferer – especially if he is elderly or feeling faint – should consult his GP. The doctor may numb the nose with a local anaesthetic and pack it with gauze or an inflatable balloon. He may then take the patient's blood pressure to check for hypertension, and test the blood to see if there is any underlying cause for the bleeding. He may also cauterise any blood vessels prone to bleeding.

OBESITY

In South Africa there are very many obese adults. Seriously overweight people have an above-average chance of developing any of several diseases, including high BLOOD PRESSURE, CIRCULATION PROBLEMS, DIABETES, gall bladder problems, GOUT, HEART DISORDERS and heart attack. They also may not live as long as slim people, and their excess weight may eventually damage joints, causing OSTEOARTHRITIS, particularly of the knees and hips.

Obesity is caused by eating more food and drink than the body can use up in energy. The surplus energy is then stored as fat. See SLIMMING THE NATURAL WAY.

What the therapists recommend

NATUROPATHY

Consultation Individual treatment is considered vital, because a number of factors can combine to create the problem. Differences in metabolic rates are believed to be largely responsible, but emotional, psychological and social pressures will need to be assessed.

Generally, a simple crash diet is held *not* to be the answer to obesity, as it can lead eventually to weight gain as the metabolic rate slows even further.

A naturopath's advice will be that increasing EXERCISE at the same time as changing diet is important for speeding up metabolism. Multivitamin tablets may be prescribed to help replace any lost nutrients.

HOMOEOPATHY

Consultation Practitioners stress that there is no such thing as a 'wonder cure', but that constitutional help can be of value. A change of eating habits and extra exercise will be recommended.

Self help For the type of person who is flabby and inclined to perspire a lot, *Calc. carb.* may prove helpful, especially if he is depressed and has cravings for foods, particularly eggs. If there is WATER RETENTION, try *Natrum mur.* in the 6th potency twice daily for three weeks.

DANCE MOVEMENT THERAPY

Consultation Therapy will not be aimed directly at reducing weight (though it may help) but at aiding understanding of how your body is expressing itself, and allowing you to discover and work through underlying feelings relevant to your weight problem.

Alternatively, you may be taught how to come to terms with your particular weight and your shape, and how to achieve a more harmonious, integrated relationship with your body.

Other alternative treatments

Acupuncture Treatment is aimed at reducing the heightened appetite that springs from a weakened stomach-spleen system, by restoring the 'energy' flow along the spleen meridian. Points on the stomach, spleen, heart and lung meridians may be treated. Treating ear points is said to help overcome cravings for food. MOXIBUSTION, or the healing use of burning herbs, may also be used.

T'ai-chi Ch'uan Over a period of time, the exercises should tend to streamline the body. The everyday use of T'ai-chi's principles of balance, creativity and harmony should also reduce the urge to overeat and produce feelings of well-being.

An orthodox view

Most doctors will advise obese patients to lose weight by eating a balanced diet in moderate proportions (see EATING FOR HEALTH). Weight-losing drugs are not usually prescribed as they can become addictive and have dangerous side effects. EXERCISE is another effective way of losing and keeping down weight, in conjunction with dieting.

OBSESSIVE-COMPULSIVE BEHAVIOUR

Therapy for obstinate ideas and irrational acts

Obsessions are thoughts that are persistent, intrusive and difficult to control. Compulsions are actions and habits that a person feels driven to perform, and these, too, are usually persistent, difficult to stop and often unwanted. The two are often associated, and are then known medically as obsessive-compulsive behaviour.

Most people develop particular habits or routines at an early age. Sometimes these are based on superstitions such as touching a lucky horseshoe or always stepping over cracks in the pavement. Often they become parts of daily routine – dressing in a particular order, for example.

Other actions are based on safety or security, and these include repeatedly making sure that the car doors are locked before leaving it, or checking that the cooker is switched off before going out. Sometimes a particular thought or idea, such as a certain tune or a reminder to do something, keeps running through the mind.

Most of these thoughts and behaviour patterns are acceptable because they are not unduly worrying or disruptive in daily life; they are, in fact, fairly rational and sensible – or at least harmless. However, in some people

thoughts and actions get exaggerated and out of control, and become a problem.

In most cases, obsessive-compulsive behaviour is associated with strong feelings of ANXIETY. The anxiety may be based entirely on a fear that something bad or untoward will happen if the thoughts and actions are not carried through.

The sufferer may think that if he fails to keep himself and his house scrupulously clean, he will catch some infection or disease. He may feel compelled to wash his hands, body, clothes and all surfaces in the house repeatedly and thoroughly.

If he does not do this, he becomes increasingly anxious and uncomfortable, until eventually the need to engage in these activities overwhelms him, and he gives in. Other sufferers repeatedly check that doors and windows are locked, or arrange objects and ornaments in particular order. Others avoid certain objects, places or situations, or repeatedly check that they have not dropped or mislaid something.

The fear or anxiety may be logical. For example, it is reasonable to fear that if a gas fire is left on, it may start a blaze. However, the fear may lead to an irrational action – one that is not necessary or helpful – such as constantly checking that the gas fire is off.

Obsessional thoughts are also usually based on anxiety and FEAR. The obsessional person may repeatedly recite lists or numbers. If particularly anxious about his physical well-being, he may mentally run through a lengthy and involved checklist, making sure that every part of his body is all right. Some obsessional thoughts arise from the fear that something repulsive or abhorrent may be done, such as typing swear words into a letter, or standing up in church to blaspheme, or hitting someone, or performing some indecent act in public.

If unchecked, obsessive-compulsive behaviour can lead to a very disrupted life, and even to serious illness – mental disorders such as DEPRESSION and physical maladies such as malnutrition, for example.

Treatment in severe cases is difficult and should be left to professionals. However, one or two alternative therapies have proved helpful, and PSYCHOTHERAPY – particularly BEHAVIOURAL THERAPY – has been shown to be of some benefit in alleviating and controlling the condition.

What the therapists recommend

ART THERAPY

Self help This can be helpful in enabling a patient to 'let go' of some of the underlying fear, TENSION and anger, which often can lead to ritualistic behaviour. The resulting art work, however simple, provides a channel for communication and an outlet for deeply repressed anger. Using modelling clay, or other malleable materials, can be particularly helpful in the safe release of emotion.

BEHAVIOURAL THERAPY

Consultation Repeated thoughts and actions are seen as short-term ways of dealing with fear and anxiety. The therapist aims to teach the sufferer to manage his anxiety in more productive ways – for instance, by relaxation training.

Response prevention is also an important part of the treatment: the client is encouraged not to repeat the thought or action, so discovering that nothing bad or untoward will happen – that, in fact, his irrational fears do not come true.

AUTOGENIC TRAINING

Consultation Obsessional conditions are usually difficult to overcome, but autogenic training has a lot to offer for those with this kind of problem. In the hands of an experienced practitioner, great progress is said to be made in many cases.

Other alternative treatment

Colour Therapy The practitioner may find that old, unresolved difficulties are at the root of the problem, and very careful COUNSELLING is required to go over and try to break through the patterns formed in the mind of the client. This may be difficult, since the obsessive-compulsive behaviour is often rooted in the subconscious.

It may manifest itself in small, stupid, harmless actions at which most people might laugh – or, at the other end of the scale, as serious crime.

Counselling with colour has, it is claimed, shown that a soft magenta, along with relaxation therapy, given by an experienced, professional practitioner, can turn what may be a vicious circle of negative actions into a spiral of growth. Tactful recognition of the self – through the counsellor – is vital. Relaxation, colour, music and counselling are said to prove very successful.

An orthodox view

An obsessional personality is unlikely to change and does not require treatment. But if it leads to depression, doctors can help by diagnosing and explaining the problem and, if necessary, prescribing certain antidepressant medicines. Severe obsessive-compulsive behaviour is difficult to treat, although it naturally improves in time.

The results of medicines and psychotherapy tend to be disappointing, so successful management of the condition depends upon the sufferer adjusting his particular way of life to reduce or eliminate the stresses that initially caused the problem.

ORGONE THERAPY

The idea that there is a universal energy present in all living creatures, in the atmosphere, in all matter and even in space was the theory behind orgone therapy. The treatment was developed in the first half of this century by Wilhelm Reich (1897-1958), an Austrian psychiatrist and follower of Freud, and it formed a part of REICHIAN THERAPY.

According to Reich, this force – which he called 'orgone energy' – is stored in units termed 'bions'. These, he maintained, can be trapped in machines which are known as 'orgone accumulators' and then used to help to heal diseases.

Reich achieved some remarkable results, but his controversial ideas brought him into conflict with the medical and legal authorities in the United States, where he had gone to practise – and where he died in prison. People objected to his linking of orgone energy with orgasm and sexual fulfilment, and in particular to his claims that patients placed in boxes containing orgone accumulators could be cured of CANCER and other serious diseases.

Although much of Reich's equipment and many of his papers were destroyed after his death, some European therapists have recently started to use orgone therapy again. Sometimes they include so-called 'vegetotherapy' which, like BIOENERGETICS, is a more widely accepted technique based on Reich's idea that muscular tensions – particularly of the abdomen – and unnatural breathing patterns can be signs of emotional problems. By manipulating the body, therapists aim to relieve both physical and psychological tensions.

See also HUMANISTIC PSYCHOLOGY.

ORIENTAL DIAGNOSIS

Clues in the pulse and on the tongue

Like Western doctors, traditional oriental practitioners begin every consultation by trying to identify the patient's problem. However, since they have a very different view of how the healthy body functions and of what causes disease, they rely on completely different methods of DIAGNOSIS.

Most of the oriental techniques come from traditional Chinese medicine, which views good health as a state of harmony between YIN AND YANG – stages in the processes of change that constantly occur in the body – and balance in the body's energy, or Qi (chi).

Qi is said to flow along an invisible network of pathways called MERIDIANS that link all bodily organs and systems. Any blockage or imbalance in the network is believed to cause physical or mental illness. The purpose of diagnosis in oriental therapies such as ACUPUNCTURE, ACUPRESSURE and SHIATSU is to identify any trouble spots or blockages on the meridians, so that appropriate treatment can be given.

A variety of sophisticated techniques are used to make the diagnosis, many going back in time several thousands of years. As well as asking questions about the patient's symptoms, history, habits and way of life, the practitioner makes careful notes about the sound of the voice, the texture and colour of the skin, breathing patterns, posture and even smell.

All are used together to build up a detailed picture of the person's health, but most weight is given to two particular procedures: pulse diagnosis and tongue diagnosis.

Pulse diagnosis At least 12 different pulses are usually measured in Chinese medicine, corresponding to the major organs and systems of the body.

The practitioner finds them by pressing lightly with three fingers – each of which can detect a different pulse – along the artery on the inside of the wrist. Different pulses are measured by pressing a little deeper, and the procedure is then repeated on the other wrist, giving a total of 12 pulses. Medium pressure is sometimes used to read six more pulses that are believed to reflect the energy level of the blood.

Each pulse is interpreted in terms of 28 different qualities or descriptions – such as 'rapid', 'slippery', 'choppy', 'full', 'scattered' and 'empty'. On the basis of these interpretations and the strength or weakness of each pulse, the practitioner decides where energy imbalances lie and how to correct them. Using deduction, based on their observation of signs and symptoms, skilled practitioners claim to find evidence of past diseases and can suggest the likelihood of any future health problems.

The pulses are said also to be affected by factors other than illness, such as time of day, season, nervousness and physical exertion. An experienced practitioner will be aware of all these influences and he will be able to link them to information about the patient's state of health.

Tongue diagnosis Practitioners consider the colour, shape and coating of the tongue as well as how moist or dry it is, whether it has surface markings, such as cracks or 'thorns', and whether there are any scars or ulcers on it.

Different parts of the tongue are examined to provide information about different organs. For example, a bluish-purple tip is said to show a particular energy state in the heart, and teeth marks around the edge may indicate a digestion problem.

A light white coating on the tongue is considered to be normal, but a thicker grey, yellow or white 'fur' to show some disturbance. A healthy tongue should be slightly moist, indicating that body fluids are flowing freely; if it is too dry or too moist, an imbalance is diagnosed.

The exact type of imbalance is decided by considering other signs such as whether the tongue is cracked, swollen, stiff or quivering, together with all the other information obtained from the patient.

ORTHOMOLECULAR MEDICINE

The term was first used by the American biochemist and double Nobel prizewinner Linus Pauling (1901-), to describe treatment centred on giving individuals the best possible concentrations of vitamins and minerals for their physical and mental health. Individual needs for these nutrients vary widely, he said, and doses recommended could be dozens or even hundreds of times greater than the amounts generally thought suitable. Such treatment is now popularly called MEGAVIT-AMIN THERAPY.

OSTEOARTHRITIS

Wear and tear on the joints, which eventually damages shock-absorbing cartilage between the bones, is the usual cause of this condition. Symptoms include pain, stiffness and deformed joints, and affect mainly the hips, knees, spine and fingers. See ARTHRITIS.

OSTEOPATHY

Your skeleton key to fitness ...

The body's largest system is its framework of bones, joints, muscles and ligaments. It is this framework that allows us to walk, run, drive, speak, write, build, play sports – in fact, carry out any physical activity. Osteopathy, in some countries one of the most widely used of all the complementary forms of medicine, aims to diagnose and treat various mechanical problems in the framework.

Andrew Taylor Still

Making the body's machine run smoothly

An American doctor, Andrew Taylor Still (1828-1917), founded osteopathy in the mid-1870s after he became dissatisfied with orthodox medicine. He felt that stimulating the body's natural powers of self healing would be preferable to using the often dangerous drugs of his day.

His detailed knowledge of human anatomy, combined with his earlier study of engineering, made him interested in the body as a machine. He became certain that many illnesses arise when part of the body's structure gets out of alignment. Manipulation could, he decided, restore the balance and cure the illness.

Strong initial opposition to Still's ideas gradually dwindled in the United States, and today osteopathy is an accepted part of established medicine in that country, where most modern research into the therapy has been carried out. Osteopathy came to Britain at the turn of the century, and the British School of Osteopathy was established in London in 1917.

In South Africa, by contrast, osteopathy as a profession is technically being phased out: the Pretoria-based Associated Health Service Professions Board is no longer prepared to register osteopaths – although the related therapy of CHIROPRACTIC is recognised by the board. The study of osteopathy is included in the five-year master's diploma course offered at the Natal Technikon's Department of Chiropractic (P O Box 953, Durban 4000).

These problems may be caused by injury or STRESS, for example, and they prevent the framework from functioning comfortably and efficiently. Osteopaths believe that when the structure of the body is sound, it will work just like a well-tuned engine, with the minimum of wear and tear. The body is seen in holistic terms as a unified organism, with all systems operating in concert; and a disturbance in any one particular system can alter the functions of others.

Standing upright – particularly for long periods at a time – poses a great and constant strain on the body's mechanism. The force of gravity is particularly severe on the vertebrae of the spine and the cushioning discs between them. The spinal joints and their discs have become weight-bearing in the upright position, a burden which poor posture increases, so making mechanical problems more likely to occur. Osteopaths use their hands for massaging and manipulating the framework to restore normal, more comfortable function.

Who it can help People with spinal problems, such as low BACK PAIN and NECK PAIN, account for more than half of an osteopath's workload. But practitioners also bring relief to mechanical problems in many other parts of the body – often resulting from stresses at work. Tension headaches caused by contraction of the small muscles at the base of the skull are another problem frequently treated by osteopaths.

Many patients have sustained SPORTS IN-JURIES to muscles or to the joints of the hips, knees, ankles, feet, wrists, shoulders or elbows. Older people who are suffering the onset of OSTEOARTHRITIS can also find treatment beneficial. During PREGNANCY many women develop back pain because of a change in posture, and they, too, can often be helped by osteopathic treatment.

Finding a practitioner Try to find an osteopath by personal recommendation; or else write, enclosing a stamped, self-addressed envelope, to the South African Homoeopathic Association, 20 Botanic Grove, Berea 4001, asking for the name and address of a qualified practitioner in your area.

Though your GP may be able to refer you to an osteopath it is possible that he will be unsympathetic to your request to be treated by this form of 'alternative' therapy.

Consulting a practitioner The osteopath will first want to know how your symptoms began and what makes them better or worse. Your medical history and any current treatments you may be receiving will be noted.

Then the practitioner will carry out a detailed physical examination. He will observe you standing, sitting, lying down and performing certain movements such as bending forwards, backwards and to the side. The range and quality of movement in particular joints will be assessed, and the osteopath will examine by touch the soft tissues, muscles and ligaments to see if they are abnormally tense or stressed.

During this 'structural survey' the osteopath diagnoses any abnormalities in the body's framework, which may be confirmed by other tests, such as the conventional testing of reflexes with a small hammer. In some cases an osteopath will ask for an X-ray, par-

Self help on wheels

Car drivers often have a poor and re-stricted posture behind the wheel, which can lead to back pain, stiff-ness in the neck and shoulders, and tension headaches. To help people avoid these discomforts – and so take the 'pain' out of driving – osteo-paths suggest a set of procedures which are easy to follow and put into practice.

Make sure that the car seat is ad-justed so that the steering wheel and pedals are all within easy reach. You should be sitting up straight with your knees slightly bent but not so bent that they interfere with the steering wheel. To remind you to sit up straight, every time you get in the car make sure your bottom is as far back in the seat as possible. Then straighten up and, if necess-ary, adjust the rear-view mirror.

As your hands hold the steering wheel (preferably at between nine and ten o'clock and at between two and three o'clock, if you imagine the wheel as a clock face), your arms should be slightly bent. Adjust the seat to lean slightly back, as this will make it easier for you to main-tain a well-balanced and comfort-able position for your neck and back.

If you do have a back problem, you can buy or make a simple lum-bar roll to tuck behind you and sup-port the curve of your lower back.

When you are driving, check from time to time that your shoulders are relaxed. Keep your head upright with your chin tucked in; if it juts for-ward, the muscles at the back of your neck are under strain.

There are many relaxation exer-cises you can do in a traffic jam.

1 Shrug your shoulders towards your ears and then roll them back-wards with your head bent slightly forward. Repeat two or three times.

2 Tighten and relax your sto-mach muscles two or three times – you can do this while you are driv-ing as well as at stops. It improves your posture and helps circulation in the legs.

3 Tuck your chin close to your chest and then relax it back to nor-mal. Repeat this several times and you will feel the muscles at the back of your neck stretching gently.

ticularly if there has been a recent accident or major health crisis.

If the examination shows that your condi-tion is suitable for treatment, a course will be planned. If not, the osteopath may recom-mend that you see your doctor again. Length of treatment by an osteopath varies enor-mously. It may last over several sessions for a long-standing condition, but a recent, acute problem may be relieved immediately.

A treatment session usually lasts 20-30 minutes, and most people find it relaxing and enjoyable. Several techniques may be used. MASSAGE of soft tissue relaxes taut muscles

Treating an injured knee

Sports injuries account for many joint problems, and here a patient is examined by an osteopath after twisting a knee while playing tennis. By making a 'structural survey' of the problem area, the practitioner diagnoses the extent of the injury. He also asks the patient for her full medical history – in particular, if she has previously suffered any pain or discomfort in the knee.

and improves circulation. Gentle, repetitive movement of joints increases their mobility and reduces tension in surrounding muscles. By massaging tender 'trigger' points, the os-teopath may be able to improve the function-ing of organs lying within the same reflex zone. He may also (using what is known as neuromuscular technique) probe with his thumb for tense or fibrosed areas – the physi-cal knots that have been caused by stress.

Fixed or malfunctioning joints may be re-leased by guiding the joint rapidly through its normal range of movement. This produces the clicking that many people associate with

After assessing the damage – and deciding that the patient is a suitable case for treatment – the osteopath sets to work on the injured knee. He manipulates the malfunctioning joint back into working order and guides it through its normal range of pain-free movement. In addition, the gentle manipulation of the joint eases tension that has built up in the nearby muscles.

osteopathic treatment. A dramatic relief from pain may sometimes be achieved by such startling methods. EXERCISE, advice on posture, and relaxation techniques are often recommended; patients implement these at home between treatment sessions.

For some conditions, including head and facial pain, CRANIAL OSTEOPATHY may be used. The theory behind this controversial technique was expounded by an American named William Garner Sutherland, who believed that the various bony plates forming the skull are capable of a degree of movement. With such movement, the circulation of the cerebro-spinal fluid can be improved. The technique involves applying gentle pressures to the head and upper neck. Areas where there is strain or where movement is restricted are held painlessly at the point of tension until the condition is relieved.

An orthodox view

Conventional doctors would dispute the value of osteopathy for patients with non-mechanical symptoms. They see correct diagnosis by a qualified medical practitioner as essential before it can be decided whether osteopathy is the right treatment.

However, a qualified and experienced osteopath can give a great deal of relief to patients with musculoskeletal pain where orthodox medicine can only offer pain-killers and anti-inflammatory drugs.

OSTEOPOROSIS

Thinning and weakening of the bones

Women who are past the MENOPAUSE are the principal sufferers of this disorder, in which the bones become progressively thinner, weaker and more brittle – due in part to loss of calcium in the bones. Osteoporosis can, however, begin to affect people who are in their mid-twenties.

The spine gradually becomes shorter and more curved, resulting in loss of height and the characteristic hunching of the shoulders often known as 'dowager's hump'. The brittle bones are easily broken, especially at the hip or wrist, even by minor injuries or normal everyday activities (see FRACTURES).

Although persistent BACK PAIN is common, there are often no warning symptoms and the condition is sometimes discovered in its early stages only if an X-ray is taken for some other reason. Osteoporosis can be caused by prolonged treatment by steroid drugs and is aggravated by lack of EXERCISE or insufficient care over diet.

What the therapists recommend

Yoga Practitioners believe that osteoporosis – and other bone problems – can be combated by more efficient breathing. Diaphragmatic breathing is said to help the body to deal with changes in bone structure. In addition, relaxation techniques are employed to help ease the condition.

T'ai-chi Ch'uan The graceful movements of T'ai-chi help patients to adapt to changes in their bodies and to maintain a positive and creative outlook. This is particularly important in middle age, when diseases such as osteoporosis may occur and the female body is undergoing disturbing hormonal changes. T'ai-chi is said to promote the use of mental, emotional and physical energies, helping the patient to function normally.

Naturopathy Regular exercise is thought to be essential in preventing osteoporosis, or stopping the condition worsening. Plenty of protein is recommended, and a wholefood diet with additional seeds such as sesame and sunflower, nuts, grains and pulses will probably be suggested. Calcium and vitamin D may also be prescribed.

Homoeopathy Consultation with a therapist is recommended, for individual treatment including advice on diet and exercise.

An orthodox view

Doctors recommend regular exercise to prevent the onset of osteoporosis – although once the disease has taken hold it increases slowly with age.

The most successful conventional treatment is hormone replacement therapy (HRT; see MENOPAUSE), which can alleviate osteoporosis if taken for several years. It is particularly effective for women who reach the menopause before the age of 45. However, in some cases it can have unwanted and occasionally serious side effects.

OVARIAN PROBLEMS

A woman has two ovaries in the lower abdomen, one on either side of the womb. They produce eggs (ova) almost every month from the commencement of monthly periods until periods stop at the MENOPAUSE. Sometimes the ovaries are painful at the mid-point of the menstrual cycle when they release eggs, and this is known as ovulation pain.

Growths on or in the ovaries are usually benign, but are occasionally malignant (see CANCER). Fluid-filled swellings called cysts are common. The vast majority are small and benign, and may persist for years without symptoms. Others cause intermittent pain in the lower abdomen, often during menstruation or ovulation. Some ovarian cysts become very large, and others twist, rupture or bleed, causing severe pain and sickness.

Consult your doctor immediately if there is any pain or swelling in the lower abdomen, or if pain is felt during sexual intercourse – as this could indicate the presence of cysts.

The ovaries also release female hormones into the bloodstream. Imbalance of these hormones can cause various symptoms, including INFERTILITY and PREMENSTRUAL TENSION (PMT). The organs naturally cease to produce hormones at the menopause, and this sometimes leads to OSTEOPOROSIS.

What the therapists recommend

Naturopathy Practitioners consider that poor functioning of the ovaries can be a result of poor general health, STRESS, long-term use of the contraceptive pill, and other factors. Serious disorders such as ovarian cysts require qualified help. But for general disorders which can cause PERIOD PROBLEMS, improvements to diet and EXERCISE levels are advised. These are aimed at benefiting the reproductive system and general well-being of the woman.

Herbal Medicine Many herbs have hormonal effects. A professional herbalist may use chaste tree (*agnus castus*), false unicorn root, blue cohosh or wild yam, among others, to restore ovarian activity to normal.

Aromatherapy If you suspect that the problem is hormonal, the essential oils recommended are: clary sage, true melissa, lemon, pine and orange. Mix a total of four to six drops in a tablespoon of carrier oil, and massage into the abdomen and small of the back each night and morning.

An orthodox view

The doctor can examine the ovaries and feel any growths or cysts by performing an internal pelvic examination through the vagina. He may recommend an ultrasound scan, in which very high frequency sound waves are passed through the body to build up a picture rather as an X-ray does, or a laparoscopic examination, in which internal structures are examined with a lighted instrument passed through a small cut in the abdominal wall. These will usually reveal whether a growth is benign or cancerous. If necessary, growths can then be removed by surgery.

A doctor may recommend a blood test for hormone levels at a certain point in the menstrual cycle in order to diagnose hormonal problems or the cause of infertility. Hormone treatment, usually taken by tablet or suppository, may restore fertility or relieve symptoms of PMT.

PAIN

Nature's early warning system

The first indication of an unseen malady within the body is usually pain – a natural early warning system. This unpleasant – at times agonising – sensation afflicts most people at some time as a result of injury, disease or emotional disorder. Yet pain can at times be of great benefit to the body.

It tells the brain to take avoiding action against whatever is causing the pain. This is usually an involuntary action, as when your hand jerks away when pricked by a pin, or when you touch something very hot. It thus prevents further injury.

Though the sufferer finds pain all too real, it is often difficult to describe. However, it is important to try, for a description will help a therapist or doctor to make a DIAGNOSIS.

Continuous and throbbing pain indicates swelling or inflammation in a restricted space, as in a carbuncle or tooth abscess. Intermittent stabbing pain results from the stretching or swelling of a tube-like part of the body such as the intestine. In certain cases, such as ANGINA and gangrene, disruption of the blood supply produces continuous severe pain in the affected part. Burning pain is felt when heat, friction or chemicals destroy body tissues. A dull continuous ache can signal strained muscles and ligaments.

Exactly where you feel the pain is also important in diagnosis – it may not necessarily be felt at the site of the actual injury or disease. This 'referred pain', as it is known, can be felt down the left arm and fingers in some HEART DISORDERS, for example, while an abscess under the diaphragm gives pain in the shoulder, and pain from a slipped disc may radiate down the leg.

The pain threshold Tests have shown that the 'pain threshold' – the point during the painful stimulus at which pain is first felt – is roughly the same among all ordinary, healthy people. On the other hand, the 'pain tolerance' point, when pain becomes unpleasant, varies greatly.

However, several factors, other than the immediate cause of pain, can influence the threshold. Illness, hunger, extremes of climatic temperature, swings in temperature and pain caused by another condition all work to lower the threshold, giving greater pain. For example, many arthritics find their pain worse in spring and autumn, when swings in temperature are at their greatest.

Psychological conditions, including worry, FEAR, ANXIETY, fatigue, STRESS, DEPRESSION and INSOMNIA all play a similar role. For instance, a pain often gets worse as the day progresses, and your tiredness increases.

Other psychological factors work in the opposite way to raise the threshold and ease the pain. When you believe strongly that a pain will get better, it often does; and faith in your doctor, therapist or treatment to make it better may have the same effect. And so do concentration of the mind, and emotions such as happiness and excitement. You may be so absorbed in catching your train that you fail to notice that your shoes are giving you blisters. Then there are the physical pain relievers, such as analgesics, anaesthetics, and a variety of conventional and alternative remedies and treatments.

However, all practitioners are only too aware that pain is often an early warning that something is wrong, whether it is a physical problem or an emotional condition, such as hypochondria or PSYCHOSOMATIC ILLNESS, and will aim to diagnose and treat the root cause. Sufferers should bear this in mind too – if a pain persists, see a doctor.

Killing pain the natural way The body produces its own powerful painkillers. Endorphins and encephalins are examples – proteins occurring naturally in the brain which have effects similar to those induced by opiates. The body synthesises them from amino acids in the proteins in your diet.

Dopamine and the so-called stress hormones adrenaline and noradrenaline, which are produced by the adrenal glands, are similar proteins. Their release is triggered by stress and EXERCISE, and can prove very effective. For example, a rugby player may not become aware that he has been injured until an exciting and strenuous game is over; and many wounded people have little or no pain at the time of their injury. The hormones can also relieve chronic (long-lasting) pain.

Dopamine and the hormones are produced by the body from the amino acid phenylalanine or DL-phenylalanine (DLPA). The body cannot synthesise this, and it is an 'essential amino acid' – one that must be provided by the diet. Cheese, nuts such as peanuts and almonds, avocados, bananas, lima beans, herrings, and sesame and pumpkin seeds are good dietary sources.

Like vitamins and minerals, DLPA is available as a dietary supplement from health shops. However, you should follow the manufacturer's instructions carefully, and ask your doctor about taking the supplement if you are pregnant or are being treated for high BLOOD PRESSURE. You should not take DLPA if you suffer from MIGRAINE, are taking tyrosine as a supplement, or are taking certain drugs used to treat depression.

Besides the therapies covered below, the following may also help to relieve your pain: VISUALISATION THERAPY, OSTEOPATHY, HYPNOTHERAPY, PSYCHOTHERAPY, AUTOGENIC TRAINING, BIOFEEDBACK, YOGA, RELAXATION AND BREATHING, HEALERS AND HEALING, and HOMOEOPATHY. Different ones will benefit different people and different types of pain.

What the therapists recommend

The therapists investigate and treat the condition causing the pain. For the pain itself they recommend the following:

ACUPRESSURE

Self help For general pain, apply pressure in the hollow behind the outer ankle bone, pressing inwards and a little towards the ankle bone. For pain in the upper body, apply pressure at the end of the crease in the web between the finger and thumb, pressing towards the finger bone. For pain in the lower body, you should apply pressure one hand's width above the crown of the inner ankle bone just behind the shin bone, pressing inwards beside the bone.

AROMATHERAPY

Self help For muscular pain, use six to eight drops of essential oil in a bath, and stay in it for ten minutes. Choose two or three oils from the following: camphor, cajuput, eucalyptus, ginger, juniper, lavender, marjoram, rosemary or sage, all of which warm and relax painful tissues. A most effective application lotion can be made by using a total of 15 drops in 5 dessertspoons (50 ml) of a base carrier lotion or carrier oil. Apply night and morning or as required on the affected part.

For stomach pain, apply a teaspoon of carrier oil or lotion mixed with two drops of fennel and two drops of peppermint if due to indigestion. If it is due to constipation or wind, substitute two drops of rosemary for the peppermint. A nervous stomach will respond better to aniseed and basil.

For period pains, use oils of Roman camomile, true melissa and rose otto. These are expensive, but you can use less-expensive oils mixed with them. However, if you do use them, mix a few drops of each together in a dropper bottle for ease of application and enhanced results. Alternatively, use cajuput, sage, aniseed, cypress and marjoram. Apply the mixed lotion or oil to the abdomen and small of the back twice a day, from the tenth day before the period is due to start.

Other alternative treatments

Herbal Medicine Several herbs can reduce the level of pain. Some such as meadowsweet and willow bark are similar to aspirin. Others such as wild yam and black cohosh have a steroidal effect. If an infusion of meadowsweet and camomile does not give relief, seek qualified help for the problem.

Massage It is instinctive to rub a part of the body when it hurts, so do this initially if it helps to lessen the pain. However, in some

painful situations, massage would definitely be inadvisable, and the therapist will decide whether this is so when making a diagnosis.
Acupuncture A point on the large intestine meridian and other distal points are used for the rapid relief of pain.

An orthodox view

Doctors aim to find the root cause of the pain and treat it, or refer patients to a specialist consultant. They have a battery of drugs at their disposal. Mild pain usually responds well to non-narcotic drugs such as aspirin, which can also relieve inflammation. This can cause irritation of the stomach lining, but the use of soluble aspirin and taking it with or after food – never on an empty stomach – helps to some degree. Paracetamol does not have this side effect, but it does not relieve inflammation, and an overdose – even a small one – can cause severe liver damage.

Narcotic drugs that dull the senses and induce sleep are prescribed for more severe pain. Many of them, like codeine, are opium derivatives, and most can lead to ADDICTION. They should be used with caution.

Always follow very carefully the manufacturer's instructions on dosage for over-the-counter painkillers, and tell your doctor what you have taken if you consult him later.

Anti-inflammatory drugs ease arthritic and rheumatic pain. Apart from aspirin these fall into two groups: steroids and non-steroidal anti-inflammatory drugs (NSAIDs), such as ibuprofen. One or two of these, such as ibuprofen (Nurofen), are available without prescription. The side effects of steroids include increased appetite, weight gain, digestive disorders, NAUSEA AND VOMITING and change in sleep patterns. NSAIDs may cause DIARRHOEA, gastrointestinal irritation and bleeding, and HEADACHES. If you experience any such side effects, see your doctor at once; another drug may suit you better.

A further group of drugs reduces the formation of uric acid and are prescribed for GOUT pains. Side effects include digestive upsets with stomach pains, nausea, vomiting and loss of appetite, and itching or rashes.

See also ULCERS, INDIGESTION and TOOTH AND GUM DISORDERS.

PALPITATIONS

Healthy people are usually conscious of their heartbeat after strenuous exercise – such as running for a bus, or up a flight of stairs – or while experiencing ANXIETY or FEAR. Awareness of the heart beating at other times, known as palpitations, may sometimes be a sign of heart disease. There are three main types of palpitations: rapid heartbeat, irregular heartbeat, and extra heartbeat.

If you have prolonged or persistent palpitations, you should see a doctor before undertaking any alternative therapy.

Rapid heartbeat, or tachycardia, can be a sign of an overactive thyroid gland (see THYROID DISORDERS), and may occur in short bursts called paroxysmal tachycardia. It particularly affects anxious people whose bodies produce a lot of adrenaline. Caffeine in coffee sometimes causes rapid heartbeat.

Irregular heartbeat, accompanied by an irregular pulse, is common in elderly people. It can also be caused by ALCOHOLISM, thyroid disorders, or disease of the heart valves or blood supply (see HEART DISORDERS).

Extra heartbeat affects everyone at times. A premature heartbeat is followed by a pause before the next normal beat, causing the sensation of a 'dropped' or missed heartbeat. An excessive number of extra beats may be caused by anxiety, or may be a symptom of a heart disorder.

What the therapists recommend

Massage Before undergoing massage you should consult a doctor to make sure there is no underlying disease, especially of the heart. If there is no heart disorder, however, slow stroking of the limbs may help to ease the palpitations.

An orthodox view

Most cases of palpitation can be relieved by cutting down on the consumption of non-decaffeinated coffee and alcohol. However, if another cause is suspected, a doctor will take a patient's pulse and BLOOD PRESSURE. If necessary, he will arrange for an electrocardiogram (ECG) to be taken to determine if there is any heart disorder, and blood tests to detect any thyroid disorder.

Palpitations caused by heart disease usually respond to drugs such as beta-blockers, digoxin, or verapamil.

PARANORMAL THERAPIES

This group of therapies is known to the various practitioners simply as 'healing'. It includes FAITH HEALING – a term not used by the practitioners themselves – and also some therapies in which faith in the healing method or practitioner on the part of the patient is not necessary. Indeed, in some paranormal therapies the patient may not know that therapy is taking place. See HEALERS AND HEALING.

Healers all believe in the existence of a healing force or forces. These may be supernatural forces invoked by the participants and transcending the forces of nature or able to alter them, or psychic forces of the participants which, while natural, have yet to be explained.

There are several aspects of paranormal therapies. Some people are believed to have the power to 'tune in' to the healing force(s), and to channel or 'beam' them through themselves or directly to others. Such therapies include CHARISMATIC HEALING; SPIRITUAL HEALING; LAYING ON OF HANDS, which is also known as 'hand healing'; ABSENT HEALING, or 'prayers for the sick'; THERAPEUTIC TOUCH; and Christian Science.

PARATYPHOID FEVER

This highly infectious disease – caused by the bacterium *Salmonella paratyphi* – is similar in most respects to TYPHOID, being an intestinal or 'enteric' fever. It is apt to be less severe than typhoid, however; and though some people carry the disease (often in the gallbladder) without showing any of its symptoms, such long-term carriers are less frequently encountered than with typhoid. Infection occurs when food, milk or water has been contaminated by human faeces containing the bacterium; flies are often the cause of the contamination.

Symptoms of paratyphoid fever include headache, diarrhoea (sometimes preceded by constipation) and a rash of red spots.

What the therapists recommend

Homoeopathy Treatment may include the use of *Bryonia*, *Rhus tox* and *Arsenicum alb*, among other remedies. However, the patient's clinical status is ultimately the determining factor, and any emergency must always be treated in hospital.
Herbal medicine Infuse the leaves, stems and fruit of the crane's bill ('dysentery herb') in boiling water to make a tea that should be drunk throughout the day, at two-hour intervals. A medicinal tea can also be made from the leaves and flowers of another pungent indigenous plant, the cat herb (counterpart to the European horehound).

An orthodox view

The patient should be isolated and provided with nursing care, special attention being paid to the replacement of fluids which have been lost as a result of diarrhoea. Antibiotics may prolong an acute illness rather than bring it to an end; but they are prescribed for a carrier of the disease.

PARKINSON'S DISEASE

Muscular stiffness, along with slowness and difficulty in moving about, are among the symptoms of Parkinson's disease, or parkinsonism, a disorder of the nervous system.

These symptoms become progressively worse. The muscles of the face stiffen, so that sufferers may develop a blank stare or a frowning expression. Walking becomes increasingly slow and difficult. Patients stoop and shuffle, taking short steps. Some find it easier to walk backwards than forwards.

Although many people associate the disease with a shake, or tremor, this is not always the case. If it does occur, the head may nod rhythmically and the fingers may tremble involuntarily, as if a pill were being rolled between thumb and fingers. Patients often suffer from DEPRESSION, sometimes severely, or they may have hallucinations.

Parkinson's disease is caused by degeneration of the ganglia – groups of nerve cell bodies – and shortage of dopamine, a substance which is thought to be a transmitter of nerve impulses.

What the therapists recommend

Yoga Many people suffering from Parkinson's disease allow the malfunctioning of the muscular system to seize them up and make them increasingly inactive. A well-balanced programme of yoga postures (*asanas*) is aimed at providing an effective counter to the stiffening process. Relaxation while lying down, and full attention to the most suitable posture, reduce twitching and calm the body. Visualisation of the brain repairing the dopamine deficiency is said to have been used effectively by some sufferers.

Counselling This can be important for anyone in a chronic, progressive, incurable condition, because the individual may need help to come to terms with the dysfunction and disability.

An orthodox view

If you think you have Parkinson's disease – it can develop gradually and may go unnoticed at first – consult a doctor. He may prescribe drugs containing levodopa as a substitute for the brain's dopamine deficiency, or anticholinergic drugs to reduce tremor and muscle stiffness. Another useful drug is bromocriptine, which stimulates dopamine receptors in the brain.

However, between 10 and 20 per cent of patients do not respond to drug treatment, and even when treatment is effective, the disease causes progressive disability, so that sufferers become increasingly dependent on relatives and others. For further information about this condition, and for the address of a support group in your area, write to the South African Parkinsonian Association, P O Box 10901, Aston Manor 1630.

PERIOD PROBLEMS

Every woman's menstrual cycle is different, and although symptoms such as pain or irregularity can be unpleasant, they are usually the result of natural hormone changes and not illness. Some of the most common problems are:

Painful periods (dysmenorrhoea) Sufferers tend to be girls or young women. They experience cramp-like pains in the lower abdomen at the beginning of a period and sometimes also feel ill or faint. Symptoms usually pass after one or two days, and are only rarely a sign of illness. Most often, the cause is a 'tight' cervix (the muscle at the neck of the womb), which generally loosens after the first pregnancy, putting an end to the problem. An intrauterine contraceptive device (IUD) or a menstrual cycle in which no egg is produced is also sometimes to blame.

Lack of periods (amenorrhoea) This condition is natural during PREGNANCY and MENOPAUSE. In other cases, it may follow use of the contraceptive pill (see CONTRACEPTION) or be a symptom of ANOREXIA.

Heavy periods (menorrhagia) Some women have naturally heavier periods than others, but greater than usual blood loss may also be due to a hormone imbalance, use of an IUD, small non-cancerous growths in the womb known as fibroids, or to an infection of the womb or uterine tubes.

Other problems MIGRAINE headaches are more common during a period than at other times of the month. PREMENSTRUAL TENSION (PMT) and its associated symptoms are also a common complaint.

Self help Take adequate EXERCISE and eat a well-balanced diet with plenty of iron, calcium and vitamin B_1. A traditional remedy is a hot infusion of parsley leaf tea. Herbalists also recommend a similar infusion of camomile, lemon balm, marjoram or thyme, with perhaps a little ginger added.

What the therapists recommend

AROMATHERAPY

Self help Oils of Roman camomile, true melissa and rose otto are recommended for dealing with most menstrual problems – irregular or scanty periods, painful ones, PMT, and menopause. These particular oils are expensive, but it is possible to combine them with less costly ones.

If using Roman camomile, rose otto and/or true melissa – not the compound melissa oil – mix a few drops of each in a dropper bottle, for easy use and enhanced results. To prepare an application oil or lotion, blend a total of 15 drops of the chosen essential oils in 5 dessertspoons (50 ml) of carrier oil or lotion.

For irregular and scanty periods try clary sage, fennel and thyme. Apply a mixed lotion or oil to the abdomen twice daily.

For painful periods, cajuput, sage, aniseed, cypress and marjoram are recommended. A mixed oil should be applied to the abdomen and small of the back twice daily, from the tenth day before the period is due to start.

For PMT use clary sage, geranium and lavender. A bath containing a total of six to eight drops of these essential oils should be taken daily for two weeks before the period is due. It is also said to be beneficial to inhale regularly and deeply during those two weeks, using either a few drops on a tissue (or one drop in the palm of the hand, if using Roman camomile, rose otto or melissa, cupping your hands over your nose). An application lotion or oil can be mixed and used as an after-bath lotion all the time as a preventive measure.

NATUROPATHY

Self help Painful periods may be relieved by taking more exercise and eating a wholefood diet (see EATING FOR HEALTH) rich in FIBRE-containing foods such as raw fruits and vegetables. This helps to prevent CONSTIPATION during periods. In addition, alternate hot-and-cold compresses to the lower abdomen and back may help. Leave the hot compress in place for two to three minutes and the cold for about 30 seconds, alternating them two or three times.

Consultation Treatment will depend on the individual's symptoms and the diagnosis of their cause. Supplements of calcium or oil of evening primrose, taken just before the period begins, are sometimes prescribed for painful periods.

HERBAL MEDICINE

Self help Herbalists recommend a hot infusion of camomile with perhaps a little ginger added to relieve period pain.

Consultation A range of remedies is used, depending on the problem. For instance, the herbalist may choose antispasmodics such as cramp bark, motherwort or wild yam, or uterine tonics such as false unicorn root, white deadnettle or lady's mantle.

Other alternative treatments

Homoeopathy A homoeopathic doctor may recommend the following. For scanty and late periods: *Viburnum op.* 30 when accompanied by severe cramping pains, which extend down the thigh. For painful periods: when accompanied by cramping pains similar to birth pangs and much bright red blood, *Belladonna* 6 every 15 minutes until relief is obtained; when the pain is relieved by bending double and applying pressure and warmth, *Mag. phos.* 6.

Acupuncture A wide range of gynaecological disorders can be treated after any underlying problems have been ruled out. Points on the conception channel are most commonly used, and points on the stomach, spleen, bladder and kidney meridians are also treated. For the best results with painful periods, treatment should be given about a week prior to commencement of a period.

Reflexology For menstrual problems, massage would be applied to the reflex areas related to the ovaries, Fallopian tubes and uterus, along with those relating to the pituitary, thyroid and adrenal glands, and the solar plexus (see chart, p. 295).

An orthodox view

General practitioners have routinely to deal with an assortment of problems associated with menstruation.

Most disorders have simple causes and they give no cause for concern. Nevertheless, any unexpected bleeding – whether between periods, during PREGNANCY or after the MENOPAUSE – should be reported to a doctor immediately.

At the consultation the doctor will analyse the pattern of periods, and may examine the womb and ovaries by an internal examination through the vagina. A cervical smear – a sample of cells from the cervix – may be taken to detect early signs of CANCER there. If necessary, a blood sample is taken, and its hormone levels measured.

A dilatation and curettage ('D and C') operation, in which the neck of the womb is widened and samples are taken from the lining of the womb, may help to form a diagnosis and to relieve painful and heavy periods. This should always be performed when there is vaginal bleeding or pain after the menopause. The dilatation and curettage operation is usually carried out under a general anaesthetic.

Medicines such as mefenamic acid (Ponstan) may help to relieve period pains. Progesterone tablets or suppositories, or the oral contraceptive pill, may relieve heavy periods and premenstrual tension. For women who have completed their families, a hysterectomy, or a minor surgical procedure known as TCRE (transcervical resection of the endometrium) to remove the womb lining, can provide relief from heavy periods, but leaves the patient infertile.

PERSONALITY AND DISEASE

The emerging links between mind and body

Many alternative therapists feel that there is a strong connection between the type of people we are and the sort of illnesses that we get. However, conventional doctors are generally not so sure. They find it hard to accept the idea that some people have an ARTHRITIS personality, or that others are especially prone to CANCER.

Only recently have these two views started to take account of each other. It is now known that personality does influence health to some extent, but the link is seldom obvious. The old idea of 'one type of personality – one pattern of disease' has now given way to a more holistic view.

What is personality? By 'personality' doctors and psychologists mean simply the consistent patterns of behaviour, thought and feeling that people follow throughout their lives. Some seek out company, while others would rather be alone, for example; some can handle a crisis well, while others go to pieces under pressure. The first is said to have a sociable, outgoing personality, and the second a more withdrawn or introverted one. The third is probably emotionally stable, and the last unstable or slightly neurotic.

Obviously, the way people behave depends on many factors, but you have only to observe your friends or family members to recognise that we all have persistent tendencies to respond in our own particular ways to any given situation.

Some psychologists believe that constant personality traits are genetically built in. For example, being emotionally stable or unstable might depend on the sort of sympathetic nervous system – the part of the nervous system that controls BLOOD PRESSURE, heartbeat, breathing and so on – that is inherited.

Others believe that we are not born with fixed personalities but develop them as we grow up, in response to the people and situations we encounter. Nowadays most psychologists believe that a mixture of the two views is probably correct, and that an individual's personality springs from both genetics and environment.

Personality and mental health The clearest effect of personality on disease is the link with mental health. For example, it is known that outgoing, gregarious people tend to be happier than quieter, more inward-looking ones. Individuals with an emotionally unstable personality tend to be easily upset, have a low sense of their own value, and are more likely to suffer from serious DEPRESSION than those who are more stable.

In a way, links between personality and mental health are hardly surprising. After all, instability and depression overlap to some extent, and things that upset us may equally be depressing. But even allowing for this overlap, psychologists have found that an unstable personality is still a strong predictor of who is likely to suffer from depression.

The link with physical illness Thirty years ago it was believed by some doctors that particular personality types tend to suffer from particular disorders such as arthritis, raised blood pressure or peptic ULCERS. Today the picture is thought to be more complicated, although there is evidence that the theory still holds true for problems such as HEART DISORDERS and cancer.

In recent years heart specialists have come to believe that as well as physical risk factors such as high blood pressure or raised cholesterol levels, a particular way of responding to the world can also be a cause of heart disease. People with the 'Type A' personality – ambitious, aggressive and with an exaggerated sense of time passing – are twice as likely to have a heart attack as more placid, easygoing 'Type B' personalities.

In one study, Californian psychologists successfully used COUNSELLING to reduce Type A traits in men who had already had one heart attack. The results showed that the rate of second attacks was significantly lowered, as compared with heart-attack victims who had not had counselling.

Similar links have also been found between personality and cancer, another major killer in the West. Showing the link is difficult for two reasons, however. Firstly, cancer is not one disease but many, and it is unlikely that different personality patterns have the same effect on them all. Secondly, many biological factors such as diet and exposure to dangerous substances also affect susceptibility to cancer.

Sometimes these other external influences are so strong that they override the effect of personality, although there is now evidence that people with certain personality types tend to live longer than others even when they get cancer.

Nurses who work with cancer patients often describe them as 'very nice people', meaning that they put others first and do not express strong emotions, particularly not anger. This has given rise to the idea that cancer may be at least partly due to 'anger turned inwards'.

Whether this is true or not, specialists in London have found that breast cancer patients who had had surgery survived longer if they developed a 'fighting spirit' and decided not to let the illness dominate their lives.

275

Those who felt helpless or hopeless, by contrast, tended to die sooner. Researchers in San Francisco have found a similar pattern among patients after surgery for skin cancer.

A disease-resistant personality? Although a direct link with personality is generally accepted among practitioners for heart disease and cancer, a new, more subtle version of the old 'psychosomatic' idea is now emerging for other diseases.

Rather than different personality types being associated with particular illnesses, personality traits are now seen as factors which can reduce – or enhance – the body's overall resistance to disease. The actual symptoms people go down with – HEADACHES, PALPITATIONS or HEARTBURN, for example – depend on which body systems are the weakest ones.

During the break up of a large American company, researchers studied the personality traits of middle managers, as well as their disease patterns. They discovered a personality type that they called 'hardiness'. These were people who believed that they could exert some control in the world, who were committed to what they were doing, and who welcomed change because of the opportunities it could bring.

The managers who showed this hardy personality were found to be less prone to illnesses of various kinds than those whose hardiness was lower. The researchers concluded that a hardy personality could be a general protection against physical illness.

How your personality exerts an influence There are two different ways in which personality appears to affect physical health. The first is directly related to behaviour. The way we express emotions, for example, influences the secretion of hormones which may reduce immunity or increase susceptibility to disease. Severely depressed patients, for example, are thought to have a less effective IMMUNE SYSTEM.

The second link depends on how personality affects the way in which we see and react to the world. People who are hardy can accept difficult situations and try to change them for the better. They recognise health problems early on and usually seek medical treatment in good time.

People with low levels of hardiness, however, tend to ignore – or at any rate to suppress awareness of – unpleasant situations, including symptoms of illness. As a result they remain ill for longer and seek help only when they are obliged to. Unfortunately, that may sometimes be too late.

Among this second category of persons may be those with actual personality disorders – for example, those who constantly fail to adapt appropriately to change and who suffer recurring anxieties and depressions.

PESTICIDES

The use of chemicals to kill pests, particularly insects and rodents, and the use of fungicides have escalated since the 1950s. People have become increasingly concerned that poisons find their way into our air, water, soil and food. Illnesses that have been associated with exposure to pesticides include ALLERGY and HYPERACTIVITY. Cases of miscarriages and male INFERTILITY have also been reported. Despite legal controls on what chemicals farmers use, how they use them and the amount of residues allowed in foods, many people prefer to buy 'organic' food grown without chemicals.

See HEALTH HAZARDS.

PHOBIAS

People with intense, irrational fears called phobias live in perpetual dread of things (or situations) which would not normally bother the average person. Anything from spiders, cats and mice, to riding in a lift or travelling in a railway train or aeroplane can set their hearts pounding and their breathing racing. Such people may turn dizzy and start sweating profusely with fright. Often they want to flee in panic and terror from the scene. Phobia comes from the Greek word *phobos*, meaning 'fear', or 'flight'.

It is estimated that about one person in every ten in South Africa has his own personal phobia, causing attacks of panic which can strike at any time and any place. Among the most common phobias are AGORAPHOBIA, the fear of being in open places, and CLAUSTROPHOBIA, the fear of being in confined or crowded places. In many cases the two conditions overlap.

Most phobias affect men and women equally, though in varying degrees. For example, some people suffer so badly that they cannot leave their home or lead a normal life. They often make excuses to avoid going out or joining in activities that their family and friends enjoy. They have trouble holding down their job, and may be terrified of travelling. Some people are even frightened of work itself; while others can get to work and back provided they do not have to travel in the rush hour.

A morbid fear of illness prevents some sufferers from visiting a doctor. And the most recently recorded medical phobia – rivalling that of CANCER – is the dread of contracting AIDS. In extreme cases, such phobias can drive people to suicide. See ANXIETY and NERVOUS DISORDERS.

How to beat phobias on your own

Recent research in Britain suggests that phobia victims can, in many cases, cure themselves. Tests were conducted on three groups of patients suffering from phobias, and the results published in the *British Journal of Psychiatry*.

All three groups were assessed by a psychiatrist. The first group then received exposure therapy (confronting their fears) under the guidance of the psychiatrist; the second group practised self-administered exposure therapy; and the third group received instruction from a specially programmed computer. The recovery rate among the three groups was similar – and afterwards the patients had no trouble in maintaining their progress.

Here is a guide to help you escape from your phobias. It is based on the book *Living with Fear* by Professor Isaac M Marks, whose studies formed part of the three-group test. Along with other researchers, he maintains that by exposing yourself to your fears you can learn to cope with them.

Stage one Write down exactly what form your phobia takes. For example: 'I'm frightened of cats and can't be in the same room as one!' If you suffer from more than one phobia, rate them on the following scale: 0, would not avoid the situation or object; 2, would tend to avoid it; 4, would definitely avoid it; 6, would markedly avoid it; 8, would always avoid it. Then prepare to treat the main one, or ones. If possible, get support from a relative or close friend.

Stage two Write down exactly what you want to achieve. For example: 'I'll overcome my fear and visit friends with cats. I might even get one for my children.' Set aside up to two hours a day for treatment. Remember, one two-hour session is more effective than four half-hour ones.

Stage three Expose yourself to the object or situation you fear most. Immediately after each session write down the amount of fear you experienced on the following scale: 0, no fear; 25, mild fear; 50, moderate fear; 75, severe fear; 100, total fear. Discuss your progress with someone close to you, and record what you hope to achieve next time.

Stage four Write down on cards the different sensations you generally experience when frightened, such as:

(a) I want to scream or run away.
(b) I freeze in my tracks.

Recording your fears

According to some psychiatrists, the best way to conquer your fears is to face up to them each day for weeks or even months on end. Keep a daily record of how you do this. Here is part of a record kept by a housewife with agoraphobia and claustrophobia.

The woman describes the tasks, the time spent on them, her 'anxiety score' out of a possible 100, and how she coped.

As she becomes more self-confident, the sufferer finds she can spend longer in situations which normally are full of dread for her.

The more the sufferer exposes herself to her phobia the less it begins to affect her. Her 'anxiety score' goes down.

July

9 Monday 2.30pm to 4.30pm
Walked to the local supermarket and nearby shops. Bought food and presents for the family. Had coffee in the café on the corner. Felt frightened when the shops were crowded. Felt better after practising deep breathing exercises. Anxiety score was 75 out of 100.

10 Tuesday 10.00am to 11.30am.
Walked to the local park and sat there for a while. Then caught a bus back home. Felt giddy and faint while walking. Felt better after telling myself my fear and giddiness would soon pass. Bus journey didn't affect me.
Anxiety score was 70 out of 100.

11 Wednesday 2pm to 4pm.
Took a bus to the town centre and back three times. Felt frightened at first, but told myself things could be far worse – the bus could crash, perhaps. Felt worst when the bus was crowded and did deep breathing exercises.
Anxiety score was 60 out of 100.

12 Thursday

Friday 13

Saturday 14

Sunday 15

Notes

Plan for next week
– Repeat trips on bus to park and shops
– Start going to hairdresser
– Take short train journey.

After discussing her progress with her husband, the woman decides to repeat her daily outings until her 'anxiety score' is no more than 30 out of 100. Within a few more weeks, she hopes to have conquered her fears.

(c) I tremble and shake.
(d) My stomach tightens or turns over.
(e) I can't breathe properly.
(f) My heart pounds and beats fast.
(g) I feel dizzy and faint and about to fall.
(h) I break into a cold sweat.
(i) I feel I'm going insane.

Make sure that you carry the cards always. Refer to them when you feel a panic attack coming on, to help you take the sensations for granted, and so cope with them.

Stage five Look at the following tactics carefully, then choose three that you feel will help you most:

(a) I must breathe slowly and steadily, gradually learning to deal with the situation.
(b) I'm very tense. I'll tense and relax my muscles until I gradually feel more relaxed.
(c) I'm thinking of the worst possible things that could happen to me. Perhaps they're not so bad after all.
(d) I must stay here and bear this panic, even if it takes an hour.
(e) I have to get away, but I know I must stay here.
(f) I feel awful. I could be better if I thought of something relaxing and pleasant, such as lying on a beach in the warm sun.
(g) These sensations are frightful, but I can change their meaning. My heart is pounding because I've been running in a race. I feel dizzy because I've just got out of bed.
(h) I'm terrified, but I'll get over it in time.
(i) I'll never get over this, but that is just a feeling, and in due course I'll feel better.
(j) I'm so embarrassed, but it is something I'll get used to.

Once you have chosen your three tactics, imagine that you are in the grip of your most terrifying fear and use the first tactic to deal with it. Keep this up for three minutes. Then repeat with the other two tactics in turn. Write down what happens and how you feel afterwards.

Slowly, with patience and perseverance, you should overcome the things that used to terrify you.

Five golden rules

1 Remember that although anxiety is unpleasant it is seldom harmful.
2 Stand your ground: don't flee.
3 Tell yourself to face up to your fears. They are irrational, and they prevent you from leading a normal life.
4 The longer you spend confronting your fears, the less awesome they will appear, and the better you will feel.
5 The sooner you squarely confront your fears, the sooner they will disappear. It is in your power to banish them.

What the therapists recommend
HOMOEOPATHY
Self help If you suffer from agoraphobia you should take one dose of *Aconite* 30 or 200 three times a day for ten days. If improvement is felt before the period is up, stop taking the medicine. If the condition is due to severe SHOCK, and you feel weak and faint, you should take *Arnica* in the 6th potency three times a day for seven to ten days.

For claustrophobia, the fear of being trapped, possibly by a tall building falling on you, try *Argentum nitricum* 30. If the phobia involves closed, crowded, hot places such as lifts, try *Pulsatilla* 30. Both remedies should be taken three times a day for ten days.

BEHAVIOURAL THERAPY
Consultation On seeing a therapist, you are encouraged to face up to and deal with your fears and anxieties, rather than trying to avoid them. Gradually, you are shown how to overcome your fear of a dreaded object or situation through a technique called desensitisation.

For example, if you are morbidly frightened of spiders you might start by looking at pictures of the creatures. You will then move on to looking at and handling dead spiders, and watching live ones. Finally, you will be asked to handle live spiders.

Self help As part of confronting your phobia, you may be taught some loosening-up techniques, such as deep breathing.

HYPNOTHERAPY
Consultation A hypnotist will try to take you back in time to when a particular phobia first showed itself. He will then attempt to 'will' you to conquer the fear. Alternatively, he will expose you to the phobia by visualising it stage by stage. That way you may be able to withstand and then dismiss your fear.

ART THERAPY
Consultation Therapists believe that phobias are often the result of childhood terrors – and that these can be dispelled by recalling them through drawing and painting. Once your worst fears and the panic that accompanies them have been re-created in pictorial form, an art therapist will try to help you to relax and to lead a normal and phobia-free life.

An orthodox view
Rather than prescribe tranquillisers – which give rapid, short-term relief, but which can prove addictive – some doctors recommend PSYCHOTHERAPY or BEHAVIOURAL THERAPY (see also box, pp. 276-7). Training in various social skills can benefit those handicapped by social phobias.

PHYSIOTHERAPY

Physiotherapy is the treatment of a disease or injury by 'natural' – that is, physical – means rather than by drugs. The remedies used may be as elementary as fresh air, sunlight or water (see HYDROTHERAPY). They also include ELECTROTHERAPY, MASSAGE and ACUPUNCTURE, as well as heat treatment – for example diathermy, the heating of internal parts of the body by electric current – and cold treatment (using ice packs to relieve pain, reduce swelling or ease bruising).

Another of the physiotherapist's remedies is exercise. This may be either passive, as the therapist gently manipulates an affected part of the patient's body, or active, with the patient regularly carrying out a series of prescribed movements.

Physiotherapy has a very wide range of applications which can help many different conditions. Patients who have incurred sports injuries, victims of arthritis or polio, and those who are recovering from a bone fracture, nerve damage or a stroke, are among those people who can benefit from aspects of the therapy.

Finding a therapist Ask your GP, orthopaedist, neurologist or other specialist to refer you to a physiotherapist. Or write, enclosing a stamped, self-addressed envelope, to the South African Society of Physiotherapy, P O Box 47238, Parklands 2121, asking for the names of practitioners in your area.

For more details you could also write to this society's Acupuncture Group, c/o Mr Charles Liggins, King Edward VIII Hospital, Private Bag, Congella 4013.

An orthodox view
Treatment by physiotherapy is approved by doctors and is used extensively in the treatment of skeletal and respiratory problems, and for many other ailments.

PHYTOTHERAPY

This recently coined word describes the work of medical herbalists. It refers to the healing powers of plants, which are now more widely used throughout the world than at any time in history. See HERBAL MEDICINE.

PILES

Haemorrhoids, the medical name for piles, are caused by swollen veins inside or on the outside of the anus. They can cause ITCHING and pain, and are the most common source of anal bleeding.

Internal piles may protrude from the anus during straining when passing motions – and may even stay permanently outside in the form of small, soft, purplish lumps. These external piles – which usually clear up within a week or two – often leave irritating 'skin tags' which cause further itchiness. Sometimes a blood clot, or thrombus, turns a pile into a hard, extremely painful lump.

What the therapists recommend
Naturopathy Practitioners consider that most cases of piles are a result of the way of life prevalent in the West, where diets low in FIBRE and inadequate EXERCISE are the norm, and CONSTIPATION, straining and the use of laxatives are often a part of daily life.

The naturopathic approach to piles is to deal with these basic causes by adding high-fibre foods such as linseed to the diet in order to soften the motions.

Aromatherapy The essential oils which are recommended specifically for piles include cypress, camomile, juniper, frankincense or myrrh – any two of these plus one drop of peppermint should be used.

Make a sitz bath by adding four drops of the oils to half a washing-up bowl of water and sit in it for five to ten minutes. Apply a lotion or oil both after the evening sitz bath and every morning. For the application lotion or oil, use 2 dessertspoons (20 ml) of white base lotion or vegetable oil mixed with ten drops of pure essential oil.

Herbal Medicine Herbalists aim to relieve the discomfort of piles with astringent ointments such as comfrey, horse chestnut and witch hazel. An indigenous remedy is to chop the juicy root of the mother-in-law's tongue plant ('piles bush'), boil this in water or milk, and drink a cup of the liquid daily.

An orthodox view
In cases of anal bleeding, a doctor should be seen so that he can test for any more serious, underlying cause. Medical advice should also be sought if there is a disturbing change in bowel habits, such as constipation or DIARRHOEA (see also BOWEL DISORDERS).

Piles can be avoided by regularly eating adequate amounts of dietary fibre, or roughage, and by drinking sufficient liquid to avoid constipation.

If they do occur, the itchiness and pain can be relieved by taking hot baths, using hydrocortisone ointments or suppositories, and using moist wipes instead of ordinary toilet paper. Sufferers should also avoid straining when relieving the bowels.

In severe cases, if piles persist or recur, an operation can be performed under local anaesthetic to remove them.

PIMPLES

Everyone has pimples and spots at some time, particularly during adolescence. They are small, raised, inflamed areas on the skin containing pus. They usually occur singly at the roots of hairs when natural hair oil and skin keratin (a tough, fibrous protein) clog skin pores. The blocked glands continue producing oil which can become infected or leak into the skin, causing redness and inflammation. When there is a rash of pimples, the condition is called ACNE.

In some cases, pimples and spots are caused by certain foods, cosmetics, soaps and other toiletries to which people may have an ALLERGY, and which they should therefore avoid. Pimples can also be helped by taking regular EXERCISE, and adopting a sensible and nutritious diet.

What the therapists recommend

Herbal Medicine Inflammation and further infection may be reduced by sponging the affected areas with infusions of lavender or marigold, or with diluted witch hazel.

Remedies that are given internally by herbalists – usually as tinctures – include burdock, echinacea and red clover. These preparations are thought to cleanse the body and so reduce the likelihood of pimples and spots occurring.

Naturopathy Practitioners often recommend a short, supervised fast (see FASTING) to cleanse the body of impurities. This is usually followed by a diet based mainly on fresh fruit and vegetables, and excluding sugar, fried and fatty foods, alcohol, and strong tea and coffee.

An orthodox view

Apart from possibly recommending various skin creams and lotions that are on sale at the chemist, conventional doctors have little to offer for commonplace pimples and spots. In cases of acne, however, they may advise the sufferer to avoid oily or fatty foods, and may also prescribe creams and anti-acne preparations. In some severe cases, oral antibiotics are prescribed.

PLACEBO

Before the scientific testing of drugs, a placebo was simply an inactive medication or therapy given to humour the patient. The treatment itself had no effect on the illness or complaint but the patient believed that it would cure. And it sometimes did, for the sufferer's faith in the prescription brought about a change of mental attitude to the illness, and the body's powerful self-healing potential then came into play.

Today, placebos are used in the clinical testing of new drugs. One group of patients is given the drug under test, while a similar group of 'controls' is given an inactive placebo. The drug's effect is then compared with the placebo effect to give a measure of the new drug's activity.

PLAGUE

This serious disease is confined mainly to wild rodents, but it may be transferred to man by the bite of a flea from an infected animal. Symptoms appear within five days: feverish shivering, headache, and reddened, painfully swollen lymph glands in the groin and elsewhere. (The inflamed swellings are known as 'buboes', hence the term 'bubonic plague'.)

Pneumonia, with severe bouts of coughing, may result as a complication – and this form of the disease can be spread via infected droplets coughed up by a patient.

Modern medicine has eliminated plague epidemics, but sporadic outbreaks continue to take place. Control of the urban rat population helps keep the plague at bay.

What the therapists recommend

This is not the sort of disease to respond to natural treatment.

An orthodox view

With early diagnosis and treatment by antibiotics plague can be cured. Antibiotics can also be administered as a preventive, and there is a partially effective plague vaccine.

PLEURISY

Sharp or stabbing pains in the chest or shoulder – felt with every breath – can be a sign of pleurisy. The condition is caused by inflammation of the pleura, two delicate membranes which separate the lungs from the chest wall. The pleura are lubricated by a thin film of fluid which allows them to move smoothly against each other as the lungs expand and contract during breathing. In pleurisy, the fluid becomes sticky, and a doctor may hear through his stethoscope a 'pleural rub' like two pieces of sandpaper rubbing together. The patient may have a raised temperature and feel generally unwell.

Pleurisy is usually caused by a virus infection of the pleura. But other causes can include PNEUMONIA, injury to the chest wall where there is bruising beneath the ribs, pericarditis (inflammation of the pericardial lining of the heart after a heart attack, or because of infection), a blood clot in the lung or, rarely, lung CANCER.

Warning If pleurisy is suspected, consult a doctor before undertaking any form of alternative treatment.

What the therapists recommend

Traditional Medicine A drink of home-made wheat bread is said to relieve the pain of pleurisy. Oven-dry the bread, break it up into powder, and then boil it in water with salt and butter. Drink the resulting 'toast water' while it is warm.

Naturopathy Self help alone must not be practised, and naturopaths may recommend a course of HYDROTHERAPY, with chest and back compresses to help reduce the internal inflammation.

Homoeopathy If the pain is worse when you move, and you are irritable and thirsty, try *Bryonia* 30 each hour for up to 12 hours. If the attack comes on suddenly after exposure to cold wind – and is accompanied by anxiety, restlessness and fear of dying – try *Aconite* 30 once an hour for up to 12 hours. If your face is flushed and you are very hot and thirsty with dilated pupils, a similar dosage of *Belladonna* is a better remedy.

An orthodox view

When examining a patient with suspected pleurisy a doctor may hear a pleural rub. He may then arrange for an X-ray to help to determine the cause.

If pneumonia is found, it usually clears with a course of antibiotics. If there is a blood clot in the lung (pulmonary embolism), the doctor will recommend blood-thinning drugs such as heparin and warfarin. The treatment will probably start in hospital.

PNEUMONIA

A virus or bacterial infection is the usual cause of pneumonia, when one or both lungs become inflamed. It develops with a cough and shortness of breath.

Bacterial pneumonia is considered a serious health hazard, although viral pneumonia can also be dangerous – especially in the elderly and the young. Legionnaires' disease is a form of viral pneumonia.

Acute lobar pneumonia usually affects only one lobe of one lung. It develops quickly, often in children and young people, and causes high FEVER, rapid breathing and a persistent, dry cough. There is usually little phlegm, but the patient may cough up blood.

Bronchopneumonia often affects both lungs, and the victim produces large quantities of green or yellow phlegm. It can be a complication of SMOKING or infections such as INFLUENZA, and mainly affects elderly people or those who are weakened through other illness. It is often the final cause of death in people dying of CANCER or old age.

Pneumonia is sometimes a feature of AIDS. In its viral form, it is often the result of CHICKENPOX or MEASLES.

Warning If pneumonia is suspected, consult a doctor before undertaking any of the alternative treatments.

What the therapists recommend

Herbal Medicine Herbalists advise pneumonia sufferers to seek expert medical help. But they prescribe expectorants to loosen the phlegm, including lobelia or thyme combined with anti-infective herbs such as echinacea or GARLIC. Any fever is treated by herbs such as elderflower and yarrow.

Homoeopathy When the illness begins suddenly in cold, dry weather and the patient experiences fever, ANXIETY and FEAR, *Aconite* 30 may help – give up to 12 half-hourly doses. If chest pains get worse with movement and improve when lying on the affected side, *Bryonia* 30 may give relief.

Therapists advise that you take *Phosphorus* 30 hourly or half-hourly as required for chest pains with a dry cough, blood in the sputum, and symptoms that worsen when lying on the left side.

Naturopathy Treatment should be attempted only under the supervision of a fully qualified therapist, especially in the case of elderly patients. A diet of nothing but fresh fruit and vegetable juices is usually recommended for a few days, and then fruit, vegetables, grains and a little protein are slowly added. Dairy products and sweet foods are avoided to decrease mucus production, and supplements such as vitamin C and vitamin A in fairly large doses may be prescribed to boost the IMMUNE SYSTEM.

An orthodox view

In cases of bacterial pneumonia, lifesaving antibiotics should be given as soon as possible. The patient's lungs will be sounded and a chest X-ray arranged. If the illness is present there will be a characteristic shadow across one or both lungs on the X-ray.

Many cases can be treated at home with antibiotics taken by mouth. Severely ill patients may need an intravenous drip in hospital, together with physiotherapy to help clear the lungs of phlegm.

Elderly people, particularly if they smoke, may be advised to have a follow-up chest X-ray after treatment to make sure that there is no underlying lung cancer.

POLARITY THERAPY

Balancing the body's vital energy

The basis of this wide-ranging therapy – which incorporates Eastern and Western healing techniques – is that most illness is caused by 'blockages' of the body's energy currents. By removing the blocks, and allowing the currents to flow naturally, it is said that people can overcome illness – and that once eliminated it should not recur.

The therapy was developed in the United States over a period of some 50 years by the Austrian-born Dr Randolph Stone (1890-1983), who trained in CHIROPRACTIC, NATUROPATHY and OSTEOPATHY. In addition, he studied various Eastern healing systems, including ACUPUNCTURE, AYURVEDIC MEDICINE and YOGA. Early in his career he noted that after curing patients by manipulation, there was often an underlying, residual condition that made them ill again later.

Seeking a solution, he adopted the oriental belief in a form of 'life energy' known in China as *Qi* (or *chi*), and in India as *prana*. In the West it is usually regarded as the spirit, or soul. The energy is thought to govern people's physical, emotional and mental processes. Pain and illness arise when it fails to function properly. These blockages or imbalances are also caused by bad eating habits, irrational behaviour patterns, psychological problems and STRESS.

He asserted that good health depends upon 'polarity relationships' – positive, negative and neutral – between different parts of the body and its five energy centres. According to ancient Indian thinking, these centres are: air (governing respiration and circulation); earth (bladder and rectum); ether (throat and ears); fire (bowels and stomach); and water (glands and pelvis).

The aim of Dr Stone's polarity therapy is to balance all these complex factors. To do so, it uses four basic techniques: manipulation and touch; stretching postures; diet; and thought and mental attitude (see box).

Who it can help According to its practitioners, anyone who is ill can benefit to some degree from polarity therapy. However, it concentrates on achieving balance, or polarity, in the patient – rather than dealing with specific symptoms. For polarity therapy to succeed, it calls for the patient's full co-operation, commitment and belief.

Finding a therapist Few qualified practitioners are as yet available in South Africa, but a local training centre for the therapy – under the auspices of Britain's Polarity Therapy Educational Trust – is in the planning

Four paths to health

Dr Randolph Stone, who developed polarity therapy, devised four techniques designed to help the body to balance and heal itself, which are practised by therapists today.

Manipulation and touch The therapist uses his hands to release and then 'polarise' blocked energy currents said to be a cause of ill health. Three types of pressure are applied: *positive*, involving manipulation of various parts of the patient's body, from the toes to the back of the neck; *negative*, involving deeper pressure and manipulation, particularly of the tissues; and *neutral*, involving a light, soothing touch with the fingertips.

Stretching postures Exercises such as squatting, sitting with legs crossed, and clasping hands behind the head aim to open up energy currents, tone muscles, sinews and ligaments, and strengthen the spine. To help release TENSION, the patient is asked to shout and groan while doing the exercises.

Diet To clear the system of poisons accumulated through bad eating habits and pollution, the patient will be put on a 'cleansing diet' for anything up to 14 days, depending on condition. Basically, the diet consists of fresh fruit and vegetables and plenty of natural fruit drinks (see VEGETARIANISM). In addition, there is a special 'liver flush' – a drink created by Dr Stone, made from olive oil, lemon juice, root ginger and garlic.

Once the system has been cleansed, the patient is put on an extended 'health-building' diet, followed by a 'maintenance diet', intended to maintain fitness and health.

Mental attitude Through counselling work, negative attitudes which may predispose the patient to ill health are explored and an openness to new possibilities encouraged. This is of prime importance in balancing the body and stabilising the mind.

stage. For further information write (enclosing a stamped, self-addressed envelope) to Polarity Therapy Educational Trust, 43 Ritchie Street, University Estate 8925.

Exercises to balance the body

As well as receiving instruction in polarity therapy from a qualified therapist, you can do the following basic self-help exercises at home. They are designed to let you work in depth to cure your particular forms of imbalance or energy blockage. The exercises should also help to boost your vitality and increase your general well-being.

Basic squat
Lower yourself slowly into the squatting posture. Then circle and rock gently to and fro to 'open up' and stretch your body. If necessary, support your heels with pillows or cushions.

Neutral sitting
Sit with your legs bent in front of you. Cross your hands and grasp your right ankle with your left hand; your left ankle with your right hand. Close your eyes and let your mind be at peace.

Variations on squat
First, put your hands behind neck and elbows between knees. Let your arms become heavy to stretch the spine. Second, lift up your chest, open elbows, press shoulder-blades in and take deep breaths. Simultaneously shout or groan in order to release your tension.

Woodchopper Ha!
Put your feet slightly apart, bend knees and put your hands above your head as if wielding an axe. Bring your hands down between your legs in the 'woodchopper' action, at the same time shouting 'Ha!' to release tension. Repeat the action as often as you like, providing that you are comfortable with it.

Dr Randolph Stone's *Health Building*, published by CRCS Press, provides useful facts about polarity therapy for the layman.

Consulting a therapist First you are asked for a full medical history. The therapist then analyses your energy patterns and physical structure, searching for any blocks by testing the body's pressure points and reflexes. Touch and manipulation techniques are used which are aimed at balancing these energy patterns and their physical repercussions.

The importance of being aware of the body's healing processes is also stressed. For example, during treatment for low BACK PAIN, you will be asked to concentrate on the site of the pain and to note the emotions, thoughts and mental images you experience. This, it is said, will help you to build up a complete picture of your state of health – physical, mental and emotional. In turn, this self-knowledge is claimed to hasten your return to fitness.

In addition, you may be asked to keep a record of the food you eat. From this, the therapist can assess how diet is affecting your health. In some cases, a special 'cleansing diet' devised by Dr Stone will be prescribed (see box).

If necessary, you will be offered COUNSELLING to help change any personal habits, attitudes, or ways of life that are seen as harmful to health. Some therapists may also use HERBAL MEDICINE and BACH REMEDIES to help in the overall healing process.

An orthodox view

Polarity therapy, like many alternative therapies, draws on Eastern views of 'energy' and health. Such therapies have much in common, using a combination of diet, EXERCISE, touch and MEDITATION. Little harm and much benefit can result from their use, but it is vital to get a competent DIAGNOSIS first.

POLIOMYELITIS

Early symptoms of poliomyelitis – a virus infection – are very like those of INFLUENZA. There is generally FEVER, a sore throat or HEADACHES, lasting a few days. Fortunately, most people only suffer the early symptoms and do not develop the full-blown version of the disease. They do, however, become immune to further infection.

Only a minority of those infected go on to develop encephalitis – inflammation of the brain – with its accompanying fever, severe headache, drowsiness and neck stiffness. Cramping muscle pains and spasms may develop, possibly leading to paralysis and muscle wasting, particularly affecting the muscles that were most active during the early stages of the disease.

Polio, as it is commonly called, usually strikes in epidemics – and because of wide-scale immunisation, is mostly restricted to developing countries and those areas where sanitation is inadequate. The virus is excreted in the faeces of someone infected, and infects others who come into direct – or even indirect – contact with the faeces, through sewage, contaminated drinking water or poor personal hygiene.

Note Polio is a notifiable disease and suspected cases must be seen by a doctor.

What the therapists recommend

T'AI-CHI CH'UAN

Consultation Holding the spine vertically and allowing the quiet flow of all energies is said to help the relaxation of the joints, and T'ai-chi breathing exercises (*Ch'i kung*) are said to be beneficial. They may be either in the form of meditation or the directing of mind-breath energy (Qi) through the spine and limbs, or subtle breathing-movement exercises, aimed at smooth muscle co-ordination and spinal mobility.

Correctly carried out with guidance, all of these have produced encouraging results. T'ai-chi's inspirational elements of beauty, philosophy, creativity and harmonious ease of movement are believed to give the patient vital psychological support. However, it is important that the instructor should have experience of therapy – not merely of teaching T'ai-chi movements.

Other alternative therapies

Yoga Although there is little evidence of yoga having a direct effect on polio, it can play a major part in keeping the body and mind in order – and in doing so, help in fighting infections and other conditions which may cause grave problems.

Hydrotherapy Needle spray or vortex baths are recommended, to promote or improve lower limb circulation, before specific exercise programmes and patterns in a hydrotherapy pool.

An orthodox view

Polio can be prevented by adequate sanitation and personal hygiene, and by immunisation of children and travellers. In South Africa, all children are recommended four doses of oral vaccine, usually at the ages of three months, four-and-a-half months, six months and 18 months – at the same time as vaccinations for diphtheria, WHOOPING COUGH and tetanus.

When polio develops, there is no specific cure, but rest, skilled nursing – and, if breathing muscles are affected, artificial respiration on a life-support machine – will aid the patient until recovery. If there is paralysis, it is permanent, but physiotherapy and mobility aids, such as callipers, may help a victim to lead as normal a life as possible.

PORPHYRIA

This rare inherited disorder, of which there are six types, is caused when 'porphyrins' – the breakdown products of the red blood pigment – accumulate in the liver or bone marrow. A characteristic symptom is the discoloration of the urine; when left to stand it turns pink, red or brown.

Often the skin on the body is blistered when it is exposed to the sun; wounds may be slow to heal; and there may be cramps in the limbs, abdominal pain, depression, anxiety, and the onset of more severe forms of mental disturbance.

The commoner types of this disease may be precipitated by alcohol and a wide variety of drugs, including barbiturates, the contraceptive pill and some anaesthetics.

What the therapists recommend

Homoeopathy The treatment is specific to the symptoms shown by the patient. Often it will correspond to the treatment administered for LIVER DISORDERS.

Naturopathy A cleansing diet of natural fresh foods – no fatty substances, preservatives or alcohol – is recommended.

Herbal Medicine An infusion made from any of a number of common herbs (camomile, lemon balm, yarrow) or indigenous plants (the leaves of the cancer bush, the shoots of the wild asparagus) can help to cleanse the liver.

An orthodox view

Patient awareness and education is very important. Patients must avoid sunlight and those drugs that are known to bring on attacks of porphyria.

For an acute attack a high carbohydrate intake will be prescribed, and a narcotic may be given for pain. Another form of treatment is a haematin infusion, fed intravenously.

POSTURAL INTEGRATION

Practitioners of postural integration believe that the body quite literally 'embodies' experiences as well as emotions and thought patterns. Through injuries, trauma, or prolonged stressful patterns of use, muscles and the connective tissues surrounding them will lose their natural responsiveness. The result is loss of flexibility, TENSION, and often PAIN.

Practitioners aim to restore the natural flow of energy, healthier breathing, and less stressful patterns of alignment. Physical, mental and emotional patterns are therefore encouraged to change together, reducing tension and increasing well-being. A more functional posture with better balance may be the result.

Postural integration practitioners use techniques similar to ROLFING, REICHIAN THERAPY, ACUPRESSURE and other forms of movement in an integrated manner. Their methods also have much in common with those of the ALEXANDER TECHNIQUE, for both aim to promote a harmonious state of mind and body, and the techniques employed by these therapies do not conflict with orthodox medical opinion.

PREGNANCY

Preparing for a new member of the family

Some women become pregnant as soon as they want to start a family, but others take longer, and one couple in ten may have to wait a year or more (see INFERTILITY). Most babies are conceived around the middle of the woman's menstrual cycle, following sexual intercourse taking place just before or after her ovaries produce an egg – known as ovulation. Once the egg has been fertilised by a sperm from the man, it implants itself into the lining of the womb and becomes a growing embryo.

By the time the first period is missed, the embryo is usually about two weeks old and its heart is already beginning to beat. Twelve weeks after conception, it is recognisable as a human baby and all the organs are formed. Birth usually occurs about 40 weeks after the first day of the last ordinary period, but any time from 38 to 42 weeks is normal.

Most pregnancies follow a smooth course, but all women need regular check-ups by a doctor, midwife or antenatal clinic to monitor their health and that of the baby. Alternative practitioners can provide extra help and advice, but cannot replace conventional medical care.

Preparing for pregnancy All women should have a blood test for German measles before trying to start a family – catching the disease in the first three months of pregnancy can damage the baby's hearing, eyesight, heart and mental development. Even if you believe you have had the disease or been inoculated against it, you may still

Exercises for pregnancy and birth

These gentle exercises are safe for most pregnant women, but ask your doctor's advice before beginning any exercise programme, and never push yourself beyond what feels comfortable.

For back and abdomen
Stand straight in a relaxed, natural posture with feet slightly apart and arms at your sides. Without moving your feet, twist gently, first to the right, then to the left, maintaining good posture.

For suppleness and good circulation
Practise squatting and sitting in the tailor pose, as shown, whenever you can – for example, when watching television or reading.

For supple hips
Sit or lie on the floor with your knees bent and the soles of your feet together. Gently press the knees down towards the floor, hold, and relax.

For good posture
Lie on your back with arms stretched straight above the head. Breathe in and stretch as fully as you can, pushing back and knees against the floor.

For abdominal muscles
Lie on your back or side with knees bent and hands on the abdomen. Breathe in, then exhale while pulling the abdomen in. Hold and breathe normally for a few moments, then relax.

Getting back into shape after childbirth

Begin gentle exercise as soon as you feel ready. Stop whenever you feel tired, sore or uncomfortable, and ask your doctor's advice if in doubt. Frequent short periods of exercise are better than occasional longer sessions.

First days after birth
Lie on your back with knees bent and hands resting lightly on the abdomen. Breathe in and out slowly and rhythmically; on each out-breath pull the abdomen in gently and tilt the pelvis upwards. Hold for a count of four, then relax.

Stand with feet a little apart, knees slightly bent. Place one hand on the abdomen, the other on the lower back, fingers pointing down, as shown. Breathe in, then out, and tilt the pelvis forwards and upwards, pulling the abdomen in and tucking in your bottom. Hold for a few moments while breathing normally, then relax.

After a few days
Sit on the floor with knees drawn up and arms folded, but held away from the body. Breathe in, then exhale, tilting the pelvis forwards. Allow yourself to lean back until you feel the abdominal muscles tighten. Hold and breathe normally for a short time, then sit up and relax.

Lie on your back with knees drawn up and clasped to your chest as shown. Breathe in, then out while pulling in the abdomen and pressing the knees to the chest. Breathe in again, and relax.
Other exercises to tone abdominal muscles include leg rolls (see BACK PAIN) and breathing techniques (see RELAXATION AND BREATHING).

be at risk. Only if a blood test shows that you are immune is a vaccination not necessary.

A healthy way of life is important for both partners right from the start: stop SMOKING, eat a balanced diet (see EATING FOR HEALTH), take moderate EXERCISE, and allow plenty of time for rest and relaxation. Women should preferably avoid alcohol altogether, never taking more than four units a week (see ALCOHOLISM), and should stop taking any medicines or drugs that are not essential. See your doctor as soon as you think you may be pregnant, to ensure proper care for you and your baby.

During pregnancy Most women agree that they feel 'different' when pregnant. Some feel wonderful, others miserable, and most find themselves easily tired and more emotional than usual. A healthy diet and way of life will help to reduce these problems, but it may also be necessary to reschedule daily tasks to make time for resting, without giving up regular exercise.

Minor health problems often include MORNING SICKNESS – common in the first three months, but usually better after that – CONSTIPATION, BACK PAIN, PILES, INDIGESTION and HEADACHES. Avoid taking medicines to deal with these – doctors and alternative practitioners can offer other treatments. Some breathlessness may also be encountered. A few pregnant women develop dangerously high BLOOD PRESSURE, for which medical attention is essential.

Pregnancy demands a certain amount of emotional adjustment from fathers too, and it is important that they are not left out. Involving both partners in visits to the doctor or clinic, antenatal classes, making decisions and preparing for the baby at home, will help to make men feel that they, too, have an important role to play in the event.

Sex is regarded as safe for most couples during pregnancy, although you may need to experiment to find a comfortable position that suits both partners.

Some doctors advise against sex in the first three months of pregnancy if there has been a previous miscarriage or if there are other complications – ask advice from your doctor if in doubt. In late pregnancy, an orgasm may set off contractions, but it is unlikely to induce labour.

Where to have your baby Early on in pregnancy the doctor will discuss various options for having the baby. In South Africa, most couples choose a hospital delivery by a doctor. However, hospitals vary widely in their approach to having babies. Some are very regimented and will not permit deviation from their routines. Others are much more open to accepting the mother's requests regarding such procedures as shaving, enemas, birthing position and episiotomies (cutting

the vaginal opening). It is wise to check beforehand whether the hospital will consider your views on these matters.

Some couples prefer a home birth, believing that it will be more 'natural' and less stressful. Doctors will sometimes agree to this, except for first babies or if problems are foreseen.

Choice for the home birth option may be limited by the availability of doctors and midwives willing to undertake it.

Childbirth and after See the section on NATURAL CHILDBIRTH for information on making the experience as easy and as rewarding as possible.

After giving birth, women will experience vaginal bleeding or discharge which may last for a few weeks. Afterpains, rather like period pains, can also occur as the womb shrinks back to its normal size. Piles are common, so include high-fibre foods in your diet (see FIBRE) and drink extra fluids to avoid constipation. Get plenty of rest and do postnatal exercises as soon as possible, to tone the abdominal muscles (see p. 284).

Tiredness and depression are normal in the weeks following birth, and mothers who feel unable to cope can get help from their doctor or health visitor. Readjustment can be difficult for other members of the family too, but patience, a sense of humour and tolerant attitude will overcome most problems. A special effort to give other children time and attention will help to prevent jealousy and build good family relationships.

Making time for each other, sharing feelings and listening sympathetically will also help a couple to strengthen their relationship at what can otherwise be a difficult time. Sharing baby care and household chores will help fathers to feel more involved, and mothers less exhausted.

Sexual intercourse can be resumed as soon as the woman feels comfortable. Some women may be fertile again straight away, so couples should consider using contraception. Breastfeeding reduces – but certainly does not eliminate – the chances of becoming pregnant again.

When pregnancy fails Although many problems can be treated if detected early on, as many as one in six diagnosed pregnancies – and many more unrecognised ones – may end in a miscarriage, sometimes experienced as a late, heavy period. Consult a doctor at the first sign of bleeding or lower abdominal pain in the pregnancy, since these can signal miscarriage.

Occasionally it can happen that a fertilised egg is prevented from reaching the womb and begins to grow in the uterine tube instead. This is known as an ectopic pregnancy. It causes some pain and bleeding about two weeks after the first missed period, and re-

quires urgent surgery to prevent any further internal bleeding and the possibility of fatal complications developing.

Women who lose their babies in these or other ways need time to come to terms with the loss, and a chance to express their feelings to sympathetic listeners. For more information, and for the address of a support group in your area, write (enclosing a stamped, self-addressed envelope) to SHARE Southern Africa, P O Box 18455, Wynberg 7824.

What the therapists recommend

Apart from their advice on dealing with specific conditions, described in the relevant entries, a number of alternative therapists offer suggestions for general health care during pregnancy.

NATUROPATHY

Eat well-balanced, nourishing meals at least three times a day – or as many as six smaller meals if you prefer. Smaller portions more often will also help if you suffer from nausea (see NAUSEA AND VOMITING), HEARTBURN or indigestion. Base your diet mainly on fresh vegetables, salads, whole grains, pulses and protein foods such as lean meat, chicken, fish, eggs and dairy products.

Be sure to drink plenty of spring water and avoid tea, coffee, alcohol, sweets, cakes and other products made with refined sugar and flour. If you want a snack, go for nuts or fresh or dried fruit instead.

Some women find multivitamin and multimineral supplements helpful for ongoing problems such as TIREDNESS or STRESS. Vitamin E is recommended for reducing stretch marks after the birth: take 100iu a day for up to three months.

Brown skin discoloration on the face may be helped by PABA (para-aminobenzoic acid), which is found naturally in wheatgerm, whole grains, liver, mushrooms, fresh fruit and vegetables. It can also be taken as a supplement in doses of up to 500 mg a day.

HERBAL MEDICINE

Infusions (see p. 184) of black haw root are said to help prevent miscarriage, or three drops of false unicorn root tincture taken four or five times a day from the time you start trying for a baby until the 14th week of pregnancy. Pain in the legs and feet may be helped by a decoction (see p. 184) of cramp bark, and headaches by infusions of poppy heads, or equal parts of balm (lemon balm), lavender and meadowsweet.

AROMATHERAPY

Sprinkle a few drops of lavender or peppermint essential oil onto a handkerchief or tissue and then keep it near you to smell if headaches are a problem. Do the same with lavender, camomile or rose oil to relieve nausea. For sciatic pain in the leg, mix a massage oil (see p. 36) with a few drops of lavender or wintergreen essence and rub in as often as you consider necessary.

HOMOEOPATHY

Treatment is said to help with minor problems of pregnancy. For FAINTING caused by heat try *Belladonna* 30C, for fear and nervousness *Aconite* 30C, and for a euphoric mood that interferes with sleep *Coffea* 30C. False contractions in the last few months may be helped by *Pulsatilla* 6C, *Coffea* 6C or *Nux vomica* 6C, and heartburn by *Capsicum* 6C.

Take *Sepia* 6C for brown or dark yellow skin discoloration over the bridge of the nose, and *Sulphur* 6C for dry, itchy, flaking skin. Take four doses a day for up to a week. A sweet, metallic taste in the mouth accompanied by excessive saliva production may be helped by *Mercurius* 6C, and large amounts of saliva together with feelings of nausea by *Pulsatilla* 6C.

Other alternative remedies

Moxibustion Babies in a difficult birth position may be helped to turn in the womb after the 35th week by burning moxa close to the outside edge of the nail of each little toe. Hold it close enough to feel the warmth but not burn. Repeat twice a day for ten minutes on each foot.

Traditional Medicine A drink made by pouring 600 ml of boiling water over 30 g of raspberries was traditionally believed to ensure a plentiful supply of milk and a safe delivery. Begin the treatment after the third month and continue until birth.

PREMENSTRUAL TENSION

As many as three out of four women suffer from premenstrual tension (PMT) – a troublesome but largely harmless range of symptoms whose effects become evident in the run up to a period. For some the symptoms must be endured for up to half of every month. Problems include physical ailments such as WATER RETENTION and swollen joints (especially ankles), food and alcohol cravings, weight gain, skin problems, weakness and HEADACHES. There are also psychological disturbances such as irritability, poor concentration, decreased sex drive, insomnia, tearfulness and even DEPRESSION.

The main cause of PMT is a change in the balance of female hormones during the menstrual cycle which results in an accumulation of salt and water in the system and a shortage of progesterone, the hormone that prepares the uterus to receive a fertilised egg. Lack of essential fatty acids such as linoleic acid (see EATING FOR HEALTH) can also upset this balance and lead to hormone deficiency. Vitamin B_6 is known to regulate the menstrual cycle, so lack of it may be another cause of distress.

Not every sufferer experiences all the symptoms of PMT, and degrees of suffering can vary from mild discomfort to complete misery. A few women become so disturbed that they act like a completely different person – irrationally moody and even physically violent towards those they love. So family and friends may suffer accordingly from these irrational spells.

The condition also affects judgment, and women may be prone to accidents during this time. Many industrial concerns try to avoid such accidents by temporarily transferring women employees to safer jobs during the premenstrual period.

PMT is a well-known problem – most people are aware of its effects and are sympathetic to the sufferer, making allowances for her uncharacteristic behaviour. See also PERIOD PROBLEMS.

What the therapists recommend

Aromatherapy Take a daily bath containing the essential oils of clary sage, geranium and lavender during the two weeks before a period is due. The same oils may also help if inhaled from a tissue. As a preventive measure, try mixing them with a carrier lotion and using the mixture constantly as an after-bath lotion. Oils of Roman camomile, rose otto or melissa are said also to be beneficial – inhale the scent of a single drop of any of them from the palm of the hand, cupping it over your nose.

Massage Some sufferers have found that a massage can help to relieve PMT – perhaps a full body massage for its all-round relaxation and tonic effect. A neck and shoulder massage is recommended for headaches, and a light, abdominal massage to ease discomfort in that region.

Herbal Medicine Try infusions (see p. 184) of camomile two or three times a day in the week or so before a period. It is gently calming and a diuretic, removing some of the fluid that may have been retained.

A consultant herbalist may use stronger diuretics, such as couch grass, together with hormonal treatment, especially chaste tree, to encourage progesterone secretion.

Bach Remedies Crab apple is suggested for feelings of disgust towards menstrual blood; Cherry plum for tension and for a fear of being overtaken by emotion and moodiness. Water violet is prescribed when the ten-

Do's and don'ts to reduce PMT

Do eat less salt in order to reduce your retention of water.
Do cut down on sugar to combat weight gain and depression. Control cravings for it by increasing your intake of B vitamins – try a complex with magnesium and chromium.
Do cut down on saturated fats by eating less meat and dairy produce – cheese, butter, eggs, milk – as they can inhibit your production of essential fatty acids, which can result in an imbalance of hormones.
Do relax either by gentle exercise such as YOGA, or by taking a bath.
Don't put yourself under unnecessary STRESS or set unreasonable goals.
Don't drink too much tea and coffee, as the caffeine in them reduces the body's ability to absorb certain essential nutrients and can aggravate skin problems.

sion is caused by an unfulfilled need for solitude and withdrawal; Aspen for fear of the heightened sensitivity which many women experience. Holly is advised for intense, negative emotions; Beech for feeling intolerant towards one's condition, and Rock water for those who try to deny their feelings.

Acupuncture The important meridians to treat are the kidney, liver, conception and sometimes stomach and governor (see chart, p. 14). MOXIBUSTION to points on these meridians may also help.

Homoeopathy Start taking the following remedies either morning and night or every four hours, according to severity, for the appropriate symptoms 24 hours before the symptoms are expected to appear. If the sufferer bursts into tears easily, has painful breasts and irregular periods and possibly nausea, *Pulsatilla* 30 is advised. If chilly, depressed and weepy, with indifference to sex and a tendency to turn against loved ones, try *Sepia* 30.

Naturopathy Some EXERCISE usually helps general well-being and reduces fluid retention. It is also advisable to cut down on smoking and on caffeine-containing foods and drinks. Reduce intake of salt, sugary foods and alcohol. Supplements that might be prescribed include vitamin B, especially B_6, magnesium and oil of evening primrose. MASSAGE is of great benefit in relieving TENSION and congestion.

An orthodox view

Hospital trials in London in the early 1980s and some doctors' experiences have shown that a course of evening primrose oil helps many women, and treatment is usually timed to begin a few days before symptoms are expected. Extra vitamin B_6 is also prescribed in some cases, especially for women taking oral contraceptive pills, who are more likely to lack this vitamin. Doctors can help to restore hormone levels more directly by prescribing progesterone in various forms during the second half of the menstrual cycle.

Exercise and a healthy diet may help a sufferer to 'weather the storm' if relief remains difficult to attain.

PRENATAL THERAPY

The belief that the pattern of our mental, emotional, spiritual and physical attributes is laid down during gestation underlies prenatal therapy, now usually known as the METAMORPHIC TECHNIQUE. Therapists of the technique focus on the spinal reflex areas of the head, feet and hands, claiming to unlock that pattern and so release life energy blocked in the prenatal period.

PRIMAL THERAPY

The 'scream' of release from childhood trauma

As children, many people suffer hurtful and frightening experiences which, although they may be soon forgotten or pushed into the unconscious mind, cause pain, insecurity and emotional problems such as NERVOUS DISORDERS in adulthood. This is the theory behind primal therapy, which tries to offer a way of coming to terms with such experiences.

Primal therapy was developed by the American psychiatrist Dr Arthur Janov, who was very interested in the intense cries which were produced by patients as they came face to face for the first time as adults with needs for parental love that had not been fulfilled in childhood. Janov found that the simple act of voicing this 'primal scream' was often enough to cure people.

Janov's work was influenced by the ideas of the psychoanalyst Wilhelm Reich (see REICHIAN THERAPY) – who believed that mental pain was reflected also in bodily posture, breathing patterns and muscular tensions – as well as by those of the Swiss psychotherapist Alice Miller.

Miller thought that in many societies children were brought up and educated in ways that caused great pain – they were shown too little affection, had impossible demands made of them and were ridiculed, ignored or punished when they failed to meet those demands. Sometimes children who were physically ill-treated or sexually abused could not help themselves or express their pain for fear of losing their parents' love and sympathy. The childhood traumas and suppressed feelings that resulted were thought by Miller to be the root of later emotional difficulties and unhappiness.

Primal therapy aims to help the lonely suffering child within the adult to express his long-ignored needs, hurt and anger, to grieve if necessary, and finally to come to terms with his feelings so that he can begin to live freely and fully again.

Therapy is usually intensive – generally carried out at weekends, for two to three hours, over a period of several weeks.

Dr Janov popularised his controversial therapy by the publication of such best-sellers as *The Primal Scream* and *The Feeling Child.*

PROLAPSE

The most common type of prolapse – the forward or downward displacement of part of the body – occurs in a woman's vagina after childbirth. However, the displacement may not occur for many years.

Weakness of the ligaments supporting the bladder, womb or rectum causes the patient to feel a lump in her vagina – particularly when she coughs or strains. In severe cases the lump protrudes through the vaginal opening. Even when there is no actual prolapse, the ligament weakness may affect the neck of the bladder, causing INCONTINENCE.

In both women and men, SLIPPED DISC is a frequently encountered form of prolapse.

What the therapists recommend

Acupressure For prolapse of the womb, press diagonally inwards two fingers' width above the pubic bone and one hand's width out from the centre line. For a prolapsed rectum, press firmly inwards two fingers' width below the navel on the centre line.

Naturopathy Treatment would concentrate mainly on EXERCISE and posture. Pelvic floor muscle exercises in particular are considered invaluable, and a regular class in YOGA may be advised. At the same time, it is vital to avoid lifting weights and so bearing down on the lower abdomen. Correct posture can also be maintained with sessions of the ALEXANDER TECHNIQUE.

Prevention is much better than cure, and it is advisable to give attention to these factors before, as well as after, childbirth.

An orthodox view

After childbirth, the risk of a woman developing a prolapse is increased by OBESITY. Frequent or difficult childbirth and large babies can also cause the problem. In the postnatal period, therefore, it is important to do pelvic floor exercises to strengthen the muscles supporting the bladder, womb and rectum. See also PREGNANCY and NATURAL CHILDBIRTH.

If incontinence is only a problem during times of particular strain – such as when playing sports – a tampon worn during the activity may give a woman sufficient support. Doctors sometimes fit temporary plastic ring pessaries to women at risk, or advise an operation to provide physical support for the bladder, womb and rectum.

PROSTATE PROBLEMS

Dealing sensibly with a common male condition

The chestnut-sized prostate gland lies at the neck of a man's bladder. Through the middle of it runs the urethra, which passes urine from the bladder to the penis. In men over 50, the prostate gland often grows to the size of an apple, upsetting the flow of urine.

In some cases, the sufferer passes smaller amounts of urine; in others, he passes urine more frequently, particularly during the night. There is an embarrassing tendency to dribble afterwards, and a feeling that the bladder is not completely empty. Sometimes he finds it difficult and painful to urinate – particularly during the day.

An enlarged prostate may also develop malignant growths (see CANCER). Even if the original symptoms are mild, a doctor should be seen so that routine urine and blood tests can be taken – and, if necessary, a more detailed examination made in hospital.

Inflammation of the prostate gland, or prostatitis, normally occurs in younger men, causing pain in the lower abdomen, back, testicles, or the area between the scrotum (the pouch containing the testicles) and the anus. The patient may feel unwell, with a raised temperature – and his urine, which may be cloudy, bloody or smelly, is passed more often and more urgently. Prostatitis is caused by infection, which is sometimes sexually transmitted.

What the therapists recommend

Acupuncture Practitioners claim success in relieving prostate problems by using pressure points on the bladder, large intestine, spleen, kidney, conception and governor meridians. In addition, treatment by MOXIBUSTION may be applied.

Herbal Medicine For non-cancerous enlargement of the prostate, and difficulty in passing water, herbalists may use diuretic herbs such as couch grass, horsetail or saw palmetto, to promote the discharge of urine.

Naturopathy Hot and cold compresses, or sitz baths, are a key part of naturopathic treatment of prostate disorders. Regular EXERCISE is a preventive measure for enlarged prostate symptoms, and supplements of zinc may reduce the swelling: about 15 mg a day is the usual recommended dose, or perhaps eating 30 g of pumpkin seeds daily. Plenty of fluids may also help – but be sure to cut down on such drinks as alcohol, strong tea and coffee.

Biochemic Tissue Salts Try N*at. sulph.* when it is difficult or impossible to retain urine; *Calc. phos.* for a frequent need to urinate; and *Mag. phos.* when the need is constant when walking, or even standing.

An orthodox view

Older men with an enlarged prostate often benefit from an operation allowing urine to pass more freely. If the growth is cancerous, hormone treatment may control the condition for many years. In cases of prostatitis doctors will prescribe a course of antibiotics, which could last for several weeks.

PSIONIC MEDICINE

Aimed at treating the basic cause of illness, rather than using drugs to suppress symptoms, psionic medicine was founded in the late 1960s by a retired British GP, Dr George Laurence. As well as drawing on the experience gained in some 40 years of practice, Dr Laurence based his technique on several established alternative therapies. These included DOWSING (diagnosing disease by rod and pendulum), HOMOEOPATHY and MIASM THEORY (which asserts that illness is often a symptom of a deep-rooted disease). The therapy – which involves helping the body to heal itself – takes its name from the Greek letter *psi*, generally used to denote some psychic or paranormal phenomenon. However, Dr Laurence declared that psionic medicine should be practised only by qualified and experienced doctors, who had the knowledge to diagnose and treat the imbalances which cause disease.

PSORIASIS

The raised, red scaly patches caused by psoriasis can appear anywhere on the skin, but most often affect the knees or elbows. It is a common disorder, affecting as many as one person in 50. The cause is unknown, but it sometimes runs in families. It is uncommon before the age of ten, usually erupting between the ages of 15 and 30.

The rash begins as small red spots, which may merge to form circular or oval patches 50-75 mm across. It often affects both sides of the body symmetrically – for example, if one elbow is affected, so is the other. Fingernails and toenails are frequently involved, becoming pitted and thickened, and sometimes separating from the nail bed. About one in 20 psoriasis sufferers also develop a mild form of RHEUMATOID ARTHRITIS, often in the fingers, knees and ankles.

The complaint sometimes follows two or three weeks after a throat infection and can also be triggered by drugs such as chloroquine, which may be prescribed for rheumatoid arthritis, some SKIN DISORDERS, liver infections and malaria.

Although psoriasis is not caused by STRESS, worry and ANXIETY may trigger or aggravate an attack.

What the therapists recommend

Herbal Medicine Traditionally, herbalists have prescribed blood-cleansing herbs for the condition: an infusion (see p. 184) of dandelion root, red clover flowers and burdock may help the purification process.

Bach Remedies Crab apple is suggested for feelings of disgust and shame; Willow for resentment over the condition. Rescue Remedy cream or Impatiens applied externally may help to relieve itching.

Homoeopathy Psoriasis should be treated by an experienced practitioner. However, the following remedies may be helpful, taken three or four times daily for 14 days in the 6th potency. Try *Sulphur* for dry, red, itchy patches, which are worse after taking a bath, in someone who feels the heat; and *Graphites* when the skin exudes a sticky, honey-like discharge, particularly behind the ear. *Petroleum* is prescribed when the skin is dry, rough and cracked.

Aromatherapy It is said that pure essential oils of bergamot and lavender can keep the condition at bay when used both in the bath and applied in a lotion or oil. A white lotion base is recommended if the psoriasis is not over-dry or flaky. However, if the skin is very dry and the patches very scaly, then a vegetable oil may be better (and sandalwood essential oil can also be used). If in doubt, first try a lotion.

An orthodox view

While there is no cure for psoriasis, doctors can confirm the diagnosis, give general advice and prescribe creams and ointments to give relief. Coal tar, dithranol and steroid preparations are often effective, particularly if applied under a plastic dressing. Sunlight or artificial ultraviolet light may also help. Many sufferers improve dramatically if they are able to move to a sunnier climate.

If arthritis develops, doctors can take blood samples to check if another disease such as rheumatoid arthritis is the cause. They can prescribe anti-inflammatory painkillers, which help to ease pain and stiffness.

In 1990, researchers at the Finnish National Public Health Institute in Helsinki linked alcohol consumption with psoriasis. They found that 144 men with the complaint drank an average of 42,9 g of alcohol a day compared with 21 g a day in men with other skin disorders. One unit of alcohol (see ALCOHOLISM) equals 8 g.

PSYCHODRAMA

An actress, who became much more pleasant in private life when she was able to play unpleasant roles on stage, provided the inspiration for the idea of psychodrama. Jacob Moreno, a psychiatrist who lived in Vienna at the time of Freud (see PSYCHOTHERAPY), and who had noticed the actress's behaviour, reasoned that the change occurred because acting out her true hostile feelings on stage left her free to express the more positive side of her nature in real life.

Moreno developed a theory that if people could get together in groups to act out frightening and difficult situations, they would be able to express true feelings that might never be released in real life. He turned this into a form of psychotherapy.

In psychodrama, groups of patients – guided by a therapist – take it in turns to act out each other's real-life roles and situations. Because they are acting, participants feel free to express their emotions to each other much more freely and safely than they often can in real-life encounters.

Psychodrama can be a powerful experience, exposing strong emotions, so the guidance of a qualified and experienced therapist is essential. The therapist's role is to help the group to interpret the events they act out, and to clarify participants' feelings about the real people involved. Many patients claim that psychodrama enables them to come to terms with their feelings in a constructive and supportive setting.

PSYCHOSOMATIC ILLNESS

It's not all in the mind ...

There are two extreme and contradictory schools of thought among doctors regarding psychosomatic illness – the belief that physical illness can be caused by the workings of the mind. The first school believes that *all* illness is psychosomatic, in that it affects both mind and body. The second school, on the other hand, dismisses psychosomatic illness entirely, and it is not even mentioned in their medical textbooks.

The term psychosomatic – from the Greek words *psyche*, meaning 'soul', and *soma*, meaning 'body' – became current at the beginning of this century. It replaced phrases such as 'organic neurosis' and 'cardiac neurosis', which suggested that bodily illness was the result of neurotic feelings.

According to believers in psychosomatic illness, STRESS-related ailments such as ASTHMA and MIGRAINE have two main 'self-induced' causes. These are an excessive release of hormones into the bloodstream (causing changes in various parts of the body) and hyperactivity of the nervous system releasing too much adrenaline into the bloodstream.

Both these conditions occur when strong emotions such as anger, DEPRESSION, guilt and hate are tightly bottled up or belatedly released. For example, if you cannot express your anger towards someone close to you – such as your husband, wife or boss – you may channel the unreleased tension to different parts of your body.

In turn, this can give rise to a variety of symptoms, including rapid blinking, tics, TEETH-GRINDING, HEADACHES, stomach rumblings and DIARRHOEA. If the symptoms persist they may lead to more serious complaints such as high BLOOD PRESSURE and peptic ULCERS.

Psychosomatic illness is often associated with feelings of not being 'in charge' of oneself. Many self-help therapies therefore aim to give a greater sense of control over MIND AND BODY. This is particularly useful to the small number of patients who suffer from more than one psychosomatic illness at a time. Until recently, treatment was based upon a combination of tranquillising drugs and PSYCHOTHERAPY.

These have now been augmented by numerous alternative remedies, which are said to be highly effective.

Despite an increasing acceptance of genuine pain and worry caused by psychosomatic illness, many patients object to the term – which, they think, smacks of perfectly healthy people imagining that they are ill. However, as long as we are able to remember how closely linked the mind and body are, it is relatively easy to understand how the one can affect the other. For example, suppressed GRIEF – the inability to mourn the loss of someone we loved – can lead to RESPIRATORY DISORDERS.

As the saying goes: 'If the eyes do not weep, then other organs will.'

What the therapists recommend

Autogenic Training Teachers say that physical problems caused by stress have responded extremely well to the training. However, some psychosomatic problems, for example, where there is pain without an obvious physical cause – need longer than normal periods of treatment.

Dance Movement Therapy By concentrating on the links between people's emotions and their bodies, the therapy tries to provide a helpful approach to psychosomatic problems. It claims to open up new ways of understanding the feelings that cause physical symptoms – and aims to explore more positive ways of expressing and communicating these feelings.

Hypnotherapy Numerous studies have shown the effectiveness of hypnotherapy, and the relaxation it produces is said to be particularly helpful for bronchial asthma. Therapists try to get to the source of the problem, and say that getting the patient to relive the event that triggered it is often a necessary part of the cure. Self-hypnosis is also said to be particularly beneficial.

Bach Remedies Therapists say that it is important to deal with any obvious link between physical illness and your mental or emotional state. Examine your feelings as honestly as you can, and do not ignore any emotional condition which may persist and deepen, causing physical distress. Then you should be able to choose the best remedies.

PSYCHO-SYNTHESIS

Bringing out the best in yourself

An Italian psychiatrist, Dr Roberto Assagioli (1888-1974), began to develop the principles of psychosynthesis around the time of the First World War. Although originally a follower of Sigmund Freud, Assagioli took a more optimistic view of human psychology, believing that it was in each person's nature to develop a harmonious and balanced personality, and to realise his fullest potential.

While he accepted the vital importance of the lower unconscious – those aspects of ourselves related to early childhood that we have yet to become aware of, or that we ignore because they are uncomfortable or frightening – Assagioli believed that man also has a 'higher' unconscious often ignored by psychologists. In psychosynthesis he tried to correct this by giving more weight to spiritual needs and the development of a so-called 'transpersonal self'. This was what might almost be termed a 'new identity' for each person. He would no longer be concerned just with satisfying his own immediate needs, but his actions would be guided by a sense of love, unity and co-operation with others and the whole of nature.

This process of self-development, the essence of psychosynthesis, requires imagination and will – not just in the sense of 'will-power' but also as 'goodwill' and a genuine desire to change. Assagioli believed that although man has an innate drive to develop his own potential, his behaviour is not determined but free, and each individual has to choose and take responsibility for his own development.

Who it can help Since it concentrates both on curing disorders and on developing a healthy personality, psychosynthesis tends to attract a broad range of clients, some of whom are interested in personal growth and, in particular, those suffering from a mid-life crisis of meaning. It is also said to be helpful for conditions such as STRESS, MIGRAINE, PSYCHOSOMATIC ILLNESS and PHOBIAS. Anyone suffering from troubled relationships or who simply wants to understand others and communicate better with them may also benefit from psychosynthesis.

Finding a practitioner Information about qualified practitioners may be obtained by writing to 229 Main Road, Plumstead 7800, or P O Box 1435, Rivonia 2128.

Consulting a practitioner Psychosynthesis is usually given in courses of six or more sessions, depending on individual need. A wide range of different methods can be used, depending on the needs of each individual. These can include analysis, imagining, considering yourself in different ways, movement, MEDITATION and keeping a diary.

Whatever methods are used, the goals of psychosynthesis remain the same: attaining knowledge and control of all aspects of your personality, discovering a new – and true – identity, and integrating every part of yourself into it.

An orthodox view

This approach is more educational than therapeutic, and is not usually regarded as a treatment for specific diseases. However, it may be helpful by enabling individuals to become aware of their 'higher self', which is also the aim of most religious bodies, and which leads to a change in one's basic approach to life.

PSYCHOTHERAPY

Someone to talk you out of trouble

Talking your way through problems, the basis of psychotherapy, is a natural way of coping with everyday difficulties. Everyone knows that a heart-to-heart chat with a trusted neighbour or an evening spent pouring it all out to a sympathetic friend can make you feel better. At a slightly more formal level is COUNSELLING from a trained but non-specialist counsellor. However, in their way these particular procedures are all simple forms of psychotherapy.

But psychotherapy itself does more than this and can help when problems are too difficult or too deep to be solved by normal means. Like ordinary conversation, talking to a psychotherapist can have many aspects – discussing your experiences, revealing personal feelings, trying to understand your own behaviour and that of others, receiving advice and encouragement, and even sometimes getting angry or having an argument. Where psychotherapy is different, however, is in the therapist's professional training and experience, which enable him to organise and guide each session, so that the patient makes the most out of his time with the therapist. Unlike orthodox psychiatrists, psychotherapists are not usually medically trained and cannot prescribe treatments such as drugs and shock therapy.

Whether the problem is longstanding difficulties in a marriage, coping with PHOBIAS or other forms of neurosis, or simply a feeling of being unfulfilled or unhappy, psychotherapists see symptoms such as ANXIETY, TENSION, OBSESSIVE-COMPULSIVE BEHAVIOUR and DEPRESSION as a sign of some sort of inner disharmony.

The task of psychotherapy is to help the person to understand and correct this, so that he breaks out of his pattern of destructive behaviour and thoughts, has a stronger sense of his own identity, and is happier and more in control of his life and relationships. To do this, most forms of psychotherapy rely on the patient talking to a trained therapist, but some also use other means of expression such as ART THERAPY, BIOENERGETICS, DANCE MOVEMENT THERAPY and MUSIC THERAPY.

Who it can help Anyone with personal, emotional or behavioural problems may benefit. DEPRESSION, tension, INSOMNIA, STRESS, OBSESSIVE-COMPULSIVE BEHAVIOUR and irrational fears may all be symptoms of psychological problems which could be helped by psychotherapy. In addition, many physical ailments such as ANGINA, stomach ULCERS, PSORIASIS and COLITIS may be related to emotional stresses and conflicts that psychotherapy can help.

Finally, psychotherapy is not just for the sick or troubled – many people want simply to find out more about themselves, to enrich their lives and improve their relationships.

Choosing a form of therapy Psychotherapy is a very wide field, including a great range of different approaches. Choosing the right therapist is difficult at the best of times, and more so when you are troubled. Nevertheless, the choice should be made with care, since mistakes can be costly and also time-consuming. New patients are advised to consider the following issues before opting for a particular course of therapy:

Long- or short-term therapy? People with fairly simple problems – a phobia, perhaps, or a single difficult relationship – but whose lives are otherwise satisfying, may find short-term BEHAVIOURAL THERAPY, COGNITIVE THERAPY or PRIMAL THERAPY most suitable. Sessions are directed at achieving particular goals, with the therapist taking charge and the patient following instructions.

For suitable cases, this can yield quick results. The drawbacks, however, are that once probed, seemingly simple problems can turn out to have roots that go much deeper – and which the patient is often unaware of – so short-term therapy may not be enough. There is also less time to build up a good relationship with the therapist – an important factor in determining whether treatment will be successful.

Note Short-term therapies overlap to some extent with counselling, but in general this is more suitable for problems of adjustment – to divorce or retirement, for example – while psychotherapy deals with issues that involve some aspect of the patient's personality.

Difficulties involving basic problems with attitudes and relationships – for example, conflicts over security and independence in a marriage, or long-term depression and a sense of meaninglessness – generally call for more lengthy treatment such as that offered by GESTALT THERAPY, Freudian psychoanalysis and practitioners of HUMANISTIC PSYCHOLOGY (although these often offer shorter treatment as well).

These approaches concentrate on helping you to understand why you feel and behave as you do, believing that change can only grow out of self-knowledge. The patient is expected to take responsibility for his own treatment and to play an active role. Sessions tend to be freer and less directed by the therapist than with shorter therapies, and there is plenty of time to talk about feelings and responses as they occur.

A deep and trusting relationship between the therapist and patient is essential and is widely believed to enhance and enliven the patient's own inner healing powers. In psychoanalysis, the relationship is even thought to mirror the person's original relationship with his parents, giving him an opportunity to work through early vexing problems that were never properly resolved during his or her childhood.

Lengthier therapies also enable the therapist to help analyse in depth his patient's unconscious fears and longings, suppressed emotions, past traumas, dreams, and even his hopes for the future and sense of purpose. However, this can take a long time and may not offer any immediate solutions to problems. Patients must be prepared to put a great deal into their therapy themselves, and must not look to the therapist to provide all the answers.

Thoughts, feelings or behaviour? Most psychotherapists have a holistic approach, believing that thoughts, feelings and physical actions are all expressions of the same underlying personality, and that a change in one will bring about corresponding changes in the others.

Different therapies tend to adopt different approaches, so careful thought must be given to choosing which would be most comfortable to get along with, bearing in mind that feelings can change as the treatment progresses.

Shorter therapies tend to approach problems from a single point of view. Behaviourists work with actions, cognitive therapists with ways of thinking, and primal therapists with feelings.

Lengthier treatments generally use a greater variety of approaches: both thoughts and feelings are important factors to be considered in psychoanalysis, while TRANSACTIONAL ANALYSIS concentrates on thoughts and behaviour. Gestalt therapy is broad enough to tackle all three.

How much change do you want? The longer psychotherapy of any sort goes on, the more different aspects of the patient's life can be examined, and the more challenges are presented to his view of himself and others. While short-term therapy is aimed at making just a few changes, longer types can involve fundamental shifts in attitudes, behaviour and way of life.

Deciding on the right type of treatment and how long to carry on may require the insight and wisdom of the evangelist who wrote the widely-quoted verse on the next page:

Lord, Grant me
The courage to change
What can be changed,
The serenity to accept
What cannot,
And the wisdom
To know the difference.

Finding a therapist Your GP should be able to recommend or refer you to a therapist. A personal recommendation from a friend is another option. Alternatively write (enclosing a stamped, self-addressed envelope) to the Psychological Association of South Africa, P O Box 2729, Pretoria 0001, if possible giving some indication of the sort of psychotherapy that you require.

Life Line – the counselling service, with branches throughout South Africa – will be able to put you in touch with organisations for various types of psychotherapy.

Not all psychiatrists carry out psychoanalysis, so it is essential to establish at the outset what you want. In the USA particularly, psychotherapists are much more common than they are in South Africa. Whether psychotherapy will work for you depends a lot on the confidence and trust which you have in the therapist, as it is very much a two-way process.

Seeing a therapist What happens depends on the therapy involved. You may be asked to join a group or get personal attention; therapy may involve just talking, or talking and acting out your feelings, moving, drawing or making music; you may be treated as an equal partner in a process of discovery, or simply be expected to follow instructions.

Ensure at the first session that you know which approach to expect, or you may be disappointed. However, your needs may change once a process of change begins.

Generally, at this first session, you will be asked why you have come, what your view of the problem is and what you hope to gain from treatment. This is also your chance to ask questions about the therapist's training and qualifications, his methods and how he can help you. If he cannot do this in language you can understand, beware!

Never allow yourself to be rushed or pressured into a lengthy course of psychotherapy – of all treatments, this is the one where personal feelings and compatibility with the therapist matter most. If you feel uncertain, visit two or three therapists for one session each before deciding – no more, or you may end up even more confused.

An orthodox view

Short-term psychotherapy for particular problems is accepted by many doctors as a valid, often successful treatment for conditions such as phobias, anxiety and obsessive-

compulsive behaviour. It is also generally accepted that there is a psychological or emotional factor in many illnesses (see PSYCHOSOMATIC ILLNESS; PERSONALITY and DISEASE) and that psychotherapy may be a useful additional treatment for them.

See also NERVOUS DISORDERS.

PUBERTY AND ADOLESCENCE

The period of physical and psychological changes that herald adulthood – adolescence – is often difficult. It starts with puberty, when sexual maturity begins. See COPING WITH PROBLEMS OF GROWING UP, p. 292.

PULSE DIAGNOSIS

This method is an important diagnostic aid in traditional Chinese therapies. Practitioners interpret the strength and 'quality' of the pulses in a patient's wrists as a clue to past, present and future health – and as a guide in deciding treatment. See ORIENTAL DIAGNOSIS.

PYRAMID POWER

A cat in the Great Pyramid at Giza near Cairo was the unlikely starting point for discovering the seemingly 'magical' potential of pyramids built to similar proportions. In the 1930s a French holidaymaker, Antoine Bovis, saw the cat, and was struck by the fact that it had not decayed, but dehydrated. He later experimented with small models of the Great Pyramid – itself covering over 5 hectares. He reproduced its proportions correctly and positioned his model in the same way, with the sides facing due north, south, east and west. He placed a dead cat in his pyramid and found that it also dried out – and so did fruit and vegetables.

Scientists generally regarded his findings as worthless at the time, but some remained interested. They and many lay people pursued the investigations, particularly in the United States.

There in the 1970s Bill Schul and Ed Pettit reported that the growth of sunflower seedlings in a pyramid was speeded up – but not equally throughout.

They found that the area just below the apex produced the fastest growth and that on the floor along the sides had least effect. They found that seeds kept in pyramids germinated more quickly too.

Schul and Pettit tested milk in pyramids a number of times. They reported that while control samples outside the pyramid went sour and mouldy within days, those inside turned into a creamy yoghurt-like substance with no mould after six weeks. Tomatoes, grapes, eggs, calf's liver, sirloin steak and fish were also tested.

Again controls outside the pyramid went 'off', while items inside dehydrated and shrank, but did not go mouldy. Pyramids of glass, wood, cardboard and plastic have all produced similar effects.

This lack of decay suggested that bacterial growth was halted. This was also borne out by an unusually quick healing of cuts, burns and bruises on people who spent time in a pyramid model. Toothache, headaches, cramps, rheumatic pains and tension have also been relieved in a pyramid.

Their experiments confirmed similar findings by Boris Vern, director of a pyramid research centre in Washington, DC. Two more US researchers, Bill Kerrell and Kathy Goggin, did similar tests.

In addition they found that patterns of brain activity on electroencephalographs changed markedly in people inside a pyramid, even though they wore blindfolds and did not know when or whether a pyramid was placed over them. Many reported a warm, tingling sensation when inside a pyramid. Sounder sleep, increased vitality and improved well-being have also been reported.

A peculiar energy flow, a change in IONISATION or an electromagnetic force is considered by some scientists to be involved in the mysterious powers of pyramids, but a confirmed source of those powers has yet to be pinpointed.

Researchers are testing theories that the pyramid shape creates a heightened energy field that alters the rate of physical, chemical and biological processes.

One experimenter put Bovis's findings to practical use. Karel Drbal, a Czechoslovak radio and television engineer, extended the experiments to metal, and found that minute pockets of moisture that cause weaknesses in metal dried out in a pyramid.

In the late 1940s he patented a pyramid-shaped razor-blade preserver that has sold widely, and it is said to keep a blade sharp for many weeks. The blade lies in the pyramid between shaves with its edge pointing north-south. Drbal's explanation is that minute pockets of moisture remaining along the fine edge of the blade swiftly evaporate, halting the corrosion of the edge.

An orthodox view

Most scientists in the world today view various proponents' claims for pyramid power with considerable scepticism.

Coping with problems of growing up

The teenage years are well known as a time of upheaval and stress for young people and their families alike. Girls and boys face rapid and uneven changes to every area of their lives; parents have to cope with their children's erratic behaviour and sometimes baffling choice of friends and clothes. Parental authority may be seriously questioned as happy, well-behaved children change suddenly into moody adolescents, spending more time alone or with friends than with the family.

Disruptive as adolescence can be, it is a natural and necessary part of growing up. Understanding, love and acceptance by other members of the family can do much to smooth the rocky path to adulthood.

Although the words are often used interchangeably, adolescence and puberty are not the same. Puberty refers to the physical changes – such as breast development in girls, for example, or deepening of the voice in boys – which mark the start of adolescence, and which transform the child's body into that of a sexually mature adult. Adolescence, by contrast, refers to the whole process of growing up, including all the mental, emotional and social changes that must occur before the person is accepted as an adult member of society.

Puberty   This process of development takes about two years, and is usually completed between the ages of 12 and 17. It is a period of rapid growth, boys gaining about 10 cm and 6 kg a year and girls about 8 cm and 5 kg. It is also a time of rapid sexual development.

For boys, the first sign is an increase in the size of the testicles and penis, followed by growth of hair around the genitals and in the armpits, and the beginnings of a beard. The voice box increases in size, causing the voice to 'break' and eventually to deepen to a man's pitch. By the age of 13 most boys have experienced their first ejaculation and find themselves easily aroused.

In girls, puberty begins with breast development, growth of the reproductive organs, genital and armpit hair, and an increase of fat around hips and thighs, giving a more womanly appearance. The first period usually occurs about a year later – on average, at around 12 or 13, although it can be as early as 10 or as late as 17.

Adolescence   This continues for some time after puberty, often into the twenties – and is not considered completed until the individual achieves physical maturity, emotional independence, a sense of identity (including sexual identity), education and training for a job, financial independence and a full sexual relationship.

These changes can take a long time and prove very demanding. Even so, most adolescents cope well and emerge as mature, well-adjusted adults. However, some areas can cause particular problems . . .

If puberty arrives early or late   Boys especially tend to worry if they seem to be developing more slowly than those around them. In fact, although on average puberty starts at 13 or 14, any time up to about 17 can be considered normal. Unless malnutrition or illness is interfering with normal development, reassurance and time are all that are needed. Hormonal treatment may be considered if puberty has not begun at 18, or in rare cases of hormone deficiency.

Unusual conditions such as premature hormone production may lead to puberty beginning as early as five or six. Affected children develop physically and sexually, while retaining the thoughts, emotions and social status of infants. Drugs or surgery may be needed to prevent too-rapid development from overwhelming them and causing behavioural problems.

Coping with periods   Most girls view the approach of their first period with a degree of fear and apprehension, and even those who look forward to their entry into womanhood can be frightened or embarrassed when it actually happens. However, these doubts and fears are usually short-lived and girls soon learn to cope, needing only a little extra attention and understanding from parents, and advice about using sanitary pads or tampons.

Better to be active

In some girls considerable PAIN, NAUSEA, HEADACHES, DIZZINESS, WATER RETENTION, sore breasts and irritability may be associated with their periods. These symptoms tend to lessen or disappear as the hormonal cycle becomes more regular over the years, but until then periods can often be heavy, irregular or painful. Even after the cycle has settled down, it can easily be disrupted again by STRESS, travel, illness or excessive dieting.

Period pains can usually be relieved by hot-water bottles or mild drugs available from chemists – doctors advise that it is better to take these and remain active than to stay at home feeling ill and sore. Slight tension and irritability before a period is normal and needs no treatment.

Hormonal drugs are given only if periods are extremely heavy or irregular, or cause serious feelings of illness. For less severe cases, alternative remedies such as the herbal oil of evening primrose may be helpful. See also PERIOD PROBLEMS; PREMENSTRUAL TENSION.

Spots and pimples   They can make life a misery for both boys and girls during puberty, causing them to feel self-conscious and unattractive. The problem usually disappears as puberty progresses and hormone levels settle down. For help and guidance, see ACNE; SPOTS AND PIMPLES.

Breast worries   Girls often worry if one breast appears to grow faster than the other during puberty. This problem seldom lasts,

Learning to relate

During adolescence boys and girls enjoy each other's company more than they did as children. At this stage they need frequent opportunities to get together in groups, make new friends and practise social skills without adults being present. Parents can help by providing safe places to meet and not intruding too much.

usually correcting itself as hormone production stabilises. A slight difference in size is, in fact, quite normal and needs no treatment.

Tender and slightly enlarged breasts can also affect some boys as a result of hormonal changes during puberty. The condition usually disappears without any treatment. Simple reassurance that it is not a sign of any form of 'sex-change' or homosexuality is generally all that is needed from parents.

Weight problems As the hips and breasts start to grow and take on a rounded, feminine form, teenage girls often find themselves worrying about putting on weight and getting fat. The changes happen in sudden spurts – some girls putting on as much as 9 kg around the time of the first period – which can be alarming and hard to accept.

This weight gain is normal, however – the hormone oestrogen is the cause, so although many girls start dieting, cutting down on food does little to help. Unfortunately, a few girls and boys want so desperately to stay thin that they resort to extreme dieting and end up suffering from the so-called slimmer's disease, ANOREXIA.

Most adolescents, however, tend to find that they can stay slim enough to feel and look good simply by eating a well-balanced diet every day (see EATING FOR HEALTH). Such a diet should include plenty of FIBRE; cutting down on sweets and snacks; avoiding alcohol; and taking regular, moderate exercise. Weight worries often disappear too as teenagers grow taller and start to take on their full adult proportions.

Masturbation Young people sometimes feel guilty about masturbation, or worry that it can harm them – usually because of uninformed comment or advice. In fact, masturbation is a natural form of safe sex. And not only does it relieve sexual tensions, it can help both boys and girls to understand their bodily responses and contribute to a happy sex life in adulthood.

Identity crisis The many changes that adolescence brings can be quite bewildering to teenagers. Friends and society generally may treat them as responsible and grown up, while parents still expect obedience and fitting in with rules at home. Adolescents may also reject parents' beliefs and standards, while still needing special support and guidance for they may not yet be sure of their own values.

The situation is made even more difficult by the powerful sexual feelings adolescence brings, while hormonal fluctuations mean that even sexual feelings change rapidly, adding to teenagers' uncertainty.

That sense of identity, however, becomes more and more influenced by friends and less by parents. And unlike parental love, acceptance by friends depends on ability and personality. Trying to win acceptance can be a source of stress and anxiety.

Most young people will emerge from these common difficulties with a strong sense of their own identity. However, a very small number remain unsure of themselves, unable to relate satisfactorily to others – particularly to those of the opposite sex – or lacking in confidence.

The danger always exists that these teenagers may become withdrawn, rebellious or resort to various drugs or alcohol. For them, sensitive help from a counsellor (see COUNSELLING) may be needed. Families and friends can help by giving understanding and support.

When help is needed

A stable, loving and accepting family, support from friends, and people to look up to as good examples will usually prevent teenage difficulties from becoming serious problems. Those who lack these protective factors may find themselves in trouble or needing help. Even then explanation, time and reassurance are usually enough.

Very few need medical help for conditions such as hormonal imbalances, and PSYCHOTHERAPY is recommended only for serious emotional or behavioural problems. Among other alternative therapies that may alleviate less serious problems are the BACH REMEDIES.

QUINSY

A condition marked by a red and swollen throat

Occasionally during an attack of Tonsillitis, an abscess forms behind one tonsil – an uncommon condition known as quinsy. Pain is worse on the affected side of the throat and may also be felt in the ear. There may be difficulty swallowing and speaking.

Diagnosis of quinsy is made by looking into the mouth and seeing that one side of the throat is red and swollen, so that the tonsil and the uvula – the fleshy lump that hangs down from the back of the palate – are pushed towards the other side.

What the therapists recommend

Naturopathy Plenty of fluids, especially cold fruit juices, should be taken. Herbal gargles, particularly red sage, are recommended. In addition, a cold compress around the neck may help to ease the inflammation and any swelling. Extra vitamin C is likely to be prescribed: 500 mg to 1 g a day, with zinc or vitamin A.

An orthodox view

Although an ordinary sore throat does not usually require medical attention, consult a doctor if you suspect quinsy. He can arrange for an ear, nose and throat surgeon to release the pus from the abscess under local anaesthetic, providing rapid relief. Antibiotics may be given to clear up the infection and reduce any fever.

To prevent further attacks, some surgeons advise removing the tonsils after the inflammation has cleared up.

RADIESTHESIA AND RADIONICS

The Abbé Mermet, a Swiss priest, applied the ancient art of Dowsing to medicine in the 1920s. He coined the term *radiesthesia*, 'sensitivity to radiation', for his technique. See also Paranormal Therapies.

Radionics is a method of healing at a distance using specially designed instruments in conjunction with radiesthesia. Radionics is concerned with the 'energy patterns' which are thought to be emitted by all forms of matter. Any disharmonies or distortions in these patterns, it is claimed, can be identified and measured accurately so that the practitioner who is using the instruments for analysis builds up a 'holistic blueprint' of the patient

covering his mental, emotional and physical aspects. It is said to be possible to actually determine some diseases before they are physically obvious.

When a patient applies to a practitioner, he is sent a case-history form, and a list of charges. The patient fills in the form and returns it. The practitioner then carries out an analysis, and sends treatment(s) to the patient. In giving treatment, the practitioner seeks to correct the fundamental causes of disharmony identified by the analysis by stimulating the natural healing forces inherent in all living things, and so to return the patient to good health.

An orthodox view

Although there is increasing acceptance of the 'energetic' level of human function, very few if any of the claims made by the practitioners are verifiable, and caution and scepticism are appropriate.

RAW FOOD DIET

The value of food in its 'natural' state

A naturopathic, or 'nature cure', diet that has been in use throughout the world for about 100 years is one in which 80 per cent of the food (measured by weight) is eaten raw, mainly as fruit and vegetables.

This sounds more extreme than it really is. Fruit and vegetables contain a relatively large amount of water and are usually eaten in heavier portions than more kilojoule-concentrated foods such as fish, dairy foods, eggs and meat. As a result, considerable variety can be included in even the 20 per cent of non-raw foods that are permitted in the diet.

Although fruit and vegetables provide the bulk of the diet, raw foods with a higher concentration of kilojoules – nuts, seeds (sunflower, pumpkin, sesame and poppy), uncooked cereals such as Muesli, and sprouted pulses and grains, for example – ensure that the diet provides an adequate supply of protein and energy.

No more than 66 per cent of the total number of kilojoules are obtained from fruit and vegetables, so the intake of proteins and fats can still be maintained in line with the national recommendations for healthy eating (see Eating for Health).

There are two main ideas behind the raw food diet. The first is that the human digestive tract is not designed for a high-meat diet. It is long in proportion to body size, like those of plant-eating animals. Food takes a relatively long time to pass through it, which is

ideal for the good digestion of vegetable matter, but which gives meat or fish time to start decomposing. Such unsuitable food, the theory goes, upsets the body's ability to maintain its health.

The second aim of the raw food diet is to avoid the loss of Vitamins, Minerals, enzymes and Fibre that occurs in most cooking and processing methods. In addition, supporters of the diet often divide food into two groups according to its effect on the body. Fruit and vegetables are classed as so-called 'alkali-forming' foods; and meat, egg yolk, fish and dairy products as undesirable 'acid-forming' foods. A diet with a high proportion of raw ingredients naturally promotes the eating of alkali-forming foods and reduces the amount of acid-forming ones that are eaten, since these are generally foods that require cooking.

A raw food diet can supply every nutrient except vitamin B_{12}, which is virtually confined to animal foods – although, in practice, it is added to many breakfast cereals and yeast extracts. However, to ensure a wide range of nutrients in a particular diet takes careful meal-planning, especially where children are concerned.

In practice, it is generally much easier and more sociable to ensure a suitable intake of kilojoules, iron, calcium, zinc, protein and vitamins B_{12} and D by making sure that you add small amounts of oily fish, dairy foods, meat and cooked beans, peas and lentils. The fruit and vegetables included should be as varied and fresh as possible, and eaten only when in season.

RAYNAUD'S DISEASE

'Cold hands' complaint

People who are very sensitive to the cold can be affected by this condition, in which the fingers, hands and sometimes feet suddenly turn pale and numb. In severe cases they may turn blue and there may be burning pains. Very occasionally the sufferer may develop gangrene (death and decay of the fingers or toes when the blood supply to them is cut off), or Ulcers.

About 5 per cent of people suffer from the disorder at some stage in their lives, the vast majority of them women. Attacks usually last for no more than 15 to 30 minutes, providing the cause is treated.

In most cases the disease is caused by the contraction, due to cold, of the small arteries supplying blood to the surface of the skin.

Occasionally it can result from the vibration caused by using power tools or drills; from drugs prescribed for other ailments; from the pressure of gripping or carrying something; or from cigarette SMOKING.

Raynaud's disease (or Raynaud's syndrome, as it is also known) was named after Maurice Raynaud (1834-1881), a distinguished French physician who discovered the condition in the early 1860s – when he described it as 'a case of local asphyxia of the hands and feet, leading to gangrene'.

Self help Wear long thermal socks, gloves, fleece-lined shoes and a hat in very cold or wet weather. Be sure to use warm bedding and seal the bedroom doors and windows against draughts. If necessary, wear a nightcap, bedsocks or gloves in bed and keep a vacuum flask of hot tea or coffee by you in case you wake up cold.

If possible, take some EXERCISE every day, and be sure to eat regular hot meals. Avoid smoking completely. This narrows the arteries and restricts blood flow. Cut out any activities that you find trigger attacks. For further advice on keeping warm see COLDNESS and HYPOTHERMIA.

What the therapists recommend

Biofeedback Practitioners believe that worry or nervous upset may reduce the amount of blood flowing to people's extremities – especially their fingers and toes. This is thought to apply particularly to anyone who is prone to Raynaud's disease.

Therapists recommend sufferers to train themselves to warm their extremities using a hand-held thermometer which indicates when warmth is restored to the affected areas. By relaxing and imagining being in a warm situation (such as on a sunny beach or in a warm bath), and observing the effect on the instrument, it is possible to learn quite quickly to control the condition.

An orthodox view

Generally speaking, Raynaud's disease is more of a nuisance than a serious illness, and simple measures to keep warm are usually sufficient. However, if the patient's symptoms are extreme, and do not respond to ordinary warming, a doctor may prescribe drugs to stimulate the circulation. To exclude any underlying disease, such as inflamed arteries, he may also arrange for X-rays and blood tests.

A new drug called iloprost has recently been introduced, which is given by infusion with a drip. By mimicking a natural hormone, prostacylin, in the blood vessels, it prevents blood cells from clotting and blocking the circulation.

The treatment, given to hospital outpatients, lasts for a total of 72 hours, spread over several days. Meanwhile, trials are taking place in Britain on a tablet form of the drug, taken orally at home.

REBIRTHING

A technique of bringing patients to re-live the process of birth as a form of PSYCHOTHERAPY is known as rebirthing. It is based on the idea that traumatic experiences at birth have long-lasting effects which can lead to psychological problems in later life. Therapists say that re-living the pain and anxiety of the experience helps to release patients' tensions and heal disorders in a way similar to PRIMAL THERAPY.

See also HUMANISTIC PSYCHOLOGY.

REFLEXOLOGY

Treating illness with foot massage

By massaging what they call 'reflex areas' found in the feet, reflexologists treat diseases in parts of the body they claim to be related to those areas. Exactly what happens when the reflex areas are massaged is not fully understood, and cannot be explained scientifically. But it is thought that illness occurs when 'energy channels' in the body are blocked, causing damage to one area or another. Massage is aimed at destroying these blocks, allowing the energy to flow freely again and so heal the damage.

Reflexologists regard the feet as a 'mirror' of the body, with the left foot representing the left-hand side, and the right foot the right-hand side.

Different parts of the sole connect in some way to such organs as the bladder, kidneys and lungs; the big toe connects to the head and brain; and the small toe to the sinuses. The massage alone is said to immediately prompt the body to heal itself – no drugs or instruments are used.

Reflexology is said to have originated in China some 5 000 years ago, when pressure therapies were used to correct energy fields in the body (see ACUPRESSURE; ACUPUNCTURE; SHIATSU). The ancient Egyptians also used a form of reflexology, as shown in a wall-painting in a tomb dating about 2330 BC at Saqqara, south of Cairo.

But it was not until around 1913 that the therapy was introduced to the West by an American ear, nose and throat consultant,

Major reflex areas on the soles of the feet

Reflexologists use charts like the one below to show how zones of the feet are thought to mirror various parts of the body. They believe that illnesses show up as tender spots on the reflex areas of affected organs, and that by applying special foot massage techniques to the correct points they can treat almost any organ or area of the body. Most but not all parts of the body have corresponding (though not necessarily identical) points on each foot.

Top of head/brain
Side of head/brain
Shoulder
Solar plexus
Liver
Pancreas
Gall bladder
Large intestine
Small intestine
Sciatic nerve
Spine

Pituitary gland
Sinuses
Eyes
Neck
Ears
Heart
Lungs
Stomach
Spleen
Adrenal glands
Kidney
Bladder

Dr William Fitzgerald. He devised a method termed ZONE THERAPY, which involved applying healing pressure either with the hands or with special instruments to certain parts of the body.

He divided the body into ten zones, or channels, through which, he said, flowed the person's vital energy. The zones extended from the toes, up through the body to the head, and back down again to the hands. Each of the zones was of equal width, covering each organ and part of the body.

By applying pressure to, say, an area in the same zone as the ear, he produced an anaesthetic effect which deadened any pain that might be there. It is quite similar to someone automatically gritting his teeth when in pain, or gripping the sides of the chair at the dentist's. Unwittingly, he is using a form of reflexology to deal with discomfort in an everyday situation.

In the early 1930s Dr Fitzgerald's work was followed up by another American therapist, Mrs Eunice Ingham, who published two popular books on reflexology called *Stories the Feet Can Tell* and *Stories the Feet Have Told*. Unlike Dr Fitzgerald, however, she did not work on different parts of the zones, but treated the body by concentrating on the feet.

Who it can help While not claiming to be a 'cure-all', reflexology has been used to treat a host of common ailments, including BACK PAIN, DIGESTIVE PROBLEMS, MIGRAINE, PERIOD PROBLEMS, SINUS PROBLEMS and STRESS. It has also reportedly helped patients with more serious conditions, such as HEART DISORDERS, MULTIPLE SCLEROSIS and strokes.

In addition, reflexologists claim that they can sometimes detect an impending or potential illness, then give preventive treatment, if appropriate, or advise the patient to see a specialist. By having treatment every month or two, good health may be maintained – and early warning signs spotted.

The often powerful effects of the therapy may mean it is not always suitable during PREGNANCY or for anyone suffering from ARTHRITIS in the feet, DIABETES, certain heart disorders, OSTEOPOROSIS (thinning bones), phlebitis (vein inflammation), or THYROID DISORDERS. In such cases, treatment will be given with extra care – or not at all.

Finding a therapist Treatment should be carried out by a fully trained practitioner. For a list of therapists working in your area, write (enclosing a stamped, self-addressed envelope) to the South African Reflexology Society, P O Box 28040, Malvern (Natal) 4055. The International Institute of Reflexology (30 Thomson Street, Colbyn 0083), the Reflexology Academy of South Africa (P O Box 97681, Petervale 2151) and the South African Federation of Reflexology (8 Denne Street, Weltevreden Park 1709) all offer training courses in

Basic reflexology techniques

Stimulating a reflex point (above) *The therapist applies pressure with the side and end of the thumb – in this case to a point on the side of the foot. Either the right or left thumb may be used, whichever is most comfortable, while the fingers gently hold the foot in place and the other hand provides support. The thumb joint is kept bent.*

'Kneading' the foot (left) *This involves pressing the arch area of the sole of the foot with the flat side of a clenched fist, while applying pressure from the top with the other hand. The hands are moved around the whole arch area in a kneading motion to give a generally stimulating and toning effect.*

Locating treatment points *Pressing with her thumbs, the therapist probes the reflex areas on each foot in turn, looking for spots of special sensitivity. The points are no bigger than a pinhead so movements have to be*

precise. To move from one point to another the thumb is eased back from the first point and then slid forwards to the next one, keeping in contact with the skin all the time but not exerting pressure while moving.

the therapy; and these organisations, too, will supply names and addresses of practitioners.

Consulting a therapist At your first visit you are asked for a full medical history. You are then asked to lie comfortably in a reclining chair, with feet raised. Shoes and socks are removed and the feet quickly examined for CORNS or calluses, which can interfere with the blood supply, or infections which could indicate disease.

Before starting treatment, the therapist will gently massage talcum onto your feet to get you used to the 'feel' of the technique. Reassuringly, massage does not tickle.

Whatever the ailment, all the reflex areas on both feet are massaged. Using the thumb to apply pressure, the reflexologist examines the soles, sides and tops of the feet, feeling for areas of tenderness. If one is found, then the corresponding part of the body is believed to be out of balance, or sick. Where there is no discomfort, the corresponding part is in balance and working efficiently.

Any tender areas receive extra attention, and the therapist will deal with the causes of the condition – as well as its symptoms. By treating the whole body, it is possible to treat more than just one problem at a time.

The first treatment lasts for about an hour. As well as the good that this should do, you may well benefit from just sitting back and relaxing. Six to eight sessions are usually needed to deal with a specific ailment. To begin with, the sessions will be given once a week; but later they may be spread out at intervals of every two or three weeks.

In some cases a patient may feel better after just one treatment. But at least another two treatments are recommended to prevent a relapse or recurrence of the complaint. In other cases, improvement may not occur until the second or third treatment. However, if the patient does not start to improve after three treatments, this may mean that reflexology is not going to help him, in which case he would probably be referred to another alternative therapist or to his doctor.

Usually there are no unpleasant side effects after treatment. However, some form of healing reaction may occur as the body starts to right itself. For example, treatment for a congested sinus may result in a cold; and CONSTIPATION treatment can cause increased bowel movements. However, providing the therapy has been used correctly, such reactions should not be severe.

An orthodox view

No clinical trials have been conducted to prove the claims made by reflexologists, but doctors believe that little harm can come from this therapy and many people find the massage particularly soothing.

REGRESSION THERAPY

In the common parlance of psychology 'regression' refers to a return to an earlier stage of development, as when an adult behaves like a child.

The scope of regression therapy (or past-life regression therapy, as it is also known by some people) is different. It is based on the belief that we carry memories not only of this existence but of past ones as well – and that in one of these previous incarnations something may have happened to block the normal energy flow of the 'higher conscious', with on-going consequences.

The regression therapist helps his client to draw upon these latent memories, unblocking energy so that particular problems can be overcome, emotional traumas resolved and 'dis-eases' healed. Every part of the body is said to hold a different sort of memory, and by tapping into any one part a person can release the appropriate memory.

Regression therapy has close links with the oriental conception of 'karma', the theory that actions in one life have inevitable consequences in the next. The therapist (who claims psychic power) helps his patient to release karmic patterns from the past.

Reflexology in the home

Although the best results are obtained through a complete treatment by a therapist, people can treat themselves at home by using a few simple techniques. Even so, a practitioner should advise on which techniques to use and how to perform them.

Only comparatively minor conditions are suitable for treatment, including: low back pain, catarrh, headaches, migraine, neck pain, sinus problems and tension. If you find it awkward to work on your own feet, corresponding reflex areas in the hand can be used instead.

To massage the feet, sit comfortably on the floor or on a bed in a warm, quiet room, with your back supported by cushions.

Begin by massaging the whole foot, and be sure not to overwork any reflex areas that might unbalance the body in any way, causing possible unpleasant effects.

Sinus (*left*) Massage the reflex areas found in the back and sides of the smaller toes for complaints such as catarrh, colds, hay fever and sinusitis.

Tension (*right*) Massage the solar plexus reflex as shown. Then massage the adrenal reflexes in the middle of the feet, and pituitary reflexes in centre of pads of big toes.

Headaches (*below*) Massage head reflexes on the tips of the big toes and along their outer edges.

Neck pain (*above*) Apply pressure to the neck reflex area on the base and along the inner edge of each big toe.

Back pain (*right*) Treat the spine reflexes along the inside edge of each foot sole.

Finding a therapist A small number of practitioners of regression therapy operates in South Africa. For information, write (enclosing a stamped, self-addressed envelope) to the Wellstead Resource Centre, 1 Wellington Avenue, Wynberg 7800. The Wellstead stocks books and tape-recordings by Chris Griscom, an American practitioner who has visited South Africa.

An orthodox view

In orthodox medicine there is no generally accepted framework into which to fit the theory of regression therapy.

REICHIAN THERAPY

The psychiatrist Wilhelm Reich (1897-1957) began his career as a follower of Freud, practising psychoanalysis in Vienna. Later he broke away from the Freudian school, moved to the USA, and developed the ideas and methods known as Reichian therapy.

Reich extended and challenged Freud's views, believing that when frightening or hurtful experiences and feelings are repressed into the unconscious mind this can create physical tensions as well as psychological problems. He firmly believed that certain physical movements can release these accumulated tensions while freeing repressed emotions.

In Reichian therapy, the therapist helps the patient to become objectively aware of how his posture, muscular tension – called 'body armouring' – and breathing patterns reflect his emotions.

Therapy often includes thorough physical manipulation which is aimed at relaxing body armouring and releasing tension – methods which have been further developed in BIOENERGETICS.

Later, Reich incorporated sexuality into his theory, suggesting that psychological problems stem from blockages of 'orgone energy', a life force associated with the experience of orgasm (see ORGONE THERAPY). He devised an 'orgone accumulator', a box in which patients sat, supposedly to have this energy restored.

Most psychologists and scientists rejected this theory and after conflicts with US legal and medical authorities, Reich was jailed for selling prohibited medical equipment and defying a ban on publishing his theories. He died of a heart attack in prison. However, many of his ideas are still widely respected, and his methods have undergone a revival.

See also HUMANISTIC PSYCHOLOGY.

RELAXATION AND BREATHING

Regular periods of relaxation are an essential part of physical and mental well-being, yet STRESS often prevents us from entering a naturally relaxed state. One of the simplest and most effective ways of counteracting this is by means of breathing exercises designed to ease TENSION and promote calmness. Many ancient traditions such as YOGA and MEDITATION make use of special breathing techniques to alter mental states, and West-ern medicine, too, is increasingly coming to recognise the way in which different breathing patterns are connected with general health. For example, anxious people are known to breathe more rapidly than others, using only the upper part of the chest, and talking with the lungs full of air (see HYPERVENTILATION), while depressed people sigh more and tend to talk after exhalation.

Breathing is a unique way of directly influencing the unconscious processes of the body, since of all the functions directed by the autonomic – or involuntary – nervous system it is the easiest to control by will. Some yogis and experienced meditators are said to

Relaxation and breathing techniques

Chest breathing *Lie on a firm, comfortable surface, hands lightly resting on upper chest. Breathe slowly in and out using chest muscles, so hands rise and fall with each breath.*

Diaphragmatic breathing *Lie down, hands resting on abdomen. Slowly and rhythmically fill and empty the lungs using the diaphragm, which should move up and down.*

'Corpse position' *Use this yoga posture to practise the progressive muscular relaxation exercise on p. 300. Lie with your head, neck and back aligned, feet about 450 mm apart, and hands turned up and held about 150 mm away from your body.*

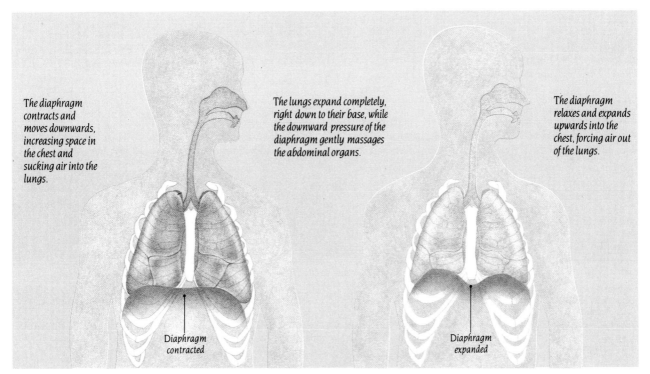

The diaphragm contracts and moves downwards, increasing space in the chest and sucking air into the lungs.

The lungs expand completely, right down to their base, while the downward pressure of the diaphragm gently massages the abdominal organs.

The diaphragm relaxes and expands upwards into the chest, forcing air out of the lungs.

Diaphragm contracted

Diaphragm expanded

INHALATION

EXHALATION

How to breathe naturally

The habit of breathing from the diaphragm, or midriff (as shown above), often has to be relearned in adult life.

be able voluntarily to lower their heart rate and BLOOD PRESSURE, but few of us realise that we possess such control over our own bodies. Everyone, however, can alter their breathing patterns and, through them, other parts of the nervous system, giving them control over their level of bodily relaxation.

The fundamental purpose of breathing is to provide the lungs with a constant supply of air from which essential oxygen can be absorbed into the blood and circulated to all the body tissues.

Breathing out empties the lungs for the next breath and allows the body to expel waste gases present such as carbon dioxide.

The respiratory rate changes naturally at different times of the day and in different situations, such as walking, sitting, or running for a bus, to accommodate changing needs for oxygen intake and carbon dioxide expulsion. These correspond to different levels of relaxation and tension, and are reflected in the two basic types of breathing that can occur: chest breathing and diaphragmatic breathing.

Chest breathing This is the fastest way of getting a quick injection of oxygen into the blood. It usually occurs during vigorous EXER-

CISE, excitement, FEAR, ANXIETY or emergency situations which call for action, but it can also be used to get the system going in the morning or give a boost when energy is low.

During chest breathing the rib muscles contract, forcing the chest to expand upwards and outwards so that air is drawn quickly into the upper chest. Breathing is shallow and fast, with the emphasis on inhalation, and a general stress response, including increased muscular tension occurs.

This is appropriate in some situations – it may even save life by allowing split-second action in an emergency on the road, for example – but if it continues for too long or becomes a regular breathing pattern, the body may enter a permanently stressed state with serious consequences for health. It may also become hysterical overbreathing, with too much carbon dioxide expelled and metabolic changes in the body, leading to feelings of faintness and 'pins and needles'.

Diaphragmatic breathing This is the normal, natural way to breathe when you are relaxed – which should be most of the time. Instead of using the rib muscles, breathing occurs by the rhythmic contraction and relaxation of the diaphragm – a dome-shaped sheet of muscle separating the chest and abdominal cavities.

As you inhale, the diaphragm contracts and flattens, increasing space in the chest and sucking air into the lungs. The lungs ex-

pand completely, right down to their base, and the movement of the diaphragm gently massages the abdominal organs. On exhaling, the diaphragm relaxes and moves up into the chest, forcing air out of the lungs. You can feel the movement of the diaphragm by lying down and placing a hand on the abdomen.

Diaphragmatic breathing is more efficient than chest breathing, promoting relaxation rather than tension. The lungs are more completely filled and emptied with each breath, so providing more oxygen for metabolism. At the same time, there is no build up of waste products such as carbon dioxide in the lungs and lactic acid in the blood, which can cause nervousness and TIREDNESS.

Why relax?

The human body, like that of other animals, is adapted to cope with brief periods of arousal or stress that occur in the natural state – for example, when danger threatens or when prey has to be caught. At such times, irregular, shallow chest breathing occurs, muscles become tense, and panicky, anxious feelings may be experienced.

In nature, stressful situations usually last only a short time, and tension is quickly dissipated in action of some sort, leaving body and mind free to return to normal.

But in modern life, with its pressures and strains and few physical outlets, aroused states can be less easy to get rid of.

Quick relaxation at work

Office workers can relieve neck and shoulder tension and correct poor posture in just a few minutes with a good stretching session. Here is how to do it in under five minutes.

Chest and back stretch (Below) Stand up straight with neck and shoulders relaxed and feet slightly apart. Slowly raise arms, bend elbows and touch fingertips to the breastbone. Next lower the arms and straighten them out behind you as high up as you can, hands clasped together and head tilted as far back as comfortably possible.

Neck turns (Left) Sit on a fairly low chair at a desk or table, and place elbows on the surface, about 6-8in (150-200mm) apart with hands clasped together at the back of the head. Slowly press the head down until your chin touches your chest. Close your eyes and hold the position for a few moments.

Unclasp hands and turn head slowly until chin rests in palm of right hand. Push slowly down with the left hand and up with the right to turn head as far as possible. Hold for a few moments, return slowly to centre and relax. Then repeat in the opposite direction.

Shoulder rolls (Right) Sit comfortably in a chair, fingers pressing down onto shoulders. Keeping shoulders down, circle elbows up away from the body, back, down and forwards several times. Repeat in opposite direction.

(Above) Stretch the back by bending forward, raising your arms up over your back and allowing your neck to relax and hang down. Hold for a few moments, then slowly straighten up, unclasp hands and drop arms to your sides.

Whole body stretch (Right) Stand up straight and take a deep breath to fill the lungs right to the bottom. Throw your arms out behind you and tilt your head back to look at the ceiling. Relax, breathe out slowly and bend forward from the waist with knees slightly bent, hands hanging loosely down and neck relaxed. Hold for a few seconds, slowly straighten up and return to first position, inhaling deeply.

Lower back and leg stretch (Above) Sit on a low chair and draw one leg up so that the foot rests on the chair seat. Keep back straight and clasp knee as close to the body as you can. Hold for a few moments, relax, lower foot and repeat with the other leg.

In continually stressful situations such as a high-pressure job or a troubled marriage, long periods of stress may be experienced, and these may eventually result in the development of ailments such as high blood pressure, heart and lung disorders, MIGRAINE headaches and anxiety.

The most effective way of combating stress and preventing these illnesses is to make time for regular relaxation. This can take the form of 'active' relaxation such as MEDITATION, taking exercise or practising rhythmic breathing techniques, or 'passive' relaxation such as listening to music.

In the relaxed state, there is regular diaphragmatic breathing, muscular relaxation and mental calmness. The body uses up less energy than usual and there is less work for major organs such as heart, lungs and brain to do. Regular relaxation exercises have been shown to lower blood pressure and improve performance at work. Participants in studies also report that they sleep better, learn new skills more easily and feel more energetic. Their stamina and fitness improve and they experience greater involvement and enjoyment in family life.

Relaxation through breathing

The first step in learning to relax is being able to recognise physical or mental tension. Breathing patterns provide one of the best indicators – shallow, uneven chest breathing is a sign of stress, and can occur in ordinary situations, such as waiting at traffic lights, making decisions or queueing for a bus.

Stress experts say that a good way to introduce relaxation into everyday life is to watch your breathing patterns so that you start to notice stressful points during the day. Whenever you find yourself breathing from the chest, take a deep breath in and then let it out slowly. You should feel tense muscles relax throughout the body as you exhale.

In addition, a daily relaxation routine of 10-15 minutes is said to improve physical and mental well-being and help to counteract many harmful effects of stress.

You can begin by finding a quiet, well-ventilated room where you will not be disturbed at all. Loosen any tight clothing and lie down on the floor with your feet about 45 cm apart. The head and neck should be aligned with the back.

Close your eyes and practise diaphragmatic breathing with one hand gently resting on the abdomen to check that the diaphragm is moving rather than the chest muscles. Concentrate on the rhythm of your breathing, letting it become smooth and regular so that there are no gaps.

As you practise slow, rhythmic breathing, focus your attention on the coolness of the air breathed in and the warmth of the air

breathed out. When thoughts come into your mind, let them go again without dwelling on them, so that you stay focused on your breathing rhythm.

After seven to ten minutes your mind should feel clear and your body relaxed. Gradually allow yourself to become aware of outside sounds and gently open your eyes. When you feel ready, slowly get up.

Progressive muscular relaxation

In times of stress the nervous system becomes overactive and stimulates the muscles more than usual, causing them to contract and become tense. The technique of progressive muscular relaxation is designed to undo the effects of stress, relax muscle groups one by one, and lead to a healthier, less stressed state if practised regularly. It works by first tensing and then relaxing each part of the body in turn.

Choose a quiet room where you will not be disturbed for about 10-15 minutes. Remove your shoes, loosen tight clothing and lie eyes closed on a bed or carpet, with head, neck and trunk in a straight line.

Begin by raising your eyebrows and tensing the forehead muscles for a count of five; then relax, feeling the difference in the muscles. Repeat, then go through the same procedure for different muscle groups, first with eyes squeezed tightly shut, then with mouth wide open, face muscles stretched and lips, eyebrows and chin puckered up. Repeat with jaw muscles tightened and teeth clenched; then with shoulders raised and neck and shoulders tense; then with left arm raised, arm muscles tensed and fist clenched; then with right arm tensed.

Now contract your rib muscles, taking careful note of how your breathing changes. Relax, then pull in and tighten the stomach muscles, hold for a count of five, relax and breathe out. Lift the left leg a little and push the foot away from you so that the muscles tense. Hold for a count of five, relax, then let the leg drop. Repeat, then do the same with the right leg.

RESPIRATORY DISORDERS

Many different conditions can affect the respiratory tract and make breathing difficult. The most common are virus and bacterial infections such as COLDS of the nose and throat, INFLUENZA, LARYNGITIS (inflamed voice box), TONSILLITIS and BRONCHITIS.

Other viruses and bacteria are responsible for tuberculosis, PNEUMONIA and PLEURISY, which affect the lungs and surrounding tissues. Recurrent infections – and exposure to

dust or cigarette smoke – can cause the lungs to become overinflated, resulting in EMPHYSEMA.

The respiratory system is particularly susceptible to ALLERGY because irritating substances such as grass pollen or house dust are easily breathed in, and may trigger HAY FEVER or ASTHMA attacks.

RESTLESS LEGS

Some people feel a constant need to move their legs, particularly when they are lying in bed. The condition is known as restless legs and is harmless, except that it disrupts sleep and leads to TIREDNESS. The cause of the condition is not known.

What the therapists recommend

Massage Provided there is no related problem, such as a skin rash or infection, or such conditions as phlebitis or VARICOSE VEINS, a general massage of the legs may help circulation and ease the restlessness.

Acupressure The point therapists recommend to be treated (known as 'gall bladder 34') is on the outer side of the knee, four fingers' width down from the kneecap, in the hollow between the skin and the smaller leg bone. You should press inwards and against the upper bone.

Naturopathy Therapists consider that the most common cause of restless legs is iron deficiency and chronic mild ANAEMIA through loss of blood – for example, in women who have heavy periods. A diet that is rich in iron, especially from green, leafy vegetables, would be advised. Naturopaths may prescribe iron and vitamin E supplements, and suggest hot and cold sitz baths (see HYDROTHERAPY) to improve the circulation.

An orthodox view

Apart from commonsense measures, such as keeping warm and avoiding coffee in the evenings, the only orthodox medical treatment that works is a dose of diazepam (Valium) at bedtime. However, like other benzodiazepine drugs, diazepam is addictive and most doctors today are reluctant to prescribe it, except in very short courses.

RHEUMATISM

Pain and stiffness of the joints and muscles are commonly referred to as rheumatism – a word more often used by laymen than doctors. It in fact covers a large number of distinct medical conditions, including fibrositis (inflammation of the connective tissues, especially those of the muscles in the back), rheumatic fever, and various forms of ARTHRITIS – in particular OSTEOARTHRITIS and RHEUMATOID ARTHRITIS.

Rheumatism is common in old age, and a significant cause in over 65s is a condition which is called polymyalgia rheumatica. This tends to comes on suddenly, with severe neck and shoulder pain, morning stiffness and HEADACHES.

A rare complication is temporal arteritis, an inflammation of arteries supplying blood to the eyes which, if not treated quickly, can lead to blindness.

What the therapists recommend

Acupuncture Practitioners claim to have cured rheumatism by treating points on the patient's gall bladder, large intestine, kidney, governor and stomach meridians. MOXIBUSTION is also said to help.

Traditional Medicine One of the most popular country remedies is garlic oil – 'devil's mustard' – which is made by crushing GARLIC with oil and lard. To relieve pain it should be rubbed firmly and deeply into the affected area.

Some people wear copper bracelets in the belief that this will relieve rheumatic pain. See COPPER THERAPY.

Massage To begin with, massage of the neck and shoulders should be applied gently. As the treatment progresses, deeper frictions and kneading, or petrissage, techniques can be employed. However, deep massage can be painful if you aren't careful. To ease any pain you should always finish with slow, soothing strokes.

Hydrotherapy Practitioners claim success when rheumatism is treated with underwater douches, relaxing needle sprays, hot or cold packs and hot paraffin wax for the hands or feet. The treatments are used in various permutations according to the patient's condition at the time.

Herbal Medicine Initially, patients can help themselves by cleansing their systems (see EATING FOR HEALTH) and reducing their consumption of alcohol, red meat and sugar. Massage with diluted oil of lavender or rosemary – two or three drops to a teaspoon of vegetable oil – may help to reduce rheumatic inflammation.

Herbalists will give dietary advice and may prescribe remedies such as buckbean, celery seed, devil's claw, lignum vitae, wild yam and willow bark, as appropriate.

Homoeopathy Where the patient has a fear of being touched, the prescription is *Arnica*; and where the rheumatism is greatly aggravated by movement, *Bryonia*. If rheumatic pain is worse on beginning to move, but im-

proves with continued gentle movement, try taking *Rhus. tox.*

Reflexology Massage is recommended to the reflex areas relating to the parts of the body affected, and also to areas relating to the solar plexus and the pituitary, parathyroid and adrenal glands (see chart, p. 295).

An orthodox view

Most cases of rheumatism respond to simple measures such as keeping warm or applying a hot-water bottle to the affected area. Anti-inflammatory painkillers such as aspirin or paracetamol may help, but should not be taken over long periods without consulting a doctor. There are many causes of rheumatic pain, and a firm diagnosis should be made by a doctor before starting lengthy and often expensive courses of treatment.

RHEUMATOID ARTHRITIS

One of the most common forms of arthritis, rheumatoid arthritis is estimated to afflict about one person in 100 in South Africa at some time in their lives. Unlike OSTEOARTHRITIS, which is progressive and irreversible, rheumatoid arthritis may come and go spontaneously – though there is as yet no sure cure, and the underlying cause is not properly understood.

Most cases start between the ages of 25 and 55, often with swelling, stiffness and pain in the knuckle joints of the hands or in the feet. The stiffness is often at its worst early in the morning. In some cases, the inflammation of rheumatoid arthritis may spread beyond the joints, to the lungs or eyes. Blood tests and X-rays may be needed to distinguish it from osteoarthritis or GOUT.

RICKETS

Rickets (or 'rachitis') is a children's disease, a bone deformity which is caused by vitamin deficiency in the body, especially the lack of vitamin D. This vitamin plays an essential part in the absorption of calcium from the intestines into the bloodstream, and hence into the skeletal system. The action of ultraviolet light (in sunlight) on skin fats produces vitamin D, which is also found in such fatty foods as dairy products, oily fish and fish-liver oils.

Despite South Africa's abundant sunshine, rickets has not been eradicated from the

country, especially in poorer areas where parents are unable to procure for their children a balanced diet. The symptoms include bow legs, knock knees, spinal curvature, a prominent forehead, and painfully deformed swelling of the bones at the wrists, ankles and knees. Affected children present an altogether unhappy picture.

What the therapists recommend

Naturopathy Sunshine and a diet rich in vitamin D provide a natural means of treating rickets.

Homoeopathy To correct this disorder of bone metabolism, calcium carbonate, calcium phosphate and silica are indicated, and these are given in homoeopathic doses.

An orthodox view

X-rays and blood tests will confirm the diagnosis of rickets. In addition to advising on a better diet the doctor will prescribe vitamin D supplements – although the latter must be taken in moderation to avoid hypercalcaemia, an abnormally high level of calcium in the body. A rickety child may be referred to hospital for corrective treatment.

RINGING IN THE EARS

In the condition known medically as tinnitus, the sufferer is conscious of a constant ringing or buzzing noise in one or both ears, which only he can hear. In some cases it is caused simply by a blockage of wax in the outer ears. But other more serious causes include DEAFNESS, HYPERTENSION, Ménière's disease (progressive deafness and dizziness caused by inner-ear disease) and otosclerosis (a type of deafness that runs in families).

In yet other cases, it is brought on by old age or by certain drugs such as aspirin or quinine. Often there seems to be no obvious cause, although the condition may be aggravated by ANXIETY or DEPRESSION.

Rarely, ringing in the ears is the result of a benign tumour of the nerve from the ear to the brain, called an acoustic neuroma. If a serious underlying cause is suspected – or if the patient is emotionally disturbed in any way – a doctor should be consulted as soon as possible.

What the therapists recommend

ACUPRESSURE

Self help Ringing in the ears may be relieved by pressing inwards with the fingers one finger's width in front of the ear at the top of the cheekbone.

ACUPUNCTURE

Consultation Traditionally, acupuncturists believe that ringing in the ears is caused by liver disorders or gall-bladder problems. They therefore treat pressure points on the liver, gall bladder and governor meridians. In addition, MOXIBUSTION – the therapeutic use of burning herbs – is applied to the bladder and kidney meridians.

Acupuncture is said to be particularly effective for treating tinnitus if previous attempts have not worked.

NATUROPATHY

Consultation Some practitioners consider CATARRH and sinus congestion (see SINUS PROBLEMS) to be common causes of tinnitus. Patients would be advised to cut down on dairy produce and refined starchy foods, and to avoid tobacco and smoky atmospheres. Steam inhalations may also prove helpful in relieving the condition.

HOMOEOPATHY

Consultation Many remedies are claimed to be effective. When there is pain in the cartilages of the ears with roaring, giddiness and deafness, *Salicylic acid* 6 may be recommended as one of the most useful. For ringing, hissing or tinkling in the ears that is worse for movement, try *China off.* 6.

An orthodox view

A doctor investigating a case of tinnitus will first examine the patient's ears and perform simple hearing tests using a tuning fork. If necessary, he will arrange for a hearing specialist to conduct a test called an audiogram. If acoustic neuroma is suspected, he will send the patient to hospital for an X-ray of the bone between the ear and the brain.

Regular drug treatment may give relief, especially in some cases of Ménière's disease. Severely affected patients may benefit by wearing a 'masker', an instrument that looks like a hearing aid but produces a low background noise to block out the ringing.

RINGWORM

The highly contagious infection of the skin known popularly as ringworm is also medically called tinea. The term ringworm is somewhat misleading, since no worm is involved – it is caused by a FUNGAL INFECTION. However, as the infection spreads, inflammation extends in a ring shape, while the centre reverts to the appearance of normal skin.

Ringworm can occur anywhere on the body, but warm, moist areas – such as the armpits, groin, beneath the breasts and the feet – are the commonest places.

Local treatment with antifungal preparations is usually very effective, combined with simple hygiene methods such as washing thoroughly, drying carefully, and applying talcum or antifungal powder.

ROGERIAN THERAPY

The work of Carl Rogers (1902-87) has been a major influence on modern PSYCHOTHERAPY since the 1950s, when he began to publish his ideas. Rogers was one of the first to begin using techniques completely different from the Freudian psychoanalysis favoured by most therapists at the time.

The new approach became known as Rogerian therapy. Rogers himself called it 'client-centred' or 'person-centred' therapy, since he wished to emphasise the active, responsible role of those people who sought therapy, refusing to view them as patients. In Rogerian therapy, the client's own point of view and experiences are given primary importance, rather than the therapist's views. This is known as 'non-directive' treatment, since instead of offering advice, the therapist helps the client develop his own view of the situation and work out the options open to him.

The aim is to strengthen the individual's sense of his own identity, to help him find a compatible way of life and to develop himself as fully as possible in all respects.

See HUMANISTIC PSYCHOLOGY.

ROLFING

According to the founder of Rolfing, the American biological chemist Dr Ida Rolf (1896-1979), many health problems are caused by poor body posture – for example, hunched shoulders and stooped backs. Sufferers are constantly striving to rectify this, and as a result they are drained of vitality and the normal working of their bodies is impaired – leaving them open to illness.

To combat this, Dr Rolf devised a complex manipulative system which she called 'structural reintegration', now known as Rolfing.

By massaging the body's connective tissue and muscles, she aimed to realign the body so that its physical structures were in a straight vertical line. She believed that only then could the earth's field of gravity properly support the body's own energy field, and physical and psychological well-being be re-established.

Who it can help Anyone whose body structure is out of line can benefit.

While there are as yet no practitioners of Rolfing in South Africa, deep massage of a similar kind is routinely practised by qualified physiotherapists and masseurs.

An orthodox view

Rolfing combines a CHIROPRACTIC/osteopathic approach with BIOENERGETICS. It is a variant of many similar mind-body therapies and should be seen more as a way of learning about the body than as a specific treatment for any particular disorder.

(Above) The therapist works on the connective tissue around the ankle joints. This aims to improve flexibility.

To relieve the strain of carrying the head too far forward, the practitioner eases the shoulder muscles towards their normal position.

ROUNDWORMS

Giant parasites that breed in unsanitary conditions

The disease caused by the common roundworm is known medically as 'ascariasis', and it is prevalent – especially among children – in unsanitary conditions where food and water become infected with the worms' eggs. This worm is a giant parasite, between 10 and 30 cm long.

Developing in the human intestine from an egg, the worm in turn lays eggs that are excreted in the faeces, which contaminate the soil. Symptoms of ascariasis are malnutrition and stunted growth.

What the therapists recommend

Naturopathy Fasting for three days starves the worms; the fast could be followed by a diet of pure vegetable juice (for example, carrot juice). Alternatively purge the bowel with Epsom salts in water.

Herbal medicine Horseradish and hyssop are among herbs that may be prescribed by a medical herbalist. Some indigenous people of South Africa tend to use the pounded root of the wild medlar, after it has been softened in water, as a purgative.

Homoeopathy Remedies include homoeopathic doses of aconite, calcium carbonate, silica, spigella and sulphur. As always with this therapy, the homoeopath pays attention to the patient's all-round state of health before prescribing.

An orthodox view

Antihistamine drugs such as mebendazole or piperazine will be prescribed, to be taken orally. This compound paralyses the roundworms, and laxatives help to expel them.

During Rolfing, clients lie, sit or stand in various positions. (Left) The client lies on her side while the practitioner works on the limbs with the aim of improving the hip joint to change the relationship of the leg and pelvis.

After the first three sessions, the practitioner moves on from the outer muscles to the deeper layers closer to the backbone. This work on the front of the body affects the back. (Above) The diaphragm is worked upon, together with the muscles that flex the hip joint. These muscles can all contribute to back and neck pain.

During the sixth session, the entire back is worked upon. In this technique (left), the practitioner is moving the client's leg to articulate the hip joint, while holding on to various other muscles, including those that are sometimes involved in causing the pain of sciatica. Advanced sessions can continue the process of improving posture.

ROYAL JELLY

Worker bees excrete this nutritious, milky substance from their salivary glands as food for the select bee larvae that are to develop into queen bees. The queens grow to be twice the size of the workers and live for up to six years, laying as many as 2 000 eggs each day of their lives. By contrast, the worker bees, which do not receive the 'wonder food', live for only about six weeks and are sterile.

Analysis of royal jelly has revealed some 20 amino acids, VITAMINS, including most of the vitamin B-complex and vitamin C, and the MINERALS iron, potassium and sodium.

The attributes of the queen bee and the presence in the jelly of several essential human nutrients is probably the basis of the claims currently made for it.

It is said to provide energy, help reduce high BLOOD PRESSURE and to relieve hardening of the arteries. It is also believed to treat DEPRESSION, dermatitis, ANOREXIA, MYALGIC ENCEPHALOMYELITIS (ME) and the pain associated with RHEUMATOID ARTHRITIS.

An orthodox view

The amount of vitamins and other nutrients that royal jelly provides is extremely small, but medical research suggests that it is their proportions which may account for its supposedly beneficial effects.

SALT-FREE DIETS

Common salt, or sodium chloride, is the body's main source of sodium. Although sodium is an essential MINERAL, the average Westerner eats 12 g of salt a day, compared with the recommended daily amount of 5 g. About 70 per cent of this intake is sodium not naturally present in food, but added in the course of manufacture and processing. For example, prepared foods such as bread, cheese, yeast extract, breakfast cereals, biscuits, soups, stock cubes, sauce mixes and tinned vegetables are all heavily salted or contain other sodium compounds. Flavour enhancers such as monosodium glutamate, bicarbonate of soda, baking powder and certain other FOOD ADDITIVES all add large amounts of sodium.

A high salt intake has been shown to encourage high BLOOD PRESSURE in those prone to it. As a result, salt-free diets are often suggested for those with a tendency to HEART DISORDERS, high blood pressure, CIRCULATION PROBLEMS or KIDNEY COMPLAINTS.

What are commonly referred to as 'salt-free diets' are really 'low-salt diets', however. A totally salt-free diet is difficult to achieve because most foods contain salt. In any case, such a diet should be followed only under the supervision of a doctor or medically qualified therapist. But food without added salt provides all the sodium the body needs.

Instead of salt, you can flavour food with citrus juice, vinegar, herbs, spices, GARLIC, onions, wine or vegetable purées. Salt substitutes are also available, but some contain potassium chloride and should not be used by people with certain heart conditions, so check with your doctor first.

SALT-WATER TREATMENTS

Bathing in salt water is recommended for people suffering from stiffness and a variety of aches and pains. The treatments are aimed at soothing the body and encouraging it to use its own healing powers.

See HYDROTHERAPY.

SAUNA BATH

Turning on the heat to get fit

When taking a steam sauna bath, bathers sit in an insulated pine cabin and are subjected to hot, moist air produced by throwing water over heated stones on a stove. The treatment is based on increased humidity rather than increased heat, and is calculated to expel moisture from the body, eliminate waste products and poisons, stimulate the circulation, and help people to relax.

It is best to take a sauna unclothed, as wearing trunks or swimsuits – or draping yourself with a towel – will impede the flow of perspiration and make you feel uncomfortably damp and sweaty.

Most saunas operate at relatively high temperatures. For safety's sake the heat is

This 19th-century etching shows bathers enjoying the benefits of the Russian sauna, or 'Bagne Russe'. Some are striking their bodies with birch twigs while others douse themselves with pails of cold water. Water thrown on the fire at left produces billows of steam.

often thermostatically controlled at an upper limit – though some establishments rely on the regular opening of the sauna door, as bathers enter and exit, to prevent excessive temperature increase.

The sauna cabins mostly contain horizontal wooden benches of differing heights, the lower benches being exposed to less heat than the higher ones. Knot-free benches are generally preferred as the resin in them does not escape and burn your skin.

Saunas originated in Scandinavia in the Middle Ages, and in Finland bathers still gently beat themselves with birch leaves in order to help cleanse the skin and get the blood flowing.

In South Africa saunas are now available at many HEALTH RESORTS, health clubs, gymnasiums and other sports centres. Some enthusiasts have small cabins, holding two or three people, installed in their homes; also available is a 'one-man sauna', running on castors, in which the bather sits with his or her head exposed. Firms supplying home saunas are listed in the *Yellow Pages*.

Once you are used to taking saunas and know that they have no bad effects on your system, you can spend up to 15 minutes at a time in the cabin. It is then advisable to emerge and take a cool shower before returning for another session. Some experts claim that a total of 30 minutes will eliminate as much waste as your kidneys normally dispose of in 24 hours. Depending on your fitness, it is possible to take gentle EXERCISE while in the sauna.

Before entering a sauna you should give your skin a preparatory cleansing with a tepid shower. After a sauna you can take an invigorating cold shower or swim, provided that you are 100 per cent fit – ask your doctor's advice if uncertain. In Scandinavia some healthy and experienced bathers roll naked in the snow after a sauna.

Beginners, however, should spend about five minutes inside the cabin to start with – preferably on the less hot, lower benches – and build up gradually from that. Anyone who feels sick, faint, dizzy, or whose heart beats uncomfortably fast while taking a sauna, should leave the cabin and rest for a while. See also HYDROTHERAPY.

Warning Be sure to wait for at least two hours after eating a large meal before you take a sauna. You should speak to your doctor before taking a sauna if you suspect that you are not in perfect health.

Avoid saunas altogether if you suffer from any of the following: ANGINA, hardening of the arteries, high or low BLOOD PRESSURE, EPILEPSY, DIABETES or SKIN DISEASES (except ACNE). Also keep away from saunas during pregnancy, or if you are in the first few days of a period.

SCABIES

Scabies is a highly contagious skin disease caused by a parasitic mite (*Sarcoptes scabiei*) that lives only on the human skin, into which it burrows and in which it lays eggs. The favourite sites for the mite are the areas between the fingers; the wrists and armpits; the palms of the hands and the soles of the feet; and the genitals. Tiny but extremely itchy pimples appear a few weeks after the initial infestation, and the almost inevitable scratching produces sores, scabs and coarsening of the skin.

What the therapists recommend

Naturopathy Calendula cream, applied to the affected areas, is a traditional and effective treatment for scabies and other skin infections.

Herbal medicine To soothe the itching, apply a strong tincture made of rosemary, thyme, nettle and fennel (both the leaves and the seeds). An indigenous remedy is a weak tea made from the leaves, stems and flowers of the wild verbena; wash the infected areas with this.

Homoeopathy *Sulphur* is often indicated for scabies.

An orthodox view

A powerful insecticide lotion (benzyl benzoate emulsion or gamma benzene hexachloride) is applied to the affected parts of the body, and surrounding areas; and once the mites have been killed an antibacterial cream is used to treat the infected pimples.

Since scabies is so easily transmitted, all other members of the household should use the insecticide lotion too, as a preventive measure. Absolute cleanliness – especially of clothing and bedding – is essential to prevent a recurrence.

SCARLET FEVER

This highly contagious disease is a severe form of streptococcal TONSILLITIS. The sore throat is accompanied by fever, sickness and a rash of tiny, bright-red spots which starts on the neck and chest, and gradually spreads over the entire body. Infection is spread by close physical contact and germ-laden air breathed out by victims. Patients should be kept in isolation for seven days from the start of the rash – by which time it has usually disappeared. Antibiotics speed recovery and prevent complications such as kidney infections. Scarlet fever is a notifiable disease, so call your doctor if you suspect it.

SCHIZOPHRENIA

Schizophrenia is a form of psychosis that strikes – often suddenly and without any warning – usually between the ages of 18 and 30, causing behaviour that seems bizarre to other people but often perfectly normal (or at worst confusing) to the sufferer.

Symptoms may include delusions (for example, that a television set is sending messages to the person, or controlling his or her mind); hallucinations (hearing imaginary voices, or seeing things that are not there); displays of irrational bad temper and violence; over-sensitivity and paranoia (a feeling of being persecuted); or catatonia (complete inability to communicate and cooperate with others). In addition, a schizophrenic's conversation may be unreal and disturbing to the listener – and his ideas seem confusing, vague, extravagant and even quite comical.

A lack of initiative and drive is also commonplace, and this sometimes results in the sufferer losing his job and becoming virtually unemployable. His emotions may become unpredictable and perverse – for example, he may laugh at bad news and weep for no apparent reason. (This, rather than the existence of two differing personalities, is the basis of the common term 'split personality'.) The schizophrenic may also suffer simultaneously from DEPRESSION.

Severe bouts of schizophrenia can last for a few weeks or longer. Some people have a single attack and no more. But usually the condition tends to recur after a sometimes prolonged period of normality. But even with treatment, schizophrenia may grow progressively worse over the years and even become permanent.

As well as being extremely distressing for the sufferer, schizophrenia can have a devastating effect on other family members – who may eventually become depressed and ill themselves owing to the victim's abnormal behaviour.

What the therapists recommend

Music Therapy By encouraging schizophrenics to listen to music, and possibly to play music themselves, therapists aim to develop a sense of self-identity in their patients. In other words, to allow them to see themselves as they really are – or should be – and to help them regain their true normality.

Art Therapy With some patients, painting or pottery is their only way of finding a personal language and of communicating with other people. Their work therefore helps to counteract the sense of isolation and confusion that schizophrenics feel. In addition, their creations may have a symbolic signific-ance and so provide an insight into their chaotic world.

Colour Therapy Even mild cases of schizophrenia require long and painstaking professional help. The use of the colour violet – along with RELAXATION AND BREATHING and MUSIC THERAPY – is said to help patients recover their mental balance.

Counselling Trained counsellors are able to help families and victims by providing support, advising on day-to-day problems, and putting them in touch with social services and self-help groups.

Psychotherapy Treatment may help in some cases but should be given as a supplement to orthodox psychiatric help. Support rather than in-depth probing is needed at first and during serious bouts of the illness, but psychological exploration may be undertaken later if appropriate. Sometimes the therapist may wish to see the whole family, not just the victim.

Homoeopathy According to homoeopathic practitioners, the following remedies may help: *Belladonna* 200 when there is violent, manic excitement with great restlessness and hallucinations; *Stramonium* 200 when the patient is talkative, uses swear words, spends time praying, hears voices, and is afraid of the dark; *Hyoscymas* 200 when there is obscene talk or behaviour, paranoid behaviour and hysterical laughter, suspicion of other people, and the desire to be naked.

An orthodox view

Before the advent of modern drugs, many schizophrenics spent long periods – in some cases most of their lives – in psychiatric hospitals. Drugs such as chlorpromazine (Largactil) and haloperidol (Serenace) now help to relieve symptoms and prevent the illness from recurring. They allow many patients – with the support of doctors, nurses, social workers, family members and friends – to lead a reasonably normal life in the community. But others, without family or continuing medical support, become outcasts sleeping rough in big cities.

SCIATICA

This pain running down the back and outside of the thigh, leg and foot is caused by irritation of the sciatic nerve at its root in the spine of the lower back. The onset may be sudden – following a twisting of the body, for instance – and is worse on bending forwards, coughing or sneezing. Common causes include a SLIPPED DISC, when the displaced disc presses on the nerve, and displacement of joints between the vertebrae of the spine. See

also the entries dealing with BACK PAIN, LUM-
BAGO, and NERVE DISORDERS.

What the therapists recommend

Acupuncture Points on the meridians relating to bladder, gall bladder, kidney, spleen
and large and small intestine governors may
be treated. MOXIBUSTION applied to the bladder and kidney meridians may also sometimes be advised.

Acupressure Apply pressure inwards on
the outside leg, one hand's width plus a
thumb above the crown of the ankle bone,
between the shin and smaller leg bone.

Osteopathy Sciatica may often be relieved
by stretching the spine in the lumbar region
– the part of the back between the lowest ribs
and the top of the pelvis – and by reducing
spasm in the local muscles. Gentle mobilisation to improve the mobility of the joints in
the lower back can also be helpful. But osteopathic treatment may not be appropriate in
very severe cases where sciatica affects both
of the legs.

Hydrotherapy If the symptoms are severe,
try an ice pack at the base of the back. For
less severe, long-standing pain, try a hot
pack. The therapist may suggest an underwater douche and teach specific postural and
remedial exercises in the hydrotherapy pool.

Heat therapy Sciatica responds well to
radiant heat. Sitting or lying under a reflective
surface lined with light bulbs, the patient
(with head kept well clear) is exposed to temperatures of about 100°C.

Herbal medicine Apply to the affected area
a warm herbal compress consisting of a wad
of material soaked in a strong infusion of
elder, rosemary or thyme. An indigenous
remedy is to bind to the painful area a pad
of knobwood (wild cardamom) bark, softened
in hot water.

An orthodox view

Doctors often advise sufferers to rest in bed
on a firm mattress or with a board under the
mattress. Back X-rays are not usually much
help, but may show narrowing of the space
between two vertebrae where the disc has
been squashed. In severe cases, special X-
rays such as a three-dimensional CT scan, a
magnetic resonance scan or a myelogram (in
which dye is injected around the spinal cord)
may be used in order to reveal displacement
of the disc.

Usually the offending portion of the disc
shrivels so that the pain disappears in time.
If it does not, a surgeon may operate to
remove it, possibly using a fibre-optic instrument to avoid major surgery.

Some conventional doctors are now
trained to use alternative treatments such as
manipulation and acupuncture to treat joint
displacement between vertebrae.

SCORPION STINGS

A scorpion sting is not to be taken lightly. All
scorpion venom is neurotoxic (affecting the
central nervous system), but one family of
scorpions, the Buthidae, is more dangerous
than the other family, the Scorpionidae.

Buthidae have thin pincers but thick tails
with a formidable poison apparatus at the tip;
in addition to severe pain, the poison will
lead to sweating, rapid breathing, vomiting
and irregular heart-beat. Fatalities are uncommon in healthy adults; young children
and the elderly are most at risk.

Scorpionidae have thick pincers and thin
tails. A sting from one of these creatures will
cause some pain and burning or tingling, but
the effects are not life threatening.

What the therapists recommend

Herbal medicine Squeeze the juice from a
sour-fig leaf onto the sting, constantly repeating this remedy. Some people apply juice
squeezed from the tuber of the flame lily. Yet
another local remedy is a strong infusion of
the flowers, leaves and stems of the wild
dagga plant (the minaret flower or lion's ear);
the infusion is dabbed on the wound.

Traditional Medicine Cover the sting with
mud or clay, and allow this to dry.

An orthodox view

Seek immediate medical help if the symptoms of a scorpion sting cause anything more
than mild discomfort. The doctor will prescribe pain-killers and may inject an antivenom. In serious cases respiratory support
may be necessary. If possible, keep the scorpion for identification.

SEXUAL PROBLEMS

The most common group of sexual problems
stems from disturbances of the normal sexual response cycle that occurs in sexual intercourse. The cycle has three quite distinct
phases: desire; excitement/arousal; and res-
olution/orgasm (climax). The stages tend to
happen in sequence, for each is designed to
trigger the next. However, they need not
necessarily do so, and a disorder may arise
in any phase.

It is possible to function sexually without
feeling desire; or to feel desire and not be
able to function; or to experience an orgasm
without the changes – erection or secretion
of lubrication – that occur in the excite-
ment/arousal phase.

The main difficulties arising from the normal sexual response cycle, each phase of
which is served by different physical, chemical, nervous and psychological systems of the
body, are as follows:

Both men and women may suffer from *inhibited sexual desire*. In this state desire is completely absent or is so weak that no sexual
behaviour is initiated and/or sexual overtures
from others are rejected. Problems connected with the excitement/arousal phase are
erectile insufficiency or IMPOTENCE in men, and
general sexual dysfunction or FRIGIDITY in women.

In the next phase of the cycle, resolu-
tion/orgasm, men may experience *premature
ejaculation or delayed/inhibited ejaculation*. In the
first, the orgasm happens too soon. However,
this is a rather subjective definition, for the
'best' time for ejaculation depends as much
on the partner's satisfaction as on that experienced by the man.

In the second problem, ejaculation is difficult to achieve and the difficulty destroys
the pleasure of intercourse. In some cases the
cause may be a specific malfunction of the
man's sexual organs. For example, there may
be the sensation of an orgasm, but the semen
is ejaculated internally into the bladder instead of out through the shaft of the penis.

The equivalent problem in women is
known as *general orgasmic dysfunction*. Orgasm
does not occur, so sexual arousal results in
a dissatisfied feeling. Sometimes there is
also dull or intense pain. This is because the
pelvic blood vessels become engorged by
arousal, but the blood is not released at orgasm. However, it usually disappears as arousal subsides.

There are two more problems that men
may experience. One, *specific loss of erection upon
attempting intercourse*, may have psychological
causes – for instance, a fear of creating a pregnancy or fear of penetration itself. However,
it is more likely to stem from a physical cause.
For example, the man may become more active as he prepares for penetration; blood
then flows away from the penile tissue to
other muscles, consequently depriving the
man of his erection.

The other problem is *pain upon intercourse*, a
condition known medically as *dyspareunia*. The
cause is nearly always physical in origin. The
pain may only occur at ejaculation, and in a
few rare cases of this kind the cause is a psychological one.

Women may experience *vaginismus*, a condition equivalent to the male specific loss of
erection. The lower (outer) third of the vagina
contracts very sharply when the vulva (vaginal
lips) or vagina are touched – as in any attempt
at intercourse – making penetration impossible. It is often caused by adverse sexual
experiences or clumsy internal medical
examination through the vagina. However,

women who experience vaginismus may achieve an orgasm by other means, such as stroking of the clitoris (the rudimentary female penis).

Many physical conditions such as ulceration or inflammation result in vaginal pain, and the sudden contractions of the vagina may be an avoidance response to such pain.

Women can also experience dyspareunia. There are even more possible causes than in men, and they are mostly physical. Common conditions that may cause painful intercourse include ulceration of the sex organs, pelvic or vaginal inflammation or infection (see CYSTITIS), vaginal injury, and dryness or shrinking of the membrane lining the vagina. In a few cases the condition may have a psychological cause.

Self help There is a great deal that individuals can do to counter inhibited sexual desire, impotence, frigidity and other sexual problems. First of all realise that these problems can affect even the best of relationships, and can do so at any time. So try not to worry, for ANXIETY is one of the main causes of the difficulties; often fear of failure results in failure. DEPRESSION, STRESS and fatigue also play a part.

Try to talk freely and listen sympathetically to your partner. Express your needs and preferences and try to understand your partner's. For example, men often underestimate the importance of foreplay in female arousal, and hiding sexual dissatisfaction often aggravates the problem.

Try not to expect too much from sex. At certain times, for example, after illness, an orgasm may not be 'necessary'; kissing, cuddling, hugging, comforting, gentle massage, concern and attention for your partner – even simply holding hands – may be equally satisfying. They are also an aid to discovery of a partner's needs and preferences.

One of the main problems in sexual relationships is the differing libidos (sexual drives) of the partners. And in both sexes, the sex drive may be different at different times. Again, couples need to work out their own understanding and compromise. For instance, women often experience less interest in sex at certain times in their menstrual cycle, after childbirth and at the menopause. Partners should try to realise that this is not a rejection of them, but of sex generally.

The ability to relax is all important (see RELAXATION AND BREATHING). Allow yourself time to 'unwind' from the cares of daily life – office work, travel, looking after children, housework, for example. Get 'in the mood'. You may find dimmed lights, soft music or dancing helpful, but again, each couple must find its own preferences.

Cut out alcohol, smoking and any drugs such as tranquillisers, antihistamines and

the like, that are not essential for your well-being. All impair desire and performance, often causing impotence. Eating a heavy meal just before lovemaking often has the same effect.

Take EXERCISE – you will soon find how much you need – and eat a healthy diet (see EATING FOR HEALTH). Loss of desire and ability to perform sexually are some of the earliest effects of malnutrition. Zinc is a particularly important MINERAL, as both the female and male body need it to produce testosterone, a hormone necessary for sexual desire. Try a daily supplement of 20-30 mg for a month or two. Men also need it for the healthy functioning of the prostate gland, which produces the liquid in which sperm are carried out of the body.

Iodine and thiamine are essential for a healthy thyroid gland, which produces a hormone that controls metabolism; deficiency leads to lethargy, tiredness, lack of desire and lowered interest in sex. And all glands need the amino-acid constituents of proteins. Choline is another essential, and its precursor is found in egg yolks, meat, maize and soya beans.

Brewer's yeast tablets may also be a helpful supplement. The yeast contains the glucose tolerance factor, without which the body develops glucose intolerance, which is believed to be another cause of impotence. However, if you are diabetic, you should consult your doctor before taking this supplement (see DIABETES).

Finally, discount the numerous myths about sex that have arisen. Perhaps the commonest is that 'good sex' is the right of all, and that it is entirely a question of performance and technique. And with changes in moral attitudes over the last 30 years, increased availability of birth control, and despite the spread of AIDS, a myth persists that people who do not indulge freely in sex are freaks. Both these attitudes can place intolerable stress on individuals.

Another common misconception is that interest in sex is absent in older people, and that sex is actually bad for them. This is not true. You may not be able to do at 65 what you did at 25, but a happy, rewarding sex life can be enjoyed by the over-60s.

Another myth is that sexual intercourse puts undue strain on the heart. Tests in Britain and the USA have shown that the amount of physical energy spent during the sex act is below the energy required for most jobs. Even after a heart attack, by the time most patients return home they are ready for sex – but consult your doctor to make sure that this is true in your particular case. Usually a heart attack that occurs during or immediately after sex is due to some other factor, such as excessive indulgence in alco-

hol or food, or the stress associated with an extramarital affair.

Getting advice Should you feel that you need outside help for your problem and do not want to consult your doctor, you could find a therapist or counsellor through FAMSA (Family and Marriage Society of South Africa) or GASA (Gay Association of South Africa), both of which have branches throughout the country. If unable to help you themselves, these organisations can refer you to other specialists. The same applies to the personal counselling service Life Line.

Another source of help are the sex therapy clinics that are attached to some general hospitals. Or direct your enquiry to the Sex Education and Dysfunction Unit of South Africa, P O Box 2342, Clareinch 7740. All these organisations will advise you in strict confidence.

What the therapists recommend
BEHAVIOURAL THERAPY
Consultation The course of therapy depends on the exact nature of the problem(s) involved. Basically, treatment consists of education (providing information about sex); communication (encouraging partners to discuss and agree on their sexual contact); sensate focusing (concentrating on the physical sensations of various aspects of foreplay and intercourse); and desensitisation (ensuring a relaxed and pleasurable sexual union by progressing through various stages of intimacy).

BACH REMEDIES
Self help Therapists suggest: Clematis if the problem is obsessive sexual fantasy with no action; Honeysuckle for being over-sentimental and romantic; Mimulus for fear of experiencing intense sexual desire; Centaury for feeling one does not have a right to have sexual needs, or for feeling used, unable to say 'no'; Heather for being over-demanding in a self-obsessed way; Water violet for shyness and reluctance to make intimate contact; Crab apple for feeling the body is unclean or shameful; Pine for guilt; Chicory for jealousy and possessiveness.

HYPNOTHERAPY
Consultation Once organic disease is ruled out, investigation is carried out by hypnoanalysis. If the problem is based on anxiety, then relaxation techniques are used. Patients may be taught ego-strengthening techniques to be used at home.

An orthodox view
The causes of problems related to the normal sexual response cycle may be physical; drug-induced or caused by nervous or psychological disorders. The doctor may ask to see both

partners at the same time, or separately, for a full discussion of the problem.

A physical examination will be made. A diagnosis may be difficult, as in the case of pain that occurs only on arousal or ejaculation. If this is so, try to describe exactly what happens at these times. The doctor may then refer the patient(s) to a sexual function specialist. Physical conditions such as a dry vagina or cystitis will be treated, or the patient(s) may be referred to a consultant.

Certain drugs impair sexual performance, so the doctor will review any that have been prescribed. Drugs that may have such a side effect include phenelzine, used to treat depression and anxiety, and beta blockers, prescribed for high BLOOD PRESSURE.

If the difficulty persists, the patient(s) may well be referred to a neurologist (nerve specialist) or psychotherapist.

See also CONTRACEPTION.

SHIATSU

Pressing the vital points for health

Although the Japanese name *shiatsu* means literally 'finger pressure', this stimulating form of massage is given by much more than fingers. The palms and heels of the hands, forearms, elbows, knees and feet are used, but thumbs most of all. Like ACUPRESSURE, shiatsu uses pressure on hundreds of surface points (*tsubo*) along the body's meridians (energy paths) to stimulate the flow of the Qi (life force) through the paths.

Shiatsu-style therapies have been practised in Japan for centuries and developed (as did the Chinese acupressure) from *amna*, an ancient oriental massage system of rubbing and manipulating the hands and feet. Unlike the later development ACUPUNCTURE, shiatsu and acupressure were used as home treatments handed down the generations and practised by one family member on another.

Despite its long history, shiatsu was not formulated as a comprehensive therapy until early this century. Tokujiro Namikoshi was among the first to popularise the system. Now it has become rather more widely used than acupressure in the West.

It is a safe and effective technique, largely preventive but also used as a form of physiotherapy for specific ailments. It is said to act on the subtle electromagnetic forces of the body, which are particularly high or low in the areas used as pressure points. By stimulating or calming these points, shiatsu aims at rebalancing the quantity and quality of electromagnetic energy being distributed along the meridians – benefiting not only the body but also the mind, feelings and spirit.

Who it can help Practitioners claim that a wide variety of everyday ailments can be relieved by shiatsu – including HEADACHES and MIGRAINE, BACK PAIN and toothache. Treatment is said to be effective also for DIGESTIVE PROBLEMS, CONSTIPATION and DIARRHOEA. Convalescents and others have found their vitality and stamina restored. People suffering from STRESS and TENSION, DEPRESSION or INSOMNIA are believed to benefit. The general mobility and comfort of joints and muscles has been found to increase in people with chronic stiffness, and injuries resulting from sport or other physical exertion have responded well to treatment. Shiatsu is also a whole-body programme designed to prevent these conditions, to tone up the circulation, nervous system and IMMUNE SYSTEM, to promote the elimination of poisons, and to help to strengthen bones.

Finding a therapist While no association of shiatsu practitioners exists in South Africa, individual therapists are to be found throughout the country. Some also conduct workshops in shiatsu. For example, in Johannesburg, it is possible to take a 60-hour basic course held over three consecutive weekends. For the name of a therapist in your area you can write (enclosing a stamped, self-addressed envelope) to P O Box 1709, Houghton 2041. Alternatively, scan the advertising columns of magazines that promote alternative health and healing therapies.

Consulting a therapist Diagnosis comes before any treatment – and determines its exact form. The therapist will watch you, listen to your medical history, ask questions and perhaps touch affected areas to test their condition. Symptoms that affect you in everyday life will be of particular interest and allow the therapist to tailor the treatment specifically to your needs.

Treatment sessions last about an hour. No instruments or equipment are used. The only requirements are a firm surface and a warm

Manipulating back and leg to stimulate the flow of 'life force'

A shiatsu therapist sometimes begins a treatment with a preparation technique, such as this one, to loosen and relax the back. A broad pressure is applied by using the palms with focus on the heels of the hands. No set order is laid down for shiatsu sessions.

The 'Hara' (or abdomen) is thought to be the centre of the body energy or life force, and important in both diagnosis and treatment. Below, the therapist seeks to activate the flow of life force along the inside leg meridians to stimulate its flow to the Hara.

Later in the session, the therapist applies more direct pressure to the back using the thumb pads (above). This is done in order to penetrate deeper and provide more focus to the treatment. It is said to stimulate the flow of Qi – or life force – along the bladder meridian close to the spinal column.

Exercises that you can do

Treatment of certain 'tsubo' (points) is said to relieve the symptoms of specific disorders, and here a shiatsu therapist shows you how to treat some of them. The exercises are part of the system known as Do-In, and are claimed to improve general well-being as well.

Apply pressure on the palm where the tip of a completely flexed middle finger touches it. Press for 10-15 seconds, then repeat three times. This is claimed to relieve exhaustion, low vitality, stomach disease, high blood pressure.

When nauseous or to prevent travel sickness, try pressing hard and inwards with one thumb two thumbs' width above the wrist, in the fold between the two tendons in the middle of the wrist. Press for 7-10 seconds three times.

Press hard and inwards with the thumb for 7-10 seconds, three times on the point on the inside of the lower leg, four fingers' width up from the tip of the ankle bone, just behind the shin bone. Therapists claim that this relieves period pains, insomnia and digestive problems. Don't do this if pregnant.

Press in and upwards on the points directly below the pupils when looking straight ahead, in the spaces under the cheekbones. This is said to relieve sinus and nasal congestion, facial tension and paralysis and toothache.

Lightly, then gradually more firmly, tap the top of the shoulder, side of the neck, and down the back as far as you can. Do this for 15-20 seconds, then repeat on the other side. The method is said to relieve stiffness and aches anywhere when used on the affected area.

For revival, shock, epilepsy, period pains and dizziness, try the point on the sole of the foot about one-third the distance from the middle toe tip to the heel, midway across the ball of the foot. Press hard and inwards with two thumbs for 10-15 seconds, three times.

room. You need to wear loose, comfortable clothing during the session. Make sure that you do not have a large meal or drink any alcohol beforehand.

The session sometimes begins with stretching, turning and stimulating exercises. These are designed to set the energy flowing. You may be advised to practise them at certain intervals between sessions; they are routines used in Do-In. One example is to curl your hand into a loose fist and, with the wrist relaxed, tap along the inside of your other arm from armpit to hand. Then tap along the outside of the arm from hand to shoulder. Repeat this three or four times and compare the sensation in the treated arm with that in the untreated side.

Continue the tapping all over the body including the head, and the back as far as possible. As a general rule, the tapping should move upwards on the front of the body and inside the legs and arms, and downwards on the back and the outside of the legs and arms.

When the therapist treats pressure points, the pressure will be deep but pleasant, though there may sometimes be pain. This signals energy blockage, and subsides with treatment. The strength will differ for different points, and the duration of pressure is determined by the energy flow response. It is applied as you breathe out, because the body is most relaxed then.

Pressure is applied mostly by the thumbs – not the tips but the pads of the top joints. This is the most sensitive part used to give therapy, so is the easiest to control. Control is increased by bracing the rest of the hand lightly on the client's body. You may be asked to sit, or lie face down, face up or on your side as various points are treated.

As the energy flow changes you may feel elated or depressed for a time, either during or after the session. Seemingly adverse reactions such as 'cold' symptoms are common, but are part of the healing process and usually disappear within a day or two as energy blockages dissolve. Treatment may be once a week to start with, then at fortnightly or longer intervals to maintain the correct energy balance.

An orthodox view

This is a useful home technique, particularly for relieving pain. It may be that the strongly applied pressure stimulates the body to produce endorphins, its own painkillers. The therapy is unlikely to cause harm in most people – especially if only the thumbs, fingers and palms are used – but it should not be used on inflamed, infected or damaged areas or on a person who has a FRACTURE or SLIPPED DISC, or anyone who is taking steroids such as cortisone.

SHINGLES

This painful, blistered rash can develop only in people who have had CHICKENPOX at some time in their lives. The chickenpox virus lies dormant in a nerve root for years, only to be reactivated later in life. As a result, shingles develops on the area of skin supplied by the particular nerve. The reactivation can sometimes be the result of contact with someone – usually a child – who has chickenpox; or it can arise from STRESS following, say, the death of a husband or wife.

Shingles is known medically as *herpes zoster*, from the Greek words *herpes*, meaning 'to creep', and *zoster*, meaning 'girdle' or 'belt'. There is a mistaken belief that if the rash stretches all the way around the body and meets in the middle, the patient will die.

The first symptom of shingles is severe pain, without any apparent reason, on one side of the body – usually the chest or back. A few days later this is followed by a skin eruption, or rash, in the painful area. The rash normally goes after two or three weeks – often leaving scars where crusts have formed. However, the pain – which is known as post-herpetic NEURALGIA – can persist for months if not years afterwards.

Always see a doctor if you think you have shingles – and as soon as possible if it affects the forehead near the eyes, as sight can be damaged if treatment comes too late.

What the therapists recommend

Homoeopathy If shingles is caught in its early stages, homoeopaths claim the attack can usually be cut short. If the skin is blistered, red and itchy *Rhus tox*. 6 should be used. If the skin burns and stings, apply a cold application such as *Apis mel*. For severe pain and itching, use *Mezereum*. If the patient finds it uncomfortable to move, and his appetite declines, *Ranunculus* may help.

Aromatherapy To be at all effective, treatment should start as soon as the symptoms occur. Three drops each of geranium, sage and thyme in 20 ml of carrier oil or lotion may be rubbed onto the affected area. If the skin is sensitive to the touch, the oil should be dabbed on gently. Alternatively, the same number of drops in a small glass of water may be helpful when poured onto the shingles, or applied as a compress.

Acupuncture This therapy is effective both for the acute phase of shingles and for the post-herpetic neuralgia. The sooner treatment begins after the discovery of the rash, the better the outcome. After the initial rash has subsided, the neuralgic pain can be treated by strong manual stimulation at points on the following meridians: stomach, large and small intestine, and governor. Pain

points next to the rash may also be used to relieve the neuralgia.

Naturopathy As sufferers are often in a run-down condition, and the illness itself can be extremely weakening, treatment aims to restore vigour. Therapists may advise a high-dosage of the vitamin B-complex. In addition, up to 1 g a day of the essential amino acid L-lysine may be prescribed. Post-shingles pain can linger for a long time, often causing depression, and natural therapies are claimed to be very effective against this.

An orthodox view

If shingles is diagnosed early and treatment begins within 24 hours or so of the rash appearing, antiviral drugs will shorten the course of the illness and reduce the risk of post-herpetic neuralgia. If necessary, strong painkillers will be prescribed – although these can result in side effects, including CONSTIPATION.

The patient should wear loose clothing such as a large shirt or pyjama jacket, so that the blisters are not rubbed and irritated. Two or three cool baths a day may help relieve the pain. Do not shake talcum powder onto the affected area, as it will irritate any places where the blisters have broken.

If shingles affects the forehead, a doctor will examine the patient's eyes to make sure that the cornea (the transparent membrane covering the eye) has not been harmed. Special eyedrops will be prescribed to protect the eyesight.

SHOCK

It is important to distinguish between emotional fright, which can be caused by sudden bad news, panic or minor injuries, and clinical shock, a dangerous condition which can even kill.

Clinical shock usually has a physical rather than a psychological cause, and results when insufficient blood is circulating to vital organs, particularly the brain and kidneys. It can be caused by bad burns or by an accident where there is serious external or internal bleeding.

Extreme PAIN or distress, severe vomiting (see NAUSEA AND VOMITING) or DIARRHOEA, near drowning, a blood infection and severe ALLERGY (such as to a vaccine) can also cause clinical shock. The patient is pale or grey, and has a weak pulse which is rapid and may be irregular. Breathing is rapid and shallow, and the skin may be clammy.

Warning The use of alternative remedies applies only to cases of emotional fright not involving clinical shock.

What the therapists recommend

Homoeopathy For emotional shock, after bad news, *Ignatia* 30 or 200 is recommended every five minutes until calm is restored.

Massage Effleurage technique (when the hands are passed continuously and rhythmically over the skin in one direction only) and petrissage (kneading of the skin) should be used, and not percussive movements.

Bach Remedies Star of Bethlehem may ease shock and trauma. The Rescue Remedy (a combination of five separate remedies) can be applied if there are intense feelings or fainting fits.

An orthodox view

People may quickly recover from emotional fright. Comfort and attention are the best remedies. However, it is important to remember that extreme distress can sometimes lead to clinical shock.

In the event of clinical shock, seek medical assistance immediately. Lie the patient down so that the head is below the level of the heart, to ensure that sufficient blood goes to the patient's brain to prevent unconsciousness. Make sure that his airway is clear and that he is breathing. Give artificial respiration if necessary. Unless it interferes with breathing, raise the patient's legs to drain blood to vital organs. On no account give anything to eat or drink.

If he is unconscious, place him on his stomach with his face on one side in the recovery position. This prevents his tongue from falling into the back of his throat and choking him, and allows fluid – such as blood or vomit – to drain from his mouth. If the patient is bleeding badly, press firmly on the wound to slow or stop the loss of blood.

A doctor or paramedic can help the patient by giving oxygen, fluids through an intravenous drip and, in cases of allergic shock, possibly an injection of a stimulant drug such as adrenaline.

SHOWERS

Water jets and sprays can be used to treat a whole range of ailments, from HEADACHES and GALLSTONES to ARTHRITIS and DIABETES. Even an ordinary bathroom shower or hand-held shower attachment can be therapeutic if used correctly.

Alternating hot and cold jets of water cause the blood vessels to dilate and contract. This has a pumping effect on the blood, and congestion inside the blood vessels is reduced. (Note: Such treatment is unsuitable for the very young.)

See also HYDROTHERAPY.

Trying to measure a therapy's success

Many patients are worried that technology seems to be taking over more and more in conventional medicine. As it does so, the general practitioner's role is often reduced merely to deciding which clinic or consultant to pass patients on to. Further, patients are worried that busy doctors have so little time to talk to them that the traditional relationship of trust between doctor and patient does not develop.

Faced with this situation, many people have turned to alternative practitioners and have been helped – which has created in orthodox medicine a greater readiness to consider alternatives to its science-based approach. The readiness has been reinforced by orthodox doctors' recognition of shortcomings in their system. There are qualms about its 'infallibility'. If the removal of tonsils and radical mastectomies – once standard treatment – are no longer thought necessary, the scientific method that advocated them is not infallible. So questions arise: are there flaws in other orthodox treatments? Should alternatives be considered?

The medical establishment is now beginning to show more interest in them. In 1983, a survey of general practice trainees in Britain found that 80 per cent of them wanted to train also in at least one alternative therapy, and 21 per cent had already used one. If alternative therapies were to be wholeheartedly embraced and monitored by the establishment, one difficulty for patients would end – judging whether or not a therapist is properly trained. In South Africa, an increasing number of therapies have associations that accredit practitioners, but it is still possible for untrained people to practise.

Also in 1983, the British Medical Association (BMA) set up a committee to look into alternative medicine. One of the committee's aims was to see whether there were acceptable ways to measure the effects of alternative therapies. This has always been the greatest barrier to co-operation between orthodox and alternative medicine.

Science-based orthodoxy demands of its system of medicine measurable proof that a patient's condition has been changed for the better, and an understanding of why the change has happened. Advanced technology is used to aid DIAGNOSIS, and lengthy trials are held to test the effects of orthodox treatments. Diagnosis and treatment have altered as more has been discovered about the natural laws governing the body's biology and chemistry.

Much of alternative medicine, however, is built on completely different beliefs about what disease is and what causes it. Stimulating the life force or restoring the body's proper balance is at the core of many alternative therapies. Science finds such approaches unacceptable, since they are not always based on its knowledge of how the body works.

During its enquiry, the BMA committee saw more than 600 submissions from doctors and lay alternative therapists, plus replies to questionnaires sent to organisations. Some alternative disciplines chose not to participate, feeling that the committee's purpose was not appropriate to their methods. The ALEXANDER TECHNIQUE, IRIDOLOGY, ACUPRESSURE, SHIATSU and T'AI-CHI CH'UAN were among these. Perhaps not surprisingly, the doctors stuck strictly to the criteria demanded in their own discipline, and gave no credence to alternatives based on assumptions contrary to conventional knowledge of the body – classical ACUPUNCTURE and REFLEXOLOGY, for example.

The committee did not itself try to measure the effectiveness of alternatives, but noted what evidence there was and regretted that the alternative disciplines themselves had not reviewed their practices in the light of current scientific knowledge. The doctors also pointed to dangers that were being overlooked – in HERBAL MEDICINE, for example (see opposite) – because scientific tests were not being held.

Clinical trials

To be convinced of the value of alternative medicine, doctors demand the kind of clinical trials their own treatments are judged by – including a clear definition and diagnosis of the condition being treated. There must be a sufficient number of cases, widely distributed, to provide valid statistics relating to the general population.

In one type of trial, those being given treatment are split into two randomly chosen groups, one to be given a genuine treatment, the other a PLACEBO (a substance containing no active drug). The results of both treatments are carefully noted, and allowances made for errors in procedure and coincidence. If enough of those getting genuine treatment show measurable improvement, the treatment is counted effective.

Just feeling better is not considered proof enough – you may feel better after taking a painkiller, for example, but the cause of pain remains. Some of those given a placebo also show improvement – the placebo effect is powerful. So clinical trials do not *guarantee* effectiveness. Even when the overall findings are favourable, some individuals tested – and patients treated later – do not respond to the treatment.

Alternative medicine has an ambivalent attitude to clinical trials. It questions their usefulness, finds them impracticable and points out that only mainstream medicine or drug manufacturers have laboratories equipped to carry out large-scale trials. Yet alternative practitioners are often eager to cite findings favouring their own therapies.

Therapists usually deal with patients who have chosen their own treatment, and so are not a random group. Symptoms are often unspecific and the therapist's diagnostic method may not follow orthodox procedures. The results of treatment also are often generalised – an improved sense of well-being rather than a measurable change in a blood count, for example.

The doctors' findings

The British Medical Association committee findings, published in 1986, showed odd anomalies: some therapies gave measurable benefits, and had even been adopted by doctors, but sprang from unacceptable theories about the body and disease. OSTEOPATHY and acupuncture, for example, were found effective for some purposes. On the other hand, practitioners of HOMOEOPATHY and medical herbalists, whose training in diagnosis, anatomy and physiology was along lines of orthodox training, were said by the BMA to be giving many useless – and even some dangerous – treatments.

Many homoeopaths have also had conventional medical training. They treat the same range of conditions as orthodox medicine, and 80 per cent of those treated are satisfied. The scientific view is that homoeopathic remedies are given in such tiny doses and are so diluted that little or no trace of the original substance remains. 'Cures' are considered to be due entirely to the placebo effect; conditions treated successfully would usually have followed the same course with no treatment at all, say doctors. Practitioners argue that homoeopathy does not lend itself to clinical research, because diagnosis and treatment have no norms, being tailored to the individual.

Herbs have been the source of many drugs used in orthodox medicine, which has isolated their active constituents. However, the report said that medical herbalists, while traditionally paying attention to the time of day a plant is picked and to its exact place of origin, have not been so meticulous in analysing its constituents, and that some herbal remedies can be both beneficial and dangerous.

For example, herbal teas such as Maté, senecio and heliotrope can cause liver damage, and so can extracts or oils of comfrey, sassafras, mistletoe and pennyroyal. Amygdalin, from apricot and peach kernels, can cause cyanide poisoning, and some herbal mixtures contain lead or arsenic. Further, some herbal remedies interact dangerously with drugs prescribed by orthodox doctors. Lily of the valley, for example, increases the effect of digitalis, which is prescribed for heart conditions but is dangerous in excess.

Acupuncture has been adopted by many doctors as an extra tool – but only to support modern Western concepts of medicine, not to affect energy flow along meridians as held by traditional oriental medicine. Doctors use it simply for pain relief whereas most acupuncturists regard their therapy as a comprehensive treatment for all disorders. Scientific research has shown that it works by stimulating nerve fibres to send pain-blocking messages. It also stimulates production of endorphins and encephalins, the body's natural painkillers. Acupressure may well work in the same way.

MASSAGE, HELLERWORK and AROMATHERAPY may also stimulate in ways similar to acupuncture, but there is little scientific proof of what they do. Some electrocardiogram and electroencephalogram readings suggest that the rhythmic massage strokes have a sedating effect.

Of all the 'touch' therapies, osteopathy and CHIROPRACTIC are the most acceptable to doctors – but only for properly diagnosed muscle and joint disorders, not as comprehensive therapeutic systems, as some practitioners claim. Even so, they have given swift relief of long-term pain for many patients when orthodox medicine has failed. A UK Medical Research Council trial, reported in 1990, showed chiropractic to be significantly better than conventional physiotherapy for patients who were suffering from low back pain.

Osteopaths claim that their sensitive hands feel sources of pain that science cannot measure. A possible explanation has been discovered by Professor I M Korr, of Kirksville College of Osteopathy and Surgery, in Missouri, USA. He found a higher measure of electrical resistance than is normally present on the skin over painful areas. The measure also became higher or lower according to the load put on the painful area, and was detectable before orthodox medicine could detect the injury.

One therapy that seemed unlikely to produce scientific proof has nevertheless allowed tests to be made. SPIRITUAL HEALING has been the subject of several small trials in the USA. Among them was one conducted among heart disease patients and another which used headache sufferers. Patients were treated either by healers or by people only seeming to give healing, while actually concentrating on something else. In these, as in other tests, the genuine treatments gave significantly greater improvements. In Britain a controlled trial with RHEUMATOID ARTHRITIS sufferers has been in progress at Leeds General Infirmary.

Healing in the mind

Sympathetic talk and touch may not be scientific treatment, but are undoubtedly beneficial to patients – and often what patients seek when they turn to alternative medicine. The fact that a patient who feels better still shows the same degree of disease in tests may be unsatisfactory from a scientific standpoint; but for the patient, feeling better is of prime importance. Relief from PAIN, ANXIETY or other symptoms boosts confidence and builds a positive attitude in the mind. The placebo effect itself testifies to the power of a believing mind to bring about actual improvement in the body.

Scientific medicine has been reminded recently of what a potent health factor the mind can be. Follow-up studies of patients treated by orthodox methods for breast CANCER found that despite having the same treatment, those least likely to survive were the resigned and hopeless ones. Those who survived longest – at least 15 years – were the fighters who refused to accept that their life was threatened, and who showed a fierce determination to live. Is this the unmeasurable life force that alternative therapies are all about?

SILVA METHOD

The power of mind over matter

By consciously taking control of the mind, followers of the Silva Method – a form of dynamic MEDITATION – claim to cure conditions such as STRESS and TENSION.

The method compares the brain to a vast computer, which is controlled by the mind. The brain emits electrical impulses called brainwaves, which operate at different frequencies and are linked to different states of consciousness. The method works on the assumption that most people are aware only of the surface, everyday level of the mind. The Silva technique is said to put them in touch with deeper, more creative levels.

The therapy was launched in 1966 by José Silva, a self-educated Mexican American.

Who it can help According to its teachers, the method can assist people of almost any age or profession. However, it may not be suitable for anyone with severe emotional or mental problems. In such cases, always check with a doctor or psychiatrist first.

Finding a teacher Courses in the Silva Method are held regularly in Johannesburg and Cape Town. For details, write to Silva Mind Control Training either at P O Box 7877, Johannesburg 2000, or at P O Box 4622, Cape Town 8000.

Consulting a teacher Each course consists of a four-day seminar, held over two consecutive weekends.

An orthodox view

The method is an approach to integrating the body and the mind, using techniques taken from other therapies.

SINUS PROBLEMS

The sinuses are air-filled spaces lined with mucous membrane in the bones of the face. Normally, mucus is channelled through tiny air ducts from the spaces to the nose, but during COLDS the ducts can become congested and the circulation of air and mucus impeded. If mucus builds up in the sinuses and they become inflamed, sinusitis results.

HAY FEVER can also cause sinusitis, and ALLERGY or exposure to dust and irritants such as tobacco smoke can cause persistent symptoms, or chronic sinusitis.

Symptoms include pain in the forehead and cheeks, which worsens on stooping, lying down or coughing. There may be a green, yellow or bloody discharge from the nose, and the nostril on the affected side is blocked.

The patient may suffer HEADACHES and the sense of smell is diminished. If the sinus is infected by bacteria the bone over it is tender, the skin may be red or swollen and the patient may have a raised temperature.

What the therapists recommend

Acupuncture Points on the governor and the large and small intestine meridians are treated, and on the spleen meridian when allergy is the cause.

Aromatherapy You are advised to inhale a drop or two of eucalyptus oil and/or peppermint oil, together with either lavender, bergamot or lemon, from a kitchen tissue for immediate effect.

To improve the sinus condition in the long term, apply a lotion every night made up of 60 ml white base lotion and 15 drops of any one or more of the same oils. If congestion is severe, press with the fingertips along the cheekbone from the nose to the temple, after applying the lotion. Repeat a little lower down on the same bone. Also try six to eight drops of oil in the bath.

Herbal Medicine Steam inhalations with essential oils of eucalyptus, pine, lavender, camomile, cinnamon, thyme, peppermint or cypress may be beneficial. You may also take infusions (see p.184) of elderflower, ginger, peppermint or eyebright.

GARLIC is recommended as a general preventive against sinus problems, as well as being effective against colds, CHILL, INFLUENZA and bronchial complaints.

Homoeopathy For chronic sinusitis a therapist should always be consulted. He may recommend the following remedies taken every two hours for two days – less if relief is quickly obtained.

When there is yellow, stringy catarrh and heavy congestion try *Kali bich.* 6. If the face is very sensitive and tender, the patient is chilly and irritable, with yellow discharge, try H*epar sulph.* 6. If the area of pain keeps changing, the symptoms are worse when indoors, there is a tendency to weep, the nose is sometimes stuffed up and there is yellow catarrh, you should try *Pulsatilla* 6.

Ionisation Dust makes mucus more viscous, and so ionisers are said to help mucus to drain more easily.

Reflexology You are advised to massage areas relating to the sinuses, head, nose, eyes, upper lymph nodes, neck, upper spine and adrenal glands (see chart, p. 295).

An orthodox view

Acute sinusitis usually clears up quite quickly with antibiotics and decongestants. More chronic cases can be treated by washing the sinuses out. In severe cases, an operation may be necessary to improve drainage from the sinuses.

SKIN DISORDERS

The skin is a vital body organ which protects everything inside it from the elements, allows us to sense touch, pain, heat and cold, and, through variations in blood supply and sweating, helps to control our body temperature and fluid loss.

Skin disorders may reflect various diseases of the skin itself (see, for example, ACNE; ECZEMA; PIMPLES and SPOTS; SHINGLES; COLD SORES; IMPETIGO) or they may result from disorders affecting other parts of the body (for example, PSORIASIS, ALLERGY, BEE STINGS, excessive BRUISING or CHICKENPOX). Areas of skin can also become malignant (see CANCER), may develop CIRCULATION PROBLEMS, or form ULCERS.

See also NATURAL AIDS TO BEAUTY.

SLEEP DISORDERS

Overcoming problems

In an anxious world, full of pressures, challenges and stresses, sleep should be a restoring antidote to daytime cares – a chance to rest the mind, repair the body and prepare for each new day. Yet many thousands of South Africans suffer regular night-time disturbances such as sleeplessness, restlessness, or troubled dreams.

Scientists still do not fully understand what makes us sleep, but certain 'sleep centres' have been found in the brain – a sort of 'body clock' which is thought to control the timing of rest and wakefulness. A number of natural sleep-promoting chemicals in the body also appear to play a role. See also INSOMNIA; JET LAG.

Individuals need different amounts of sleep and, throughout our lives, as well as from day to day, each person's needs are constantly changing. Many people – especially as they grow older – worry about not getting enough sleep. But as we age it becomes normal to sleep less, to take longer to get to sleep, and to tend to wake more often during the night.

It is thought that with age the body's processes slow down naturally, reducing the need for long rests at night. In the same way, people who practise deep relaxation exercises – which can slow down bodily processes even more than deep sleep itself – may also get by with less. On the other hand, if you are ill or under STRESS, your need for sleep is likely to increase.

The natural pattern of sleep can be disturbed for many reasons, but the most common problems are as follows:

Insomnia Difficulty in falling asleep, frequent waking and restlessness during the night, and early waking that leaves you feeling tired are common problems that can have many causes.

Hypersomnia Sleeping too much and continually feeling tired can be as troublesome as not being able to sleep. These symptoms may be a sign of DEPRESSION, and often go hand in hand with lack of ENERGY during the day. See also TIREDNESS.

Nightmares and troubled dreams Usually a sign of ANXIETY, strange or frightening dreams occur to nearly everyone at some time and are only a problem if they continue for prolonged periods. Restoring peaceful sleep depends on coming to terms with the underlying worries.

Nightmares sometimes make children afraid to go to sleep, while other children wake suddenly during the night in a state of fear and may cry, scream, speak incoherently or simply stare into space. The best response is to stay calm and give comfort at the time. Later you can discuss the child's fears with him and offer reassurance and help – often anxieties about separation from parents or problems at school are responsible for the troubled nights.

Restlessness Many sleepless nights are due to tossing and turning, and feeling unable to find a comfortable position in bed. The cause can be anything from illness to an uncomfortable bed or being too hot or too cold. See BEDS AND BEDDING.

Sleepwalking This is a rare problem that affects mainly children. Anxiety is sometimes to blame, but often there is no identifiable cause. Guide the victim gently back to bed without waking him if possible, but there is no danger if he does wake up. It should not be necessary to consult a doctor.

Snoring People who snore habitually sometimes stop breathing altogether for short intervals – a symptom of some HEART DISORDERS. See SNORING.

What the therapists recommend

Massage This should be given last thing at night in a warm room with dimmed lights. First, lie on your back while your partner applies soothing effleurage strokes to the legs, then gentle, rhythmic petrissage to the abdominal area.

Next lie face downwards, while your partner gives gentle effleurage to your whole back, followed by rhythmic wringing, rolling and squeezing petrissage over the shoulders – if possible in time with your breathing – slowing gently to a finish, allowing you to roll over again and drift into sleep.

Herbal Medicine For mild sleeplessness due to minor worry or stress, a bedtime infusion (see p. 184) of lavender, lime blossom, lemon balm or camomile is often all that may be needed.

A hot bath with a few drops of essential oil of lavender added may help you to unwind after a tense day. Individual advice from a practitioner will depend on the causes and symptoms of the problem. Herbs such as valerian, skullcap, cowslip or hops may be used to reduce high anxiety levels.

Homoeopathy If sleep is disturbed by fear, panic or the aftermath of a shock, *Aconitum* is recommended; or *Arnica* if overtired physically or mentally and the bed seems too hard. When your mind will not rest – after sudden good news, for example – and you feel wide awake, *Coffea* may help. For 3 am sleeplessness due to strain or overindulgence of any kind, when you drop off only to wake up irritable and unrefreshed, try *Nux vomica*. Take a dose of the indicated remedy half an hour before going to bed, and repeat the remedy half hourly as necessary. In each case, try taking potency 6 or 30.

Hypnotherapy Practitioners can teach methods of relaxation which are said to be very effective for inducing sleep. Analysis while under hypnosis may also be used to help poor sleepers who have underlying emotional problems.

Behavioural Therapy A good sleep pattern should be based on good sleeping habits and routines. Where a disturbed sleep pattern is a symptom of some greater problem, such as depression or severe anxiety, the therapist will aim to deal with this as well as re-establishing good sleep routines.

Biofeedback When insomnia is related to stress, training in biofeedback can help the user to learn relaxation and stress-reducing techniques that should be of benefit.

An orthodox view

Doctors are able to treat some causes of sleep disturbances such as sickness, pain and depression. In other cases, you are likely simply to be offered sleeping pills or tranquillisers. Taking these occasionally does no harm and many people find them a great help, particularly at times of stress. But they are not recommended as a long-term solution and some can disrupt the natural sleep cycle, adding to your problems.

To free yourself from reliance on sleeping pills, try to reduce your dosage gradually, even though this may mean more restless sleep than usual in the short term. Anyone with a heavy dependence on drugs for sleep should seek further advice from a doctor, however. (See also ADDICTION.)

Physical exercise is often a simple but effective promoter of sleep.

Getting a good night's rest

First find the cause of your sleeplessness. It can be any kind of physical or emotional strain – illness, PAIN, heat, noise, a new or uncomfortable bed, depression, overeating or drinking.

Many sleep problems can be avoided simply by taking steps to cope with these problems – for example, doctors can provide medication to relieve pain, depression and unpleasant symptoms such as a blocked nose if they keep you awake. Installing double glazing will cut down street noise. However, this is an expensive business, and wearing wax ear-plugs is economical and fairly effective.

A calming bedtime routine should also help anyone with sleep problems. Listen to music, take a walk, or read a book before bed, to help you to unwind and forget daytime tensions. Avoid late meals and arguments or serious discussions late at night. If something is on your mind, try writing it down, or making a list of your worries, so that you recognise them as problems to be set aside and dealt with at another time.

You could also practise RELAXATION AND BREATHING exercises, take a hot bath or ask a partner to give you a MASSAGE. In addition, you could try herbal TISANES such as camomile, rose hip or cinnamon, perhaps with a little honey added; or a milky drink. Avoid tea, coffee and cocoa, however – they contain caffeine which may keep you awake. Do not take any drinks at bedtime if you tend to wake during the night to go to the lavatory.

If you do find yourself lying awake in bed, again practising breathing exercises, or concentrating on a pleasant, detailed image or memory, may help. Or try listening to soothing music or a relaxation tape.

If sleep difficulties continue for any length of time, think about whether you are getting enough EXERCISE and eating a good diet (see EATING FOR HEALTH). If you have serious marital problems, money worries, depression or other emotional strains, try talking to a close friend, who may at least be able to offer comfort, and possibly advice. Or consider seeking professional guidance through COUNSELLING or consulting a doctor or psychologist.

Painless ways to lose weight

The slim body beautiful is the goal of many today, and undoubtedly thinner people suffer less illness and live longer than those who are overweight. Fads and fancy diets often fail; slimming the natural way is a good alternative.

From high-protein to low-fat diets, from fibre diets and single-food regimes to strange combinations and milkshake meals, people who want to lose weight come in for a great deal of bewildering – and sometimes bizarre – advice.

Mostly the advice is harmless enough – much of it so impractical or unsociable that no one can stick to it for long – but in a few cases it could be dangerous or even make you put on more weight in the end. And for seasoned slimmers who have already tried other regimes there is the guilt and despair of yet another failure, as unrealistic eating gradually drives them back to their old, bad ways yet again.

Fortunately, slimming need not involve fad diets or peculiar eating patterns. On a sensible, balanced diet of natural foods low in fat and sugar it is possible for most people to lose weight safely and simply – and establish healthy eating patterns that should last a lifetime.

Note This is not true for people taking certain drugs – steroids and some antidepressants, for example. In any case, anyone receiving any form of treatment should consult his doctor before embarking on a reducing diet. The same applies if you suffer from emotional illness, for dieting could cause added stress.

For some people the change to a low-fat, low-sugar diet needs only small adjustments to their eating habits; for others it could mean changing their whole way of life if the results are to be permanent. The changes can take time to get used to, but the effects in terms of better health, increased vitality as well as weight loss are strong incentives for persevering, even if occasional lapses do occur. Like all slimming diets, losing weight naturally depends on keeping track of kilojoules. A kilojoule is a unit of energy, and to lose weight you must take in fewer kilojoules every day than are burnt up in activities, building and repairing tissue, and carrying out essential bodily processes.

Are you overweight?

It all depends on the build of your body. To measure your natural frame size, try the wrist test below or the shoulder-arm comparison on the right, then plot the ideal weight range for your build and height on the graph opposite.

Wrist test
Measure your wrist at its narrowest point, just below the joint bone. For women, less than 14 cm indicates a small build, 14-16,5 cm a medium build, and above 16,5 cm in a large build. For men, any measurement under 16,5 cm indicates a small build, 16,5-18 cm a medium build, and above 18 cm a large build.

Length Width

Shoulder-arm comparison
Small frame *The width of the shoulders is less than the length of the upper arm.*

Medium frame *The width of the shoulders is about the length of the upper arm.*

Large frame *The width of the shoulders is greater than the length of the upper arm.*

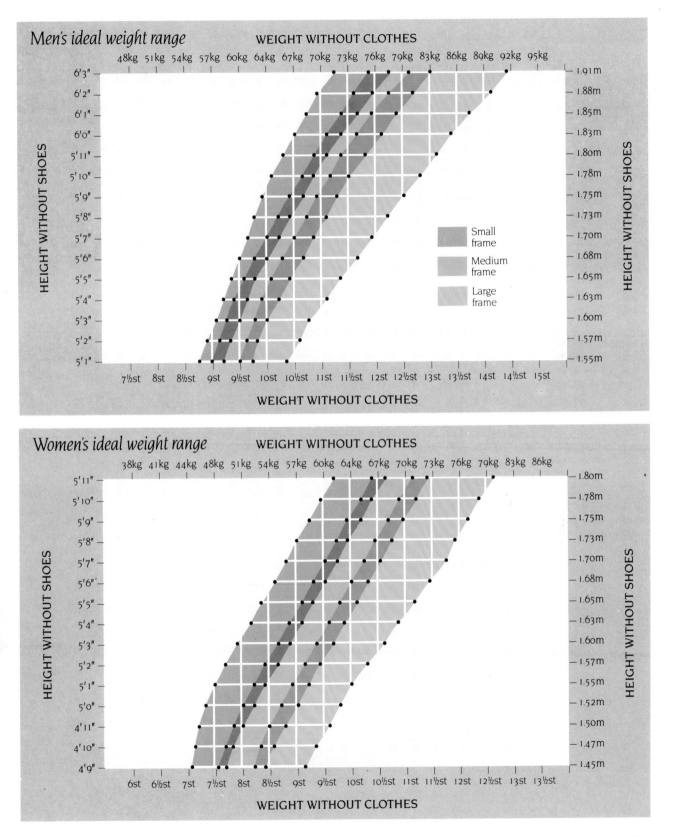

Men's ideal weight range

WEIGHT WITHOUT CLOTHES

48kg 51kg 54kg 57kg 60kg 64kg 67kg 70kg 73kg 76kg 79kg 83kg 86kg 89kg 92kg 95kg

HEIGHT WITHOUT SHOES

6'3" — 1.91m
6'2" — 1.88m
6'1" — 1.85m
6'0" — 1.83m
5'11" — 1.80m
5'10" — 1.78m
5'9" — 1.75m
5'8" — 1.73m
5'7" — 1.70m
5'6" — 1.68m
5'5" — 1.65m
5'4" — 1.63m
5'3" — 1.60m
5'2" — 1.57m
5'1" — 1.55m

Small frame
Medium frame
Large frame

7½st 8st 8½st 9st 9½st 10st 10½st 11st 11½st 12st 12½st 13st 13½st 14st 14½st 15st

WEIGHT WITHOUT CLOTHES

HEIGHT WITHOUT SHOES

Women's ideal weight range

WEIGHT WITHOUT CLOTHES

38kg 41kg 44kg 48kg 51kg 54kg 57kg 60kg 64kg 67kg 70kg 73kg 76kg 79kg 83kg 86kg

HEIGHT WITHOUT SHOES

5'11" — 1.80m
5'10" — 1.78m
5'9" — 1.75m
5'8" — 1.73m
5'7" — 1.70m
5'6" — 1.68m
5'5" — 1.65m
5'4" — 1.63m
5'3" — 1.60m
5'2" — 1.57m
5'1" — 1.55m
5'0" — 1.52m
4'11" — 1.50m
4'10" — 1.47m
4'9" — 1.45m

6st 6½st 7st 7½st 8st 8½st 9st 9½st 10st 10½st 11st 11½st 12st 12½st 13st 13½st

WEIGHT WITHOUT CLOTHES

HEIGHT WITHOUT SHOES

Energy is stored in the body as fat, each kilogram representing 32 200 kilojoules. So to lose one kilogram of body weight you have to eat about 32 200 kilojoules less than you burn up. The amount of energy you use each day depends on your metabolism, way of life and type of work. A slightly built woman who travels to work by car or bus and spends the day sitting at a desk may use up as little as about 7 600 kilojoules a day, while an active, 76 kg miner or manual labourer may burn up twice as much. (However, it is not necessarily entirely dependent on size and weight, since people with a very fast metabolic rate may burn up a greater number of kilojoules.)

This means that different people will lose weight on different dietary regimes – the miner, for example, would lose weight if he reduced his intake to 8 400 kilojoules a day, while the office worker would actually gain weight if she ate this much. While bearing this in mind, nutritionists generally tend to recommend diets in the region of 4 200 to 5 000 kilojoules a day for anyone wishing to slim.

A total amount of 4 200 kilojoules is thought to be about the lowest safe daily intake for any length of time, as less is unlikely to provide the body with adequate nourishment. Crash diets of 3 400 kilojoules or even fewer are unhealthy and often do not work any faster since the body reacts by conserving energy, slowing you down and making you feel tired rather than active and fit.

Making your daily intake as satisfying and nutritious as possible is the secret of natural slimming. Nutritionists agree that 4 200 kilojoules a day is not a lot if you eat mainly junk food and snacks – one 100 g bar of chocolate alone may be 2 200 kilojoules, half of your whole allowance. On the other hand, if you choose wisely, 4 200 kilojoules will go much further – an apple is only about 250 kilojoules and a slice of bread about 300.

Eating normal, healthy foods like these means ultimately that slimmers can have the same meals as the rest of the family, but that they will have to take smaller portions. No one need even know you are following a reducing diet.

By avoiding processed and refined foods, your body will get more vitamins and minerals too, boosting your health even though you eat a smaller amount. And when you feel well it is a lot easier to carry on eating less. In addition, your new way of eating teaches good habits that will go a long way to helping you stay slim in the future, even when you are no longer on a reducing diet.

Dieting do's and don'ts

Do try to work out why you overeat. If it is for emotional reasons – to make up for DEPRESSION, unhappiness or boredom, for example – you could consider joining a slimming club or self-help group, or even having PSYCHOTHERAPY.

Do leave the table as soon as you have finished to avoid the temptation of second helpings or nibbling away without noticing.

Do use a smaller plate to suit your smaller helpings.

Do make sure you are getting enough EXERCISE. It boosts your metabolic rate and burns up kilojoules, makes you look better and feel better about your body, and also provides an alternative emotional outlet to eating.

Do eat slowly and always chew your food well.

Don't eat while watching television or concentrating on something else – it is all too easy to eat more than you mean to without noticing.

Don't be tempted by very low-energy meal-in-a-glass diets. They don't provide the same balance of nutrients as ordinary healthy food, and most of the weight you lose is thought to be lean tissue and fluid, not fat. If you put on weight again later it will be as fat, making weight loss more difficult.

Do plan your meals ahead.

What you can eat

The natural slimming diet is based on the same foods that make up any healthy diet: fruit, salads, vegetables, wholegrains, pulses and small quantities of fish, lean meat and dairy products (see EATING FOR HEALTH). You eat more high-fibre foods such as wholewheat bread, oats and potatoes (see FIBRE) and more fresh foods, while cutting down on sugary and fatty ones.

The average daily westernised South African diet contains about 80 g of sugar and 100 g of fat. Cutting each by half will not take away any essential nutrients – provided the rest of your diet is balanced – but it will save about 2 560 kilojoules a day, or half a kilogram of body weight every week. You could cut out all added sugar without losing *any* nutrients. But no one should ever try to cut out all fat, since it 'carries' essential fatty acids and vitamins A and D. But eating only half as much fat leaves you with enough of these, provided you get vitamin D from sunlight.

Do not be afraid of so-called 'starchy' foods such as bread, pasta, rice and potatoes – they are low in fat and because they are filling you are less likely to top up with unhealthy snacks. Choose wholegrain varieties for their extra fibre, vitamins and minerals. You should be careful what you put on top of these foods. The margarine and cheese on a slice of bread contain far more kilojoules than the slice of bread itself.

Eat plenty of fresh fruit and vegetables. They are low in kilojoules and rich in nutrients, and the variety of colours, flavours and textures available means that your diet need never be boring. Including something fresh in every meal leaves less space for sweets and fatty foods, and adds vitamins and minerals which prevent the 'rundown' feeling that makes so many slimmers give up before the diet has time to succeed.

Dressings and mayonnaise are traps for slimmers eating salads. Just two tablespoons of mayonnaise can add up to 950 kilojoules – far more than the salad contains – so experiment with low-fat dressings instead. Low-fat plain yoghurt makes a good substitute – flavour it with fresh herbs, pepper, garlic, mustard, tomato purée and lemon or orange juice.

Eat meat only sparingly – even the leanest is about one-tenth fat – and choose fish, chicken, turkey or game in preference to red meat. Try not to fry food, but bake, steam, poach, grill or roast it instead, and add no more than a light brush of oil. Avoid pastry products, even wholewheat ones – they can be up to one-third fat.

Starting the diet: The Unit System

Use the following daily for a balanced, natural way of losing weight.
The food is divided into six groups, and you are allowed to eat a
certain number of units of each food group daily.

Food group	No. of units per day	Size of 1 unit	Average energy-value of 1 unit	Total energy value	Points to bear in mind
1. Milk (skimmed) for protein and calcium	2	250 ml skim milk 250 ml fat-free yoghurt 180 ml 2 per cent fat milk 250 ml buttermilk	340 kJ	680 kJ	30 g cheese can replace 200 ml of milk. 5 ml milk powder = 25 ml milk. Avoid sweetened yoghurt, ice cream, condensed milk, milk-based puddings. Use low-fat plain yoghurt as a salad dressing.
2. Cereal/ bread/starchy vegetables for fibre, vitamins and minerals	4	3 Provitas 1 slice brown/wholewheat bread (1 cm thick) 125 ml cereal 125 ml cooked porridge 1 Weetbix 125 ml cooked rice/pasta 1 medium potato (100 g) 125 ml mealies 180 ml (3/4 cup) peas 125 ml cooked legumes 250 ml butternut/Hubbard squash	300 kJ	1 200 kJ	Concentrate on high fibre, unrefined products. Fibre intake can be increased by 1-3 tablespoons of digestive bran. Avoid cake, biscuits, rusks, pancakes, tarts, cakes, pastries.
3. Fruit for fibre, vitamins and minerals	3	1 small fruit (slightly smaller than a tennis ball) 125 ml unsweetened fruit juice 125 ml fruit salad 1 heaped tablespoon dried fruit, cooked without sugar	250 kJ	750 kJ	Eat 1 citrus fruit every day for vitamin C. Eat 1 yellow fruit every day for vitamin A. Avoid sweetened fruit juices.
4. Vegetables for fibre, vitamins and minerals	4	250 ml raw vegetables 125 ml cooked vegetables 125 ml raw carrots	105 kJ	420 kJ	The following vegetables can be eaten freely: lettuce, cucumber, radishes, celery and green peppers. Avoid salad dressings and mayonnaise. Do not add margarine, butter or sugar to vegetables. Eat vegetables raw where possible. Eat one green and one yellow vegetable every day.
5. Protein-rich food for protein, vitamins and minerals	4	30 g cooked lean red meat (size of a match box) 45 g cooked chicken without the skin 60 g cooked fish 1 large egg 20g hard cheese 2 tablespoons cottage cheese 125 ml cooked legumes	315 kJ	1 260 kJ	Remove visible fat before cooking. Eggs: not more than 3-4 per week. Limit intake of red meat. Avoid sausages, viennas, cold meats, meat pies and sausage rolls, frankfurters and salami. Do not fry food, but grill, bake, steam and poach.
6. Fats and oils for essential fatty acids and absorption of fat-soluble vitamins	3	5 ml soft margarine 5 ml sunflower oil 10 ml low-oil salad dressing 1 rasher of bacon 3 half pecan nuts 1/8 medium avocado	190 kJ	570 kJ	Use polyunsaturated (soft) margarine.

SLIPPED DISC

The discs are the shock absorbers of the spine, pieces of cartilage which separate the top 24 vertebrae and help to cushion them from impact. Normal discs have a fibrous outer casing surrounding a soft pulpy centre, but occasionally the tough outer section is damaged, allowing part of the soft centre to bulge or burst out. This condition is known as a prolapsed or slipped disc.

The protrusion may irritate adjacent ligaments or the outer membrane of the spinal cord. It may also constrict the root of a spinal nerve. Symptoms include severe, dull, aching pain, and muscle spasm, nerve irritation and sometimes numbness in the leg or foot.

Pain may be felt at the site of the problem or 'referred' to some other area served by the affected nerve. A slipped disc in the lower back, for example, often irritates or traps the sciatic nerve, causing pain down the back of the leg which worsens when the patient stretches the nerve by bending, coughing or sneezing (see SCIATICA; NERVE DISORDERS).

Pulpy centre of disc — Spinal cord

Prolapsed disc

Compressed nerve

Nerve root

Disc

Vertebra

The severe pain from a slipped disc can be caused when the disc 'pinches' the root of a nerve as it leaves the spinal column. Pain may also occur in the area served by the nerve – down an arm, for example.

A prolapsed disc most often occurs in the lower back. It sometimes results from strenuous activity, especially if this is sudden, as when you lift something heavy or twist around violently. However, it more often comes about gradually, and generally occurs between the ages of about 20 and 50. Before 20 the discs are so strong that – except for some severe neck injuries – pressure will fracture the bony vertebrae before damaging the discs. In late middle age the soft disc centres begin to harden and again become resistant to damage.

Note The term 'slipped disc' is often incorrectly used to refer to BACK PAIN caused by joint displacement or muscle or ligament strain, properly known as LUMBAGO.

What the therapists recommend

Osteopathy Only some cases of disc damage can be treated by osteopathy. If pain is severe, practitioners advise bed rest and possibly traction.

In other cases, gentle MASSAGE and techniques designed to relax the contracted back muscles may be used, as well as treatment to improve mobility and reduce pressure on the affected disc.

Acupuncture The bladder, kidney, spleen, gall bladder and large and small intestine meridians are treated to ease pain.

Acupressure Press inwards on the 'bladder 11' point, on the back at the top of the rib cage, two finger widths out from the spine.

An orthodox view

A true slipped disc can heal only when the piece of soft disc centre that has escaped either shrivels up or is surgically removed. A doctor usually advises bed rest to take pressure off the disc and promote healing, which usually takes about six weeks.

However, 'slipped disc', rather like 'flu', is one of the commonest misdiagnoses in medicine, and it is absolutely essential to make an accurate diagnosis before trying to treat back pain. Simple X-rays are often not helpful, and it may be necessary to carry out a myelogram, CT scan or magnetic resonance (MR) scan. True prolapsed discs causing symptoms can then be treated by surgery.

SMOKING

In spite of overwhelming evidence worldwide of its detrimental health effects, smoking continues to be one of our most popular addictions. For those who want to stop smoking, however, help is readily available from natural medicine. See HOW TO GIVE UP SMOKING – FOR GOOD, p. 326.

SNAKE BITE

It is important whenever possible to identify the snake responsible for a bite. Most of South Africa's 164 snake species and subspecies are harmless; but 16 are capable of inflicting fatal bites, and treatment after a bite depends partly on the nature of the venom injected.

The venom of adders (excluding the berg adder) and spitting cobras is mainly cytotoxic; that is, it attacks the cells of body tissue and disrupts the blood system. Symptoms include intense pain, swelling and bruising. Cobras, mambas, the rinkhals and the berg adder inject a neurotoxic, or nerve-acting, venom. The pain at the site of the bite is often minimal, but a paralysis of the nervous system leads to the onset of drowsiness, slurred speech, difficulty in swallowing and laboured breathing.

Both these groups of snakes have fangs at the front of the mouth. The back-fanged boomslang produces a haemotoxic, blood-affecting venom that prevents blood-clotting, leading to extensive bleeding. This damage is slow to take effect, and the bite itself may give little pain.

What the therapists recommend

Snake bite is potentially extremely serious and antivenom may be essential to save life. However, there is place for natural remedies in non-emergency situations.

Herbal Medicine To soothe a snake bite, apply gently to the wound the leaf-pulp of the davyana aloe; or a lotion made by steeping in boiling water the leaves and stems of the dysentery herb (crane's bill); or a strong infusion of wild dagga (leaves, twigs, flowers) in boiling water. The bark of the knobwood (wild cardamom) tree provides another indigenous remedy. Apply it, crushed and pounded, to the bite; the victim can also chew and swallow it at regular intervals.

Homoeopathy 'Mother tinctures' of *Cedron*, *Guaco* and *Calendula*, swallowed as soon as possible after the bite, are believed to help neutralise the poison.

An orthodox view

Victims should receive medical attention immediately; if necessary a serum will then be injected.

Keep the victim quiet, wipe any venom from the bite and apply a sterile dressing. Apply a pressure bandage to the entire limb, leaving the extremities free. Should there be any discoloration of the extremities, loosen the bandage and reapply. Venom that has entered the eyes must be washed out immediately with a bland liquid – milk or even water will do.

SNEEZING

Sneezing – an involuntary expulsion of air from the nose and mouth – is the result of irritation or inflammation in the nasal passages. The most common causes of inflammation are COLDS, INFLUENZA and HAY FEVER. Irritation can come from accidentally breathing in such things as pepper or dust.

What the therapists recommend

Herbal Medicine In some cases, herbalists believe that sneezing may be, like hay fever, the result of an ALLERGY. If this proves to be so, try infusions of camomile, eyebright or plantain. Other remedies that may be useful include ephedra, ground ivy and hyssop.

Aromatherapy The following remedy may be of use when inhaled or put in bath water: one drop of peppermint oil in six to eight drops of cedarwood, cypress or hyssop.

Naturopathy Therapists concentrate on the cause of sneezing, such as colds or allergic rhinitis (inflammation of the lining of the nose). Eating less dairy produce, such as butter and milk, is believed to reduce the amount of mucus produced, which could reduce sneezing to some extent.

Allergic irritants such as pollen can be effectively washed out of the nose by sniffing water. A short but high-level course of vitamin C – 3-4 g a day – is also sometimes prescribed. It is thought to act in the same way as an antihistamine.

An orthodox view

Sneezing can be a sign of colds, allergy or emotional TENSION. It requires no specific treatment unless the sufferer is unable to stop. In most such cases, sedation with a mild tranquilliser should be enough.

SNORING

About one in every five adults snores at some time or other – breathing through the open mouth in such a way that the soft palate of the roof of the mouth vibrates, making a harsh noise. Until recently, snoring was regarded simply as a social nuisance rather than a medical problem.

Sometimes, however, it can be a symptom of 'sleep apnoea', in which someone stops breathing – sometimes for as long as 90 seconds – when asleep. As a result, the body is deprived of oxygen and it produces too much adrenaline (a hormone which stimulates the system). In turn, this can lead to high BLOOD PRESSURE and increase the risk of ANGINA and other HEART DISORDERS.

Other major causes of snoring are OBESITY, alcohol abuse (see ALCOHOLISM), SMOKING and lack of EXERCISE.

What the therapists recommend

YOGA

Self help As there are several different causes of snoring, no single approach will necessarily be effective. However, you should always try to go to bed in a reasonably calm and tranquil state – especially if you have been to a party, had a hectic night out, or have been eating or drinking late.

Ideally, before going to bed you should relax on the bedroom floor, on a carpet or rug, with your arms and legs comfortably apart. Alternatively, lie on a firm bed. Become aware of your breathing and make sure it is fairly slow and rhythmical – and that you exhale for longer than you inhale.

Exhaling correctly is a vital part of relaxation. Concentrate on breathing out in a relaxed way to the exclusion of all other thoughts. Keep this up for no more than five minutes. Then, when you get into bed, think about the peaceful way in which you have been breathing – and the tranquillity it has brought. The breathing exercise will not banish snoring immediately, but practised nightly it should soon bring an improvement to the condition.

HYPNOTHERAPY

Once obvious causes of snoring have been dealt with – such as alcohol intake, which may also benefit from this therapy – hypnosis can then be used to help reduce excess weight, and to enable the patient to go to sleep gently in a relaxed frame of mind.

TRADITIONAL MEDICINE

If snoring is caused by sleeping on your back, it may help to attach an object such as a small rubber ball to the back of your pyjamas, where it will cause discomfort when you turn onto your back.

An orthodox view

If obesity or smoking is making you snore, it will help if you lose weight and cut down on or stop smoking altogether. In addition, do not drink large amounts of alcohol in the evenings. You should also ask your doctor to check your blood pressure.

Children who snore a lot may be suffering from a blockage in the back of the nose, due to enlarged adenoids or tonsils. If this blockage leads to sleep apnoea, they may need an operation to relieve the obstruction. Consult your doctor if you believe your child has a snoring problem.

If snoring becomes an embarrassment, special 'snore alarms' can awaken sufferers when they begin to snore.

SOUND THERAPY

Gaining health from good vibrations

In many ancient cultures the power of sound was considered an intimate part of the healing process, and had a central role in religious practices aimed at developing spiritual and physical well-being. In more recent times, growing interest in alternative therapies has revived some traditions such as healing chants and prayers; and modern 'sound therapists' say that they can relieve certain conditions by directing sound waves at affected parts of the body.

In everyday life the effects of different sounds are plain to see: singing before a soccer match heightens emotions and reinforces a sense of group unity; low-flying jets and rush-hour traffic cause ANXIETY, irritation and TENSION; and piped music in supermarkets is designed to make shopping more enjoyable so that people stay longer and spend more.

Sound is also a way of expressing yourself and communicating with others. Its quality often reflects the state of relationships between people. For example, it is natural to shout when angry, sing when happy, or murmur softly to express affection. Mothers all recognise the cries of their own babies, and most people are sensitive even to subtle variations in the timbre of familiar voices.

Sound waves from the outside reach the ear as vibrations that are converted into nerve impulses and transmitted to the brain, which interprets them as the sounds we hear. The waves also reach other parts of the body which, although they cannot 'hear' like the ear, are still affected by being rhythmically compressed and expanded at a microscopic level by the vibrations.

Sound therapy is based on the theory that organs and cells of the body respond in particular ways to particular patterns of compression and expansion. Each part of the body is thought to have a natural resonance and to respond well to sounds that vibrate in harmony with it. Dissonant vibrations, by contrast, may have harmful results.

Poor health and disease are believed to affect the frequency at which organs and cells vibrate, and in the most common form of sound therapy, practitioners try to restore and strengthen 'healthy' frequencies by directing harmonious waves at trouble spots.

Sound can be used therapeutically in a variety of other ways as well. It plays an important part in MUSIC THERAPY and DANCE THERAPY, and some practitioners teach singing and chanting as a way of altering breathing patterns, promoting relaxation and stimulating the body's own healing powers –

similar to the effects of YOGA or MEDITATION. Done in groups or couples, it is said to strengthen bonds between people and help them to 'tune in' to each other.

If the body is 'in tune with itself' all will be well, say sound therapists; and they believe that the human voice can itself be regarded as an instrument for toning the body and for providing it with an 'internal massage'. The vowel sounds are particularly effective for this purpose. Clients are encouraged to resonate 'from the spine', the sound being uttered with either an open or a closed mouth, and the pitch ranging from a low growl to a fairly high hum.

The spiritual significance of sound

The power of sound has long been recognised by spiritual and mystical traditions the world over. In the East, meditative, spiritual exercises based on sound go back thousands of years, and many have been taken up by religions such as Buddhism and Islam. Today, chanting and rhythmic breathing and movements are still widely used in the East as a path to self-development and spiritual enlightenment.

Sound also plays a central part in Western religions. Experts say that intoning the liturgy, chanting prayers and singing hymns in church may all help to put people in touch with the spiritual side of life.

The way in which sound affects people's states of mind is not fully understood, but it is thought that certain vibrations and rhythmic breathing techniques may alter electrical brainwave patterns, inducing relaxation or heightening awareness.

Another clue may be provided by the work of the Swiss doctor and scientist Hans Jenny, who developed an instrument called a 'tonoscope' which can depict any sound as a three-dimensional image. On the tonoscope the sound 'O' made by the human voice produces a perfect sphere.

It may be that this is the basis of the *om* or *aum*, one of the best-known MANTRAS that is chanted in many Eastern traditions as the expression of everything that is, as well as of the Christian and Jewish 'amen' and the Muslim 'amin'.

One therapist, Fabien Maman, a musician, believes that by listening to the sound of the voice and the resonance of energy centres in the body he can find a particular sound to suit each individual and enhance his well-being. Maman also claims that carefully chosen sound waves may be able to attack diseased cells and strengthen healthy ones, helping to heal some illnesses. Yet another use of sound is in massage. The practitioner uses the resonance of a gong to detect areas where, for example, endocrine glands may be blocked, and is then able to clear the obstruction by means of massage.

Who it can help Sound therapy, using electronically generated waves, is being researched in the orthopaedic departments of some hospitals overseas, where it is also used as an aid to bone regeneration and the healing of FRACTURES. It is also generally thought to be useful for other muscle and bone conditions such as FIBROSITIS, RHEUMATISM, ARTHRITIS, BACK PAIN, strains and SPRAINS. NEURALGIA, MIGRAINE and sinusitis may also be helped.

Pre-surgical treatment is said to make hip replacement operations more effective, and the pain of a slipped disc may be reduced enough to allow manipulative treatment to take place.

Teachers of rhythmic singing and chanting say that anyone may benefit, particularly if suffering from STRESS or related disorders. By changing patterns of consciousness, controlled sound can also be extraordinarily effective as an aid to MEDITATION.

Finding a therapist For detailed information about chanting and using sound as a form of meditation, write (enclosing a stamped, self-addressed envelope) to the Wellstead, 1 Wellington Avenue, Wynberg 7800. The Wellstead also sells an assortment of tape-recordings – for example, of forest sounds and Himalayan bells – calculated to promote relaxation and meditation.

Detailed information about the use of gongs in healing therapy, and for meditation, can be obtained by writing to Inner Resonances, P O Box 34044, Rhodes Gift 7707. For further addresses you can refer to the entry on MUSIC THERAPY.

Consulting a therapist The best-known form of sound therapy is the use of electronically generated wave signals directed at particular parts of the body in order to heal them. Before treatment can be given, a proper diagnosis of the problem is essential. It would probably be advisable to consult an orthodox practitioner first.

The therapist uses a machine to generate waves believed to be of the correct frequency to heal the patient's condition. Many different wave patterns can be generated, and choosing the right one requires skill.

The waves are transmitted to the body by means of a small hand-held 'applicator' placed over the affected region. A gel is smeared on the skin first to improve transmission of waves to the body. The applicator focuses the waves so that they supposedly home in on the problem area and leave healthy tissue unaffected. While treatment is in progress you may hear a sound or feel vibrations, but this does not always happen – sometimes the frequencies are too high or too low to be detected.

Other forms of sound therapy involve group or individual sessions where participants are taught to produce healing sounds by using their own voices. No singing ability or musical knowledge is needed, as sounds are generally chanted, hummed or 'vibrated' in a way that anyone can master.

An orthodox view

The basic principles of sound therapy are compatible with modern physics, according to which all matter is in a constant state of vibration, even at the smallest subatomic level. Conventional doctors accept that disturbances in electrical wave patterns produced by the heart can show if it has been damaged, but it is not generally agreed that other organs react in the same way, or that sound can be used to treat, as well as to diagnose, disorders.

While accepting also that chanting can have a soothing and relaxing effect, modern medicine has not developed the understanding which would allow it to evaluate the detailed claims made by those practitioners versed in this ancient therapy. So anyone seeking this form of therapy would be wise to approach it with caution.

See also ULTRASONICS.

SPAS AND HYDROS

Taking the waters . . .

The word 'spa' is taken from the east Belgian resort of Spa, noted for centuries for its therapeutic hot springs. 'Hydro' is an abbreviation of 'hydropathic establishment' – originally a hotel, with special baths, at which water played a predominant part in the treatment of illnesses (see HYDROTHERAPY).

South Africa has some 90 thermal springs with temperatures exceeding 25°C, and spas have been established at many of them.

The therapeutic value of spa waters is attributed to their warmth, their mineral content and (if it exists) their radioactivity.

Through skin contact, the waters stimulate the bather's nervous and glandular systems. (A mud bath operates on the same principle.)

Some spring waters are thought to be especially beneficial when they are drunk; and a variety of these waters have been bottled and sold commercially. See MINERAL WATERS.

South Africa's hot springs may be classified according to their chemical content:

Simple (or 'indifferent') thermal waters are low in dissolved solids, with no more than 1 part in 5 000 parts of water. Such waters are found, among other places, at Citrusdal, Goudini, Montagu, Baden and Cradock, in the Cape Province, and at Loubad (near Nylstroom) in the Transvaal. The waters at Loubad are thought to be unique in South Africa for their content of calcium and magnesium bicarbonates.

Chalybeate waters contain iron salts in solution. Manganese is also found in South Africa's chalybeate springs. Some of these springs are located near Caledon, Calitzdorp, Willowmore and Barrydale, all in the Cape.

Salt waters contain appreciable quantities of sodium chloride or common salt. Saline spring waters emerge at Malmesbury and Aliwal North (Cape Province); Baden-Baden and Florisbad (Orange Free State); and Christiana, Evangelina and Letaba (Transvaal). Unusually, the spring at Christiana is cold, while those at Malmesbury and Letaba contain sulphates and bicarbonates in addition to salt.

Sulphate waters are also found at Tugela and the Sabie River, in the Transvaal.

Alkaline waters are rich in sodium bicarbonate and sodium carbonate. Examples of springs of this kind are found at (or near) Badplaas, Piet Retief, Machadodorp, Naboomspruit, Warmbaths, Thabazimbi, Groblersdal, Ohrigstad, Delmas and Tshipise, all in the Transvaal; and near Greytown, in Natal.

Triple waters – as at Evangelina, Transvaal, and near Vryheid, Natal – contain roughly equal amounts of chlorides, sulphates and bicarbonates.

Sulphur springs contain quite small but therapeutically important amounts of dissolved hydrogen sulphide. Examples are the spring waters at Malmesbury, Fort Beaufort, Cradock and Aliwal North (Cape); Christiana, Piet Retief and Tshipise (Transvaal); and Lilani (Natal).

The hydro, too, has taken on a new lease of life – as well as a wider meaning, the word now being used for HEALTH FARMS and other health establishments where hydrotherapy is only one of many forms of treatment available. Water-related facilities include jacuzzis, sitz-baths and swimming-pools (in which aerobics may be performed).

For addresses and other details of spas and hydros, contact a branch of the South African Tourism Board (SATOUR).

SPASTIC COLON

This distressing, but not serious, condition is caused by the abnormal action of the colon muscles, and is generally known as IRRITABLE BOWEL SYNDROME. Symptoms include pain, DIARRHOEA and CONSTIPATION.

SPIDER BITES

There are about 4 000 spider species in South Africa, and almost all of them secrete venom and have a pair of fangs for injecting it – both a defence mechanism and a means of capturing prey. Yet very few South African spiders are potentially harmful to man, and only one of them is life-threatening. This is the black button spider (also erroneously called the 'black widow spider'); its venom is neurotoxic, affecting the nervous system and causing dizziness, muscle cramps, nausea and difficulty in breathing.

The violin spider is another species to be avoided. Its poison is cytotoxic – attacking cell tissue – and can lead to an unpleasant, ulcerating wound. The bite is initially painless, symptoms setting in only some two to eight hours later.

Most spiders, by contrast, inflict bites that are at worst no more troublesome than a beesting.

What the therapists recommend

Herbal Medicine To relieve itching at the site of the bite, squeeze onto the skin the juice of a sour-fig leaf.

Homoeopathy *Ledum* is one of the common remedies used.

An orthodox view

Seek immediate medical assistance if you suspect that a button spider or other harmful species is responsible for the bite. Meanwhile, apply an ice-pack to the skin to restrict dispersal of the venom. Applying this ice-pack for too lengthy a period will result in serious tissue damage – great care should therefore be exercised. Don't apply an ice-pack for longer than 2-3 hours, and remove it periodically until a certain amount of feeling has returned. The bite victim should be kept quiet. Always try to identify the spider.

Button spider antivenom is available (but there is no specific antivenom to treat a bite by a violin spider). For an ulcerating wound, apply an antiseptic dressing.

Some people may have a serious allergic reaction to the bite of even a relatively harmless spider. In such a case, call a doctor immediately. See also STINGS AND BITES.

SPIRITUAL HEALING

This form of healing – not to be confused with Spiritualism – uses a holistic approach, helping a person to return to the 'wholeness of being' – harmony of body, mind and spirit. By prayer and meditation healers channel divine healing energies, which are said to change the patient's personal life force for the better. The therapy can be a form of ABSENT HEALING or LAYING ON OF HANDS.

For more information contact a branch of the South African Federation of Spiritual Healers – at 10 Corvette Avenue, Sun Valley, Fish Hoek 7975; 18 Ebony Drive, Glen Anil, Durban 4051; or 6 Roos Street, Monument, Krugersdorp 1739.

See also ABSENT HEALING and HEALERS AND HEALING.

SPORTS INJURIES

Coping with and avoiding damage to your body

Sport strengthens muscles, increases stamina, improves sleep patterns and helps to control OBESITY. However, sport and EXERCISE are only a part of good health, and contribute to fitness only when taken regularly in conjunction with a healthy lifestyle. Practised unwisely or to excess, sport and other physical activity can result in injury.

Fractured bones These common injuries usually follow accidents in which the bone is put under sudden strain. Skiers often break legs in this way, and cricket and hockey players their fingers.

Other fractures, known as stress fractures, occur without sudden impact. They usually take the form of a hairline crack that eventually causes so much pain that it interferes with movement. For example, as a result of repeated use, a long-distance runner may fracture a foot bone, or a high jumper his fibula (outer bone of the lower leg).

Sprains and dislocations Ligaments that hold joints together may tear, causing SPRAINS. An affected joint becomes painful and weak, and if the ligament is completely severed or torn, the joint becomes unstable.

A severe sprain may cause the joint to dislocate so that its surfaces are no longer aligned, the shoulder being the most prone to this type of injury. Repeated injury may cause the ligaments to become so lax that the joint becomes unstable and dislocates easily. See also JOINT PROBLEMS.

Muscle strains and bruises These account for ten to 30 per cent of all sports injuries.

They occur when a muscle is damaged by impact – for example, a kick to a footballer's leg – or as a result of overloading when a player does not warm up properly. Reduced coordination and overextension due to fatigue, or deliberate efforts to overextend muscles, may also increase the risk of strain. There is bleeding into the muscle and the muscle fibres may be torn. The muscle feels tender and painful on movement.

Tendon problems Muscles are attached to bones by tendons, which may also be damaged in sport. Most commonly they become inflamed. In severe cases, the tendon may rupture fully or partially so that the muscle becomes disconnected from the bone and is ineffective. A fully ruptured tendon may require surgery, but if the rupture is partial, the damage eventually repairs itself. Tendons with a relatively poor blood supply such as the Achilles' tendon at the back of the ankle may be slow to heal.

'Overuse syndrome' This is the name given to inflammation of tendons and other soft tissues as a result of being subjected to repeated strain, aggravated by training errors such as warm-up periods that are too short, together with faulty technique, incorrect equipment and prolonged training sessions. Overuse syndrome may also be more common in tissues that are not so strong, due to hereditary factors. There is the belief that some runners develop tendon injuries because their tendons are genetically weaker than other runners. This certainly applies to bone injuries which occur with greater frequency in weak bones.

One example of an overuse injury is TENNIS ELBOW, an inflammation of the outer elbow, where forearm tendons join the bone. Athletes, particularly when changing from one playing surface to another, may experience shin pain caused by another overuse syndrome called *periostitis* – inflammation of the covering membrane of a bone.

Bursitis Bursae are small sacs of fluid that are normally found around joints and where ligaments and tendons pass over bones. Their purpose is to reduce friction between the moving parts, especially around the hip, knee, foot, shoulder and elbow joints. When a bursa becomes inflamed, the condition is known as BURSITIS.

A bursa may also become infected to produce a fluctuant swelling – one in which wave motion of the liquid inside occurs when the swelling is pressed. Redness, pain and tenderness accompany the infection.

Cartilage injury This usually affects the knee joint, which is designed to move only in one plane, back and forth. However, in sports such as soccer, hockey, rugby and tennis, it is often forced to move from left to right as well. The rotation of the thigh bone acts like a wrench on the tough but relatively soft cartilage (packing tissue) in the knee, causing it to tear and giving rise to pain and swelling. Because cartilage is poorly supplied with blood, it is often unable to repair itself, and surgery may be the only solution.

Back injuries Damage to the back is usually the result of poor lifting technique in sports such as weightlifting and during weight training, but it may also result from sports accidents. Most injuries involve damage only to soft tissues such as muscles and ligaments, and will heal themselves in time. Occasionally, however, the vertebrae may be damaged, causing spinal injuries which require immediate, specialist medical attention because of the risk of paralysis. Such injuries have occurred with some frequency in rugby and gymnastics over the years. In fact, gymnastics is responsible for more back problems than any other sport.

Other problems Blisters, CRAMP and stitches – pains in the upper abdomen, caused by spasm (unrelieved contraction) of the diaphragm – are common among sportsmen.

Preventing sports injuries

Never start playing a sport suddenly; rather go for regular, progressive training which gradually increases the strength and flexibility of your joints, bones and muscles. This includes always allowing time for an adequate warm-up period before each session of sport. Learn and practise good technique so that you avoid unnecessary strain.

A well-balanced diet (see EATING FOR HEALTH), plus adequate fluid replacement during and after exercise will help; so will suitable clothing – especially footwear. Stop SMOKING, and avoid alcohol completely – it is not part of a healthy lifestyle. Use appropriate protective clothing; for example, a helmet for cycling and horse riding.

Ask a doctor who has a thorough knowledge of sport and sports injuries for advice before taking up a new sport or greatly increasing the amount of exercise you take. Regular health checks will also help.

What the therapists recommend

Massage It has not been categorically established that massage is a good form of treatment for sports injuries, but many Olympic and international sports and athletics teams use trained remedial masseurs for toning muscles and joints before events and for treating them afterwards.

Homoeopathy For aching muscles after overexertion at sport, as well as bruises and shock, try *Arnica* 30. Pulled tendons and sprains should first be treated with *Arnica* and then with *Rhus tox.* or *Ruta*, according to symptoms. For cases of tennis elbow try *Ruta* 30 four times a day for a week.

Acupuncture Points local to the injury are treated. Points on the large intestine meridian are used for the rapid relief of pain. Treatment is also given at points on the governor meridian, which has a controlling effect on all the channels and points, in addition to its calming and sedative action.

Hydrotherapy Some injuries – but not severe lacerations, which need stitching – are treated by ice or at least cold packs initially, followed by special hydrotherapy massage, water jets, whirlpool baths, hot or cold packs, appropriate remedial exercises or combinations of these.

Acupressure Gentle pressure is applied at local points about 15 cm away from the site of an injury, and not directly on the problem area itself.

An orthodox view

See your doctor or go to a hospital accident and emergency department if you think you may have sustained a head injury, fractured a bone, dislocated a joint, completely ruptured a tendon or have any other acute injury. A fracture will be revealed on an X-ray. It is treated by reduction of the fracture into the correct position ('setting') and immobilisation of the affected limb or part.

First aid for sprains and strains is to apply ice, and then compress and elevate the injured limb.

Anti-inflammatory painkillers such as aspirin or paracetamol can relieve pain, or if necessary a doctor may advise the use of a stronger painkiller.

Take care, however, that lack of pain does not encourage you to continue with harmful exercise and so do further damage – in particular, avoid repeating the movement that induced the injury. And remember that painkillers and many other drugs are banned in some competitions and may result in disqualification or suspension if detected.

Recovery from overuse syndromes can be slow. In the early phase, ice reduces swelling and inflammation. Once the acute phase – the period of severe pain – has passed, use local heat in the form of a heat lamp or hot-water bottle to speed recovery. Support the affected part with strapping or taping, and avoid activities that aggravate the pain. In general, analyse why the injury occurred and take steps to prevent a recurrence.

Your doctor may help with a local anaesthetic and steroid injection, or refer you to a physiotherapist for massage, local short-wave or ultrasound treatment (see SOUND THERAPY; ULTRASONICS), and an exercise programme to aid recovery. The risk of sustaining a sports injury can be reduced by correct preparation ('warming up') and by the choice of appropriate equipment and clothing. Seek expert advice about these.

SPRAINS

Injury to a ligament which occurs when a joint is suddenly stretched beyond its normal range of movement is known as a sprain. Fibres within the ligament – which helps to hold the joint together – tear, causing pain and weakness of the joint. In a severe case, the ligament may tear completely, causing the joint to become unstable. See JOINT PROBLEMS; SPORTS INJURIES.

As well as causing bruising of the ligament itself, a sprain may also cause bleeding into the joint, and may be accompanied by other injuries such as cartilage damage. Symptoms of a sprain include swelling, tenderness and bruising around the joint, and pain on stretching the ligament – for example, by gently repeating the movement that caused the injury.

The ankle joint is commonly sprained during sports activities. Ligaments between the vertebrae in the neck may be sprained by a 'whiplash' injury, such as that caused to a car occupant when the car is suddenly shunted from behind.

What the therapists recommend
MASSAGE
Consultation Although firm strapping and padding may be necessary at first, massage should be commenced at the earliest opportunity to disperse swellings and prevent the formation of adhesions – the joining of internal surfaces that are normally separate – and also to encourage the normal free range of movement of the injured joint.

In the early stages of treatment, massage should be restricted to a firm effleurage stroking movement above and below the injured joint. At subsequent treatments, when the pain and swelling have subsided, the depth of treatment should be gradually increased and a gentle petrissage around the joint with the thumb and fingers introduced. Eventually, it will be possible to apply massage to the injured joint itself.

HOMOEOPATHY
Self help As soon as possible after the accident try Arnica 30, taken hourly for six hours. This should be followed by Rhus tox. 6, taken three times a day for about ten days. If the injury is close to the bone, Ruta 6 may be more effective.

If there is much swelling, distension and pain on the slightest movement, you should try Bryonia 30 three times a day until the condition improves. Then use Rhus tox. to complete the treatment.

For a moist compress apply Arnica mother tincture – ten drops in about 300 ml of water – and support with a firm bandage.

AROMATHERAPY
Self help As soon as possible after the injury has occurred, apply hyssop and marjoram oils to the area and massage gently: use two drops of each oil in a teaspoon of vegetable carrier oil. Then apply a compress held in position with cling film and leave for a few hours. Make the compress with five drops of each oil and just enough water to soak all through the compress. (Old cotton vests, handkerchiefs and tea towels make good compress material.)

Other alternative treatment
Acupuncture Treatment is applied at local points. Points on the gall bladder, lung, bladder, and large and small intestine meridians are also used.

An orthodox view
First aid for sprains starts with applying ice, if available, or a cold compress to the affected area as soon as possible to reduce internal bleeding and inflammation. Compress the affected part with an elastic or crêpe bandage or elastic tubular bandage, and raise it to reduce swelling.

A damaged ligament must be protected from repeated overstretching. So avoid weight-bearing or unnecessary use of the affected part – for example by supporting an injured arm in a sling. Consult a doctor or physiotherapist as soon as possible.

In severe sprains, particularly of the ankle joint, the doctor may advise immobilising the joint in a plaster cast. However, when possible, prompt, active use of damaged joints and ligaments speeds recovery and reduces the likelihood both of stiffness and muscle wasting.

Sprains generally heal more slowly than fractures, and recovery often takes as much as six to eight weeks.

STAMMERING
Coping with a common speech problem

Stammering is a relatively common speech disorder, particularly in men, for which there are several possible causes, including an emotional shock or a distressing experience in childhood; a delay in the brain's mechanism for checking what it has heard; slow development of the co-ordination of tongue, palate and lips needed for speech; and, mostly among people over 50, partial paralysis of the mouth and face following a stroke.

In a child aged between two and five, stammering can be the result of overanxious parents making him feel that something is wrong if he has difficulty in speaking.

What the therapists recommend
YOGA
Self help Stammering can be treated by the regular practice of slow, relaxed breathing. For instance, a minute spent controlling your breath before making a speech may be helpful. Many people may find that breathing practice combined with co-ordinated movement is also useful. Sit upright in a chair and raise your arms while breathing in. Hold your breath while stretching upwards, and breathe slowly out while bringing your arms down. Now try speaking.

BACH REMEDIES
Self help People who stammer and are frightened of speaking could try Cherry plum. For frustration and anger about stammering try Holly. Chestnut bud is advised if you speak too fast and fail to complete words. Take Vervain if you work too hard to overcome stammering and find it difficult to relax. If you are too self-critical over stammering try Rock water. Beech may help if you are too intolerant of the condition.

Parents of a child who stammers should take Vine if they are overauthoritative, and Beech if they are intolerant and harsh. Pine is said to help relieve feelings of self-blame.

HYPNOTHERAPY
Consultation Where appropriate, a patient can be taken back in time – regressed – to try to discover, and sometimes relive, the onset of the problem. In all cases, ego-strengthening techniques are used while the patient is in a hypnotic, relaxed state. Autohypnosis can, with the aid of prerecorded tapes, be applicable for speech and voice problems. Visualising difficult social situations under hypnosis, while at the same time receiving positive suggestions, may also help to desensitise some stammerers.

ACUPRESSURE
Self help Voice problems may be relieved by pressing down on the bottom, outside corner of the thumbnail.

An orthodox view
Although stammering cannot be cured by any single treatment, there are various techniques and aids which can improve fluency. A GP may send someone who stammers to see a speech therapist, who will select a method suited to the patient's personality and the cause of his condition. Techniques include speech exercises, ways of relaxing, and the use of headphones to stop the stammerer hearing his own voice.

See also VOICE THERAPY.

How to give up smoking – for good

Deaths related to smoking are estimated at about 12 000 a year in South Africa, and some two million worldwide. The dangers come mainly from chemicals inhaled in cigarette smoke – an astonishing 4 000 of them, including tar, nicotine, carbon monoxide, hydrogen cyanide and ammonia.

Nicotine is the addictive agent in cigarette smoke, and makes it hard to quit the habit (see ADDICTION). It is a stimulating drug which elevates your mood, making you a little more confident with each puff – and a little more addicted to it. Nicotine and other chemicals in the smoke are responsible for three of the most deadly smoking-related diseases: lung CANCER, HEART DISORDERS and EMPHYSEMA.

Lung cancer is nearly always fatal. More than 3 100 people die from it each year in South Africa, and 90 per cent of them are smokers. In fact smokers stand a 1-in-12 chance of dying from this disease. Chemicals in cigarette smoke attack the lung cells, causing them to multiply out of control. The resulting growths eventually prevent the lungs from absorbing enough oxygen for the body's needs.

Smoking has a more complex effect on the heart and circulation. Although this is still not fully understood, doctors estimate that about 4 000 fatal heart attacks annually in South Africa can be attributed to smoking.

It is believed that nicotine and carbon monoxide make the heart beat faster while at the same time thickening the blood and increasing the chances of clotting. This puts a great strain on the heart and, together with the narrowed arteries caused by cholesterol deposits on artery walls also caused by smoking, is responsible for heart disorders that eventually kill one in eight smokers. Add another risk factor such as OBESITY, too little EXERCISE, raised blood cholesterol levels or taking the contraceptive pill, and a smoker's chances of developing some form of heart disease rise dramatically.

Chronic obstructive lung diseases – including emphysema and BRONCHITIS – account for about 6 500 deaths in South Africa every year, about eight out of ten of them caused by smoking.

Other risks include cancer of the mouth, throat and larynx – up to five times more common even among those who do not inhale, such as pipe and cigar smokers. Smokers also suffer more from strokes, blood clots, ULCERS, high BLOOD PRESSURE and, if they are women, cervical cancer.

The longer you smoke and the more heavily, the greater are your chances of getting one or more of these diseases. On average, smoking takes 12 years off a life, sometimes far more. The good news is that from the day you stop the risks begin to go down, and the longer you don't smoke the further they drop. If you stop smoking before developing a serious lung or heart condition, your chance of developing one in the future immediately drops by half. After five years without smoking, your risk of heart disease is about the same as if you had never started.

Dangers from other people's smoke

Estimates vary about exactly how much damage breathing in other people's cigarette smoke – passive smoking – can do to a non-smoker, but it is thought that the chances of lung cancer increase by about one-third. Compared with the risks to smokers, this is small, but it still amounts to scores of lives lost every year in South Africa. A recent study has shown that even if they do not develop a serious illness, non-smokers exposed to smoke at work show significantly reduced lung function.

One of the most worrying aspects of passive smoking is its effect on babies and children. Smoking during pregnancy increases the chances of a miscarriage, stillbirth, premature birth or death of the baby in the first week after birth – by about one-fifth if the mother smokes fewer than 20 cigarettes a day, and by one-third if she has more. Effects continue after birth too, since nicotine is concentrated in breast milk to two or three times its level in the blood. Women who do not stop smoking in early pregnancy should not give up hope, however. Stopping at any point, particularly before the sixteenth week of pregnancy, lessens the dangers.

Older children are also at risk. Studies have shown that the smoke they breathe is equivalent to smoking an average of 80 to 150 cigarettes a year. As a result, they suffer more attacks of ASTHMA, PNEUMONIA and bronchitis.

Strategies for stopping

The story goes that the American author Mark Twain found it easy to stop smoking: 'I've done it hundreds of times,' he is reputed to have said. Luckily not everyone finds it so hard to break the habit for good. Some simply make the decision and never look back; for others there may be setbacks. Here are some helpful tips to remember:

Make the decision If you are not yet sure that you really want to stop, remind yourself of the health risks. Imagine what life would be like with heart disease or lung cancer, dependent on others for the rest of your – probably shortened – life, and how that would affect your family. Add up what you spend on smoking and think what you could do with the money if you stopped. The advantages of stopping must outweigh the transient pleasure of a cigarette.

Choose a good time to stop Do not put yourself under extra strain by trying to stop smoking at times of stress – for example, when changing jobs, or facing a divorce or money problems. On the other hand, do not put it off too long; if everyday life is stressful, a holiday may be the best time.

Name the day Set a fixed day to stop smoking altogether rather than trying to cut down gradually. Make it a stress-free day, mark it on the calendar, and tell family, friends and colleagues the date. If you cannot face going 'cold turkey', plan a strict programme of 'tapering off': cut out at least one cigarette a day, and more if you smoke heavily.

Be prepared Start keeping a diary showing every cigarette you smoke, when you smoked it, what you were doing, whether you also ate or drank anything, and how badly you wanted each cigarette. As your pattern of smoking becomes evident, you will recognise danger times and be able to plan other activities or reschedule your day to avoid them.

If, for example, you smoke most when relaxing after a meal, start going for a walk instead, doing RELAXATION AND BREATHING or YOGA, or using the time for a hobby such as knitting or DIY. These both keep your hands busy and take your mind off cigarettes.

Eat a healthy diet Base meals on fresh fruit, vegetables and salads to help cleanse your system of impurities. Don't skip meals, and allow yourself healthy snacks if you want them. Be sure to get plenty of liquids such as fruit juice, herbal TISANES and water. Avoid tea, coffee, alcohol, cola, red meat and chocolate, which can all increase your craving. Supplements of vitamins A, B-complex, C and E, and zinc, are also said to help the body to cleanse itself, and reduce the desire to smoke.

Don't worry if you put on a little weight at first – this is best dealt with later, and should not be a problem.

Get others to help Tell friends, family and colleagues that you don't smoke any more. Ask them to help by not offering you cigarettes and by sitting with you in non-smoking areas of restaurants, buses and other public places.

Think positively Tell yourself constantly that you no longer want to smoke, and that you feel better every day. Remember that it will get easier all the time, and after four to six weeks, *not* smoking starts to become a habit.

Reward yourself Use the money you save on cigarettes to treat yourself occasionally. Spending it on a hobby or activity is a good idea – it will take your mind off smoking.

Say no Avoid odd puffs or having a cigarette now and again; this is the fastest way to undo all your efforts. Do not give up if you do slip occasionally, but learn from your mistakes and say no next time.

Take action Write to the Council Against Smoking, P O Box 23244, Joubert Park 2044, for its pamphlet on 'How to Stop Smoking' or its 'DIY No Smoking Course'. If you live in Johannesburg you can attend one of the stop-smoking courses organised by the council; a course runs for 6 to 8 weeks. In Cape Town stop-smoking programmes are run by the Heart Foundation of South Africa, P O Box 7091, Roggebaai 8012.

Nicotine alternatives Smokers have successfully been 'weaned' of their addiction by using alternative sources of nicotine – either in the form of chewing-gum, or in a transdermal patch applied to the skin. The patch allows nicotine to pass through the skin in small regular doses.

Ask your General Practitioner about these alternatives to smoking. Ultimately, of course, the ex-smoker must be encouraged to dispense with the alternatives too.

How alternative therapies can help

Acupuncture Provided you really want to stop, this can work well. Needles are usually inserted into the ear, on the addiction and lung points. Practitioners can also insert small needles which are left in the ear for a certain period of time so that you can stimulate the points yourself every time you find yourself craving a cigarette.

Behavioural Therapy This can often be very successful. Various methods are used, including rewards, better planning of your time, relaxation, habit-breaking techniques and AVERSION THERAPY.

Naturopathy A practitioner can help you by drawing up a diet, exercise and relaxation programme suited to you. This often includes dietary supplements, such as a daily 500 mg dose of vitamin C, which is destroyed when you smoke.

Hypnotherapy The patient is put into a relaxed and receptive state, and given various suggestions designed to strengthen his resolve to stop, remind him of the harm smoking does, and help him to change his behaviour. Post-hypnotic suggestions are also used to take effect afterwards.

Youth tempted

The temptation to smoke can be very strong for children and young people. Advertising associates cigarettes with sophistication, independence and sex appeal. Prohibitions at school and home can encourage the habit by making it seem daring.

Ten things to do when you want a cigarette

1 Consult your smoking diary – is this a danger time? Are you doing something or in a situation that always calls for a cigarette? If possible, do something else. If not, put your craving down to circumstances and try to change these circumstances.

2 Go outside, stand up straight and practise deep breathing (see RELAXATION AND BREATHING). This gets more air into the lungs, and after a few minutes the craving should weaken.

3 Remind yourself of your reasons for stopping, one by one. Do you really need a puff enough to forgo all these?

4 Move to a non-smoking work area.

5 Tell yourself that you are saying no to just this cigarette. Don't look ahead – think only of the immediate situation.

6 Write a letter or make a telephone call you have been putting off.

7 Drink a large glass of fruit juice or water. If you like, have a high-protein snack such as a cheese sandwich.

8 Chew a piece of sugar-free gum. Some people find tranquillisers or anti-smoking tablets help too, but not everyone. Ask your doctor's advice.

9 Remember that just one cigarette will narrow your arteries, raise your blood pressure and put an extra strain on your heart for an hour and a half.

10 Remind yourself that there are hundreds of thousands of ex-smokers in South Africa. *If they can do it, you can!*

STINGS AND BITES

As a natural form of defence, insects such as bees and wasps, marine creatures such as jellyfish and bluebottles ('Portuguese men-of-war'), and plants such as the blister bush ('bergseldery') and the nettle produce poisonous proteins which cause pain in human skin. The site of the sting or bite becomes red, painful and itchy. See BEE STINGS, MOSQUITO BITES, WASP STINGS.

Traditional remedies abound for dealing with stings of all kinds. For example, it is well known that the rash from a bluebottle sting can be alleviated by applying laundry blue, wetted. Vinegar, methylated spirits and meat tenderiser are alternative treatments – as is the juice squeezed from a sour-fig leaf.

To kill a tick attached to the skin, douse it in paraffin or turpentine, and after gently removing the creature disinfect the bite with alcohol. (If you suspect a tick-transmitted infection, however, consult a doctor. See TICK BITE FEVER.)

In rare cases, insect bites and stings cause a dangerous allergic reaction called anaphylactic shock: the victim's blood pressure falls, and he becomes light-headed and short of breath, with a rapid, weak pulse and a widespread, itchy rash. Seek immediate medical attention if any of these symptoms appear. Potentially life-threatening, too, are the venomous bites from certain species of snakes, spiders and scorpions. See SNAKE BITES, SPIDER BITES and SCORPION STINGS.

An orthodox view

Anaphylactic shock is treated by an adrenaline injection, followed by an injection of antihistamine, together with basic life support if the patient is unconscious. If you are allergic to stings, your doctor may provide you with your own pre-filled syringe of adrenaline to inject in an emergency. Injections of antivenom are given to counter the bite (or sting) of a dangerously poisonous snake, spider or scorpion.

STOMACH COMPLAINTS

The stomach is a bag-shaped organ in the upper abdomen where food is churned and the main processes of chemical digestion begin. The most common complaint of the stomach and the rest of the digestive system is INDIGESTION, which can have various causes ranging from over-eating and CONSTIPATION to feelings of STRESS and ANXIETY (see also DIGESTIVE PROBLEMS). Other common digestive complaints include COLITIS (inflammation of the large bowel), COLIC (spasmodic pain in the abdomen), NAUSEA AND VOMITING, and WIND.

Occasionally patients may suffer from ULCERS, often caused by an excess of acid in the stomach. (Ulcers in the stomach are called gastric ulcers; those of the first part of the small intestine are duodenal ulcers.) More rarely there may be an attack of COELIAC DISEASE, in which the patient – usually a child – is unable to absorb essential foods from the intestines.

Persistent and painful stomach complaints should always be seen to by a doctor.

STRESS

Anything that is a threat to bodily health or which affects the body's functioning adversely is known as stress. Disease, injury and worry are the main causes. See LIVING WITH STRESS AND STAYING WELL, p. 330.

STYE

Bacterial infection of eyelash roots is the cause of styes – small boils on the glands that lubricate eyelashes. Symptoms are redness and a swelling on the eyelid, which comes to a head after a few days and discharges pus. Styes are common, irritating and unsightly, but do not affect the eye itself, so eyesight is not at risk.

What the therapists recommend

Naturopathy As far as possible, avoid rubbing the eye. Hot compresses, with cotton wool or perhaps grated carrot wrapped in muslin or clean cloth, should help bring the stye to a head. Recurring styes are generally believed to indicate lowered vitality, so multivitamin and mineral supplements may be prescribed.

Herbal Medicine A decoction (see p.184) of eyebright or camomile used as an eyebath may help to reduce inflammation. A herbalist may also use remedies such as marigold or poke root taken orally, aiming to stimulate the lymphatic system and the body's defences (see IMMUNE SYSTEM).

Homoeopathy A remedy often used for styes is *staphysagria*.

An orthodox view

A stye usually heals on its own, but you can speed the process and help it to discharge by 'drawing' it with a hot compress every two or three hours. Take care not to scald it! Antibiotics may be prescribed if the stye is particularly severe or slow to heal.

A persistent lump on an eyelid may be a meibomian cyst which, though never cancerous, may prove troublesome and can be removed by minor surgery. It can, however, become infected and look like a stye: treatment is the same as for a stye, but the cyst discharges through the inner surface of the eyelid, rather than the rim.

SUNBURN

Prolonged or unaccustomed exposure to the ultraviolet (UV) radiation in sunlight produces this burning sensation of the skin. There are three types of UV radiation: UVA is the gentlest; while it may cause a suntan, it rarely burns. However, it does penetrate deeply, and may contribute to premature ageing of the skin and increased risk of skin CANCER. UVB radiation is more dangerous; it tans and can cause severe burning. UVC can cause ageing and skin cancer.

Minor sunburn causes red skin, with tenderness and itching. This is followed a few days later by a suntan, when more of the dark-brown to black pigment called melanin is produced by the skin as protection against further radiation.

More severe sunburn can cause pain and fluid-filled blisters, followed by peeling of the outer layer of the skin.

Excessive exposure to any form of UV radiation adds to your risk of developing skin cancer. Worldwide the incidence of this type of cancer is increasing by 4-5 per cent a year, with Australian sun-worshippers suffering the highest rate of increase. In South Africa 8 000 new cases are reported yearly.

Self help Follow the advice in the *Do's and don'ts for avoiding sunburn* box.

Choose sun lotions and creams carefully, and read the information given on the pack before buying; different products filter out different amounts of radiation. The strongest protection comes from the opaque 'sunshade' creams containing zinc oxide or titanium dioxide, which block out most UVB and UVC, and much UVA radiation. They can be messy to apply, so are best for small, sensitive areas such as the nose and lips.

Next come 'sunblock' and 'sunscreen' preparations which are graded in factors up to 20 or more according to how much protection they supply. The amount of sunlight you can take without burning is multiplied by the factor of the cream, lotion or oil – for example, a factor three means that you can take three times more than you could without protection, while with one of factor 20 you can take 20 times as much, provided you reapply the preparation regularly.

Your skin can never have too much protection, and even those who want to tan should use a sunblock. Low factors are suitable only for easy tanners; higher factors should be used for fair complexions which do not produce as much melanin. If you simply want to protect your skin, avoid lengthy exposure to strong sunlight as much as possible, wear protective clothing and use a high-factor sunblock whenever you are in the sun. The best preparations are the rub-in lotions and creams, which are said to remain on the skin longer than oils and mousses.

Products designed to promote tanning and creams which do not state a factor often offer very little protection and should be avoided unless you are going to be in the sun for only a short while or your skin is already tanned.

The skin of your lips is very thin, with little melanin and few moisturising glands, so it is very vulnerable to UV radiation. Use a special lip screen to prevent painful burning.

Remember that cold air, especially winds, on your face and other exposed parts can counteract any burning sensation and disguise the fact that you are getting sunburnt.

Do's and don'ts for avoiding sunburn

Do avoid excessive exposure to sunlight – more than 20-30 minutes a day – at the beginning of your holiday before your skin has produced extra melanin.

Do increase your exposure to the sun only gradually.

Do use a protective sunscreen lotion or cream, and reapply it regularly, particularly if you swim or perspire a lot.

Do remember that the fairer your skin (the less pigment it has) and the sunnier the location, the greater the protection you will need from sun lotion or cream.

Do remember that autumn and spring sun can also do damage to your skin.

Don't sunbathe for more than 1-2 hours a day during the period from mid-morning to mid-afternoon, particularly if you have a fair skin and particularly in tropical or subtropical regions.

Don't use tanning preparations if your skin is fair – go for medium to high factor sunblocks instead.

What the therapists recommend

Herbal Medicine Treat as a burn, applying cold water initially; addition of one or two drops of oil of lavender can be helpful. Or apply a cold compress of marigold infusion. Herbs with fleshy leaves, such as houseleeks or plantain, are cooling if applied when fresh. A little comfrey or marigold cream will soothe large areas of mild sunburn.

Naturopathy Treat small areas as minor burns: immerse them in cold water for two to three minutes, then carefully dab dry. For large areas, a cold bath may help, followed by application of rich moisturising creams, such as vitamin E creams. The vitamin taken internally will help to heal damaged skin.

Traditional Medicine Folk remedies include a soothing mixture of water and vinegar, and a lotion made from dock roots.

An orthodox view

Treat sunburn as you would any other burn. Soothe the skin with a cool shower, take painkillers such as paracetamol, and have extra drinks to replace fluid loss. Do not burst blisters, and avoid clothes that chafe, and further damaging exposure to the sun.

SWEATING

Losing moisture through the skin is a vital part of the body's self-regulating mechanism and, although it can be troublesome at times, seldom indicates a medical problem.

There are two kinds of sweat glands: the apocrine glands, found mainly in the armpits and genital areas, and stimulated by emotional and nervous changes; and the eccrine glands, which cover the whole body and are stimulated by heat to keep you cool.

Excessive sweating is usually harmless and affects mainly the armpits, hands and feet. It often begins at puberty and may last for life. Clothing becomes wet, but the main problem is the unpleasant body odour that accompanies this, mostly in areas where clothing prevents fresh air from circulating. Occasionally, heavy sweating is a symptom of THYROID DISORDERS. It can be made worse by ANXIETY, EXERCISE, OBESITY and heat.

What the therapists recommend

Naturopathy Therapists shun commercial antiperspirants, as one function of sweating is to eliminate body wastes. They believe that deodorants permit, but antiperspirants prevent sweating, forcing wastes to find another way out of the body – often causing PIMPLES AND SPOTS. They also hold that the aluminium salts used in some antiperspirants can prove poisonous, causing dermatitis or blocking pores and perpetuating odours.

Naturopaths also believe that strong body odour can be due to a zinc deficiency, which can cause KIDNEY COMPLAINTS, with excess urea being excreted by the skin. This may be indicated by white marks on the nails and a cracked tongue. They may suggest a supplement of 20-30 mg a day for a few months.

Aromatherapy Certain essential oils such as rose oil, clary sage, ginger, lemon and nutmeg may be applied – diluted in a carrier lotion (see AROMATHERAPY) – as a natural perfume to disguise body odour. Cypress and nutmeg are recommended for bad cases. For sweaty feet, try rubbing a few drops of neat cypress oil into the soles and between the toes once a day until the condition improves.

Homoeopathy General remedies that may help are: *Hepar sulph.* for profuse, sour, sticky sweat during the day or night, where the skin feels very sensitive to touch – take in 6X potency, morning and night for two weeks, but stop before two weeks if there is an improvement; *Sepia* for profuse sweating of the chest, back and thighs at night, particularly during the MENOPAUSE.

Take *Sulphur* for body odour that is accompanied by unhealthy looking skin, and where sweaty feet are a problem. Take in 6X potency morning and night for two weeks, but stop before two weeks if there is an improvement.

Acupressure Press inwards on the thumb side of either hand, at a point three fingers' width up from the wrist crease, and in line with the thumbnail.

Autogenic Training Excessive sweating is often a symptom of anxiety, and the mentally calming effects of the training can be helpful. Night sweats are also often said to be relieved by this method.

Behavioural Therapy Anxiety is known to cause heavy sweating, and the therapy teaches people how to try and relax and avoid this. Apart from special relaxation techniques, sufferers are advised to slow down both physically and mentally.

An orthodox view

Anyone who sweats excessively will be advised by his doctor to lose weight if necessary, and try and improve his general level of health. The GP may prescribe antiperspirants to be applied at night and then washed off the following morning. He will also probably give advice on frequent washing and changes of clothing to keep the condition in check.

In severe cases, a surgeon can remove some of the skin in the armpit, so reducing the number of sweat glands.

Doctors do not approve of commercial vaginal deodorant sprays as these can cause allergic reactions, including itching, burning and blisters (see also VAGINAL DISORDERS).

Living with stress and staying well

The jet-setting executive with dangerously high blood pressure or the competitive businessman nursing his ulcer through endless working lunches are popular images of stress victims. Seldom do we think of a young couple excitedly planning their wedding, a new mother at home with her baby, or someone just retired and looking forward to freedom and leisure after a lifetime that has been devoted to hard work.

Yet all these people – in fact, anyone who is faced with important changes or new demands – may be at risk from stress and related disorders.

Stress in itself is not bad or dangerous. It is part of the wear and tear of everyday life and cannot – indeed, should not – be avoided. Challenges and changes add spice to life, fire the imagination and spur us on to new achievements – if handled in the right way. Many of the happiest and most successful people are those who have learned to respond to high levels of stress in a balanced way.

A stress victim, by contrast, fails to adapt to pressures and problems as well as he might. We all have a vast reservoir of 'adaptive energy' to draw on, but if our response to stressful situations is rigid, not flexible, we block that energy flow and are robbed of our ability to act creatively and imaginatively. (The blocks may, in fact, have been put in place very early on in our lives by well-intentioned but incorrect parental advice – what psychologists call 'negative programming'. A child may, for example, have been encouraged to be excessively perfectionist, and as a result he or she grows up forever unsatisfied and a prey to stressful ANXIETY.)

Stress actually ages the body and it can, if prolonged, foster physical illness. It also manifests itself in innumerable lesser ways. The victim may, for instance, habitually bundle unpaid bills into a drawer and try to forget about them, or lose his temper and call his wife extravagant – or even obsessively write out a cheque the minute each new bill arrives.

Each response may sometimes be appropriate, but when one of them becomes a general way of coping with an awkward situation, the result can be a serious stress problem. Luckily help lies largely in the victim's own hands.

Self help for stress victims

Coping with stress is a continual task of trying to respond in the best possible way to each new situation. There is no single, simple method, but stress experts have recommended the following four-step approach:

Recognise the signs Stress affects the whole person – body, mind, feelings and behaviour – and symptoms can take many forms. Most result from increased tension in the muscles – NECK PAIN, lower BACK PAIN, HEADACHES, TEETH-GRINDING, feeling a 'lump in the throat', high-pitched or nervous laughter, trembling, shaking, a nervous TIC and blinking. If untreated, muscular tension can also lead to more serious symptoms and disorders such as high BLOOD PRESSURE, MIGRAINE, and DIGESTIVE PROBLEMS such as IRRITABLE BOWEL SYNDROME.

Other symptoms include a fast pulse, thumping heart, HYPER-VENTILATION, PALPITATIONS, SWEATING, dryness of the throat and mouth, and difficulty in swallowing. INSOMNIA and other SLEEP DISORDERS are common, and there may also be FAINTING, DIZZINESS, a feeling of weakness and lack of ENERGY.

Mind, feelings and behaviour can also be affected – poor concentration, vague ANXIETY or FEAR for no apparent reason, and periods of irritability and perfectionism followed by DEPRESSION and lethargy are all signs of stress. Other warning signs include self-destructive behaviour such as eating and drinking too much, SMOKING excessively, relying on tranquillisers and even being unusually accident-prone.

Identify the causes If you recognise symptoms of stress, the next step is to become aware of the causes – called 'stressors' by doctors. These can be anything that throws you off balance, makes demands or initiates change – even for a short while.

Some stressors are internal – for example, worrying about how you are going to pay the mortgage or get to work on time, eating something that disagrees with you, or even being physically ill. Others come from outside – a noisy environment or a badly polluted one, a constantly ringing telephone, pressure at work or a baby that will not stop crying can all cause strain.

Modern life itself is often severely stressful – we move house, change jobs and end marriages more, we travel farther, are bombarded with more information, buy more and throw away more. At the same time, we worry about the effect on the environment of using up the earth's natural resources faster than ever and producing increasing amounts of waste and pollution.

Draw up a list of all the major stressors you currently experience, not forgetting that happy events can be just as stressful as unpleasant ones. As well as bringing joy into a home, a new baby, for example, can also bring broken nights, changed family relationships, new expenses and worries, and altered domestic routines. Even a get-away-from-it-all holiday can be demanding, as you cope with foreign money, worry about travel delays and deal with unfamiliar faces and languages.

Watch your reactions The same stressor can provoke different responses in different individuals; even one person may react differently at different times. There are three basic ways of reacting to stress – the so-called 'fight', 'flight' and 'flow' responses. Each works in some situations – none should be considered good or bad in itself – but trouble can start when you habitually rely on just one type of response, even when another might be able to achieve better results.

Use the descriptions below to identify the ways in which you tend to respond to each of the stressors on your list. If you find that you nearly always respond in the same way, try writing down other ways.

Fight response This has two forms, external and internal. The external one involves assertively meeting problems head-on – sometimes even before they arise.

Those who rely on this type of reaction tend to be energetic, ambitious and competitive. Often they are high achievers, constantly pushing themselves to do better, and easily irritated or made impatient by others with a different approach. Typically, such people may find it hard to relax and can be at risk from HEART DISORDERS.

Problems can be dealt with equally directly by the internal fight response, but people who use it appear unemotional, organised and in control, rather than outwardly aggressive. They tend to have particular, fixed ways of doing things and may object if anyone suggests a change. Imbalance in this direction can result in digestive disorders such as irritable bowel syndrome (spastic colon) or a stomach ULCER.

Flight response Problems are avoided whenever possible, by pretending that they do not exist or by giving up and letting someone else deal with them. At best, this can make us careful and cautious; at worst, not in control of our lives and dependent on others.

Those who use the flight response too often may never realise their full potential or learn to express their feelings to others. Dangers include a sense of isolation, withdrawal and, in extreme cases, feelings of despair which some practitioners link with increased risks of CANCER.

Flow response This involves accepting the stressor without either fighting or running away from it. The idea is to 'flow with the tide', letting the feelings of the moment guide you.

The danger here is one of appearing to be vague, without fixed values and beliefs. You may find it hard to make firm decisions and take action; you may even come to feel that nothing really matters. People who tend to just 'flow' can be susceptible to accidents and mild illnesses, and easily fall for passing health fads and fringe cults.

Develop a holistic approach Once your stress responses are under control, consider a wider, more long-term approach to the problem. Overall harmony and well-being is something to work for throughout life and is never complete, but stress experts suggest these first steps:

Be constantly aware of the many stressors and stress responses in everyday life. Look after yourself by eating a balanced diet (see EATING FOR HEALTH), taking regular exercise and getting a good night's sleep.

It is important to opt for compromises rather than extreme or one-sided solutions to problems. Get help from other people and suitable groups when you need it. Practise a form of RELAXATION

Will changes make you ill?

In the early 1970s two stress experts at Washington University, Thomas Holmes and Richard Rahe, found that stress due to important 'life changes' was an accurate predictor of future illness. They drew up an index of 43 possible changes and rated each one for stressfulness on a scale from 1 to 100. (Financial factors have been generalised here to allow for inflation.)

To rate yourself on the scale, add up the scores for all the events listed that you have experienced during the past year. A total of over 150 gives a 50 per cent chance of a health change occurring in the near future, and over 300 a 90 per cent chance – unless effective antistress measures are taken.

Death of spouse	100
Divorce	73
Marital separation	65
Jail term	63
Death of close family member	63
Personal injury or illness	53
Marriage	50
Loss of job	47
Marital reconciliation	45
Retirement	45
Change in health of family member	44
Pregnancy	40
Sexual problems	39
Gain of new family member	39
Business readjustment	39
Change in financial state	38
Death of close friend	37
Change to different type of work	36
Change in number of arguments with spouse	35
High mortgage	31
Foreclosure of mortgage or loan	30
Change in responsibilities at work	29
Son or daughter leaving home	29
Trouble with in-laws	29
Outstanding personal achievement	28
Spouse begins or stops work	26
Beginning or ending education	26
Change in living conditions	25
Changed personal habits	24
Trouble with boss	23
Change in working hours or conditions	20
Moving house	20
Changing schools	20
Change in leisure pursuits	19
Change in church activities	19
Change in social activities	18
Low to medium mortgage or loan	17
Altered sleeping habits	16
Change in number of family get-togethers	15
Change in eating habits	15
Going on holiday	13
Approaching Christmas season	12
Minor violations of the law	11

You can also use the index to predict and plan changes in the future such as moving house, taking out a loan or starting a new job so that stressful events do not all happen at once or build up to a crisis.

AND Breathing, Yoga or Meditation every day. Express your feelings to others – and if this is difficult, Psychotherapy, Art Therapy or Bioenergetics may help.

What the therapists recommend

NATUROPATHY
You are advised to eat a healthy diet, possibly supplemented by multivitamin and mineral tablets to replenish nutrients which are used up more quickly when under stress. Try not to look to cigarettes, alcohol, coffee or tranquillisers to make you feel better – take exercise or practise relaxation techniques or meditation instead, and give yourself regular 'time out' completely free of work pressures.

HERBAL MEDICINE
To help you unwind, try infusions (see p.184) of lemon balm, camomile, catmint or lime blossom. Include oats in your diet – unless you suffer from Gluten Intolerance. Practitioners may prescribe stronger relaxants such as skullcap, valerian or cowslip, or the restoring herbs vervain and St John's wort, as well as recommending changes in your way of life. An indigenous remedy for stress is a tea brewed from the whitish, aromatic leaves of the everlasting (*Heliochrysum peteolatum*).

BEHAVIOURAL THERAPY
Practitioners say you should learn to relax – either through a specific technique such as yoga, or generally finding time to unwind and enjoy yourself by good use of your leisure time. Set limits on the amount and type of work you do. Learn to say 'no'. Take a break – a tea break or five minutes' rest – every hour. Face up to and deal with your problems. There is a difference between worrying about a problem and thinking it through. Don't attempt to set your standards too high.

HOMOEOPATHY
Ignatia 30 is prescribed for stress due to shock, bereavement, or an unhappy experience. If overwork, entertaining or eating and drinking too much lead to digestive troubles and irritability, try *Nux vomica* 40. For students under pressure, or anyone who feels weak and depressed as a result of stress, *Ac. phos.* may help.

ART THERAPY
Patients are given the opportunity to release tension and express their frustration in a creative way. Self-expression in art also helps to put people in touch with thoughts and feelings they may be unaware of, in an environment where there is no pressure on them to 'perform' or 'get it right'.

T'AI-CHI CH'UAN
The slow, flowing movements are aimed at balancing body, mind and emotions, releasing tensions and adjusting the energy flow. Correct breathing is taught, particularly a way of breathing out fully which promotes relaxation and calmness. Practitioners say that T'ai-chi improves posture as well as creating inner harmony in an uncompetitive, stress-free atmosphere.

Other alternative therapies

Dance Movement Therapy   Individually or in a group, this can relieve tension and aid relaxation, while at the same time helping you to express pent-up emotions. The therapy can also benefit children whose behaviour problems are the result of stresses within the family.

Colour Therapy   Practitioners suggest that replacing fluorescent light at work with flicker-free, natural daylight bulbs may help to reduce stress. Certain colours (blue, for example) are thought to be especially calming, and can produce a beneficial response.

Massage   In cases where stress is due to physical discomfort and, on occasions, emotional disturbances, a gentle, caressing, 'caring' general massage may well help to bring about a more balanced state. The recipient of the massage is then able to cope with his worries more constructively.

Reflexology   The overall approach of the treatment is to induce relaxation, but reflexology can also treat physical symptoms by working on the relevant reflex areas. It may take up to three sessions for symptoms of stress to be eliminated.

Music Therapy   Simply listening to music at home is often a good way to unwind after a stressful day. Attending therapy sessions can also help. Those with shy, withdrawn personalities may derive especial benefit from the congenial presence of others taking part in a group session.

Ayurvedic medicine   In Ayurvedic teaching stress indicates that the patient has strayed from the path of nature, and a general review of lifestyle and eating habits is required. Go to bed early, rise early, and take one's main meal at midday. Massage, aromatherapy, yoga and music therapy are among Ayurvedic means of eliminating stress.

Autogenic Training   Patients can be taught to relieve existing tensions and stresses, and to cope better with stressful situations in the future. This simple relaxation therapy helps the body to cure itself.

Hypnotherapy   Suggestions are made under hypnosis which continue to be effective later, and techniques of self-hypnosis to aid relaxation are taught. Self-hypnosis can be used to alleviate a wide variety of stress-related symptoms.

Yoga   Postures and breathing patterns are taught to promote relaxation and balance of body and mind. Yoga is particularly effective in eliminating stress-related tension.

An orthodox view

Doctors can offer patients general advice on how to set about reducing stress – by cutting down their workload, playing sport or learning relaxation methods, for example – and may also prescribe tranquillisers for short-term relief. One well-established relaxation technique consists in alternately tensing and relaxing all the muscles of the body. Begin with the toes, then work gradually all the way up the body to the head. Breathe rhythmically and deeply during this process, inhaling through the nose, expanding the chest and then exhaling fully through the mouth. A passive form of relaxation is achieved by clearing the mind, to concentrate on a single, simple phrase.

Adding up your chances of becoming a victim

The physical and mental effects of stress are due not only to the amount of stress you experience, but also to how good your defences are and how well they enable you to cope with stressful situations. The tests below are designed to measure both factors, and are based on questionnaires *developed by the American stress psychologists Lyle H Miller and Alma Dell Smith of the University of Boston's Medical Centre. Test 1 measures the overall level of stress you are subjected to at the moment, and test 2 your ability to cope with it.*

Test 1: Rate yourself for stress

The list on the right gives ten responses often made by people under pressure. Each response can be rated for stress from 1 (not stressful) to 5 (very stressful). If you can remember responding in any of these ways in the last six months, circle the number under the 'past' column that represents the amount of stress you experienced at the time. Under the 'future' column, circle numbers to represent the amount of stress you expect to experience from responses that may occur during the next six months. Add up both past and future scores, then add them together. A score over 30 indicates a potential stress problem, while more than 53 calls for a worked-out programme to fight stress.

Response		Past					Future				
1 Depression		1	2	3	4	5	1	2	3	4	5
2 Frustration		1	2	3	4	5	1	2	3	4	5
3 Guilt		1	2	3	4	5	1	2	3	4	5
4 Anxiety or panic		1	2	3	4	5	1	2	3	4	5
5 Desperation or hopelessness		1	2	3	4	5	1	2	3	4	5
6 Feeling out of control		1	2	3	4	5	1	2	3	4	5
7 Selfconsciousness		1	2	3	4	5	1	2	3	4	5
8 Irritation and anger		1	2	3	4	5	1	2	3	4	5
9 Restlessness		1	2	3	4	5	1	2	3	4	5
10 Feeling trapped or helpless		1	2	3	4	5	1	2	3	4	5

Test 2:
Measure your resistance

This test measures how much your way of life supports you and bolsters resistance to stress. Rate yourself for each of the 20 items on the scale from 1 (almost always) to 5 (never) according to how often they apply.
Add up your total score. A score of 45 or less shows high resistance to stress and a healthy way of life; 45 to 55 indicates that you may be susceptible to the effects of stress and could benefit from adjusting certain aspects of your daily life; over 55 and stress could be a serious risk, calling for a reappraisal of your general way of life.

How much of the time are these statements true for you?	Almost always	Most times	Some-times	Rarely	Never
1 My health is good (including eyesight, teeth, etc.)	1	2	3	4	5
2 My income meets my basic expenses	1	2	3	4	5
3 I am about the right weight for my build and height	1	2	3	4	5
4 I give and receive affection regularly	1	2	3	4	5
5 I express my feelings when angry or worried	1	2	3	4	5
6 I have fewer than three caffeine-containing drinks (coffee, cocoa or cola) a day	1	2	3	4	5
7 I take part in regular social activities	1	2	3	4	5
8 I eat at least one full, well-balanced meal a day	1	2	3	4	5
9 I do something just for pleasure at least once a week	1	2	3	4	5
10 There is at least one relative within 50 miles (80km) of home on whom I can rely	1	2	3	4	5
11 I have some time alone during the day	1		3	4	5
12 I get seven or eight hours of sleep at least four nights a week	1	2	3	4	5
13 My religious beliefs give me strength	1	2	3	4	5
14 I exercise hard enough to work up a sweat at least twice a week	1	2	3	4	5
15 I have a network of friends and acquaintances	1	2	3	4	5
16 I discuss problems such as housework and money with other members of the household	1	2	3	4	5
17 I have at least one friend I can talk to about personal affairs	1	2	3	4	5
18 I smoke no more than 10 cigarettes a day	1	2	3	4	5
19 I organise my time well	1	2	3	4	5
20 I have fewer than five alcoholic drinks a week	1	2	3	4	5

T'AI-CHI CH'UAN

Meditation in motion . . .

The art of T'ai-chi Ch'uan – usually shortened to simply T'ai-chi, meaning 'wholeness' – is based on a series of slow-moving, circular, dance-like movements which are best performed in the open air. It aims to get people to focus on their mental and emotional state as well as their body.

Its practitioners say that, provided it is taught with insight, and studied responsibly, it is probably the most complete, natural and effective of all holistic therapies. It is a highly complex art form involving patience, perseverance and the ability to simplify, adapt and change – and should not be looked upon merely as a means of 'working out'.

T'ai-chi is based on the belief that, following emotional and/or mental disturbance, illness stems from imbalances such as energy (known as Qi) moving too quickly or too slowly through the body – or too much energy gathering in one particular area (for example, the head and chest) and too little elsewhere (such as the legs), so that the sufferer is 'top heavy'. Such imbalances may be corrected by mental focusing through the various movements of the therapy.

Deeply rooted in Chinese culture (see box, p. 336), T'ai-chi came to wider public attention in the West following US President Richard Nixon's visit to China in 1972, when the outdoor practice of T'ai-chi was shown on television programmes. In South Africa T'ai-chi was until recently largely confined to Chinese families (among whom it remained a secret system); and it has been taught here by qualified Western practitioners only since the mid-1980s.

Practitioners say that the therapy cannot be self-taught, and you should receive instruction from a qualified teacher.

Who it can help As a natural process of healing, T'ai-chi has for centuries been considered both curative and preventive. Its graceful, flowing movements are particularly effective against such conditions as ANXIETY and STRESS, because they encourage people to relax and 'let go'. The movements can also help to improve breathing and posture considerably, generally tone up the body, and stimulate circulation. In many cases – particularly for people leading high-pressure

In China even young children often join in T'ai-chi sessions – for many of them the beginning of a lifelong habit.

Parks such as this one in Beijing (right) are favoured among many thousands of ordinary Chinese as open-air venues for morning and evening T'ai-chi practice.

How the movements of T'ai-chi are performed

The movements illustrated below and on p. 336 make up just one small sequence in the 'long form' of T'ai-chi. They begin with

the posture known as 'the bird's beak' (below left), which evolves subtly into 'strumming the lute' (below far right).

1 The bird's beak

2

3

4

5

6

Strumming the lute

7

lives – T'ai-chi is prescribed as an effective alternative to tranquillisers.

T'ai-chi can be practised at almost any age, and in China it is popular among young and old, who are said to find it physically, mentally and spiritually rewarding.

Finding a teacher For information about teachers and classes write to the British T'ai-chi and Shaolin Kung Fu Association, P O Box 1686, Cape Town 8000. Alternatively make inquiries at your local library; or scan noticeboards in health shops and health clubs, and the advertising columns of magazines that cater for alternative lifestyles.

Wherever possible, enrol with a teacher who has had sound training and at least four years' experience with the therapy's 'long form' (see below).

Consulting a teacher Once you have contacted a teacher, you should ask to watch him – or her – conducting a class before enrolling. Classes should be peaceful, well-organised, and not crowded. Students dress in light, loose-fitting shirts and trousers, and wear socks or thin slippers which allow full use of the foot muscles. The teacher should be calm and perceptive. There should be plenty of opportunities for discussion of what is being

Riding the tiger and resisting the monkey

According to Chinese legend, the beginnings of T'ai-chi Ch'uan date back to the 11th century and a Taoist thinker named Chang San-feng. The aggressive nature of martial arts were of some concern to him, and he sought a softer form which would help spiritual development.

One day while watching a magpie pecking at a snake, he was impressed by the way the snake moved slowly and continuously as it tried to evade its attacker. Its neat, circular movements and 'yielding' quality later formed the basis of a new form of *ch'uan*, or 'fist' – an exercise for developing self-mastery.

With this were incorporated the characteristic qualities of different animals, as developed by Taoist physicians such as Hua T'o in the 3rd century AD. These included the tiger (symbol of the ego), which had to be 'ridden' or 'mastered'; the monkey (symbol of mischievousness), which had to be 'resisted'; as well as the bear, the stag, the crane and others.

In about the 14th century, the more advanced form of this *ch'uan* acquired the name of T'ai-chi Ch'uan ('supreme ultimate fist') and was aimed at mastery of the whole self. It was adopted by Taoist monks in their monasteries and temple schools as a way of integrating body, mind and spirit by combining movement with breathing. The monks found that performing the movements focused their bodies and minds, and T'ai-chi was gradually transformed into a meditative healing process in which anyone who wanted to could take part.

It is based largely on achieving a balance between YIN AND YANG, the two complementary life forces in Chinese philosophy: yin, the gentle, yielding and peaceful feminine force; yang, the firm, active and creative masculine force.

T'ai-chi was first performed by the public in the mid-19th century – and today millions of Chinese practise it in the early mornings and early evenings.

One movement flows into another as the T'ai-chi sequence begun on p. 334 progresses to 'holding the circle' (centre left, below) and 'the stork cools its wings' (far right, below).

Holding the circle

The stork cools its wings

8 9 10 11

experienced, studied and achieved. From the start, you are taught that T'ai-chi is a 'growing' therapy which unfolds its benefits gradually. As such, it requires regular attendance – preferably in a class with group teaching – for at least 1½ hours a week.

You should beware of teachers who progress too quickly. Insist on repeating and refining what you have been taught. Personal guidance is essential for correct body alignment (such as keeping your spine vertical, your hips level and your head upright), relaxation, and maintaining an active but peaceful mind – a prerequisite for a balanced personality and healthy body.

There are two forms of T'ai-chi movement, the long form and the short form, both of which should be performed slowly and with a tranquil mind – in the open air wherever this is possible.

The short form This has about 40 movements without repetitions, and takes from five to ten minutes. Although it is beneficial, practitioners believe that this more recent adaptation does not provide the full therapeutic value of the long form.

The long form There are more than 100 movements involved, and this complete exercise takes from 20 to 40 minutes, depending on its structure. This includes repetitions, which – in reflecting the rhythms of life – are considered essential to physical and psychological balance.

An orthodox view

T'ai-chi is a beautiful and elegant form of physical 'routine' which encourages body awareness and helps with balance and confidence. As a therapy, it can reduce much anxiety and stress.

TAPEWORM

Tapeworms – so-called because of their long, flat, ribbon-like bodies – are parasites living in the intestines of human beings and many other animals. Some species can grow up to 9 m long. The worm, which consists of a head, a neck and a segmented body, attaches itself to the inner lining of the gut by suckers and hooks on the head; and it absorbs food through its whole surface.

Segments full of eggs detach themselves from the worm and pass out of the body with the faeces. If the eggs are eaten by an intermediate host – for example, a cow, pig or fish – they develop into cysts in its body tissues. Human beings become infected by eating such cysts in raw or inadequately cooked food. Tapeworms cannot be passed directly from person to person, however.

Many people with a tapeworm show no symptoms. Others suffer from weight loss, nausea, upper abdominal discomfort, DIAR-RHOEA and irritability. Because of its large size the beef tapeworm (*Taenia saginata*) may cause an intestinal obstruction.

A person can act as the intermediary host for pork tapeworms, and this leads to a serious condition known as cysticercosis. Cysts develop in the muscles, eyes and brain, causing muscle pains, weakness, fever, blindness or symptoms resembling those of EPILEPSY or a brain tumour.

What the therapists recommend

Naturopathy Garlic and raw carrots can weaken tapeworms. However, strong treatment is necessary to paralyse and expel the worms, so a qualified naturopath must therefore be consulted.

Herbal Medicine A consultation is advised, as the remedies for paralysing and expelling the worms are potentially toxic. They include wormwood, tansy and male fern, which are usually given together with powdered purgatives.

An orthodox view

A single oral dose of a drug such as niclosamide will eradicate the worm. Cysticercosis is treated with praziquantel.

TEETH-GRINDING

Dealing with abnormal pressure on the jaw

Misaligned or missing teeth, an uneven bite, or some other source of abnormal pressure on the jaw joints is often responsible for this night-time symptom.

The two jaw joints are located in front of the mid-points of the ears, and connect the jawbone (or mandible) to the temporal bones of the skull. The principal movements of the joints are up and down, allowing the mouth to open and close, but the jaw can also move from side to side to some extent – as happens when chewing food. When the joints are under strain the jaw muscles contract and tense up, grinding the teeth together during sleep.

Teeth-grinding, like other problems such as ARTHRITIS and injuries to the jaw, may eventually lead to disorders of the jaw joint – known as temporomandibular joint dysfunction. Symptoms may include clicking and pain in the jaw, and sometimes referred pain, felt as HEADACHES, earache, painful sinuses, soreness of the throat or neck glands, or even shoulder pain.

If strain due to teeth-grinding persists without treatment, arthritis in the temporomandibular joints may eventually develop. Occasionally the jaw may even become dislocated, but this is most often the result of sudden violence, such as a blow to the jaw when the mouth is open, 'whiplash' produced in a car accident, or even a sudden muscular spasm when yawning. When this happens, the jaw becomes locked in an abnormal position, the mouth will not fully open or close, and the head of the jaw can be felt in front of its usual position.

A dislocated jaw needs to be treated by a doctor or dentist, but alternative therapies may help to overcome the cause and subsequent pain.

What the therapists recommend

Acupuncture Treatment is given on the large intestine and stomach meridians to relieve pain; heart and bladder meridians as sedative points; points on the governor, stomach, heart, large intestine and bladder meridians as general treatment.

Autogenic Training This is said to be helpful in relieving excessive muscular tension in the region of the face and jaw. Grinding the teeth during sleep and facial pain resulting from tension in the jaw muscles are frequently eased or eliminated.

Osteopathy Often all that is required is for the osteopath to exert gentle but sustained pressure downwards on each side of the jaw. This has the effect of releasing contracted muscles and the osteopath can then gently guide the jaw into a better position.

Acupressure Apply pressure at a point two fingers' width in front of the ear in the hollow under the cheekbone, pressing inwards.

Massage The role of massage in this condition is largely to provide supportive extra treatment to the 'adjustment' performed by an osteopath.

An orthodox view

If you dislocate your jaw, your doctor or dentist can manipulate it back by pressing downwards on your molar teeth with his thumbs while lifting your chin with his other fingers. This overcomes muscle spasms and tension, and allows the joint to return to a normal position. Dislocation weakens the ligaments which hold the joints in place, so that recurrence is a possibility.

If you develop pain in one or both jaw joints, or a headache when chewing, you should see your dentist to check that your teeth and bite are even. If they are not, he can build up your teeth to protect you from arthritis in the joints and to relieve headaches and other associated pains you may have. If the pain is severe, an anti-inflammatory painkiller may be of some help.

TENNIS ELBOW

Inflammation of the tendon joining the muscles of the forearm to the lower end of the upper arm bone is known as tennis elbow. The muscles at the back of the forearm straighten and bend back the fingers and wrist, and they are all connected to the same point on the outer side of the humerus. It is not surprising therefore that vigorous use of those muscles produces inflammation and pain, which may radiate down the forearm and upwards towards the shoulder.

Tennis is only one of many activities such as typing that can provoke the condition.

What the therapists recommend

Osteopathy In the early, very acute, inflammatory stage, ice packs and rest are recommended. However, osteopathic treatment is claimed to be very effective for this condition, which often lasts for months. Deep friction massage is given to the painful points in the muscles surrounding the joint. Restricted mobility of the joint may be corrected by gentle mobilisation.

Massage In the early stage, following an initial period of rest – particularly from the activity responsible for the condition – gentle effleurage and petrissage kneadings may serve to relieve the pain. They can also help to prevent adhesions (the growing together of normally separate surfaces) and the softening of tissue.

After the acute inflammatory stage has passed, deeper finger friction and kneading are usually applied.

An orthodox view

Despite treatment, tennis elbow can be a persistent and troublesome complaint, particularly if the sufferer continues the activity that caused it in the first place. Sometimes this is inevitable if the patient's livelihood depends on it.

Massage, painkilling tablets, steroid (cortisone) injections, injections of local anaesthetic, and strapping or elastic support around the elbow may all help. Various exercises, manipulation and local short-wave or ultrasound treatment given by a qualified physiotherapist may also be recommended (see ULTRASONICS).

Forearm bones and muscles

Humerus – upper arm bone

Tendon tying forearm muscles to humerus

Muscles of the forearm

Ulna – bone in forearm

Radius – second forearm bone

Tennis elbow strikes when overuse of the forearm muscles inflames the tendon that anchors them to the bottom of the humerus, or upper arm bone, causing pain on the outer elbow.

Poor technique is responsible for many tennis injuries. The player on the left risks straining his forearm muscles by locking the elbow joint in this backhand stroke. The young woman below has a common beginner's fault: getting so close to the ball that she is forced to play a cramped and awkward forehand. Not only her game suffers – the manoeuvre strains both arm and elbow muscles.

TENSION

Designed to prime muscles for action, bodily tension was intended by nature to have a quick release. However, in the modern world, stresses and strains seldom find an immediate physical outlet, and tension easily builds up to a dangerous level. Never ignore warning signals such as HEADACHES, NECK PAIN, BACK PAIN, DIGESTIVE DISORDERS and raised BLOOD PRESSURE, or more serious disorders may develop.

Treatment and self-help measures for tension are the same as for STRESS.

TERMINAL ILLNESS

Breaking the final taboo

A terminal illness is, by definition, incurable – but this does not mean that it is untreatable. Most patients' fears are less to do with death itself than with the process of dying. They may be afraid of being in pain, of becoming dependent, of losing control over their bodily functions, or of being a burden to their relatives.

The best modern terminal care – whether at home, in hospital, or in a hospice – provides a supportive atmosphere for patients to come to terms with their illness. They have the reassurance that they will not suffer, that pain will be well controlled with drugs, and that they will die with dignity.

Nowadays fewer and fewer people die at home. Many die in hospitals, sometimes surrounded by high-technology equipment and often feeling frightened, alone and cut off from their families. They may even feel ignored, as if everyone has given them up and is concentrating on people who will get better – and sometimes this feeling is justified. If others are avoiding talking about death, the patient may feel that they are hiding some awful truth, and these fears may be replayed in the imagination until they assume horrific proportions.

Relatives too may lose the reassurance of being able to keep their loved one comfortable, and of knowing they will be on hand to help and to hold when the end comes. It can also be difficult for relatives to come to terms with a death when they have been unable to see the person and say their final goodbyes. Indeed, because dying and death seldom occur at home, comparatively few of us have ever seen anyone die, and may imagine what happens to be far worse than it really is.

Children especially are usually 'shielded' from the processes of birth and death, so most of us grow up with little sense of the continuity of the life cycle, and its beginning and end become shadowy, mysterious events, somehow removed from real life. This can help to produce an atmosphere of denial surrounding terminally ill patients, where medical staff and relatives feel that it may be cruel or unnecessarily traumatic to talk to them about facing impending death.

However, patients are often very aware that they have an incurable condition without being told so directly, and they too may shy away from mentioning it because they in turn do not want to upset their relatives. When the subject is broached, almost everyone is greatly relieved to be able to talk openly about it, rather than constantly steering conversations away from the situation.

Talking about dying It is often said that dying has become the final taboo. Not only do people find it difficult and even embarrassing to talk about death and dying with those who are terminally ill, even doctors and nurses often feel uncomfortable about discussing it in a direct manner.

Because conventional medicine is mostly concerned with making people better and battling against disease, some doctors feel a sense of failure when they are no longer able to offer any hope of a cure. Some terminally ill patients do not want to know the truth; others welcome time to come to terms with their own feelings without having to discuss the prospect of death. But for many the 'conspiracy of silence' about death which is maintained by their families and those who care for them can be deeply distressing.

Many patients feel the need to talk about what is happening to them, to ask questions to relieve their fears and uncertainties, and to discuss both practical and emotional matters with their nearest and dearest.

Coming to terms Dr Elizabeth Kubler-Ross, a physician working at the University of Chicago, has done work aimed at dispelling the myths surrounding death and dying for patients and doctors alike. She describes five stages in the emotional response of patients with a terminal illness:

Denial On suspecting or being told the diagnosis, the patient's reaction is often 'This can't be happening to me', and a refusal to accept the verdict. Often doctors and relatives will collude in or even encourage this denial, leaving the patient unable to acknowledge what is really happening.

Anger The patient may now become angry at what is happening. This anger may be directed against himself ('Why didn't I stop smoking?'), or his doctors ('Why can't they cure me?'), or his relatives ('If I hadn't been so busy looking after them I would have seen the doctor more quickly'), or even against fate ('Why me?').

Bargaining At this stage patients try to extend the time left to them. They stick to treatments and diets, and may press for drastic surgery or extreme drug treatments. Some start seeking a miracle cure, visiting numerous doctors or alternative practitioners, or trying religious healers or shrines. Some try to strike a bargain with fate – 'If I am good and atone for my sins, I might get better'.

Sadness As patients start to accept the inevitability of their own death they begin to grieve for what they will lose – family, friends, possessions, years of life they might have had. Sometimes severe DEPRESSION will set in for a time.

Acceptance Many patients are lucky enough to come to terms with their illness before they die. They experience peace and tranquillity combined with a certain joy in what life still has to offer. Often, if they have been able to share their feelings, they experience an emotional attachment to their family which many describe as being closer than at any time in their lives.

Final stages The choice of where to spend the final stages of a terminal illness – at home, in hospital or in a hospice – will be determined by the nature of the illness, the degree of support relatives and friends are able to give, and the local facilities available. Many hospitals have specialists in terminal care, or there may be a hospice nearby. Alternatively, the hospital or hospice may be able to provide a home-care service, supplying doctors and nurses who can make regular visits to patients.

Some patients stay in hospital for a while, then go home when their symptoms are well under control, while others stay at home for as long as possible, then go into a hospice.

TETANUS

Tetanus is a serious and sometimes fatal infectious disease of the central nervous system. The disease is also known as 'lockjaw' from one of its commonest symptoms: the jaw and neck stiffen, and opening the mouth becomes difficult. The mouth may set in a mirthless smile (technically known as 'risus sardonicus').

The disease occurs when the body is infected with the spores of the bacterium *Clostridium tetani*. These exist in soil and in animal faeces, and they can develop in human tissue only where oxygenated blood is in poor supply or lacking, as in a flesh wound. Once installed, they multiply, producing a powerful toxin that acts on the nerves controlling the muscles.

Other symptoms of tetanus include a high temperature and fast pulse, sweating, a headache, stiffness of abdominal and back muscles, and sudden muscular spasms.

Newborn infants may acquire tetanus (and almost invariably die from it) as a result of the practice, in some rural areas, of 'cleansing' the umbilical stump with earth.

Tetanus, an infection, should not be confused with the less serious 'tetany' – muscular twitching and spasms caused by a low level of calcium in the blood (or some other biochemical disturbance in the body).

What the therapists recommend

A patient with tetanus should be hospitalised, for this is an emergency. Alternative therapies can be of benefit in the recovery stage. Nursing in a quiet, darkened, well-ventilated room is essential.

An orthodox view

Suspected tetanus should be treated at a hospital. Any infected wound is thoroughly cleaned, and the patient is given an anti-toxin injection to neutralise the effects of the bacterial poison. Drugs will be prescribed to help alleviate any stiffness and control muscle contractions. If the symptoms seem to be far advanced and the patient has difficulty in breathing, a tracheostomy – the insertion of a breathing tube through an opening in the windpipe – may be necessary.

Tetanus can be prevented by immunisation, with booster injections, every ten years. Infants are routinely vaccinated against tetanus (along with DIPHTHERIA and WHOOPING COUGH).

T-GROUPS

The growth of group PSYCHOTHERAPY has led to similar techniques being exploited to extend its use from solving personal problems to improving people's relationships with others, both socially and at work.

T-groups – or training groups – are formed to improve relationships within large organisations. ENCOUNTER GROUPS and SENSITIVITY TRAINING use similar methods, but have different objectives depending on members' needs and the context in which therapy occurs. See also HUMANISTIC PSYCHOLOGY.

T-groups are usually made up of about 12 to 20 members who meet either for regular sessions over a period of weeks or for a single intensive weekend session. The group leader, who is sometimes called a 'facilitator', encourages participants to express attitudes, feelings and motives which they are usually unaware of or which they feel they have to conceal from others.

Often T-groups adapt to their own use the principles of ROGERIAN THERAPY, in which more importance is attached to the experiences and points of view of the clients than to those of the therapist.

Although some people find T-group sessions extremely useful, many report deriving little benefit, and others find the experience unpleasant and disturbing. For this reason, responsible therapists recommend that individuals should be carefully assessed by a group leader or other psychotherapist before participating in a group.

THERAPEUTIC TOUCH

Healing with the hands

Before attempting to locate and cure illness by therapeutic touch, those who consider themselves gifted with the power of healing, usually 'centre', or concentrate, their mind on a calm and beautiful visual image, such as a tranquil country scene. This, they say, lets

them clear their mind of inessentials and harness psychic energy for their work.

They then run their hands over or near the patient's head or body seeking out any area of sickness. If anything is found to be wrong, the healer places his hands on the area so that the healing energy can flow through him to the patient, or so that any imbalances in the patient can be corrected (see LAYING ON OF HANDS). The treatment – which, ideally, should be done in a quiet atmosphere – takes about 10-15 minutes, after which the patient should start to feel better.

Therapeutic touch is particularly popular in the USA, and is practised mostly by trained nurses. See HEALERS AND HEALING.

THROAT PROBLEMS

The average sore throat lasts about three to four days, and is the commonest of throat problems. A virus or bacterium is generally the cause, and the throat is often the first area of the body to respond to the infection. See LARYNGITIS; NOSE AND THROAT AILMENTS; QUINSY; TONSILLITIS.

Some people are particularly prone to sore throats, but the likelihood of getting one does decrease with age. Several factors can lessen resistance to such infection, including TIREDNESS, an unhealthy diet, SMOKING, overindulgence in alcohol, or any form of STRESS – which often results from emotional problems, such as the loss of a partner or job.

Warning If a sore throat lasts more than four days, consult a doctor. It may be an early symptom of an illness such as GLANDULAR FEVER, MUMPS or SCARLET FEVER.

Self help Make sure that you get enough sleep, and follow a healthy diet (see EATING FOR HEALTH). Do not smoke or take alcohol.

A soothing drink can be made by adding the juice of half a fresh lemon, 1 teaspoon of honey and 1 tablespoon of glycerine to a glass of hot water. Alternatively, drink agrimony tea (available at health-food shops). Hot, damp air is also helpful, so put 1 teaspoon of friar's balsam in 600 ml of hot water in a bowl, and inhale the steam under a towel for ten minutes, up to three times a day.

What the therapists recommend
NATUROPATHY
Self help Plenty of fresh fruit juices are usually helpful for throat problems. Avoid dairy products, sweets, cakes and similar foods. Sucking zinc lozenges is believed to be a good way to fight any throat infection directly, and this can be backed up by a vit-

amin C supplement. Steam inhalations ease congestion, and gargles with lemon juice or cider vinegar may be recommended.

HERBAL MEDICINE
Self help Sore throats and minor infections can be helped at home with regular gargles of sage or thyme, especially if fresh lemon juice is added. An indigenous remedy is a gargle made from diluting with warm water a mixture of honey, lemon juice and ripe, black nastergal (common nightshade) berries, soaked in brandy and then crushed and sieved. If you are prone to sore throats, it may be advisable to take one or two garlic capsules a day, particularly during the winter months.

Consultation For severe or recurrent throat infections, herbalists use gargles, notably tinctures of myrrh, sage, wild indigo or thyme. Remedies such as echinacea or wild indigo, to be taken internally, may be prescribed to boost the immune system. If your case is considered to be particularly serious, you will be advised also to see a doctor.

HOMOEOPATHY
Self help For a sore throat which is swollen, shiny and soggy looking, and which is worse with increasing heat, but when there is no thirst, therapists recommend Apis mel. 30. Burning pain in a raw throat, when the sufferer must keep swallowing and hoarseness is relieved by coughing, is usually treated with Causticum 30.

Hepar sulph. 30 is used for a sore throat with an established cold, when the patient has a sensation of something stuck in the throat, and pain shoots to the ears on swallowing, and when the sufferer is very irritable and sensitive to the least draught. For a congested, sore, dark red throat, when the patient cannot swallow even water and his neck muscles feel stiff, homoeopaths recommend a dose of Phytolacca 30 every two hours for a day, followed by four doses daily for two days.

An orthodox view

Most sore throats go away of their own accord. If necessary, a doctor may prescribe antibiotics to clear up bacterial infections, and in severe cases, painkillers such as paracetamol or aspirin.

THRUSH

This condition, also called candida, is caused by Candida albicans or Monilia, a yeast-like fungus which thrives in warm, moist areas and may form white flaky patches. It may be present for long periods without causing symptoms, especially in men, but may then become troublesome due to hormonal changes, STRESS or an unbalanced diet.

Thrush is particularly prevalent in babies, elderly people, fat people (see OBESITY), DIABETES sufferers, pregnant women and those taking antibiotics. It is also common where the IMMUNE SYSTEM is not functioning properly – for example, in people with AIDS or LEUKAEMIA, or those taking steroid drugs.

The thrush organism normally lives on the skin, so an infection can flare up without contact with another person. Such skin infection is common, particularly in the warm, moist skin folds of fat people. The groins, armpits and the skin under the breasts are most commonly affected, becoming inflamed and itchy. People whose work involves frequent wetting of the hands are susceptible to infection of the fingers. There is tender swelling and sometimes pus in the skin around the fingernails and, in chronic cases, deformed nails.

Babies frequently have white patches of thrush in the mouth or a red 'nappy rash' on their bottom, often with separate red spots around the rash and on their thighs. Adults sometimes get thrush in the mouth, especially if they wear dentures. If the immune system is not functioning properly, the thrush infection may spread down the oesophagus or gullet, causing pain and burning when the person eats or drinks.

Thrush infection of the vulva and vagina is common, recurrent and troublesome. It causes itching and soreness, with a white vaginal discharge, which may be thick, like curds. Although it is not necessarily sexually transmitted, a sexual partner may develop the infection, with redness and soreness of the end of the penis and under the foreskin. Any clothing that limits the circulation of air around the body will make infection more likely, and will aggravate the condition once it is established. This is particularly true of tights, tight jeans, and underwear made from synthetic fibres.

What the therapists recommend
NATUROPATHY
Consultation Mouth and vaginal thrush responds very well to natural treatments, and a practitioner may also aim to prevent a more widespread fungal invasion – of the digestive tract, for example. You may be recommended to cut out all sugars and refined starches, alcohol, tea, coffee and chocolate drinks immediately, but to eat plenty of vegetables, pulses and whole grains.

Suggested supplements are likely to include garlic and acidophilus, in order to suppress excess fungal growth and to restore the normal micro-organisms in the digestive tract. Live, natural yoghurt or frequent salt washes are recommended for vaginal thrush.

HERBAL MEDICINE
Self help Tinctures of myrrh or marigold are recommended mouthwashes. A soothing vaginal wash can be made by dissolving up to 1 tablespoon of salt in 600 ml of water. Alternatively, apply live, natural yoghurt on a sanitary pad.

An old rural remedy for vaginal thrush is a douche made by steeping finely chopped sour-fig leaves in vinegar, then straining the liquid and adding warm water.

Antibiotics are thought to upset the balance of micro-organisms in the gut, allowing the *Candida* fungus to thrive. So, after a course of antibiotics, take three to four garlic capsules a day for a week. If the thrush recurs, seek professional advice, for it may seriously damage your health.

AROMATHERAPY
Self help For oral thrush, try a mouthwash of three drops of tea tree essential oil and one drop of essential oil of myrrh in half a glass of water. Stir vigorously before use, swishing around the gums three times a day.

For vaginal thrush, dampen the tip of a tampon, add three to four drops of tea tree essential oil and insert it for one to two hours. Alternatively, use the oil in an application oil or lotion, and apply each night and morning. Regular sitz baths (see HYDROTHERAPY) with three to four drops of the above essential oils, or conventional baths with six to eight drops are also recommended.

Other alternative treatment
Biochemic Tissue Salts If cold sores on the lips accompany oral thrush, Nat. *mur.* 6 is often recommended.

An orthodox view
A doctor may check that there is no underlying cause for thrush. For example, he may test for high sugar in the urine which could indicate diabetes.

Oral thrush responds favourably to nystatin or miconazole drops, and skin thrush to nystatin, clotrimazole or imidazole cream or ointment. If, as frequently happens, the thrush infection causes an ECZEMA-like reaction on the person's skin, the doctor may prescribe a cream or ointment containing both an antifungal agent to combat the infection and a steroid such as hydrocortisone to reduce the inflammation and itching.

Nail infections may require incisions to release the pus and prolonged treatment with antifungal agents. However, the most important measure is to avoid repeated soaking of the fingers, by wearing rubber gloves, for example.

Conventional treatments for vaginal thrush include pessaries or cream inserted high into the vagina, even during a period.

Nystatin must be used for fourteen days, but newer drugs such as clotrimazole or imidazole may be effective in shorter courses – even in a single high dose. A single oral dose of fluconazole (Diflucan) is often effective when vaginal pessaries or creams fail, but it must not be used during pregnancy.

Recurrent vaginal infection is common, particularly if a sexual partner is harbouring the infection on his penis, and he too must be treated.

THYROID DISORDERS

The thyroid gland is situated in the lower part of the neck, immediately in front of the windpipe and just below the Adam's apple. This gland produces the thyroid hormones, iodine-containing substances that control the rate of metabolism (the body's chemical reactions and processes) and therefore our mental and physical growth and development. The thyroid is in turn controlled by the pituitary gland at the base of the skull, which secretes thyroid-stimulating hormone.

The main thyroid hormones are called T3 and T4 (also known as thyroxine). The main disorders of the gland are swelling, and under and overactivity, which can affect the body in disturbing ways.

Swelling of the gland is known as goitre. It may be caused by a lack of iodine in the diet, but this condition, known as endemic goitre, is now rare (see GOITRE). Swelling may also be due simply to overgrowth, or to a tumour, which in very rare cases may be cancerous. Unlike LEUKAEMIA, CANCER of the thyroid gland seems to be less common around nuclear installations.

Underactivity of the thyroid gland (called hypothyroidism) can begin at any age. Some babies are born with it. They have difficulty in feeding and sleeping, and suffer from CONSTIPATION and delayed mental and physical development.

If it is not detected, sufferers develop coarse features. They grow short and fat, with a protruding tongue and sparse hair, and are known as cretins. However, a blood test a few days after birth can detect the disease and ensure prompt treatment.

If the gland becomes underactive later in life, the symptoms develop gradually and may not be obvious at first. The patient becomes lethargic, sleeps more and unaccountably puts on weight. The hair and skin become dry, and the hair may fall out (see HAIR PROBLEMS). The eyes become puffy and the voice deepens.

In some cases, thyroid underactivity may be caused by inflammation of the gland (thyroiditis). The symptoms are similar to those of a sore throat (see THROAT PROBLEMS), but the gland is tender and swollen. The underactivity begins after an interval of weeks or months following the inflammation. Usually, however, the cause of an underactive thyroid is unknown.

Overactivity of the thyroid gland (called hyperthyroidism) results in too much of the thyroid hormones in the blood (thyrotoxicosis), the effects of which are the opposite to those of underactivity. The body's metabolism speeds up and, despite a good appetite, the sufferer loses weight, becomes restless and fidgety, and cannot sleep. There may also be a tremor – most obvious when the sufferer's hands are outstretched – along with PALPITATIONS and SWEATING. In addition, goitre may develop, and the eyes may protrude and appear to be staring.

What the therapists recommend

Acupuncture Treatment for thyroid disorders is given on the large intestine (neck area), gall bladder and governing meridians.

Herbal Medicine Iodine-rich foods such as kelp and other seaweeds may help mild thyroid disorders. As a tonic, herbalists may prescribe bladderwrack.

Severe thyroid disorders should always be diagnosed by means of blood tests and professionally treated.

Homoeopathy Overweight people with an enlarged thyroid should try *Fucus vesiculosus* 3, four times a day. Patients with an overactive thyroid should try *Iodum* 30 twice a day for two weeks. If the thyroid is swollen, feels hard, and the patient is constantly clearing his throat, try *Spongia* 30 twice a day for two weeks.

Reflexology Massage the reflex areas relating to the thyroid gland, and also those which relate to the adrenal, pituitary and reproductive glands (see chart, p. 295).

An orthodox view

When it does occur, endemic goitre is treated with iodine supplements to the diet, but the use of iodised table salt has made this unnecessary in many countries.

A blood test in which low levels of thyroid hormones are found in the sample confirms diagnosis of underactivity of the thyroid gland. Doctors treat the condition in all ages with T4 (thyroxine) tablets. Patients usually have to take the tablets daily for the rest of their lives. The symptoms gradually disappear and there are no after-effects as long as the treatment is kept up.

A blood test that reveals antibodies confirms diagnosis of thyroid inflammation.

For overactivity of the thyroid gland, doctors usually prescribe a course of antithyroid tablets called carbimazole (Neo-Mercazole). Alternatively, a dose of radioactive iodine may be given to destroy part of the gland, or part of it may be removed by surgery.

As long as the patient's blood is tested regularly and any necessary treatment is given, the outlook for sufferers of both hypothyroidism and hyperthyroidism is now generally excellent.

TIC

People with a tic may repeatedly blink their eyes, clear their throat, twitch their mouth, or nod their head for no obvious reason. This nervous muscle twitch – also known as habit spasm – is a common complaint which can develop at any age.

It particularly affects children, who often are not aware there is anything 'wrong' with them. In their case it may be caused by strong feelings of insecurity, which should be understood and sympathised with.

Calling attention to the child, or scolding him or her in any way, will only tend to make the condition worse. The best policy is to completely ignore the tic, which will disappear of its own accord, usually within a month or two. Sometimes, however, it may last into adulthood.

What the therapists recommend

Behavioural Therapy Family and friends are asked to avoid paying undue attention to the tic. The sufferer will be asked to try to achieve control over the tic by relaxation training at the times and in the situations when it is most pronounced. Another recommended technique might be to develop other physical responses that compete with the tic – for example, if the head twitches to the left, an alternative response could be to move the head to the right.

An orthodox view

There is no conventional drug treatment for tics, and no need to consult a doctor unless the condition causes undue distress or embarrassment. In some rare, extreme cases psychiatric treatment may be called for.

TICK-BITE FEVER

While most tick bites are innocuous, occasionally a bite can spread an infection known as tick-bite fever (or tick typhus), caused by bacteria-like micro-organisms known as rickettsiae. The fever, which is not life-threatening, is characterised by severe headaches, in addition to feverish symptoms. A bluish-black scab covers the site of the bite.

What the therapists recommend

Homoeopathy The treatment prescribed by the therapist will depend on a detailed assessment of the patient's health.

Herbal medicine Many herbal teas can help reduce the fever. Try any of the following, infused in boiling water: wild basil, catnip, camomile, feverfew, lemon bush ('fever tea') or stork's bill geranium. Drink the tea at regular intervals, either hot or cold.

Naturopathy The patient needs rest and plenty of fluids. Diet should be high in fruit and vegetable juices, and include steamed vegetables.

An orthodox view

After some days tick-bite fever often subsides of its own without the need for medical treatment other than pain-relieving drugs for headache. Antibiotics are normally prescribed, however, in particular tetracyclines or erythromycin.

TIREDNESS

Combating that tired-all-the-time feeling

All of us go through periods in our lives when we are always tired. We lose our zest for life, have no energy and are easily fatigued. We are tired when we wake up in the morning. It is hard to concentrate on daily tasks and to maintain interest in loved ones, friends and leisure activities. And we often become exceptionally irritable.

For some people, this unhappy state of affairs becomes a chronic, permanent condition. It may become overwhelming, leading to debilitating despair – and even to suicide. Doctors sometimes call it the TATT (tired-all-the-time) syndrome.

Chronic tiredness is one of the most common reasons why people visit a general practitioner or alternative therapist. It is also one of the most difficult problems to treat, because many factors can be involved in the condition, and both doctors and therapists find that the best results come from a truly holistic system of treatment – one in which the physical, psychological, spiritual and emotional facets of the sufferer and his lifestyle are considered.

Diagnosing the cause of tiredness A full case history will include details of the patient's past, particularly information about any recent traumas, such as a death in the family, the loss of a job, or a divorce. The practitioner will want to know if the tiredness occurs in regular bouts, and whether these can be related to any traumas or periods of 'feeling low'.

Physical aspects are also important. The practitioner will investigate the patient's diet, for one high in sugar can lead to HYPOGLYCAEMIA, which could be the cause of the tiredness. Similarly, a lack of iron can lead to ANAEMIA, one of whose symptoms is tiredness, and which in women can also be caused by heavy periods.

Chronic tiredness can also be a symptom of PREMENSTRUAL TENSION or the MENOPAUSE, both of which are associated with hormonal imbalances. Some women experience a 'new lease of life' when put on hormone replacement therapy (see p. 238).

Other hormonal imbalances may be involved – for instance, hypothyroidism, in which the thyroid gland produces too little thyroid hormone (see THYROID DISORDERS), or Addison's disease, in which the body has too little adrenal hormone. These are rare conditions, but are easily treated.

On the other hand, MYALGIC ENCEPHALOMYELITIS (ME) is difficult both to diagnose and to treat. Besides prolonged tiredness, patients also suffer from extreme exhaustion and muscle aches and pains, particularly after physical exertion. However, recent research has shown that a virus may be implicated in ME, and that information should at least aid diagnosis.

Doctors and therapists all recognise that one of the main causes of chronic tiredness is not a physical condition at all, but personal problems – often problems at work or at home that the patient cannot face and has 'hidden'. Once physical causes have been eliminated, practitioners will help patients to explore their personal lives, in order to uncover the cause.

Unexpressed GRIEF can also result in chronic tiredness. In such cases, people fail to mourn properly after a loss. This can be the loss of a loved one, or even a part of themselves – in the case of a woman, a breast or an unborn child; or in a man, IMPOTENCE. Grief over the loss of a job or a home can also be a cause of tiredness.

Unexpressed anger often has the same effects as unexpressed grief. Many people are trapped in an intolerable life situation, and bottle up their rage. This repression uses up much of their energy, and they have little left for other things. Women are particularly prone to this condition. Many are trapped in a marriage or job where they are unable to make full use of their abilities, or their skills are not recognised. A partner may completely dominate them or fail to recognise their need to express their feelings.

In such situations, women lose their self-confidence and become prone to DEPRESSION, of which tiredness can be a symptom. Eventually they may become dependent on tranquillisers and sleeping pills. Assertiveness training will probably be able to help such patients. Women's groups are often of benefit too, for they help sufferers to talk through their problems and feelings, and to think more positively about themselves and their situation.

Today, many people face unemployment, money problems and poor, overcrowded living conditions. For example, a young family may have to share a home with their in-laws. These situations all put a strain on individuals, and they can all lead to depression. This may manifest itself as chronic tiredness, and in such cases the practitioner needs a great deal of skill to get to the heart of the matter.

The same is true of another condition in which sufferers have lost their faith or sense of purpose in life. They may be perfectly healthy, yet they feel that something is missing. Their life becomes empty of meaning, and chronic tiredness results. This frequently leads them to consult some type of therapist.

Chronic tiredness can, in itself, be both debilitating and a cause of worry – which in turn aggravates the condition. Great patience and effort on the part of both practitioner and sufferer are needed to find an effective cure.

Self help Ensure that you have adequate sleep (see SLEEP DISORDERS; INSOMNIA) and, if possible, practise relaxation and breathing exercises. Learn to express your feelings – to let go – and not keep them bottled up.

Make sure that your day-to-day diet is well-balanced (see EATING FOR HEALTH), with regular meals. Light, high-protein snacks between meals will probably help you to combat the tiredness. Cut down on sugar and avoid stimulants such as caffeine (in coffee, tea and cola drinks).

Make sure that your intake of MINERALS and VITAMINS is adequate – zinc, magnesium, potassium, vitamin C and folic acid are particularly important.

What the therapists recommend
HOMOEOPATHY
Self help If, following too much physical effort, you are unable to sleep and the bed feels too hard, try two or three doses of Arnica 30. After a long period of strain or study, Phosphoric ac. 6 three times a day for 21 days may help to restore lost energy. Two or three doses of Kali phos. may help when there is lack of nerve power, or a feeling of mental and physical depression.

HERBAL MEDICINE
Self help Make your own invigorating 'bath salts' by mixing together equal quantities of coarse salt and oat flakes, and a double quantity of fresh lavender leaves and twigs. Tie a handful of this mixture in muslin, and place it in a hot bath. Use the bag to gently massage your body.

ACUPUNCTURE
Consultation Tiredness is believed often to be caused by some dysfunction of the internal organs, and treatment to those organs is given. General basic treatment consists of MOXIBUSTION combined with acupuncture to points on the bladder, gall bladder, conception, governing, large and small intestine, lung, kidney, spleen and/or stomach meridians.

MASSAGE
Self help When the tiredness is only temporary, and not a symptom of a medical condition or the companion of muscular fatigue or exhaustion, then a brisk, light tonic, general massage is often the answer, and the means of sparking some new life into the various body systems.

A really vitalising massage could consist of rapid effleurage strokes in the direction of the venous return (towards the heart), working up the legs and arms, and over the entire back, from the lumbar to shoulder area. This is followed by stimulating petrissage wringing and squeezing techniques, and the clapping and finger hacking procedures for tapotement – all made at a brisk pace.

ACUPRESSURE
Self help Apply pressure at a point three thumbs' width from under the kneecap, in the hollow on the outer edge of the skin, pressing inwards. As an alternative, apply pressure to the centre of the palm at the point where the middle finger rests when the hand is folded inwards.

AROMATHERAPY
Self help If the tiredness is due to a physical cause, then try stimulating essential oils, such as black pepper, lemon, lemongrass and rosemary. Either inhale from a tissue, or put six to ten drops into a bath, and stay in the water for ten minutes. For mental exhaustion, use clary sage, savory or rosemary in the same ways.

For general tiredness due to ME or post-viral symptoms, the regular use of essential oils of geranium, thyme, lemon or sage is strongly recommended. Inhale them from a tissue or put them in a bath as above. Alternatively, you can make a tea by putting two or three drops of oil on a tea bag, and infusing in 600 ml of boiling water; stir, remove the tea bag, and drink slowly without milk as needed. Be sure to keep the surplus in the fridge, and reheat as required.

An orthodox view

The doctor will first seek any physical cause of the tiredness, and treat it accordingly. If this fails, he will help the patient to review his lifestyle, and help him to talk through any stress-causing situations. The doctor may then refer the patient to a psychotherapist or another specialist.

TOFU

Bean curd or tofu is used extensively in oriental cuisine. The word comes from the Mandarin Chinese *dòu*, meaning 'bean', and *fu*, 'curdled' or 'rotten'.

The curd is made by washing and rinsing soya beans, soaking them in water, then grinding them and boiling them for 15 minutes, after which the fibre is extracted by straining. The result is soya milk, which is further cooked and allowed to coagulate, calcium sulphate being added to curdle the milk. The curd is then pressed, separating the curdled milk into whey and tofu.

TONSILLITIS

Children are the most common victims of tonsillitis, a highly infectious inflammation of the tonsils – two masses of tissue at the back of the throat. The complaint causes a sore throat and FEVER, sometimes accompanied by a HEADACHE and stomach ache. In addition, the neck glands are frequently swollen and there may be a dry cough.

Tonsillitis is usually caused by a virus against which children have not had time to develop a resistance. However, it may also be the result of bacteria called streptococci, of which some people are 'carriers' – even though they themselves may be perfectly healthy. Streptococcal tonsillitis with a rash which first appears on the neck and chest is called SCARLET FEVER.

Whatever the cause, tonsillitis tends to strike suddenly, and the worst of the illness is normally over within 48 hours. If the symptoms last for more than three days – or if the sufferer starts coughing up green or yellow phlegm – seek medical attention.

What the therapists recommend

Herbal Medicine Herbalists consider recurring infection and inflammation of the tonsils to be a key factor in illness in later life. They therefore treat the entire IMMUNE SYSTEM, aiming to eliminate this risk. For example, they may advise gargles made with myrrh, sage, thyme or wild indigo. Taking extra vitamin C may also help to boost the body's defence system, especially in the winter months.

Homoeopathy If the tonsils are inflamed and bright red, and there is difficulty in swallowing, try *Belladonna* 30. If the throat is dark red and swollen, with unpleasant breath and thirst – and if the symptoms are worse when talking and at night – try *Merc. sol.* 30. Take one dose each hour for up to 12 hours; then three times a day for two days.

Naturopathy In cases of nasal congestion, and if the ADENOIDS are also affected, avoid dairy products. Naturopaths may prescribe sage or thyme gargles, with fresh lemon juice. One or two GARLIC capsules taken each day, especially in the winter, may also help.

An orthodox view

If tonsillitis has been caused by bacteria, and the symptoms are prolonged or the patient is ill with a raised temperature, a GP may prescribe an antibiotic such as penicillin. However, if there is no fever, and the patient is not ill – as is often the case – penicillin is unlikely to help and may provoke ALLERGY or THRUSH. If the disease is the result of a virus, antibiotics will not be effective.

For treatment at home, doctors will advise patients to drink plenty of fluids, not to worry if they don't feel like eating, take painkillers such as aspirin or paracetamol, and go to bed when the symptoms are at their height.

TOOTH AND GUM DISORDERS

We all suffer from toothache at some time or other – often because we have not been taking proper care of our teeth and gums. The two most common mouth disorders are dental caries (decay) and periodontal disease. This disease takes the form of GINGIVITIS (inflammation of the gums in which they turn red and bleed easily) or – if the gingivitis is neglected – the more serious periodontitis, when the inflammation extends into the bone surrounding the teeth, and the bone is partly destroyed. Gum abscesses may form during this process.

Dental decay can start in infancy and last through life. Periodontal disease can occur at as early an age as five years, and it can reach an advanced stage without tell-tale symptoms of pain or discomfort.

These conditions can usually be avoided, or relieved, by having a dental check-up twice a year – and by taking thorough care of your teeth in between check-ups.

Self help A cheap and effective toothpowder that you can make up easily at home is a mixture of two parts of sodium bicarbonate to one part of table salt. Alternatively, simply clean your teeth with pure lemon juice. First dip the toothbrush in warm water, then squeeze a few drops of the juice onto it. Be sure to rinse your mouth thoroughly after brushing with lemon juice.

What the therapists recommend
HOMOEOPATHY

Self help For an acute tooth abscess which is red, swollen and throbbing, try *Belladonna* 200 hourly. Once the pus begins to drain away, take *Silicea*. For a less serious or a chronic abscess, *Hepar sulph.* 30 or 200 may help. *Silicea* is recommended when the abscess starts to drain.

Before and after a tooth is extracted *Arnica* 30 is suggested to try and reduce shock, bleeding and the risk of blood-poisoning. Take the remedy hourly for three hours before the extraction and for three or four hours after the extraction.

If splinters of tooth or bone are left in the gum after an extraction, *Silicea* 6 taken four times daily may help to bring them to the surface. If there is still pain, *Hypericum* 30 is said to be effective. In addition, a mouthwash of *Hypericum* mother tincture – ten drops in half a wine glass of boiled warm water – is said to help ease discomfort and speed up healing. The mouthwash can also be used for inflamed and sore gums.

For teeth which are painful and sensitive to cold after extensive dental work, try *Chamomilla* 6 four times a day for two or three days. In the case of dental haemorrhage, when there is a lot of bright red blood, try *Phosphorus* 30. Take three doses, one every ten minutes, and then hourly as needed.

HERBAL MEDICINE

Consultation You will be told that decayed teeth should be treated by a dentist by means of fillings, or other dental work. However, herbalists believe that mouth disorders can be a sign of general ill health, and may recommend changes of diet – such as eating less sugar and fewer sweet things such as puddings, cakes and biscuits. Mouthwashes or tinctures of marigold, myrrh and wild indigo may be prescribed to strengthen the gums and disinfect the mouth generally.

An orthodox view

Teeth should be cleaned regularly as shown in *Brushing and flossing your way to dental health*, p. 345. Always see your dentist if your teeth or gums hurt, or if your gums begin to bleed. If necessary he will refer you to a periodontist, and surgery under local anaesthetic may then be required.

Brushing and flossing your way to dental health

One of the most effective ways of taking care of people's teeth was devised in the 1950s by an American pathologist, Dr Charles C Bass. The Bass method of brushing and flossing is concentrated against plaque, a thin film containing bacteria that forms between the teeth and where the teeth meet the gums — and which is a major cause of gum diseases. To remove plaque, teeth should be brushed for five minutes morning or night with fluoride toothpaste, and for two to three minutes at other times during the day. Put a dab of paste on a nylon-tufted toothbrush with a small, flat head. Do not put water on the brush; the saliva in your mouth provides all the moisture you need — too much paste and froth only hampers cleaning.

Even regular brushing, however, will not get rid of all the plaque that builds up between teeth and gums. As a supplement, run dental floss — a strong, unspun, nylon thread — between your teeth once a day for a few minutes. Some people may find flossing difficult to do and they should use wooden sticks instead — especially if they have gaps between their teeth. Although plaque is almost invisible, it can be seen by chewing a disclosing tablet. These tablets contain a dye that stains areas of plaque.

Everything you need for regular dental care can be bought at a good chemist.

Brushing
1   Start with the upper, left-hand side of your mouth. Put the toothbrush at an angle of 45° against the top of your teeth and the bottom of your gum. Brush the outside surface of the teeth by moving the toothbrush head from side to side with short, vibratory strokes. The aim is to keep the bristles in the same area and so demolish the plaque. Then work the brush along the other side of your mouth. Take care not to brush too hard and bruise the gums.

2   Brush the inside surface of the teeth in the same side-to-side way, tilting the brush to make access easier.

3   Brush along the biting surface of the teeth holding the brush steady and using firm, horizontal strokes.
Finish the procedure — which should be carried out twice a day — by brushing your lower teeth in a similar manner.

Flossing
1   Take an unused length of floss about 1½ times the span of your hand.

2   Make a loop of the floss and secure with a double-knot. Put the loop over the last three fingers of each hand in a cat's cradle. Leave your forefingers and thumbs free for controlling the floss.

3   Fit the floss in a straight line between the centre of your two upper front teeth. Draw the floss firmly between the sides of the teeth with a sawing action. When the floss moves easily take it to where the teeth join the gum. Hold the floss tightly against the sides of the teeth and wipe downwards. Take care not to damage the gum between the teeth. Floss all the way around your upper teeth.

4   Repeat the process on lower teeth, wiping upwards. Afterwards, rinse your mouth, drawing the water through your teeth.

345

The healing powers of traditional medicine

Natural medicine – the 'alternative' remedies that complement conventional medicine in the West – has its counterpart in traditional healing methods that have been practised for centuries by indigenous Southern African peoples. In fact, remarkable parallels exist between 'Western' and African healing systems in such alternative categories as herbalism, holistic medicine, naturopathy and faith healing.

The early Dutch settlers practised their own system of folk medicine, and some of these home remedies (*boererate*) are used to this day (see p. 348). Devout members of South Africa's Islamic community have their own system of healing, first introduced to the Cape by slaves brought from the East Indies. This too forms part of the traditional heritage.

Traditional healing is more holistic in its approach than allopathic medicine, which has been accused of emphasising the cure of symptoms rather than the underlying causes, and of dividing illnesses too rigorously into 'physical' and 'mental' categories. In indigenous southern African communities illness tends to be regarded, by contrast, as a misfortune that involves the whole person. It is often by the combined effort of the community that the individual is healed.

Healing dances of the San   Nowhere is this better illustrated than among the hunter-gatherer San people of the Kalahari, whose elaborate 'healing dances', held as often as four times a month, are marathons lasting from dusk till dawn.

In this ancient ceremony the men dance around a group of women, who in turn sit in a circle round a fire clapping and rhythmically calling out. As the night proceeds, 'num' – a powerful spiritual, healing energy emanating from the gods – is activated in the participants, who experience enhanced consciousness. The healing power is thus released to the community, to everyone's benefit.

The San also believe that 'num' is contained in certain plant substances. These are gathered, ground to a powder and then mixed with fat that is set alight; the smoke which is released has its own properties – not only healing, but preventing the incipient illness that the San believe resides in everyone.

African medical tradition   African healing is closely allied to traditional religion, and to the idea that a perpetual communication exists between the living and the spirits of departed ancestors (the 'living dead').

While it is wrong to speak of ancestor 'worship', the departed spirits are certainly regarded with reverence; and it is believed that if the spirits withdraw their protection, evil powers are able to bring about illness and ill-fortune.

Ancestors are also able directly to cause illness, in order to make the victim aware of the error of his ways. Another belief is that dreams are ancestral communications; the meaning of these messages needs therefore to be understood. Interpreting dreams and restoring broken contact with the ancestors are specialist skills.

A Zulu Sangoma or uTwasa (diviner's apprentice). There are several different kinds of sangoma, using different methods of divination.

Sangomas   Such tasks may be performed by a diviner or 'sangoma', one of the main categories of doctors in the black community. Sangomas are diagnosticians. Usually, but not always, they are women. Several different kinds exist, each with their own methods of divination. Some throw bones (mixed with the roots and barks of certain trees), and make their interpretation from the lie of the bones cast on the ground.

Other sangomas enlist the participation of those who have come for advice, by asking them to clap their hands during the divination session.

Sometimes those people seeking advice bring with them short sticks (divining rods), and pound these on the ground during the sangoma's lively performance. The enthusiasm of the clapping, or of the pounding, is believed to help the sangoma to gauge to what extent the audience approves of her disclosures.

Often the gift possessed by a sangoma is said to be hereditary. Nevertheless the novice must be tutored by a master of the craft, and then undergo a colourful 'graduation' ceremony, before he or she can practise in earnest.

Inyangas   The other major category of doctors in traditional African medicine is the 'inyanga' or healer. The true inyanga has a sense of dedication to his calling, which he performs in the service of the ancestral spirits whose instructions he follows. His world is undoubtedly more intuitive, less rational, than that of the Western doctor.

The healing arts of Islam

Religion pervades all the fundamental aspects of the Islamic world, including the field of medicine. In the Koran (the Muslim holy scripture) and in the writings of the Prophet Muhammad, strict dietary and hygienic rules are set out. They are adhered to by the faithful and represent, in effect, a system of 'preventive medicine'.

Thus pork, alcohol and other intoxicants are forbidden, while lawful ('Halaal') food is a prerequisite for the maintenance of good health. Male circumcision is practised; and the ritual of bathing always follows sexual union.

The traditional Muslim physician or 'hakim' is not only a herbalist but something of a psychotherapist too. (He may also indulge in non-medical pursuits such as numerology, the study of the occult significance of numbers.) He is familiar with the holistic notion that the patient's health in its entirety must be attended to. Those who are spiritually whole are not in need of a physician; and there is little purpose in dealing with symptoms alone, when the root of all sickness is elsewhere. Emotional illness and physical illness are linked.

Muslims firmly believe that healing is possible by faith; the more powerful a person's spirit, the greater the likelihood of cure. Recited to the patient on a daily basis, particular verses or a particular chapter of the Koran – for example, chapter 36, the Ya Sin – bring a sense of calm. Ailments such as a snake bite or scorpion bite can be alleviated by such means.

An imam (mosque prayer-leader).

To the faithful, water can effect a cure too. An imam (mosque prayer-leader) may blow on water and then ask the patient to drink it.

Primarily he is a herbalist. He gathers the raw materials for his *mutis* (medicines) on errands through the countryside, where herbs and flowers are collected, roots dug up and bark stripped from trees (often to the disapproval of nature conservationists). Some of these items are pounded into powder form. Mineral matter (such as potassium permanganate) also forms part of the inyanga's medicine-chest.

Like the Western herbalist, the inyanga may prescribe medicine to be taken whole, or to be diluted as an infusion, decoction or inhalant. Medicinal powders may also be fed directly into the bloodstream by means of a small skin incision.

Other *mutis* perform a more esoteric 'medical' function. For example, they may be prescribed to enhance a client's dignity, to prepare a warrior for battle, or to provide protection against lightning or witchcraft – in which case the medicine is not swallowed but scattered over the endangered area.

The traditional black healer is generally highly skilled in his art and has a detailed knowledge and acquaintance with botany. However, some practitioners in South Africa do not pretend to all-round knowledge but specialise in a particular disease, or a particular area of the body such as the heart, lungs or gastrointestinal tract.

What the inyangas recommend

Here are a selection of common complaints and some of the remedies that an inyanga might recommend for them:

Colic and diarrhoea The patient is given a decoction of the roots of the yellow star flower (Hypoxis species) to drink.

Constipation The morning glory (Ipomoea purpurea) provides a strong purgative. For the same complaint, an infusion of the parsley tree (Heteromorpha arborescens) is given as an enema.

Coughs A decoction of the leaves of the ginger bush (Iboza riparis), or an infusion of the leaves and stems of the wild dagga plant (Leonotis leonurus), is prescribed for a cough.

Flatulence This condition may be relieved by eating the thick tubers of one species of spurflower (Plectranthus esculentus). The tubers can be consumed raw or roasted.

Impotence To combat this, or simply as an aphrodisiac to promote a strong sexual appetite, a man drinks a decoction of crushed roots of the besembossie (Corchorus asplenifolius).

Labour pains These are eased by an infusion of cow's tongue leaves (Streptocarpus speciosum). Taken for some days before the confinement, an infusion of yellow starwort roots and leaves (Senecio buplieriodes) ensures an easy delivery.

A muti shop displays its wares in Johannesburg. Many of the traditional medicines on sale in these shops are collected from the countryside.

Septic sores Juice squeezed from fungus-covered wild plums (*Ximenia caffra*) that have fallen to the ground and begun to rot, is applied to the sore. The remedy represents an indigenous use of penicillin.

Sprains Pain is eased by a fomentation made from infusing in hot water the leaves of the miniature iris (*Aristea cognata*).

Worms Tapeworms are expelled by drinking a bitter brew of mountain aloe leaves (*Aloe marlothii*) boiled in water; or by chewing the dried root of the male fern (*Filicis masculinus*). Roundworms are eliminated by drinking an infusion of the leaves and bark of the tinderwood tree (*Clerodendrum glabrum*). Children infested with threadworm are given an enema strained from an infusion of Michaelmas daisy leaves (*Ranunculus pinatus*).

Midwifery More than half the deliveries of black South African children take place away from either hospital or clinic. Playing an essential part on such occasions, as well as during the later stages of the pregnancy, is the traditional birth attendant ('TBA'). She has a store of knowledge equal to that of the midwife of orthodox medical practice, and is well versed in herbal remedies to prepare the mother for labour. When this happens, the TBA will have no lack of women helpers from among the community. Delivery takes place with the mother in the NATURAL CHILDBIRTH squatting position.

Wizards and witches Applied to sangomas and inyangas the popular term 'witch-doctor' is inappropriate and inaccurate. Nevertheless wizards (male) and witches (female) have their traditional place in the rural black community – or at any rate they once did so. They were the exploiters of evil powers – 'black magic' – and therefore they were greatly feared. They caused ill-health and death, and they could be hired by unscrupulous persons to do so.

To further his sinister aims a wizard used poisonous plants, portions of the human anatomy, and even human excreta. He also used a 'familiar' to carry out his orders: a baboon, snake, hornbill, owl or other creature over which he had cast a spell. The 'tokoloshe' or hairy river dwarf was another such familiar.

It was customary for a sangoma to identify a wizard or witch (although more public 'tests' were used too, with the chief and entire community witnessing the event). Traditional punishment for the identified wizard or witch was death by one or other gruesome means.

An orthodox view

There is agreement that traditional medicine plays a vital part in the black community: as many as 80 per cent of South African blacks choose to consult a traditional diviner or healer before resorting to the consulting-rooms of a qualified practitioner of orthodox Western medicine. No reliable head-count is available of sangomas and inyangas practising in the country, but the figure may be as high as 200 000, of which probably no more than half are trained. And while there are as many as 100 voluntary associations of traditional doctors in this country, none have official status. There is no single professional body with which qualified traditional healers can register. At present they can be legally registered only in Natal; registration takes place with the

Natural medicines of the early Dutch settlers

The household remedies long favoured in South Africa's country districts were known as 'Dutch medicines', for they were the traditional cures resorted to by the Voortrekkers and *trekboers* when professional medical help was unavailable. Despite the rough and ready nature of many of the remedies, the early settlers led apparently healthy lives – thanks in part to strict hygiene, for example in protecting water supplies from contamination.

Among the items packed in the farmer's sturdy wooden medicine-chest or *trommel* were preparations made from indigenous herbs and other plants. There were purgatives (purging being standard treatment for a whole range of illnesses), poultices, blood-cleansers, gargles, hair-conditioners and much else. Some herbs (such as buchu and wild dagga) were credited with an astonishingly wide range of healing properties.

Interestingly, the store of wisdom built up by the white settler herbalists closely matched that of the San and the black 'inyangas' in many respects.

Another category of remedies was prepared from the body fluids (or excreta) of wild animals. Thus, an infusion of goat's dung was drunk by a patient with measles, while vulture fat was applied to muscles and fibrous tissue affected by lumbago.

Also in the *trommel* were a variety of patent medicines. Many had colourful names, including *pampoensalf* (ointment of yellow ozide of mercury) and the foul-smelling *duiwelsdrek* (asafoetida). Keen to sell such preparations were itinerant peddlers or *wonderdoeners*, who gained a high reputation among members of the rural community.

Evidence of the enduring value placed on folk remedies is seen in old South African cookbooks, in which supplementary chapters include homely – sometimes harrowing – hints on treating all kinds of ailments, from boils and burns to piles and quinsy.

KwaZulu Ministry of Health in Ulundi, and the qualification is recognised throughout South Africa.

Today the obnoxious practices which are sometimes associated with witchcraft – including the denunciation of any person with supernatural powers as a wizard or witch – are banned by South African statute; but the law-courts still have to deal with such cases on occasions.

TUBERCULOSIS

Tuberculosis (TB) is a serious infectious disease still prevalent in poorer areas of South Africa, but also sporadically in the affluent population. It is caused by the bacillus *Mycobacterium tuberculosis*. With infection, small, destructive nodules known as tubercles form in body tissue. They may do so anywhere in the body, though the organs most often affected are the lungs, leading to pulmonary TB, once known as 'consumption'.

The lymph glands may also become infected, while if the bacteria enter the bloodstream the disease can spread throughout the body to cause 'miliary tuberculosis', characterised by the growth of many tiny tubercles. Yet another form of the disease, tuberculous meningitis, affects the membrane covering the brain.

Generalised symptoms of TB include loss of appetite, loss of weight, weakness, fever and sweating. The main symptoms of lung TB are persistent coughing (in which the sputum may be blood-flecked), chest pains and breathlessness. Bones infected with TB grow soft and deformed, with localised pain.

Tuberculosis is most easily spread via infected droplets of moisture expelled when a patient coughs or sneezes.

What the therapists recommend

Herbal medicine Honeybush tea, now sold commercially as a healthy, caffeine-free tea, is also a rural treatment for TB as well as coughs, colds and other lung infections. Other indigenous South African remedies include a tea infused from the leaves of the pennywort or wild violet.

Homoeopathy A notifiable disease, tuberculosis must be treated in the first instance by orthodox medicine. Homoeopathic treatment can, however, be useful at a later stage. (*Silica* should be avoided as it can reactivate the TB.)

Naturopathy A carefully controlled diet combined with much rest – but some regular *light* exercise for the lungs and the muscles – is recommended. The high, dry air of the Karoo and the Transvaal is beneficial.

An orthodox view

The patient will be referred to a specialist, who will prescribe daily drug treatment to kill the TB bacteria. The treatment usually lasts for several months and may have to be continued for a year or two if the body's response is slow. Most patients can eventually be restored to full health.

Mass screening by X-ray keeps a check on the broad incidence of TB in the population, and is a means of detecting the disease earlier. It is recommended that all South African infants be immunised against TB. As a preventive measure, antibiotic drugs should be prescribed for anyone having contact with a TB patient – for example, those who form part of the same household.

TURNER SYNDROME

Turner Syndrome – named after the American doctor who reported on the condition in 1938, Dr Henry Turner – is a chromosomal abnormality that affects females only; approximately one in 2 500 girls are born with it. While the normal complement of chromosomes in each cell of the body is 46, most Turner females have only 45, one of the two X sex-chromosomes being missing.

Sometimes the second X chromosome is present but defective. And occasionally the body contains both normal cells and those with a missing X chromosome – a condition known as 'mosaicism', which may mean that the symptoms of Turner Syndrome are fewer or less marked.

A symptom common to all affected by the syndrome is short stature: the average adult height is 141 cm. Other noticeable external features may include swelling of the front of the hands and feet at birth; a short neck, with a low hairline; loose folds of skin at the back of the neck; a broad chest; and arms that turn out a little at the elbow.

Many babies and young children with Turner Syndrome experience recurrent bouts of middle-ear infection (otitis media) which, unless diagnosed and treated early, can be a source of discomfort and distress to both children and parents.

A 10-20 per cent minority of children have some cardiovascular abnormality, in particular a narrowing ('coarctation') of the aorta, which can be corrected by surgery.

In adolescence secondary sexual characteristics such as breast development are retarded or absent, and menstruation fails to take place. The person is infertile and will be unable to bear children.

The intelligence of those with Turner Syndrome is normal.

What the therapists recommend

Anthroposophical Medicine Despite the absence of a physical 'cure' for the condition, much lies within the range of this holistic system to help girls and women with Turner Syndrome lead normal, happy lives – including RELAXATION and YOGA, and informed parental or professional advice to help achieve a healthy self-image and sexual identity.

An orthodox view

A surgical operation can correct the coarctation of the aorta. Loose folds of skin at the neck can be treated by plastic surgery.

Dosages of the female sex hormones oestrogen and progesterone are given to promote sexual development at puberty (and also to stop premature ageing, and the onset of OSTEOPOROSIS). However, this medication is unable to render the patient fertile. Hormonal therapy – with small doses of anabolic steroids or growth hormone – may also be given, to increase growth.

A network of active Turner Syndrome support groups exists in South Africa. For information about these, and to find out more about the syndrome itself, you can write to the Turner Syndrome Contact Group, 8 Adrienne Avenue, Glendower, Edenvale 1610 (telephone 011-537574).

TYPHOID FEVER

A potentially serious illness

Typhoid fever is an infectious disease transmitted via food or water contaminated with the bacterium *Salmonella typhi*. Carriers of the disease excrete the bacteria in their faeces – and may continue to do so for years after recovering from the disease itself. The illness is also known as enteric fever because it affects the intestines.

Symptoms include a severe headache followed by fever; abdominal pain; constipation that may be followed by diarrhoea; and a rash of small, raised, pink spots on the chest and abdomen.

What the therapists recommend

The condition may be so serious – or deteriorate so quickly – that hospitalisation is required.

Naturopathy The patient must be kept well hydrated. Remedy potassium loss with a diet of root vegetables such as carrots, turnips and potatoes, washed but not peeled.

Homoeopathy Remedies include podophyllin, *Bryonia* and *Rhus tox*.

Herbal Medicine Make a tea from the fruit, leaves and stems of the dysentery herb (or 'crane's bill'), and sip this at regular two-hour intervals.

An orthodox view

If treatment is delayed, typhoid can be life-threatening. A patient may therefore be placed in hospital. Antibiotic drugs are usually sufficient to quell the disease, which should clear up in a month.

ULCERS

There are many different kinds of ulcer – the medical term for a break in the skin or the mucous lining of the gut or mouth that does not heal. They range from peptic ulcers – painful and potentially serious ones in the digestive tract – to small mouth ulcers. Elderly people in particular can suffer extensive skin ulcers, caused by CIRCULATION PROBLEMS or VARICOSE VEINS.

Gastric (stomach) ulcers, duodenal ulcers (in the small intestine) and oesophageal (gullet) ulcers are caused by excess acid and/or the digestive enzyme pepsin. Small ones often develop, but cause no symptoms and heal without treatment. More serious stomach ulcers occur most often in men of 60 to 80, and result in recurrent upper abdominal pain and vomiting. A severe attack may last up to eight weeks.

On the other hand, duodenal ulcers occur mostly in young men subject to STRESS, and produce dull recurrent pain in the upper and central abdomen.

The pain of peptic ulcers is relieved by milk and alkalis, but aggravated by stress, excess stomach acid (see ACID STOMACH) and SMOKING, which increases acid production. The pain occurs after meals and there is tenderness below the breastbone.

Rarely, peptic ulcers bleed, causing bloody vomiting and black faeces. They may also perforate – rupture – and let the gut contents, including bacteria, into the abdomen, causing peritonitis, with severe pain and perhaps shock and a rigid abdominal wall.

Warning Any severe abdominal pain should be investigated by a doctor, and a perforated ulcer in particular demands immediate medical treatment. Leg ulcers, which are notoriously slow and difficult to heal, should also receive medical attention.

What the therapists recommend
HOMOEOPATHY
Peptic ulcers Argent. nit. is recommended when there is FLATULENCE and gnawing pain in the pit of the stomach, which is worse when pressure is applied and after food, and the sufferer craves sweet things that aggravate the pain. Try Arsen. alb. if the sufferer is anxious and meticulous, experiences DIARRHOEA and burning pain immediately after food, and has no appetite.

Lycopodium is generally recommended for flatulence, and the sufferer feels full after the smallest amount of food, desires sweet foods and cannot bear tight clothing.

When the sufferer has pain half an hour after eating a meal, headache and constipation, feels better after vomiting, and is irritable, especially in the morning, Nux vomica

may help. These preparations should each be taken in the 6th potency.

Leg (varicose) ulcers The following remedies are said to promote healing (use the 6th potency and take three or four times daily for 21 days – or less if improvement occurs sooner): Kali bich. if the ulcer looks as if cut out with a punch and there is a white discharge; Hamamelis if varicose veins are prevalent; Nitric acid if the ulcers bleed easily and there are pains similar to those caused by splinters; Merc. sol. if the discharge is smelly; Carbo veg. if the sufferer is elderly with poor circulation and respiratory problems; Lachesis if the ulcer is deep and bleeds easily, there is a putrid discharge and the surrounding skin is purplish-blue.

NATUROPATHY
Peptic ulcers The advice is to eat little and often, gradually building on an initial bland diet by including more vegetables, especially cooked ones, pulses and grains. Avoid tobacco, alcohol and sugar. It is also important to find ways of relaxing and releasing tension (see RELAXATION AND BREATHING).

Leg ulcers Practitioners often suggest a vitamin E supplement to promote healing, for example 400 iu a day.

ACUPUNCTURE
Gastric and duodenal ulcers Points on the liver, stomach, spleen, conception, bladder and governing meridians are treated.

Leg ulcers Local points are treated, and also the corresponding points on the other side of the body. Points on the meridians passing through the affected area – usually the lung and spleen meridians – and the large intestine and governing meridians are also treated.

Other alternative treatment
Herbal Medicine For peptic and gastric ulcers drink a comfrey or mallow tea. Smooth a herb ointment such as calendula cream on the skin around an external ulcer, then apply to the ulcer a comfrey root powder poultice. See also MOUTH ULCERS.

An orthodox view
Doctors can usually diagnose peptic ulcers from their symptoms. However, further tests are usually necessary for an accurate diagnosis to be made. Many gastric and duodenal ulcers can be diagnosed by means of barium meal X-rays.

A more accurate diagnosis can be made by introducing a flexible tube into the stomach with an optical viewing device which allows the ulcer to be clearly identified.

Modern drugs such as cimetidine (Tagamet) and ranitidine (Zantac) reduce the output of stomach acid and permit healing.

Do's and don'ts for peptic ulcers

Do eat a wholefood diet (see EATING FOR HEALTH).
Do try to relax and control your stress.
Do make sure that you have enough sleep (see SLEEP DISORDERS).
Do take regular EXERCISE.
Don't smoke.
Don't drink coffee, tea, alcohol or cola.
Don't eat refined sugar, refined flour or their products, or junk food.
Don't eat hot, spicy foods, or highly acid items such as apples.
Don't take aspirin or anti-inflammatory drugs if possible, especially on an empty stomach; they irritate the gut.

Surgery for peptic ulcers has become unusual since the introduction of such drugs.

Skin ulcers can be prevented by regular exercise, wearing support socks, stockings or tights if you have varicose veins, and by avoiding injury to a fragile skin (see SKIN DISORDERS). Skin ulcers, particularly varicose ulcers, need skilled nursing. Regular dressings and compression bandages, which improve blood circulation, help, but healing can take a long time, perhaps years. In severe cases, skin grafts may be advised.

ULTRASOUND

The therapeutic use of ultrasound – sound waves too high-pitched to be detected by the human ear – is known as ultrasonics. The waves are produced by placing a quartz crystal in an electric field, which causes it to vibrate at a high frequency.

Ultrasonics is a form of SOUND THERAPY, and is said to be particularly effective for treating SPORTS INJURIES, SPRAINS and strained muscles. It is thought to work by producing heat when used in higher doses, and by bringing about direct changes in body cells at lower doses. Therapists who use the technique say that the effect is to speed up healing in soft tissues and bones, and to relieve pain by changing the way in which nerve impulses are conducted.

In orthodox medicine, ultrasonic waves are used to build up pictures of organs and tissues inside the body, for example, to diagnose the state of a patient's heart or check on the progress of a baby in the womb. High-frequency sound waves are directed at the appropriate part of the body and an image of its internal appearance is then created from the echo that comes back.

VAGINAL DISORDERS

Some discharge from the vagina is normal, but when it itches and the discharge is excessive and there is an unpleasant odour, there may be an infection. This is most frequently due to *Candida albicans*, the fungus that causes THRUSH. Alternatively, *Trichomonas*, a small oval micro-organism, or a bacterium such as that causing gonorrhoea may be the cause. A tampon left in after a period has finished can also cause an unpleasant vaginal discharge, as can threadworm infection (see WORMS).

After the MENOPAUSE, lack of hormones may cause a dry, irritated, sore vagina, and there is often pain during sexual intercourse.

A tender swelling of the small mucus-excreting glands – known as Bartholin's glands – near the vaginal opening is known as Bartholinitis. The glands may become infected but will not become cancerous.

CANCER of the vagina is rare, but cancer can spread to the vagina from the cervix, the mouth of the womb. Regular cervical smear tests should detect any irregularity long before this stage, however.

What the therapists recommend
HOMOEOPATHY
Self help Several remedies are offered:
Itching vulva When the area is itchy with an unpleasant odour, and these symptoms are worse when the sufferer is hot and after washing, try *Sulphur* 6. For an itchy, red eruption which is relieved by heat, use *Rhus tox.* 6. Continue to take these remedies three times daily for 14 days.
Menopausal dryness Apply *Calendula* cream to soothe and lubricate. *Bryonia* 30 is said to help the dryness in women who also tend to be constipated and have chest problems. *Nat. mur.* may be better for women who have tearful depression. In both cases, take the remedy morning and night for 14 days. If the condition continues, you should seek homoeopathic medical help.
Bartholinitis Use *Belladonna* 30 during the early stages of the infection when the area is hot, red and swollen. If there is a discharge of yellow pus and the area is very tender, use *Hepar sulph.* 30. Take either remedy four times daily for three to four days.

Other alternative treatments
Naturopathy A consultation is recommended, but local salt washes or applications of live yoghurt are often helpful.
Herbal Medicine A consultation is recommended. Herbalists give local douches and washes, and use eliminative and/or hormonal remedies internally to restore the natural vaginal defences.

An orthodox view
If the discharge is caused by an infection, the cause will be revealed by laboratory examination of a swab taken from the vagina. Antibiotic or antifungal tablets or pessaries are then prescribed. Unfortunately, vaginal infections such as thrush tend to recur, and it is often necessary to treat the sexual partner. Alternative remedies are often just as helpful as conventional medicine in the prevention of recurrent vaginal discharges, but if you do have one, consult your doctor to check that you are not suffering from DIABETES.

For menopausal vaginitis, doctors prescribe oestrogen cream to be applied regularly to the vagina, or oral hormone replacement therapy (HRT; see p. 238).

VARICOSE VEINS
When blood flow is obstructed

In this often painful, uncomfortable condition, veins become distended, lengthened and 'knotted'. The surface veins of the legs are most commonly affected, but veins inside the rectum may also become varicose (see PILES), and varicose veins may also occur around the vulva – the female external sex organs – in PREGNANCY.

Obstruction of the blood flow is the prime cause of varicose veins, and this usually occurs when an organ presses on nearby blood vessels. In the case of leg veins, the problem usually arises in the rectum. The obstructed blood flow causes the veins' one-way valves to lose their efficiency, allowing blood to flow backwards, away from the heart. The result of this is distension of the veins.

Varicose leg veins are common from the teens, and are frequent in pregnancy. If only small they may cause no noticeable symptoms, but if extensive they result in aching legs – particularly after standing – and sometimes swollen ankles. People who spend long periods standing, such as housewives and police officers, are particularly susceptible. OBESITY can also be a contributory factor.

A varicose vein may become inflamed, causing pain and redness – a condition

Valve in a healthy vein (left) halts the backward flow of blood. Faulty valve in a varicose vein (right) lets blood run back.

known as phlebitis. Sometimes blood clots form, and are felt as hard lumps in the veins. If the circulation is severely impaired, the blood supply to the skin may be inadequate and varicose (skin) ULCERS develop.

What the therapists recommend
NATUROPATHY
Self help Hot and cold baths or splashes are useful. Sufferers are advised to take plenty of EXERCISE. They should avoid standing for long periods, and try to relax for short spells with legs raised on a cushion.
Consultation Dietary changes may be recommended, particularly if the sufferer is overweight. Supplements such as vitamins C and E, rutin and lecithin may be suggested.

An orthodox view
It is not possible to repair damaged blood-vessel valves, but doctors invariably advise sufferers to help their circulation by taking regular exercise and wearing support socks, stockings or tights. They should try to avoid standing for long periods, and also sitting with their legs crossed. A diet that is high in FIBRE will help to avoid constipation, and so relieve any obstruction of the blood flow in the pelvic region, where the rectum presses on the blood vessels.

A doctor may suggest injection of troublesome veins with a chemical such as ethanolamine to shrink or close them. In more severe cases, surgery may be necessary to strip out the veins through incisions in the leg. Once veins have been blocked by injection or stripped out, the blood will reroute through other veins, which, under pressure, may in time also become varicose. Legs from which varicose veins have been stripped must remain bandaged for some weeks.

VEGANISM

The diet that vegans follow contains no animal produce. All their food is entirely of vegetable origin (see p.352).

Sensible ways to 'go vegetarian'

People become vegetarians for a variety of reasons, from simple concern for animals or for their own health, to complex religious beliefs. A meatless diet is neither a cure-all nor an obstacle to health – which may be improved or damaged according to how the diet is managed.

True vegetarians do not eat meat or fish, but many will eat animal produce other than flesh, such as eggs, milk and cheese. Vegans do not eat any animal produce at all, so their diet consists entirely of foods of plant origin. A third group might be called partial vegetarians – people who have eliminated all or most meat from their diet, but who eat fish. All types of diet from regular meat-eating to wholly vegan can provide a basis for a healthy life – if properly managed. There are nutritional benefits but also risks associated with each style of eating. See Eating for Health.

Eating lots of red meats, eggs and dairy foods may overload the diet with fat, though this need not be so if lean meats and reduced-fat cheeses are selected. The diet will ensure ample intake of iron and calcium; on the other hand, its content of starch and fibre may be low.

Vegans will not have fat, starch or fibre problems, but need to take care over vitamin B_{12}, iron, calcium and zinc. Vegetarians who rely too much on eggs and cheese will, like big meat eaters, run the risk of too many kilojoules and saturated fats. They will not, however, share the vegans' potential shortage of calcium, iron or vitamin B_{12}. See the tables of foods rich in various nutrients on p. 357.

Vegetarian sources of vital nutrients

Protein   Meeting protein needs is rarely a problem for vegetarians. Many foods contain only small amounts of protein in themselves but together they make a useful contribution to overall protein intake. Beans, lentils, peas, bread, potatoes, porridge, rice and vegetables all contribute protein to the diet.

Vegetarians who also eat cheese, milk and eggs get ample protein, but vegans need to take a little care. Dried beans and other pulses are likely to figure prominently in their diet. Beans contain as much protein per pound as meat when dry, but when rehydrated and cooked they contain much less – about a third as much per serving as meat. This is about the same protein content as bread has.

There are differences between the proteins in various foods. They all contain a mixture of more than 20 amino acids, but in varying proportions. The amino-acid profiles of some proteins make them easier for the body to use. Sometimes, combining different foods makes the protein easier to use. Pulse-and-cereal combinations such as beans and bread have a protein value that matches meat.

Vitamin B_{12}   Only animal foods and micro-organisms such as moulds contain vitamin B_{12}. Vegans, therefore, have to take particular care to ensure their supply. Many decide to take vitamin pills. Breast-fed infants of vegan mothers will suffer a deficiency unless they are given a supplement; be sure to consult a doctor about what is suitable.

Many foods contain harmless traces of mould that yield some B_{12}. Indeed, for the millions of vegans throughout the world these, together with fermented foods and drinks, are the source of their B_{12}. Because vegetarian food in this country is much cleaner now than it once was, it provides less of the vital B_{12} via moulds. Vegans can increase their intake by spreading their bread with yeast extract.

Vegetarians will get ample B_{12} from milk and eggs.

Iron   Meat, especially red meat and offal, is the food that contains most iron. The iron in meat – reduced ferrous iron – is also easy for the body to absorb.

Fibre-rich foods such as vegetables, cereals and, to a lesser extent, fruits contain some iron, but as oxidised ferric iron which is not readily absorbed. To convert it to an easy-to-absorb form, you should eat vitamin C (in oranges or tomatoes, for example) at the same meal.

It is not only vegetarians and vegans who need to take care about this. Now that health promotion is urging people to eat less red meat to help reduce fat consumption, there is the accompanying risk of iron deficiency. Many people are already on a marginal iron intake that is barely sufficient to meet the body's needs. Women who experience heavy blood loss (hence iron loss) at menstruation should pay particular attention to boosting their iron intake.

Calcium   Milk and its derivatives butter, cream, cheese and Yoghurt are the main sources of calcium in a non-vegan diet; they provide more than half of most people's calcium. White bread, to which calcium is added to help ensure sufficient intake, accounts for a further one-fifth of most people's calcium. The remainder comes from greens and beans, fish bones – in tinned sardines and salmon, for example – and hard tap water.

It is vegans who may have difficulty maintaining an adequate calcium level. They do not eat milk products and their difficulty is even worse because fibre-rich foods – a mainstay of the vegan diet – tend to make calcium more difficult for the body to absorb. Hence, vegans need to eat even more of the source foods they find acceptable to get enough calcium. Eating plenty of greens, beans and white bread will help.

Zinc   Zinc is found more in animal than in vegetable foods, and is usually associated with protein. Vegetarians get most of their zinc from wholegrain cereals which will normally be consumed in generous amounts. As with calcium and iron, dietary fibre makes zinc more difficult for the body to absorb, so a vegetarian's diet must include a plentiful supply of zinc before enough of it will be absorbed.

Making the change

Turning vegetarian does not necessarily solve all nutritional problems; it may solve some, but it raises others. What happens all too often is that would-be vegetarians simply switch from meat and fish to eggs and cheese; nuts too become a favourite food. The likely increase in kilojoules, fat and body weight is quite the opposite of what they hope.

When you change to a new style of eating, your body will have to adapt. It does not like to change. Its metabolism and control systems are designed to maintain the status quo no matter what may be going on in the outside world. If you suddenly eat much more fibre, you will probably suffer from gas, abdominal bloating and discomfort. If you suddenly eat less saturated fat and more polyunsaturates, your liver has to make major changes in its working to cope with the new situation. Take up a new eating pattern gradually, just as you would a major exercise programme.

Adaptation takes time. Change your diet bit by bit, and your body will be able to retune without difficulty. Start with a few vegetarian dishes a week. Then have two or three entirely vegetarian days a week before you convert full-time. In this way you will make your mistakes while you can still rely on your meat and fish to provide essential nutrients.

Learn about true vegetarian recipes as well as egg and cheese dishes. Indian cookery includes a wide range of original and nourishing vegetarian recipes – as do Thai, Malay and Chinese cookery (see pp. 354-6).

If you prefer simple Anglo-Saxon dishes, start with beans on toast, a meal or snack which is nutritionally excellent. Do not worry about reports of the sugar content in tinned beans; the amount is small and unlikely to harm your teeth. You could then move on to bean and vegetable casseroles, preferably eaten with a cereal food such as bread, rice or sweetcorn. As you extend your range, try to mix as many ingredients as possible to ensure a good nutritional balance.

Any diet should include a wide variety of different foods to ensure a sufficient supply of all the nutrients, and to reduce the risk of excesses. This is even more important for vegetarians than for meat eaters.

Food combining has been made into a dietary cult by some food pundits, often with no logical basis. The best-known combining system – the HAY DIET – is, however, nutritionally sound. Some others are unwise fads that abandon common sense and can be downright dangerous.

Vegetarians are as much a prey to fads and fashions in eating as anyone else – but must resist them. Bran with everything, especially concentrated bran or bran-fortified foods, can create nutritional imbalance. Too much bran is every bit as bad as too little, and could in time cause mineral deficiencies as well as intestinal discomfort.

Polyunsaturates too are being overvalued. The vegetable origin of most such oils makes them acceptable to vegetarians, but as yet we cannot predict the long-term effects of overloading the body with them. CANCER and GALLSTONES have been suggested as possible consequences.

In its report *Diet and Cardiovascular Disease* (1984), the British Department of Health's Committee on Medical Aspects of Food Policy (COMA) urged a decrease in total fat consumption with an increase in the proportion of polyunsaturates. This was widely reported. What received little mention was that COMA also set an upper limit for the polyunsaturates. Uncontrolled consumption of safflower, sunflower and soya oils or margarines made from them can provide an excess of polyunsaturates. Olive oil is thought to be safer.

Not peeling potatoes is another current fashion. It is believed this will improve nutrition by retaining more vitamin C and dietary fibre. In fact, the nutritional benefit is minimal or non-existent. More important, though, is that not peeling increases the consumption of solanine, the natural pesticide in potatoes, which is poisonous to humans in large amounts. So, on the whole, peeling is preferable.

When other factors count

Taking up a vegetarian or vegan diet should not be seen as a guarantee of health. Some people have been misled by scientific surveys that suggest good health is more frequent in vegetarian communities than in the population as a whole. Trappist monks and Seventh Day Adventists are often quoted as examples. They have long life, low incidence of cancer and HEART DISORDERS, and good BLOOD PRESSURE. However, they also have well-ordered lives that differ in other ways: strong religious beliefs, secure family or other supportive social groups, little or no SMOKING or drinking of alcohol contribute as much as – or more than – diet to their health. At the other extreme, the majority of the world's population is, of necessity, vegetarian and many of them are malnourished and sick. However, their health is poor not because they are vegetarian but because they cannot get enough food and their drinking water is unclean.

Eating the vegetarian way clearly demands special skill. It has to be done properly if dietary balance is to be achieved. There are new shopping and cooking habits to be learned, as well as new arts in menu planning to be acquired. But once the necessary skills are mastered, the diet will be as nourishing and easy to manage as any other.

A varied diet containing ample vegetables, fruits and cereals is a good basis for health whether or not meat, fish or dairy foods are eaten as well. Vegetarians and vegans need the same nutrients as others and will easily obtain them if they have four helpings a day of staple foods (potato, bread, pasta, rice, for example); four of vegetables or fruits; and four of protein foods such as beans, peas, lentils, nuts, fresh milk, cheese or eggs. The ingredients should be as varied as possible and eaten in just sufficient quantities to maintain a healthy body weight.

Health food shops stock a wide variety of vegetarian and vegan cookery books. For more information on the vegetarian way of life you can contact the Vegetarian Society of South Africa, P O Box 23567, Joubert Park 2044 (telephone 011-6780164).

Five vegetable feasts from around the world

Black-eyed beans and mushrooms from India (1)

180 g dried, soaked
   black-eyed beans
180 g fresh
   mushrooms
4 ½ tablespoons
   vegetable oil
1 teaspoon cumin seeds
1 stick cinnamon
120 g peeled and
   chopped onions
3 peeled and chopped
   garlic cloves

300 g peeled and
   chopped tomatoes
1 ½ teaspoons ground
   coriander
1 teaspoon ground cumin
   seeds
¼ teaspoon cayenne
   pepper
½ teaspoon powdered
   turmeric
2 tablespoons parsley
Salt and black pepper

Bring the beans to the boil in a large pan of water. Cover and simmer gently on a low heat for 2 minutes. Then turn off the heat and leave the pan covered for 1 hour.

Chop the mushrooms lengthwise into thin slices. Heat the vegetable oil in a large frying pan over medium heat. When hot add the cumin seeds and cinnamon, and fry for 5-6 seconds. Add the chopped onions and garlic and stir-fry until the onions begin to brown. Next, add the mushrooms and fry until soft, stirring all the time. Add the tomatoes, coriander, ground cumin, cayenne, turmeric and parsley, and stir-fry for 1 minute. Cover and leave on a low heat for 10 minutes, then turn off the heat.

Boil the beans again, turn down the heat and simmer until soft. Add the mushrooms and other ingredients, and season. Simmer for 30 minutes, stirring occasionally. Remove the cinnamon and serve with boiled or fried rice and Indian bread such as roti. Serves four.

Spicy Thai salad (2)

2 large or 3 small limes
1 level teaspoon caster
   sugar
1 teaspoon anchovy
   essence
2 ripe mangoes
2 ripe pawpaws
1 bunch spring onions,
   trimmed and sliced
1 red or green chilli,
   deseeded and chopped

1 large tomato, cut
   into 25 mm cubes
½ cucumber, diced into
   25 mm cubes
4 sprigs of coriander
   leaves
8 fresh basil leaves,
   roughly chopped
2 small lettuces for
   garnish
Salt to taste

Squeeze the lime juice into a large bowl and mix in the sugar and anchovy essence. Peel the mangoes and pawpaws and cut into 50 mm strips, discarding the mango stones and the pawpaw pips. Put the strips into the bowl with the lime juice. Then add the sliced spring onions, finely chopped chilli, diced tomato and cucumber. Reserving a few coriander leaves for garnishing, wash and chop the rest, and the basil, and add to the bowl.

Wash and arrange the larger lettuce leaves on individual plates. Chop the lettuce hearts, add to the salad, season with salt, toss well and spoon onto the plates. Garnish with the remaining coriander leaves and serve immediately. Serves four.

Italian tagliatelle with mushroom and walnut sauce (3)

360 g fresh tagliatelle	15 g butter
120 g shelled walnuts	1 clove garlic, crushed
2 tablespoons virgin olive oil or walnut oil	240 g carton Greek strained yoghurt
½ medium onion, finely chopped	2 tablespoons fresh parsley, chopped (Italian flat-leaved parsley, if possible)
240 g field mushrooms, sliced	Salt and freshly ground black pepper to taste

Bring a saucepan of salted water to the boil. While you are waiting, wrap the shelled walnuts in a clean tea towel and partially crush them with a rolling pin, making sure that you leave some large pieces. Melt the butter gently in a large, nonstick pan. Add the walnuts and cook them over a gentle heat for about 2-3 minutes, stirring frequently and taking care not to burn them. Add the tagliatelle to the boiling water and cook as instructed until it is 'al dente'.

Remove the walnuts and wipe the pan clean. Add the oil and chopped onion to the pan and cook over moderate heat for 7-8 minutes until soft and golden, stirring occasionally. Add the sliced mushrooms and crushed garlic, turn to a high heat and cook for 5 minutes, stirring continually, until the juices run and the mushrooms are tender.

Remove the pan from the heat and add the walnuts and the yoghurt, 1 tablespoonful at a time, beating well to mix after each addition. Return the pan to a very low heat and stir until the yoghurt is heated through. Do not allow the yoghurt to boil or it will separate. Add half the chopped parsley and season with salt and pepper.

Drain the pasta and mix with the sauce immediately. Taste and adjust the seasoning, then transfer onto heated individual plates. Sprinkle with the remaining parsley and serve with a light red wine and a mixed salad. Serves four.

Note This recipe is unsuitable for vegans, who may like to experiment with soya yoghurt instead of Greek yoghurt.

Ratatouille from France (4)

3 large baby marrows	1 large onion
3 large aubergines	4 cloves garlic
6 large tomatoes	6 tablespoons olive oil
1 large green pepper	Salt and black pepper to taste
1 small red pepper	

Cut the stalks off the baby marrows and aubergines, wash them and chop into 13-25 mm slices. Place the slices in a colander with a weighted plate on top and leave for 1 hour to press out excess moisture. Skin the tomatoes and chop them into chunks. Wash the green and red peppers, remove the seeds and white ribs inside, and dice the flesh. Peel and slice the onion, and coarsely chop the garlic.

Heat the olive oil in a large saucepan and fry the chopped onion and garlic for 5 minutes on a low heat until transparent. Add the peppers, cook for 10 minutes more, then add the re-maining ingredients and season to taste. Cover the pan and cook over a low heat for 35 minutes, stirring from time to time. Season further if required.

Serve hot with rice, pasta or a jacket potato for a filling meal, or cold with salads for a lighter one. Serves four.

Stir-fried Chinese vegetables (5)

4 carrots	2 tablespoons sherry
240 g cauliflower florets	2 tablespoons brown sugar
Two 240 g tins bamboo shoots	4 tablespoons soya sauce
300 g tofu	240 g mangetout
150 ml vegetable oil	240 g bean sprouts
1 thinly sliced onion	1 red pepper, cut into thin strips
50 mm fresh ginger, finely chopped	Salt and black pepper
2 cloves garlic, crushed	2 tablespoons sesame oil

Cut the carrots into thin matchstick strips, and divide the cauliflower florets into small pieces. Blanch both vegetables in boiling water for 1-2 minutes. Drain the bamboo shoots and reserve 120 ml of the liquid. Cut the shoots into small strips and set aside together with the blanched carrots and cauliflower.

Drain the tofu, dry it with a piece of paper towelling and cut it into squares. Heat the vegetable oil in a deep frying pan over moderate heat and fry the tofu pieces until crisp and slightly brown. Remove them from the pan and dry off excess oil with paper towelling.

Pour off all except 1 tablespoon of oil from the frying pan. Add the onion, ginger and garlic to the pan and fry gently for 5 minutes. In the meantime, mix together in a jug the bamboo shoot liquid, sherry, sugar and soya sauce.

Slice the tips off the mangetout, and add mangetout, bean sprouts, carrots, cauliflower, red pepper and bamboo shoots to the pan. Turn up the heat and stir-fry the vegetables for 5 minutes. Add the mixed liquid ingredients and bring to the boil, stirring all the time.

Reduce the heat and add the fried tofu pieces, with salt and pepper to season. Simmer for 1-2 minutes, stirring continuously, then place in a heated serving dish and sprinkle with sesame oil. Serve immediately, with rice or noodles. Serves four to six.

(Facing page) Food tables such as these contain valuable information that can help vegans and vegetarians to plan a healthy diet and make sure that they do not go short of protein or important vitamins and minerals. When using the tables, bear in mind that the nutrient quantities are given per 100 g of food, so the amount you get depends on the weight of your portion. While 100 g of pasta or eggs is not a big serving, it would be a lot of brewer's yeast or Marmite to consume, even over a period of several days. So although brewer's yeast and Marmite come higher up on the protein table, eggs and pasta will probably make a much greater contribution to your overall daily intake.
The more concentrated sources of nutrients are best used as supplements to enrich other foods – as when you sprinkle wheatgerm or brewer's yeast on a bowl of breakfast cereal – or as alternatives to less healthy foods also eaten in small quantities – by spreading Marmite instead of jam on bread, for example.

Vegetarian sources of essential nutrients

PROTEIN
grams per 100 g

Brewer's yeast	46,1
Marmite	39,7
Peanuts	26,9
Wheatgerm	25,2
Split peas	24,5
Cheddar cheese	23,9
Lima beans	20,7
Cottage cheese	19,2
Almonds	18,6
Walnuts	15,0
Oatmeal	14,2
Pasta	14,0
Eggs	12,8
Wholewheat bread	9,5
White bread	8,5
Cornflakes	7,9
White rice	7,5
Cream cheese	7,1
Peas	6,7
Baked beans	5,7
Dried apricots	5,2
Brussels sprouts	4,4
Sweetcorn	3,7
Milk	3,5
Broccoli	3,3
Raisins	2,3
Potatoes	2,0
Avocados	1,7
Cabbage	1,4
Bananas	1,2
Fresh apricots	1,0

By comparison, tinned tuna contains 23,9 g, tinned sardines 21,1, chicken 20,2, calf's or lamb's liver 20,1, beef and lamb 18,5.

CALCIUM
milligrams per 100 g

Cheese, Cheddar	873
Cheese, processed	716
Almonds	254
Kale	225
Egg yolks	147
Broccoli	130
Milk	118
Brewer's yeast	106
Marmite	95
Dried apricots	86
Wheatgerm	84
Walnuts	83
Cottage cheese	82
Raisins	78
Peanuts	74
Split peas	73
Lima beans	68
Lettuce	62
Bread, wholewheat	60
Bread, white	56
Oatmeal	54
Eggs	54
Baked beans	49
Cabbage	46
Radishes	44
Brown rice	39
Brussels sprouts	34
Oranges	33
Onions	32
Strawberries	28
Dried apples	24
Pasta	22
Peas	22
Asparagus	21
Grapes	17
Fresh apricots	16
Tomatoes	11
Potatoes	11
Green peppers	11
Cornflakes	10
White rice	9
Bananas	8

By comparison, tinned salmon contains 67 mg, tinned tuna 30, tinned sardines 29, liver and chicken 16, and beef and lamb 11.

IRON
milligrams per 100 g

Brewer's yeast	18,2
Wheatgerm	8,1
Lima beans	7,5
Egg yolks	7,2
Split peas	6,0
Brown rice	5,5
Oatmeal	5,2
Dried apricots	4,9
Almonds	4,4
Dried apples	4,1
Marmite	3,7
Baked beans	3,4
Raisins	3,3
Spinach	3,0
Eggs	2,7
Wholewheat bread	2,6
Cornflakes	2,5
Walnuts	2,1
White bread	2,0
Peanuts	1,9
Peas	1,9
Pasta	1,5
Broccoli	1,3
Lettuce	1,1
Processed cheese	0,8
Potatoes	0,7
Milk	0,7
White rice	0,7
Tomatoes	0,6
Cheddar cheese	0,6
Cabbage	0,5
Fresh apricots	0,5
Oranges	0,4
Green peppers	0,4
Fresh apples	0,3
Cream	0,2

By comparison, liver contains 12,1 mg, beef and lamb contains 2,8, chicken 1,9, tinned sardines and tinned tuna contain 1,5.

ZINC
milligrams per 100 g

All-Bran	8,4
Cheddar cheese	4,0
Split peas	4,0
Processed cheese	3,2
Almonds	3,1
Oatmeal	3,0
Walnuts	3,0
Peanuts	3,0
Brewer's yeast	2,6
Marmite	2,1
Wholewheat bread	2,0
Eggs	1,5
White rice	1,3
Sweetcorn	1,0
Pasta	1,0
White bread	0,8
Baked beans	0,7
Peas	0,5
Cottage cheese	0,5
Milk	0,4
Cabbage	0,4
Broccoli	0,4
Cornflakes	0,3
Bananas	0,2
Oranges	0,2
Potatoes	0,2
Tomatoes	0,2
Lettuce	0,2

By comparison, beef and lamb contain 5,0 mg, chicken 1,0, tinned salmon 0,9 and tinned tuna 0,8.

VITAMIN B$_{12}$
micrograms per 100 g

Grapenuts	5,0
Egg yolks	4,9
Fortified cornflakes	1,7
Whole eggs	1,7
Cheddar cheese	1,5
Camembert cheese	1,2
Marmite	0,5
Cottage cheese	0,5
Processed cheese	0,3
Milk, whole	0,3
Milk, skimmed	0,3
Beer	0,2

By comparison, calf's liver contains 87,0 micrograms, tinned sardines 28,0, tinned tuna 5,0, pork 3,0, and beef and lamb 2,0.

VITAMIN C
milligrams per 100 mg

Green peppers	120
Broccoli	118
Kale	115
Strawberries	60
Spinach	59
Cabbage	52
Oranges	49
Lemons	45
Grapefruit	40
Asparagus	33
Peas	26
Tomatoes	23
Lettuce	18
Potatoes	17
Apricots, fresh	16
Apricots, dried	12
Sweetcorn	12
Dried apples	11
Bananas	10
Rhubarb	9
Carrots	6
Fresh apples	5
Baked beans	4
Grapes	4
Walnuts	3
Milk	3
Fruit cocktail	2
Lima beans	2
Split peas	2
Peanuts	2

By comparison, calf's and lamb's liver contains 10 mg and meat none.

VERTIGO

A sensation that the head is moving or spinning, when in fact it is still, is known as vertigo. The condition is often associated with NAUSEA AND VOMITING, and can be triggered by fear of falling from a height.

Vertigo can be caused by inflammation of the balance organ (the semicircular canals) in the inner ear or by MOTION SICKNESS. It can also result from Ménière's disease, in which attacks of vertigo are associated with RINGING IN THE EARS and increasing deafness; the cause is unknown.

Rarely, vertigo and deafness result from a benign (non-cancerous) growth on the acoustic (or auditory) nerve, or – if it develops suddenly in an elderly person – from a stroke. High BLOOD PRESSURE, hardening of the arteries (see ARTERIES [HARDENING]) and ear disorders can also cause vertigo. See also DIZZINESS.

What the therapists recommend

Acupuncture The equilibrium of the body is affected, and the condition is treated by stimulating points on the governor, gall bladder and kidney meridians, and also by giving MOXIBUSTION to points on the governor, gall bladder and bladder meridians.
Acupressure Apply pressure at a point one finger's width under the outer ankle bone and press inwards.

An orthodox view

If you develop persistent vertigo, consult your doctor. He will measure your blood pressure, examine your ears and look for signs of an underlying cause. If your hearing is deteriorating the cause may be a growth on the acoustic nerve, and your doctor may arrange for you to have a CAT scan, or magnetic resonance scan to pinpoint the exact location of the growth.

Conventional drugs such as betahistine (Serc) and cinnarizine (Stugeron) may relieve vertigo. However, they do not improve the hearing of Ménière's disease patients.

VIRUS INFECTIONS

A virus is a submicroscopic organism consisting essentially of a core of a single nucleic acid surrounded by a coating of protein. Viruses are on the borderline between living and non-living things. They can multiply only inside living cells, and in the process cause a wide variety of infections, from mild COLDS to life-threatening AIDS or POLIOMYELITIS. Virus infections also give rise to INFLUENZA,

some kinds of hepatitis (see LIVER DISORDERS), YELLOW FEVER, CHICKENPOX, SHINGLES and COLD SORES.

When vast numbers of a virus invade, the human body reacts, producing symptoms and signs of disease until its IMMUNE SYSTEM can produce enough antibodies – special kinds of proteins in the blood – to destroy the viruses. The antibodies then remain in the bloodstream as protection against another invasion by the same virus.

However, some viruses, such as those that cause the common cold, have the ability to mutate (change) so that the antibodies produced during one illness fail to give protection against future infections.

Other viruses, including those which cause MEASLES and MUMPS, very rarely mutate so that immunity usually lasts for a person's lifetime.

The human papilloma viruses (HPV) cause GENITAL HERPES, and may cause CANCER of the cervix (the neck of the womb). Another virus is thought to cause GLANDULAR FEVER.

What the therapists recommend

Homoeopathy The therapist will give remedies that, when correctly matched to the patient's symptoms, are said to enhance his body's ability to fight the particular infection.
Naturopathy Practitioners believe that natural therapies encourage the immune system, and that attention to overall health is of great value in combating virus infections. A vitamin C supplement and two or three garlic capsules a day are generally recommended. However, consultation is always advised.
Herbal Medicine If you are prone to frequent colds or influenza, try taking one to three garlic capsules daily as a preventive; double the dose if the infections occur very frequently. However, a consultation is recommended for all virus infections.

An orthodox view

Antibiotics are ineffective against virus infections, but they can alleviate accompanying bacterial infections. For example, if you develop a secondary bacterial infection such as BRONCHITIS or sinusitis (see SINUS PROBLEMS), penicillin will help you to recover.

Doctors now prescribe antiviral drugs for certain viral infections. For example, acyclovir (Zovirax) is effective against genital herpes, cold sores and chickenpox if given early enough in the course of the illness. Retrovir (Zidovudine or AZT) slows the progress of HIV infection and the resultant AIDS, but it does not cure the disease.

Conventional medicine cannot offer a cure for the majority of virus infections, though many – such as smallpox and measles – can be prevented by vaccination.

VISUALISATION THERAPY

Picturing your way to health

Mental pictures can be a powerful force for good or ill, depending on how they are used. In visualisation therapy, patients are taught imaginative techniques to benefit their health, to help along natural healing processes, and to reinforce positive feelings, behaviour and images of themselves.

In everyday life, people often concentrate on fears and problems rather than on how they might improve things. For example, a

How Ben, aged 8, solved his problem

The almost nightly BEDWETTING of eight-year-old Ben had not responded to several treatments when the doctor suggested visualisation might help.

The doctor asked Ben where he thought the water was coming from. Ben replied that it came from a big river. So, guided by the doctor, he was asked to imagine going for a walk along the river and coming to a large dam which stopped the water from flowing any farther. The doctor asked Ben what happened at night, and Ben told him that there was a door in the dam which was a bit leaky.

The doctor then helped Ben to imagine ways in which the leak could be stopped. Together they visualised using Superglue to waterproof the door and then padlocking it. But Ben could open the lock with a key and remove the glue with a penknife.

Every night at bedtime Ben and his mother imagined going for a walk down the river, coming to the dam and making the door watertight. Then he gave the imaginary key to his mother to put under her pillow for the night.

In the first three weeks of treatment Ben wet his bed only three times, on nights when he said the water was particularly stormy. With the doctor's help he was able to overcome even this problem, by imagining in a visualisation session that there was a hole in the river bank which occasionally let water through. Once he had visualised filling it in, his nights became completely dry.

young man going to a party may fear that no one will want to talk to him. He visualises himself entering a room full of guests and being totally ignored. And when he gets to the real party this image is so strong that he inevitably seeks out those people most likely to turn the imagined situation into reality.

Contrast this man's actions with those of someone who goes to the party believing that at least one guest will want to talk to him, and then seeks out that person.

Such imagined situations and the underlying beliefs that precipitate them tend to become self-fulfilling prophecies that influence mind, body and feelings. In the same way, people who practise creative visualisation believe that positive, health-promoting images will eventually help them to create the sort of life they want.

Making images is a natural mental process that occurs every night during dreams. Visualisation is similar to dreaming, but involves making a deliberate attempt with the conscious mind to imagine particularly beneficial events. It is based on the belief that mind and body are not separate but affect each other directly, so that thoughts can have physical effects as well as mental ones.

A number of theories have been suggested to explain how visualisation works, mostly based on the idea that there is a close link between emotions, images and sensations. Just as emotions are accompanied by physical sensations such as deep sighs and a long face when you are unhappy, so images call up emotions, and emotions are experienced in terms of images. For example, angry people are often said to 'see red'. By altering images, visualisation is believed to affect feelings and physical sensations.

It has also been suggested that visualisation may help to balance and integrate the hemispheres of the brain. The left side is believed to be concerned with logical thinking

To help people create mental pictures, visualisation therapists use paintings such as this scene by Pieter Brueghel the Elder (c1515-69). A person would be asked to look at it for two or three minutes, and then, with eyes shut, to recall it in his mind's eye. With practice, he would be able to re-create the picture in detail. He would 'see' a man sharpening a scythe, a mounted lady carrying a basket, two horses feeding, three girls carrying rakes and five porters with baskets on their heads. He would then progress to imagining a real-life scene.

Rediscovery of an ancient art

The use of mental images to cure disease has played an important part in healing traditions from earliest times. It was used by witchdoctors or 'shamans' in Africa and South America, and viewed as an integral part of most early oriental therapies. In Western medicine its origins reach back to ancient Greece, and it exerted a powerful influence until the mid-1600s, sometimes being considered the single most important factor in healing illness.

With the birth of modern science in the 17th century, holistic therapies such as visualisation began to be replaced by more specialised medical approaches, which viewed mind and body as separate. For hundreds of years this view prevailed and consequently most orthodox doctors considered there to be no rational basis for visualisation.

Recently, however, evidence of a link between body and mind has accumulated from observations and experiments in many different areas. Together with concern about the limitations and side effects of conventional treatments, this has led to a reawakening of interest in holistic approaches such as visualisation.

One of the earliest pieces of research was done in the 1920s by Edmund Jacobson, an American who discovered that when a subject visualised himself running, his leg muscles would twitch involuntarily. Other influential work on visualisation was done by Carl Simonton, a doctor at Fort Worth in Texas, and his wife Stephanie. They got cancer patients to create mental images of healthy cells attacking and destroying cancer cells. The results were startling: patients who took part in the visualisation programme lived on average twice as long as others, and in some cases the illness stopped spreading, enabling them to lead normal lives once again.

Another American doctor, Bernard Siegel, a surgeon at Yale-New Haven Hospital and an assistant professor at Yale University Medical School, works with visual images produced by patients in dreams and paintings, which he believes often show that the patient unconsciously knows what is wrong with him.

Dr Siegel's work has led him to the conclusion that many sick people have the ability to heal themselves, but that often they lack the will to live or else expect something outside themselves – a doctor, drugs or some other treatment – to cure them. For these patients he believes that visualisation therapy may be of little use, but for those who are prepared to take on the responsibility for their own restoration to health it may help to activate the inner healing processes.

toes along the spine to the top of the head, and each out-breath as travelling down from the head to the toes.

To enhance the effect of the progressive muscular relaxation exercise on p. 301, try to imagine some special, peaceful place once you are fully relaxed. Notice as many details about the scene as you can and examine each part of it with care. Try to imagine sounds, smells and sensations as well as sights if you can. After five to ten minutes, let the image slowly dissolve.

For the relief of severe pain, visualisation is said to require practice and be best learned from a therapist, but the following simple technique may be effective in less serious cases: Close your eyes, try to relax, and concentrate on slow diaphragmatic breathing. Visualise your breathing as coming in and out of the painful region, bringing a warm glow as you inhale and expelling pain with each exhalation.

Finding a therapist Visualisation is used by therapists of all types, almost always in combination with other treatments. Many practitioners are found in fields such as BIOFEEDBACK, AUTOGENIC TRAINING, PSYCHOSYNTHESIS, REBIRTHING, HYPNOTHERAPY and PSYCHOTHERAPY. A number of conventional doctors are also beginning to recognise its value, spurred on by the work of Carl and Stephanie Simonton and Bernard Siegel (see box, this page).

Consulting a therapist The practitioner begins by listening carefully to your description of the problem, and then encouraging you to relax in a comfortable position with head, neck and trunk aligned. Most people like to sit in a firm chair, but you can lie down or sit crosslegged. The therapist may also teach breathing exercises to aid relaxation.

When you are fully relaxed you will be asked to imagine a scene that in some way relates to your problem. This may be a still from a film, a photograph, a painting or a scene from the remembered past, and the therapist will ask you to describe details of what you see, perhaps making changes to the original suggestion.

While you are exploring the scene, the therapist will help you to become aware of any feelings or bodily sensations that you experience. Subtle changes to what you visualise can then be used gradually to alter your responses in ways that will help you to solve your particular problem.

An orthodox view

Visualisation is a perfectly acceptable way to aid relaxation and reduce STRESS. Its use in specific conditions, especially cancer, is still controversial, although some studies have now established the benefits in a wide range of other conditions.

and tends to predominate in many people, while the more creative and intuitive right side is relatively little used. Thinking in images is believed to involve the right hemisphere and so help to correct the imbalance.

Who it can help Therapists say that visualisation is suitable for just about any sort of physical or emotional problem. In particular, it has been used to help patients with ASTHMA, HEART DISORDERS, CANCER and PHOBIAS, and is said to be an effective form of PAIN relief. It may also help in achieving personal goals such as an improved relationship or a more positive self-image.

Children make particularly good subjects (see box, p. 358) since they have vivid imaginations and find it easy to create mental pictures. Many children live in rich fantasy worlds of dragons, knights, heroes and other mythical beings that can be used to help them overcome problems and express themselves, as well as to strengthen bonds with their parents.

Self help Therapists advise that it is usually best to learn the technique of visualisation from an expert and then practise it at home. Most people learn quickly, but for a few it can take longer, sometimes because they tend to process information in terms of sounds or sensations rather than pictures.

If you find it difficult to build visual images at first, this simple exercise may help: Look at a picture or photograph for two or three minutes, then shut your eyes and try to recreate it in your mind in as much detail as possible. Once you can do this easily, repeat the exercise using a room instead of a picture, and then finally with a moving scene from real life.

Visualisation can also be an aid to RELAXATION AND BREATHING exercises. When you practise diaphragmatic breathing (see p. 299) try to visualise a circle right in front of you. Without moving, imagine that you are drawing one half of the circle with your breath as you inhale, and the other half as you exhale. Repeat several times until the circle seems as round and smooth as you can make it. Then spend a few minutes visualising each in-breath as travelling from the tips of your

VITAMINS

Providing the body with the essentials for life

These vital substances, present in most foods in minute amounts, are needed for proper growth and development, body maintenance and general health. They control how your body makes use of other nutrients, and a serious deficiency of them can lead to a host of complaints, ranging from HEADACHES and loss of appetite to rickets and sterility. Fortunately a well-balanced diet (see EATING FOR HEALTH) provides all the vitamins that the body normally needs.

There are 13 major vitamins, all essential to health. Only one – possibly two – of them can be made in the necessary amounts by the body itself. Vitamin D is produced by the action of sunlight on the skin, and vitamin K may be synthesised by bacteria in the large intestine. The other 11, and these two if not enough of them is produced by the body, must be obtained from an outside source: the food we eat.

Some vitamins are soluble in water and others are soluble in fat, and this makes an important difference to how they are used. The water-soluble vitamins (vitamin C and those belonging to the vitamin B-complex) can easily be lost in cooking, especially if the water in which the food source has been boiled is thrown away. It may pay to steam vegetables, or to follow the example of the Chinese and stir-fry them rapidly.

Our bodies cannot store water-soluble vitamins. Any excess not taken up and used by the body is passed out in the urine. This means that the C and B vitamins must be eaten daily. The fat-soluble vitamins A, D, E and K, on the other hand, can be stored in the liver, sometimes for weeks. There is no need to eat them daily, but the intake must be regular, to ensure that the supply in the body remains topped up.

The fresher the produce, and the nearer it is to its natural state, the higher its vitamin content. Vitamins can be lost by any form of cooking (because of the heat), by exposure to light or cold, by storage, and by many of the processes of food manufacture. Water-soluble vitamins are particularly 'fragile', deteriorating at high or low temperatures and in strong sunlight. Potatoes, for example, are a valuable source of vitamin C when fresh, but can lose about half of it when kept for five months. So store fresh foods carefully, and keep vitamin tablets or capsules in a cool, dry place, preferably in the dark.

If you are in good health and your diet is right, vitamin supplements are not normally needed. Indeed, an excess of some vitamins can be just as dangerous as a deficiency. Those that are fat soluble, and particularly

Vitamins: what they do and how we obtain them

VITAMIN AND NATURAL SOURCES	RECOMMENDED DAILY AMOUNT (RDA) AND BENEFICIAL EFFECTS	EFFECTS OF DEFICIENCY
Vitamin A (retinol) Fat soluble.	RDA: 0,75 mg; 1,2 mg for nursing mothers.	
Found in: yellow/orange vegetables, especially carrots; green vegetables; tomatoes; full-fat dairy produce; liver; kidney; eggs; fish-liver oils; apricots and peaches (fresh or dried).	Vision, especially in dim light; healthy skin and mucous membranes; resistance to infection. Sometimes used to treat ACNE. **Warning:** Large doses can be toxic.	Night blindness (inability to see in dim light); damage to cornea and eventual blindness; ear, eye and respiratory infections; dry skin; dull hair and hair loss (see HAIR PROBLEMS); weight loss, and stunted growth.
Vitamin B₁ (thiamin, aneurin) Water soluble.	RDA: 1-1,3 mg	
Found in: wheat germ and wholegrain cereals, including brown rice; fortified white flour and products; brewer's yeast/yeast extract; seafood; liver, meat, poultry; pulses; nuts; potatoes; milk.	Metabolises (breaks down) carbohydrates to provide energy; healthy muscles and nervous system; countering pain; possibly learning ability.	Loss of appetite, nausea (see NAUSEA AND VOMITING), CONSTIPATION; fatigue, weakness; DEPRESSION, irritability, lack of concentration; shortness of breath, slow heart. Severe: beriberi and eventual death.
Vitamin B₂ (riboflavin, lactoflavin, vitamin G) Water soluble.	RDA: 1,3-1,6 mg	
Found in: liver, kidney, meat, poultry; eggs, cheese, yoghurt; wholegrain cereals; fortified cereals; brewer's yeast/yeast extract; fish; green vegetables; pulses.	Metabolism of carbohydrates, fats and proteins; healthy skin and mucous membranes.	Inflammation of tongue and lips, lip sores; scaly scalp and hair loss (see HAIR PROBLEMS); sensitivity to light; trembling, DIZZINESS, insomnia.
Niacin (vitamin B₃, nicotinic acid) Water soluble.	RDA: 18 mg	
Found in: some cereals including rice, but not maize; fortified white flour and products; meat, liver, poultry, kidney; yeast extract/brewer's yeast; eggs; fish; nuts, especially peanuts; cheese; peas and beans; artichokes; dried fruit.	Efficient blood circulation; control of blood cholesterol; healthy adrenal glands; healthy skin and nervous system; healthy appetite.	Loss of appetite, nausea (see NAUSEA AND VOMITING), gastrointestinal ULCERS, DIARRHOEA; dermatitis; fatigue, HEADACHES; INSOMNIA, irritability, DEPRESSION. Severe: pellagra (dementia with dermatitis and DIARRHOEA). *Continued on p. 362*

Vitamins: what they do and how we obtain them (continued)

VITAMIN AND NATURAL SOURCES	RECOMMENDED DAILY AMOUNT (RDA) AND BENEFICIAL EFFECTS	EFFECTS OF DEFICIENCY
Pantothenic acid (vitamin B₅) Water soluble. Found in all living matter and most foods, but especially beans, egg yolk, legumes, liver, oranges, peanuts, wheat germ, wholegrain cereals; also made in the gut.	RDA: 4-7 mg Use of fats and carbohydrates; healthy skin and hair; healthy nervous system; production of antibodies against infection.	Deficiency is unlikely in humans. Rare symptoms may include increased susceptibility to ALLERGY and infections; ASTHMA; CRAMP; fatigue; . INSOMNIA.
Vitamin B₆ (pyridoxine) Water soluble. Found in: most foods, but especially green vegetables, brewer's yeast, yeast extracts, fish, pulses, prunes, raisins, soya beans and flour, nuts, wholegrain cereals, milk.	RDA: 1,5-2 mg Production of antibodies against infection; red blood cell formation; metabolism of protein.	Deficiency not reported in humans.
Folic acid (vitamin B₉, folate, vitamin B_C, pteroylglutamic acid) Water soluble. Found in: liver, kidney, meat; green vegetables; fresh fruit; brewer's yeast/ yeast extract; wheat germ; pulses.	RDA: 0,3 mg Proper functioning of vitamin B₁₂; formation of red blood cells; use of proteins, fats and carbohydrates.	Lack of vitamin B₁₂; ANAEMIA; fatigue, WEAKNESS, shortness of breath, irritability, INSOMNIA, FORGETFULNESS, confusion.
Vitamin B₁₂ (cyanocobalamin) Water soluble. Found in: foods of animal origin, especially liver, meat, kidney; fish; egg yolk; dairy products, especially cheese; fortified cereals; brewer's yeast/yeast extracts (traces only).	RDA: 2 micrograms; 4 micrograms for pregnant women and nursing mothers. Proper functioning of folic acid; red blood cell formation; healthy nervous system; synthesis of nucleic acids and proteins; metabolism of fats, proteins and carbohydrates; prevention of cell degeneration.	Deficiency of folic acid; loss of appetite; fatigue, irritability; ANAEMIA. Severe: degeneration of nervous system leading to moving and speaking difficulties.
Biotin (also one of vitamin B-complex) Water soluble. Found in: egg yolk; liver, kidney; wheat germ; nuts; oats; yeast/yeast extract.	RDA: 0,1-0,2 mg Metabolism of fats; synthesis of glucose when diet is low in carbohydrates.	Very rare.
Vitamin C (ascorbic acid) Water soluble. Found in (best raw): fruits and fruit juices, especially citrus fruits and blackcurrants; rose hips and syrup; vegetables, including potatoes; chillies and peppers.	RDA: 30 mg; 60 mg for pregnant women. Healthy skin, bone, tendons, cartilage, ligaments, blood vessels, gums, teeth; energy production and growth; resistance to infection; wound healing; iron absorption: control of blood cholesterol.	Bleeding and/or soft gums, loose teeth; low resistance to infections; tender joints, muscle degeneration; fatigue, weakness irritability; ANAEMIA. Severe: scurvy, which can be fatal.
Vitamin D (cholecalciferol) Fat soluble. Produced by action of sunlight on human skin. Found in: liver; fish-liver oils and oily fish such as kippers, mackerel, sardines, tuna, tinned salmon; margarine; egg yolk; evaporated milk, full-fat dairy products; malted milk drinks; sprouted seeds.	RDA: 10 micrograms Absorption of calcium and phosphorus for healthy bones and teeth. **Warning:** Large doses can be toxic.	Bone deformities, dental caries; CRAMP; muscle weakness. Severe: rickets and osteomalacia (equivalent of rickets in adults).
Vitamin E (tocopherol) Fat soluble. Found in most foods, but especially vegetable oils, egg yolks, wholegrain cereals, wheat germ, green vegetables, nuts and seeds, pulses, margarine.	RDA: 10 micrograms or 12-15iu Healthy cell membranes, so may retard effects of ageing; healthy blood cells; blood clotting; resistance to infection; possibly: fertility.	Rare: dull hair; muscle weakness; possibly: enlarged prostate gland (see PROSTATE PROBLEMS); miscarriage.
Vitamin K (menadione) Fat soluble. Synthesised by bacteria in large intestine. Found in: green vegetables; seaweed (kelp); liver; potatoes; eggs; wheat germ.	RDA: 70-140 micrograms Blood clotting.	Very rare, but may be caused by long-term use of antibiotics: bleeding beneath the skin, NOSEBLEED, DIARRHOEA.

vitamins A and D, can build up in the body to toxic levels. If you do take supplements, be sure to keep to the recommended dosage.

The times when supplements may be necessary are when there are extra demands or stresses on the body – during PREGNANCY, for example. Women taking contraceptive pills may need extra vitamins, as may post-menopausal women, elderly people, and anybody who drinks much alcohol. Followers of VEGETARIANISM, and especially veganism, run the risk of becoming deficient in vitamin B12, which helps to maintain the nervous system in good working order. Vitamin supplements or brewer's yeast should be taken to make up the shortfall.

A theory was put forward in the 1980s that vitamin supplements could improve a child's IQ. This led to heated controversy in medical circles, but in the early 1990s the claim was still unproven. Scientific tests were carried out but the results were conflicting.

See also MEGAVITAMIN THERAPY.

VOICE THERAPY
Retraining the vocal cords

The human voice reveals a great deal about our essential character or personality, not only through the way we speak, but also through the tone, pitch and rhythm of our voice. In addition to words, we express ourselves by how loud or soft, how high or low our voice is when we laugh, cry or become angry or apologetic. Our voice also reveals much about the way in which we deal with extreme situations involving ANXIETY, GRIEF, STRESS and frustration.

Some people are let down by their voice when seeking to express anger, or assert their authority. These 'betrayals' sometimes arise because they cannot change their tone of voice to suit the occasion.

For example, a young woman who has been brought up to be sweet, generous and accommodating, may develop a voice which is stuck in a high pitch with a soft and comforting tone. She therefore may find it extremely difficult – if not impossible – to have herself taken seriously when expressing more 'dominating' emotions.

Equally, a man who has been educated to believe he should be domineering and 'protective' may develop a low, booming voice which is incapable of expressing gentler and more sympathetic feelings.

A voice therapist aims to overcome these and other related problems through special vocal and breathing exercises, MASSAGE and psychological methods.

Who it can help People suffering from DE-PRESSION may have difficulty in expressing themselves as their voice has become low, quiet and sad. Also, anyone beset with anxiety may find himself more or less gasping for breath, and his voice will be strained and unnatural. Even though the sufferers may be undergoing PSYCHOTHERAPY, their voice often needs separate attention.

Other problems with the voice may arise as a result of physical impairment or restriction, and the physically disabled can also sometimes benefit from the therapy. For example, someone confined to a wheelchair may have difficulty in being heard without getting a sore throat or experiencing TENSION. This is due to the often uncomfortable way in which he is forced to sit.

Difficulties of self-expression such as these do not necessarily mean there is a problem with talking itself. However, voice therapists may treat someone suffering from, say, STAMMERING, whom other therapists have been unable to help.

Finding a therapist While there are no South African practitioners of the particular voice therapy pioneered by Alfred Wolfsohn (see 'Sounds of war and peace' in next column), speech therapists make use of similar techniques in helping their pupils to overcome barriers to self-expression – as do teachers at speech and drama schools. To find a speech therapist, consult your general practitioner. See also SOUND THERAPY.

Consulting a therapist The aim of the therapist is to release feelings and emotions in the patient which may have become blocked or submerged. In addition, he will try to 'liberate' the voice from the effects of extreme moods – such as depression – or ease the tension caused by any physical impediment. He does this by trying to improve the actual *sounds* made by the patient, rather than by working on his pronunciation and manner of speaking as a speech therapist does.

The patient is asked to make a sound, or possibly sing a note which is played on the piano. The therapist listens carefully to the sound and then attempts to remove any physical factor which he thinks is restricting the voice.

The way this is done depends both on the individual therapist's approach and the patient's specific problem. Usually, however, the therapist tries to help the patient to breathe freely and easily. This may involve massaging the patient's back to realign the posture and the shape of the spine, and to relax muscles which are used in making sounds, in a manner similar to that used in the ALEXANDER TECHNIQUE.

In addition, the therapist listens to the moods and feelings which he says lie beneath any given sound. These are usually not ap-

parent to the patient, who is not accustomed to listening to the subtle intonations of his own voice.

The therapist encourages the patient's underlying emotions or 'deeper images' to emerge, often by making the patient imagine that he is experiencing different emotions, or pretending that he is a totally different person. In turn, this is said to change the sounds he makes.

The process has been compared to taking the patient's voice on a journey through his or her imagination. The mind contains a mixture of images, emotions, ideas, thoughts and feelings. These are often expressed in dreams and fantasies, or in the pictures we paint and the stories we tell.

Voice therapy aims at giving vocal expression to these notions, so that we can better understand the deeper workings of our minds – and therefore use our voice in a true and beneficial way.

An orthodox view

Voice therapy is regarded as a perfectly acceptable approach to the treatment of stress-related disorders. It is especially useful for those conditions in which breathing problems and emotional distress play a large part.

Sounds of war and peace

The first person to use alternative voice therapy was Alfred Wolfsohn (1896-1962), a German medical orderly who served in the First World War. He was horrified by the screams of wounded soldiers, and the moans of the dying – and these sounds came back to haunt him in peacetime.

He suffered a nervous breakdown and sought ways to express vocally the deep psychological injuries he had suffered. Gradually, he healed himself by exploring the sound of his own voice. He considered the human voice to be the 'muscle of the soul'.

Wolfsohn was a Jew, and in the 1930s he fled to England to escape persecution by the Nazis. Once there he taught emotionally disturbed people how to use their voice to overcome psychological problems and inhibitions. He founded a voice research centre in north London, and his success encouraged other healers to take up his work. Today he is acknowledged by many voice therapists to be the master of their unorthodox art.

WARTS

Viruses cause the small, non-cancerous, solid growths on the skin which are known as warts. They are composed mostly of enlarged skin cells, and occur typically on the hands and feet. There are several types and most disappear of their own accord.

Common warts are rough, horny and skin-coloured or brownish. They occur mostly in children, usually on the hands. Scratching them spreads the virus and causes more warts to appear.

Plantar warts are also known as verrucas. They occur on the sole of the foot, and are similar to common warts. However, they grow into the skin instead of outwards and are therefore more painful. They spread rapidly from person to person in communal changing rooms for swimming and other sports, where people go barefoot.

Filiform warts appear as short, hard threads, and are often seen on a person's face, neck, chin and eyelids. They are harmless and tend to disappear with time, but can be unsightly.

Plane warts are flat and pale or light brown, and are also common on the face. They are very small, generally growing in clusters – often along the line of a scratch.

Warning Have a brown wart checked by your doctor if it feels soft, suddenly changes its shape, itches and/or bleeds, or produces a discharge. It may not be a wart at all, but a melanoma – a skin CANCER.

What the therapists recommend

Acupuncture In traditional Chinese medicine, the skin is related to the lungs and the large intestine, so treatment is given to points surrounding the wart(s), and also to points on the lung and large intestine meridians. Points on the governor and spleen meridians are also used for acupuncture as they are believed to produce anti-inflammatory and immune effects.

Hypnotherapy Under hypnosis the sufferer is given suggestions that the warts will gradually lose their food supply, fade away and eventually drop off.

Aromatherapy Onion and garlic oils are held to be effective, but because of their powerful aroma they are taken in capsule form. Raw, chopped onion or garlic applied regularly as an overnight compress is said also to remove warts.

Herbal Medicine The juice or sap of garlic, celandine or cotyledon has caustic properties and should be squeezed on the wart at frequent intervals until it disappears. Or slice one of the cotyledon's fleshy leaves and bind it, slice side down, on the wart with adhesive plaster.

Charming warts away

Traditional and folklore remedies for warts are legion, and some are ancient. Here are just a few:

Tie a hair from the tail of a pie-bald pony or from the mane of a grown horse around each one.

Rub each wart with seven white stones in turn.

Rub on bacon or raw meat and then bury the meat – but do not let anyone know where it is buried.

Saliva is a popular remedy. So, lick the wart with your tongue the moment you wake up. If you cannot reach the wart with your tongue, use your forefinger to transfer saliva to the wart.

An orthodox view

Most warts can be destroyed by carefully applying an acid, such as salicylic acid, or podophyllin (Posalfilin) – a resin obtained from the dried root of the May apple – and then covering the area with a plaster. If necessary, a thin layer of petroleum jelly is first applied to the surrounding healthy skin in order to protect it. Before each treatment, dead skin resulting from the previous application is removed by rubbing the wart gently with a pumice stone.

These treatments may cause scarring, so they should not be used on the face. Both acid treatment and podophyllin should be avoided during pregnancy.

Warts are also sometimes removed by treatment with a heated instrument (cautery) or a very cold instrument (cryosurgery). The procedures require great skill.

WASP STINGS

Unlike bees, which leave their stings firmly embedded in the skin, wasps simply inject poisonous protein into their unfortunate victims and can go on to sting again. The poison causes redness, pain and itching, but wasp stings are seldom dangerous except when, in rare cases, a sting to the mouth or throat causes the throat to swell rapidly, blocking the air passage.

Wasp stings may also cause a rare and serious allergic reaction called anaphylactic SHOCK. The victim's blood pressure suddenly falls, and he becomes light headed and short of breath, with a rapid 'thready' pulse and a widespread, itching rash. Call a doctor as quickly as possible if you suspect anaphylactic shock.

What the therapists recommend

Traditional Medicine Vinegar dabbed on the sting was a traditional remedy; moistened or chewed tobacco was believed to relieve pain and any swelling. Crushed plantain or marigold leaves were used to soothe all sorts of stings.

Herbal Medicine Ice-cold water (or even an ice cube) can be applied to the sting – a few drops of lemon juice in the water is said to help neutralise the alkaline nature of the sting. Marigold ointment is then applied, reducing the inflammation. An effective rural remedy is to dab onto the sting a strong infusion of the wild dagga ('minaret flower') plant, made by pouring boiling water over the flowers, leaves and twigs. Or pick a bulbinella leaf and squeeze the juice on the sting; this yellow-flowering plant is often found in South African rock-gardens.

An orthodox view

A doctor may suggest calamine lotion or antihistamine cream, or tablets to relieve the symptoms. If the throat swells after a sting in that area, give the victim ice to suck, or ice-cold water to drink, to lessen the swelling; and seek medical help immediately. If anaphylactic shock develops, a doctor or paramedic will give basic life support if the patient is unconscious, with injections of adrenaline and antihistamine.

If you are allergic to wasp stings, your doctor may provide you with a syringe of adrenaline to inject in an emergency.

WATER RETENTION

Swelling of parts of the body can occur when water leaks from the blood and accumulates in the tissues. Puffiness of the feet and ankles is the most common sign of it. The medical term for the condition is oedema; it used to be called dropsy.

Mild water retention, with swollen ankles and a bloated feeling, occurs when the circulation is slow – for example, after a long period of sitting or standing in the same position. The circulation may also be slow because of VARICOSE VEINS – or even due to the tight elastic top of socks.

Women who suffer from PREMENSTRUAL TENSION may notice weight gain, puffy ankles and swollen breasts during the week or so before a period. Water retention is common during PREGNANCY; it is sometimes severe and may be associated with high BLOOD PRESSURE and toxaemia.

Severe water retention may be caused by some KIDNEY COMPLAINTS, HEART DISORDERS or LIVER DISORDERS. In such cases the sufferer is clearly ill and needs medical attention. Symptoms may include severe breathlessness and swelling of the ankles, legs, buttocks and abdomen. The blood pressure may be extremely high and JAUNDICE may develop.

What the therapists recommend

Naturopathy You are advised to cut out salt from your diet; it encourages water retention. Stimulate the circulation with EXERCISE and lose weight if necessary (see SLIMMING THE NATURAL WAY).

Herbal Medicine Dandelion is a natural diuretic. You can add fresh young leaves to salads, or drink an infusion of the leaves or take dandelion extract.

Acupuncture Stimulation of the kidney and bladder meridians may help.

Traditional Medicine Try taking a pinch of ground broom seeds in a spoonful of honey.

An orthodox view

Diuretic extracts or herbs will get rid of water by making you pass more urine, but they give only temporary relief and can lead to DIABETES, GOUT and potassium deficiency. Diuretic drugs (water pills) carry the same risks but are taken under supervision, for they are available only on prescription.

See your doctor if water retention is severe, taking a urine sample to be tested for signs of kidney disease. You may also be examined for signs of heart or liver disease and your blood pressure will be measured.

WEATHER AND HEALTH

Climate affects more than your moods . . .

We seldom think of the expression 'being under the weather' as literally true, but in fact doctors and alternative practitioners believe that climate and weather conditions do exert an important influence on our health and sense of well-being. Although some people appear to be more sensitive to the effects than others, nearly everyone has experienced the invigorating quality of mountain air, or knows the beneficial effects of a sunny day on his mood.

Other health effects can be less obvious and may appear only at certain times of the year. Many involve a whole range of weather factors which all influence one another, making it difficult to establish precise cause-and-effect relationships. Even so, a variety of factors is known to have definite effects. Some of the most important include:

Temperature This affects respiratory rate and the body's overall metabolic rate – the speed of the vital bodily processes. In cooler climates such as that of Britain, body heat is dissipated relatively fast, increasing metabolic rate and stimulating feelings of vitality. The high temperatures of tropical climates, by contrast, slow down the body's functions and decrease energy levels because heat is lost relatively slowly.

Although moderate heat and cold pose no direct health risks, people in hot countries appear to be more susceptible to intestinal disorders, and those in cold countries to respiratory problems. Exposure to extreme temperatures of either sort can have serious consequences: disorders such as prickly heat, heat exhaustion and heat stroke in the case of hot weather, and CHILBLAINS, FROSTBITE and HYPOTHERMIA in cold.

Temperature also affects health in a variety of ways. For example, cold weather tends to keep people indoors and reduces the amount of EXERCISE they take. Crowded public places such as shops, buses and trains are often poorly ventilated and they may also be overheated – perfect breeding grounds for germs of all sorts. And the temptation in cold weather to warm oneself up with extra food and drink – often in the form of sweet snacks, rich meals, coffee and alcohol – easily gives rise to bad habits.

Rainfall and humidity Amounts of rain vary enormously in different areas of South Africa: about 30 per cent of the country receives less than 250 mm a year, while about 11 per cent receives more than three times that annual total. Despite the popular view that damp weather gives rise to COLDS, there is no medical evidence that this is so; but most doctors accept that dampness and rheumatic complaints are connected.

Humidity measures the level of water vapour present in the atmosphere; in South Africa it is highest all along the coastal belt, and low in most of the interior. Some doctors believe that prolonged low humidity may cause the mucous membranes of the upper respiratory tract to dry out, leaving them vulnerable to infections. (Air-conditioning in office buildings may create an 'artificial climate' of low humidity, with similar consequences.)

'Bracing' and 'relaxing' climates Certain areas have long had reputations for being bracing or invigorating, while others are considered soothing and tranquil. A number of factors is thought to be involved, including wind, humidity, temperature, altitude, and possibly also the frequency of changes in the weather; but there is no accepted scientific definition.

Traditionally, certain coastal regions are thought of as invigorating – the breezy Western Cape seaboard undoubtedly qualifies. So, for different reasons, does the Highveld plateau. Mountainous areas, notably the foothills and higher slopes of the Drakensberg, fall into the same category.

By contrast Karoo resorts are generally reputed to have relaxing climates; several have been the sites of tuberculosis sanatoriums, and many an asthmatic patient has been sent to the Karoo for treatment. Different climatic conditions make Natal's coastal belt, and the Transvaal Lowveld, restful too.

Using the weather in alternative medicine

Many alternative practitioners believe that the way an individual responds to different weather conditions is able to give valuable information about the correct diagnosis and treatment of his problems.

In HOMOEOPATHY, remedies are often prescribed according to the conditions under which symptoms improve or grow worse. For example, asthma which is worse in damp weather may be treated with Nat sulph., while if the same symptoms improve in these conditions, Hepar sulph. may be used.

Weather is also considered important in several oriental approaches such as ACUPRESSURE, ACUPUNCTURE and MACROBIOTICS, which are based on achieving a balance of the body's YIN AND YANG forces. Yin is associated with coolness and damp, and yang with dryness and heat.

Depending on the patient's individual disposition, his way of life and the particular symptoms he is suffering from, the practitioner will offer treatment to restore the two forces to a state of harmony.

A condition that is exacerbated by cold weather, for example, or a patient who lives in a cold climate, may be treated in ways which are designed to strengthen the heating, yang principle. Someone whose main symptoms are inflammation and a high temperature, or who in some other way shows excessively yang symptoms may be in need of yin-strengthening measures.

How weather affects common ailments

SHORT-TERM EFFECTS	LONGER-TERM OR SEASONAL EFFECTS
Asthma Bronchial asthma is generally worse when the temperature drops suddenly, particularly if air pressure falls and wind speeds rise at the same time. It often improves when there is a high air pressure and fog.	Attacks are infrequent in winter, but increase from November onwards, becoming worse in late autumn.
Bronchitis Usually worsens in fog, especially if air pollution is heavy and the temperature falls at the same time.	Many attacks occur in winter, few in summer.
Hay fever Tends to be worse when the temperature drops.	Attacks increase in the flowering seasons of certain plants, especially grass. Often worse in October, November and December.
Rheumatism and arthritis Most forms worsen when exposed to falling temperatures or strong winds. Humidity alone has little effect.	Arthritis tends to be most common in autumn and early winter.
Heart disorders By constricting the arteries a sharp drop in temperature may cause problems.	In summer the discomfort felt by patients with heart disorders is aggravated by hot weather.
Colds Weather changes that affect the body's heat-regulating mechanism, the conditions of the mucous membranes, and the strength of the cold virus can all increase infections. Cold periods followed by sudden warming, for example, may increase susceptibility.	Susceptibility is apt to increase from March onwards, reaching a peak in August and September.
Influenza Conditions of low humidity and low wind speeds are associated with outbreaks.	Most cases occur between June and August, but vulnerability is high from March right through to September.

Sunshine Surveys show that both people who are ill and those in good health report feeling better on sunny days, and the tonic effects of a holiday in the sun are well known. Doctors and psychologists throughout the world now recognise a condition termed Seasonal Affective Disorder Syndrome (SADS), in which mood changes are affected by the seasons.

For example, sufferers become depressed and lethargic during winters of little natural daylight, but return again to normal when the days start to lengthen.

In addition, sunshine enables the body to manufacture vitamin D – important for the prevention of rickets in children – but since this can also be obtained from the diet, deficiencies seldom occur. More serious are the risks of SUNBURN and skin CANCER if overexposure to the sun occurs, particularly in those with fair hair and skin.

Wind The direction and speed of winds influence the way in which sounds are carried or dispersed. The sound of the wind can itself cause irritation, as can the wind's persistence (for example, a prolonged spell of the West-ern Cape's notorious south-easter). Air pollution may also be carried by wind, causing problems such as smog and acid rain.

Wind also adds greatly to the amount of body heat lost at low temperatures – known as 'wind chill'. Wind chill accounts for about 80 per cent of heat loss and is a more accurate indicator of how cold you feel than temperature alone. For example, a gale-force wind of 72 km/h at a temperature of -7°C will lower your body temperature to the same extent as a light breeze of 8 km/h at -24°C.

Air pollution In certain weather conditions industrial pollutants are trapped in the atmosphere and create an assortment of HEALTH HAZARDS. The danger of inhaling the pollutants is increased in periods of fog and mist, and respiratory illnesses are apt to show a marked increase.

Pressure systems and weather fronts Areas of high and low atmospheric pressure are created by convection (the vertical movement of air as its temperature changes), and these in turn produce what the weathermen call warm and cold 'fronts'. Some sensitive people find that such abrupt weather changes bring feelings of nervousness and mental tension. Changes in barometric pressure as a result of a cold front may be responsible for INSOMNIA, and for increasing the number of cases of blocked arteries resulting from blood clots.

Ionisation The relative proportions of electrically positive and negative particles – or ions – in the air vary from place to place and are thought to have a number of health effects. People tend to feel at their best in places with more negative ions, such as at the seaside, in the mountains or near natural running water such as rivers or waterfalls.

High concentrations of positive ions occur before storms, when pollution is heavy, and in indoor environments where electrical appliances, central heating and synthetic fabrics contribute to the problem. They can cause symptoms such as HEADACHES, TENSION and DEPRESSION, and may make breathing problems such as ASTHMA worse. People who suffer from these effects may find that a small home negative ionising machine makes a difference (see IONISATION).

WHEAT GERM

Weight for weight, this food supplement is one of the richest known sources of vitamin E. It is also rich in folic acid and biotin (VITAMINS of the B-complex). Wheat germ is the embryo of the wheat grain, and is separated during milling. The grain is ground and sieved several times to separate the wheat germ from the flour. See EATING FOR HEALTH.

WHEEZING

The noisy low-pitched breathing sounds known as wheezing are louder on breathing out, unlike CROUP, which is louder on breathing in. The symptom is caused by obstruction of the bronchial tubes (airways) in the lungs, and if severe it can be very unpleasant and frightening.

A foreign body such as an inhaled peanut can sometimes result in wheezing, which is also a symptom of BRONCHITIS, EMPHYSEMA and pulmonary oedema (fluid in the lungs). However, the commonest cause is ASTHMA. The walls of the airways start to swell and become inflamed, and the muscles around them contract.

At the same time the bronchial mucous glands may produce excessive mucus. All these result in coughing, shortness of breath and wheezing.

Warning Wheezing can be a symptom of a serious condition such as a foreign body in the lung or a potentially serious lung disease. Sufferers, especially elderly people and children, should therefore see a doctor.

What the therapists recommend

Homoeopathy For remedies, see ASTHMA, BRONCHITIS and WHOOPING COUGH.

Acupuncture The commonly used points are on the lung, conception and large intestine meridians. If body acupuncture results in little response, ear acupuncture, head needle therapy and MOXIBUSTION are used by the therapist in turn.

Herbal Medicine A professional herbalist will aim to find the underlying cause(s) of the symptom. For self help, mix two drops of oil of lavender in one teaspoon of vegetable oil and rub it into the chest. Inhalations of menthol and eucalyptus should also help.

Ionisation Many people suffering from heavy colds and persistent bronchitis find that using a negative ioniser reduces their wheezing and makes breathing easier. A humidifier in the room may also help.

An orthodox view

If there is a foreign body in an airway it must be removed before it causes partial collapse of a lung or PNEUMONIA.

When wheezing is caused by asthma, a doctor may prescribe a muscle relaxant such as salbutamol (Ventolin) to open the airways, an inhaled steroid such as beclomethasone (Becotide) to reduce swelling and inflammation, and a medicine such as cromoglycate to alleviate the allergy. Both patient and doctor can find out how well the sufferer is breathing – that is, measure the patient's 'peak flow' – when the patient blows into an inexpensive, simple peak flow meter.

WHIPWORM

Infection with whipworm (*Trichuris trichiura*) is common in tropical Africa, and is found in some wetter, hotter areas of South Africa. It occurs when food contaminated with the worm's eggs is eaten.

The adult worm that develops in the intestine is cylindrical and up to 5 cm long, with a thin, whiplike tail.

There may be no symptoms unless a large number of worms are harboured; then there will be abdominal pain, nausea, persistent diarrhoea (sometimes with blood in the stool), and eventually anaemia and malnutrition if the whipworm infestation is left untreated. AMOEBIASIS and bacterial infections are often found in association with whipworm infection.

What the therapists recommend

Herbal medicine Indigenous remedies to treat worm infestations (of all kinds) include a strong tea made from the leaves of either the carpet geranium (wild geranium), or the wild parsley tree; and a brew made by boiling pieces of mountain aloe leaf in sugar water.

Naturopathy Raw carrots, or carrot juice, are thought to be effective; but to expel the worms may require more drastic measures, and a consultation with a qualified naturopath is recommended.

An orthodox view

Diagnosis of whipworm infection is made possible only when the distinctive eggs are found in the patient's faeces. An antiworm drug (such as mebendazole) should then cure the infection.

WHOOPING COUGH

This infectious disease of childhood is also known as pertussis, and occurs in epidemics. It is caused by a bacterium, which is spread in the water droplets breathed out by an infected child, and attacks the mucous membranes lining the airways.

After an incubation period of seven to 14 days, a mild fever, cough, runny nose and loss of appetite develop. The cough starts to become progressively worse, particularly during the night, with 'whooping' – a noisy indrawing of breath – at the end of each cough. The child often vomits after a paroxysm of coughing, and may be very ill. The sufferer is infectious for 21 days after the onset of the 'whooping'. The illness may last up to four months, and the symptoms often recur when the child has a cough or cold.

Warning If a child develops a whoop, call the doctor immediately – whooping cough is a notifiable disease and the condition can in some cases prove fatal.

What the therapists recommend

Homoeopathy If a violent tickle in the throat brings on a fit of coughing, which is worse at night, and the child must hold his chest when coughing, give *Drosera* 30. When the sufferer vomits frequently, try *Ipecacuanha* 6 every six hours. If the child is red, hot, has a bursting cough and is worse at night and when lying down, give *Belladonna* 6 every hour until there is improvement.

Herbal Medicine A consultation is recommended. The herbalist will use a choice of expectorants – preparations that aid the production of saliva and mucus so that they may be coughed up more easily. These include white horehound, mullein flowers, thyme and elecampane. He may also give relaxants such as hyssop or lavender if needed. An infusion of sage leaves or klipdagga leaves makes a soothing herbal tea.

Naturopathy With other treatment, the naturopath will advise plenty of liquids, especially if the child is vomiting, and the avoidance of dairy products and large meals. He may also prescribe vitamin C.

An orthodox view

Immunisation against whooping cough is standard practice in South Africa, the possible side effects of vaccination being generally far less dangerous than the disease itself and its complications. The vaccine is combined with those for diphtheria and tetanus. A course of three injections is given between three and six months of age – with booster doses at 18 months and 4-6 years.

If ECZEMA results, the course should not be stopped. However, the doctor may advise against immunisation of a child who suffers from epilepsy or who has been brain-damaged since birth, or one whose parents suffer from epilepsy. The injections should not be given when a child is feverish or unwell, but may be given safely during a minor illness without fever. An attack of whooping cough usually gives the child immunity for life.

If a child develops whooping cough, a doctor may prescribe a course of antibiotics which, if taken early enough during the illness, may make it less severe. The child should be given extra liquids, regular doses of children's aspirin to reduce the fever and ease discomfort, and a proprietary cough medicine if it helps. Exposure to tobacco smoke will make the cough much worse. Hospital treatment may be necessary if the child starts to become very ill.

WILLPOWER

By using our willpower in a positive way we may help ourselves to recover from – if not prevent – illness and disease. Doctors and nurses are familiar with patients who, instead of willing themselves to get well, give up. On the other hand, there are many recorded instances of sick people who, instead of worsening or dying, have 'miraculously' recovered of their own accord.

Self-help techniques such as AUTOSUGGESTION, COUÉISM and VISUALISATION THERAPY can considerably help people to achieve the will to live. To this Emile Coué, the man who developed Couéism, added another important factor – the imagination. This faculty, he claimed, was even more powerful than the will. Even though people may have the will to recover, he said, they often *imagined* that they would not. 'When the will and the imagination are at war,' he stated, 'the imagination invariably wins.'

He concluded that it was vital to train the imagination – by means of a YOGA-like concentration – to work in harness with the will. Between them, he contended, they could make the nervous system throw off any physical or psychological disease.

WIND

Excessive gas – or wind – in the digestive tract is known as flatulence. It can result in considerable discomfort – and can find an embarrassingly audible means of announcing its presence and making its escape.

Do's and don'ts for wind

Do avoid any foods that you know give you wind, such as beans and sprouts.

Do eat more slowly, chewing well.

Do sit erect for meals and improve your general posture – with the ALEXANDER TECHNIQUE, for example.

Don't drink with your meals and avoid coffee and strong tea at any time.

Don't have protein and starch at the same meal – and go easy on sugars and raw vegetables.

Don't eat fat or too many pulses, especially soya.

Don't overeat.

The gas is sometimes air swallowed with hastily gulped food, so eating more slowly can reduce it. Or it can result from taking fizzy drinks, which can be cut out. A more complex cause is a failure of the digestive system to break down certain foods, leaving a residue that ferments in the bowel.

Beans are among the best known of these foods. Others which commonly give rise to the problem include Brussels sprouts, broccoli, cabbage, cauliflower, cucumbers, green peppers, lettuce, nuts, onions, peas, radishes, raw apples, melons and prunes. Sufferers should find out which foods are causing the trouble by cutting them out, then avoiding altogether those that induce wind.

A bloated feeling in the abdomen, frequent belching or breaking wind and CONSTIPATION are the usual symptoms. If wind persists or you also have pain, seek medical advice. An ULCER, hiatus hernia and other conditions can also cause similar symptoms.

What the therapists recommend
NATUROPATHY
Self help Practitioners recommend 24 hours' FASTING to clear the system, then simple meals, keeping carbohydrates (such as starches and sugars) and proteins (meat, fish, cheese) for separate meals (see HAY DIET). Use plenty of GARLIC, or take garlic capsules. Alternate hot and cold compresses on the abdomen may ease discomfort.

Consultation A diet to suit your needs will be worked out. Papain might be recommended. This enzyme, obtained from pawpaws and taken as tablets, is held to aid digestion. You may also be given advice on gentle massage of the abdomen.

Other alternative treatments
Herbal Medicine Use thyme, sage, marjoram and rosemary in cooking, and after a meal chew caraway seeds or a clove, or sip peppermint tea. Between meals sip a small cup of camomile, meadowsweet or balm tea. Add 5 g of dried camomile flowers (or 4 g of meadowsweet or 3 g of balm) to a cup of boiling water. Leave to infuse for ten minutes, strain and sip while still hot. If the flatulence persists, seek medical advice.

Homoeopathy For people who get wind after sweet food or when they are warm or worried, *Argentum nit.* is said to help. For those who suffer in damp weather, late in the day or after fatty food, *Carbo veg.* can be an alternative. One tablet every half-hour should be taken up to six doses, whenever there is discomfort. *Lycopodium* is for those with ravenous hunger that is satisfied by only a few mouthfuls, who find cabbage indigestible, or who have a strong desire for sweets.

Aromatherapy A therapist will blend essential oils to massage on your abdomen.

Blend basil, sage, peppermint and myrrh in a teaspoon of carrier oil or lotion (see p. 36) to make a mixture you can apply yourself: rub onto the abdomen in a clockwise direction.

An orthodox view
Doctors agree that a simple diet, cutting down on sugar, fat and coffee, and eating slowly, should prevent wind. Better posture also helps. Massage and compresses will ease discomfort but charcoal tablets, available from chemists, are the preferred conventional remedy for quick relief – they are thought to absorb gas from the gut.

WORMS

Infection by worms is by no means uncommon in South Africa, the worms (or their larvae) existing as parasites. The human victim may live for years without being aware of the infestation; or it may lead to chronic debilitating illness. Among the worm parasites are HOOKWORMS, ROUNDWORMS, TAPEWORMS and WHIPWORMS.

Pinworms (*Enterobius vermicularis*) are another such parasite. Also commonly known as 'threadworms', they primarily infect children, especially in temperate areas where hygiene is inadequate. The worms commonly infest the large intestine and cause inflammation and itching around the anus. They may be visible around it or in the faeces: tiny white threads no more than 13 mm long.

At night female pinworms emerge from the anus to lay up to 10 000 eggs around it. If the child victim scratches his bottom, eggs adhere to the hand or fingernails and may then be transferred to the mouth, directly or via food. Eggs lying loose in bedclothes may also be swallowed, for example when the sheets are shaken.

Pinworm infestation can lead to bacterial infection when the anal area is scratched. With girls the worms may also enter the vulva and cause a bloody vaginal discharge.

Strongyloides stercoralis is the Latin name for yet another such worm parasite. Similar in appearance to pinworms but larger and with a very different pattern of infestation, these worms are extremely common and can occur even in the cleanest homes. They can penetrate the skin, and it is in this way that infection initially takes place.

The mature worm lays its eggs in muscle tissue; once these hatch, the larvae then move into the intestine, and so to the outside via the faeces. For a time they are free-living, but when the environment starts to become unfavourable the larvae moult into their parasitic form.

This change can also take place inside the human intestine. The resulting internal auto-infection can lead to a large build-up of *S. stercoralis* worms in the intestine, causing an obstruction, as well as liver malfunction.

What the therapists recommend

Naturopathy A consultation is necessary. GARLIC, carrots and pumpkin seeds are all said to help, and herbal medicines will be suggested. For pinworm infection you will be advised to keep the fingernails short and well scrubbed, and to make sure you change your towels frequently.

Herbal Medicine A consultation is deemed necessary. Regular intake of garlic and raw carrots is recommended to weaken the worms, making it easier for stronger remedies given by the medical herbalist to take effect.

An orthodox view

Multipurpose drugs are available today to eradicate all the worm species that usually cause infections in South Africa. Early diagnosis is important, however, to forestall any secondary effects of the infestation. The victim of *Strongyloides stercoralis* should avoid constipation, as this increases the possibility of auto-infection.

As a precaution against the spread of pinworm, all members of an infected household should take anti-worm drugs. Toys and personal articles belonging to the victim should be sterilised. Meticulous hygiene must include the washing of hands and scrubbing of nails before meals and after visits to the lavatory, together with a morning bath to remove any eggs laid overnight.

restlessness, vomiting and jaundice. Other remedies are *Bryonia* and *Cadmium* for gastric symptoms; and *Crotalana* for exhaustion and haemorrhages.

An orthodox view

There is no effective drug against yellow fever, and treatment is supportive: the patient rests in bed and is given fluids to prevent dehydration, and analgesics for pain.

Vaccination against the disease is possible and provides adequate protection for travellers passing through infected regions. However, children under a year old should not be immunised.

YIN AND YANG

Ancient Chinese philosophy was based on the belief in two opposing but complementary forces, yin and yang, which together make up a balanced whole. Yin was the more passive, conserving force, yang the more positive, thrusting force. All understanding and explanation of the world, including medical science, was in terms of yin and yang.

The first treatise setting out a comprehensive system of medical symptoms and treatments according to the yin-yang principle was compiled by Chang Chung-ching about AD 200. The system was centuries old even then and is still followed.

When an individual's yin and yang are not in perfect balance, disease is said to result. Treatment is aimed not at symptoms, but at building up whichever of the two forces is deficient. Careful assessment (see ORIENTAL DIAGNOSIS) is needed to decide which is defi-

cient before treatment is given. Treatment may be by stimulation of energy-flow channels as in ACUPRESSURE, ACUPUNCTURE, MOXIBUSTION, SHIATSU, REFLEXOLOGY and T'AI-CHI CH'UAN, by self-massage (see DO-IN), or by diet (see MACROBIOTICS).

YOGA

Teaching control of mind and body

In the last few years, yoga has begun to be used more and more as a therapy to help in the management of particular ailments, especially of STRESS and stress-related problems. Because it works on body and mind together, yoga is recommended for the relief of such conditions. HEART DISORDERS and ASTHMA are among other ailments said to respond to yoga therapy.

Taken in its entirety, yoga – the word is Sanskrit for 'yoke' or 'union' – is a Hindu system of spiritual, mental and physical training designed to bring about reunion with the universal spirit or supreme being. In most Western countries it is the physical aspect – the postures and exercises called Hatha yoga – that is best known, but to the devotee other systems, such as Raja (which focuses on mind control), Jnana (which concentrates on intellect and understanding), Karma (moral

The great violinist Sir Yehudi Menuhin suffered a frozen shoulder that threatened to end his career. Yoga exercises freed it and allowed him to continue playing.

YELLOW FEVER

Like malaria, yellow fever is an infectious disease transmitted by the bite of a mosquito. However, it is caused by a virus (not a parasite); and one attack provides the victim with immunity for life. Fever, headache and sometimes nose-bleeding are symptoms of a mild attack, which need last for no more than three days. In severe cases the liver and kidneys are affected, and the skin turns yellow from jaundice (hence the name of the disease). Very severe cases may be fatal.

What the therapists recommend

Herbal Medicine Dandelion root, golden seal, milk thistle, cantharis, burberris and chelidonium are among the remedies a herbalist may prescribe to help the liver.
Homoeopathy *Camphor* is prescribed for the chill stage, *Aconite* when reaction sets in, with

Salute to the sun

The 'sun salute' – a series of 12 yoga postures – is designed to relax
and tone up the mind and body. Traditionally, it is practised facing
the sun at sunrise and sunset. However, if this is not feasible, you
can picture the sun rising or setting over a beautiful, tranquil scene,
engulfing you with its rays.

The postures can be done with perfect safety on your own. But they
should not be attempted by women who are pregnant or
menstruating, except under expert guidance. And they are not
suitable for anyone suffering from low back pain, high blood pressure,
hernia (rupture), or blood clots in the veins. The postures are
performed as illustrated, reading clockwise:

1

12

11

10

9

1 Stand upright with your knees and feet
together. Place your palms together and hold
them against your chest, with the fingers
pointing upwards.
2 As you breathe in, raise your hands above
your head and bend gently backwards. Your
palms should be facing up and your head
reaching back.
3 Breathe out and lean forward without
bending your knees. With practice you will be
able to touch the floor with your fingertips, or
even rest your palms on the floor.
4 Breathe in, bending your knees and putting
your palms flat on the floor. Push your right leg
back, and rest the knee on the floor. Look up
and push your hips forward.
5 Holding your breath, put your left leg
back, next to the right. Use your arms to keep
your body raised, with the palms still kept flat
on the floor.
6 Breathe out and move your body
backwards, keeping your hands in the same
place, until your buttocks rest on your heels
and your forehead on the floor.

8

2

3

4

7 Breathing in and then out, come forward taking your weight on your hands. Rest your knees, chest and forehead on the floor. Keep your abdomen and pelvis off the floor.
8 Breathe in fully and straighten your arms. Stretch your head up as far as you comfortably can, arching your back.
9 Breathe out and push up your buttocks, keeping your hands and feet flat on the floor. Straighten your legs and your back so that your body forms a triangle with the floor.
10 Breathing in and then out, bend your knees, resting your buttocks on your heels and your forehead on the floor.
11 Breathe in, bringing your right knee up between your hands and stretching forwards and upwards. Keep your palms flat on floor.
12 Breathe out, bringing your left foot up to your right. Straighten your legs and bend from the waist. Then breathe in and stand erect. Now you can stop or repeat the salute once or several times if you like. In successive salutes, alternate the leg you take back in stage 4, and forward in stage 11.

5

6

7

action) and Bakti (a devotional aspect), are equally important.

Yoga exercises can, of course, be practised by people with all kinds of spiritual belief, or by people with none. Nevertheless, yoga's underlying philosophy stresses the influence of mind over body, and holds that mental and spiritual development are necessary to reinforce the benefits that the physical exercises can bring.

Until 30 years ago virtually the only Westerners to practise yoga were those who had lived or travelled in the East, and those who were interested in oriental philosophies. A number of classical musicians were among them. One of these was the distinguished British violinist Sir Yehudi Menuhin, whose entire career was threatened by a FROZEN SHOULDER. With the guidance of his teacher, B K S Iyengar, Sir Yehudi worked at yoga exercises, and as a result of the widespread publicity given to his recovery, yoga gained enormously in popularity.

Pop culture's flirtation with oriental philosophies in the 1960s and 1970s provided yoga with a further massive boost. Its popularity in South Africa dates back several years, and there is no lack of either teachers or practitioners here.

The ancient teachers of yoga worked out some of their postures by observing how efficiently animals move and relax.

The postures are designed to develop flexibility and controlled relaxation. The movements are done slowly and the postures held

Do's and don'ts about yoga

Do take lessons with a qualified yoga teacher, choosing one who concentrates on your particular interest.
Do practise regularly, preferably daily.
Don't compete with classmates; yoga should not be a strain.
Do consult a doctor before you take up yoga if you are taking medication, have a disability, or are experiencing abnormal physical symptoms.
Do wear loose or stretchy clothing for yoga and put a thick mat or folded blanket on the floor.
Don't practise yoga with a full bladder or bowels.
Do take a shower before and after yoga to complete the relaxation and refreshment.

Basic postures for beginners

As a means of limbering up physically and mentally, the following five postures are particularly suitable for beginners. Even so, you should not expect to perform them perfectly at first. It could take weeks or even months before you have mastered them all. But with practice, carefully following the instructions, and without straining yourself, you should be able to perform the postures — either two or three at a time, or in full sequence.

If you are overweight, have high blood pressure, are menstruating or are pregnant, check with a qualified yoga teacher before attempting the postures.

1 Spinal twist Sit with your legs stretched out. Raise your right leg and put your foot on the far side of your left knee. Breathing out, turn your trunk to the right. Reach towards your left ankle with your left hand. Rest your right hand on the floor behind you and keep your back straight. Each time you breathe out twist a little further to the right. Hold for at least one minute, then repeat, twisting to the left.

2 Bow Lie face down with your feet together. Bend your knees and bring your feet towards your head. Grasp your ankles. Then, as you breathe in, pull on your ankles to raise your thighs, chest and head off the floor. Keep your arms straight and rest on your abdomen. At first, your legs will be apart, but bring them together as you gain skill. Hold the bow for 3-10 breaths. Then breathe out and release your legs.

3 Half shoulderstand Lie on your back and raise your legs as you breathe in. Breathing out, raise your hips and move your legs back over your head. Rest your weight on your arms, shoulders and elbows. Breathing in, adjust the angle of your legs so that the strain on your hands is not too great. Hold the position for 1-3 minutes, breathing normally. Then drop your arms, and slowly roll out of the position while breathing in.

4 Bridge Lie on your back, arms by your sides, with knees bent and legs slightly apart. Breathe in and raise the mid-section of your body. Interlock your fingers and stretch your arms out straight along the floor. Tuck your shoulders under you as you lean towards one side and then the other. Push with your feet and arms to increase the bridge. Breathe in with your abdomen and hold for at least 1 minute. Lower your body and straighten legs.

5 Triangle (Above) Breathing in, raise your arms horizontally and place your legs comfortably apart. (Right) Point your left foot out and, breathing out, bend to the left without leaning forward and slide your left hand down your leg towards your ankle. At the same time, raise your right arm, palm facing forwards. Look up at your right hand. Hold the position for at least 1 minute, stretching a little further each time you breathe out. Then breathe in and return to your original position. Repeat the exercise, this time bending to the right.

for a minute or more to build up awareness of the body and its tensions and patterns of behaviour. There should be no sense of extreme exertion or display during yoga exercises; the essence is inner, concentrated awareness.

Breathing plays an important part in yoga. According to yoga philosophy breath embodies the individual's *prana*, or life force. Although breathing is an unconscious function, it can be consciously modified – with a consequent effect on well-being. Breathing also reflects closely our various emotional states, so awareness and control of breathing patterns can play a part in creating mental and emotional harmony (see HYPERVENTILATION; RELAXATION AND BREATHING). Various yoga exercises can be practised to develop different levels of breathing – diaphragm, rib cage and shoulder.

Who it can help Yoga teachers believe that anyone with patience and perseverance can benefit from taking up yoga. Provided that a realistic view is taken of physical capabilities, it can be practised from childhood into very old age. Nor is it designed just for quiet, reclusive types of people; indeed, teachers hold that the more disturbed someone's daily life becomes, the greater is the need for something that brings a compensating calm.

Until quite recently, yoga's role in the West was primarily to promote fitness of body and mind, to be a form of preventive medicine rather than a therapy for specific conditions. It has long been used to help people who suffer from TENSION. Both physical and psychological tensions are often expressed in tense muscles, which may remain contracted in a state of spasm throughout the day. Consciously stretching and releasing the muscles enables the mind to let go of the worries and stresses which originally brought about the muscle spasm.

People with problems in movement and posture benefit from the twisting and bending of yoga exercises which develop flexibility in the spine and the muscles of the back. Because the spine carries nerves from the brain to the trunk and limbs, its well-being is intimately involved in many reflex movements and in the control of PAIN. Yoga is especially useful for people whose problems result from a sedentary lifestyle. It also helps to keep the joints of the arms and legs healthy. It has helped people disabled by PO-LIOMYELITIS.

In its recent therapeutic role, yoga has been used particularly to treat ailments such as severe BACK PAIN, HEADACHES, high BLOOD PRESSURE and heart conditions, asthma and BRONCHITIS, HYSTERIA, ACID STOMACH, and PREMENSTRUAL TENSION.

It is also being tried for helping some cases of chronic illness, including RHEUMATOID

Yoga: a system for all that was once only for the few

The practice of yoga is extremely ancient. Seals made some 4 000 years ago that have been excavated in the prehistoric city of Mohenjo-Daro (in present-day Pakistan) show men sitting crosslegged in positions resembling those adopted in yoga. From early times yoga had a wideranging influence on Indian culture; simple exercises, for example, are used as a form of therapy in the subcontinent's all-embracing traditional system of AYURVEDIC MEDICINE.

One of the most influential yoga teachers, or yogis, was Patanjali, who drew up the formal classification of the discipline that is still in use today. Writing in about 300 BC, he divided the practice of yoga into eight parts. The first two parts are concerned with conduct – with living a peaceful and harmonious life devoted to study, simplicity and cleanliness, and shunning greed, excess and anything that caused harm to other creatures.

The next two of Patanjali's divisions set out the physical aspects of yoga and describe various exercises that calm and energise the body and the mind.

The last four divisions concern the development of various mental and spiritual qualities: detachment from worldly concerns; the ability to rise above the distractions of everyday life; concentration; calm expansion of the mind; and finally, realisation or *samadhi*, a spiritual transformation which brings about a deep insight into the nature of reality.

For century upon century the full practice of yoga was restricted to a small elite, to philosophers and meditators who lived apart from the world in forests or caves, sometimes entirely alone, sometimes in small groups. Each of these yogis would pass on his knowledge and methods to just a few devoted followers.

It is only during the 20th century that the situation has changed markedly. Indian teachers and doctors began to make yoga accessible to all at public centres, and now the change has been so radical that it is the policy of the Indian government that physical yoga exercises should be taught to all children in school.

And the spread of this ancient system of training has not stopped at India's boundaries; yoga is today practised by millions of devotees in countries in every part of the world.

A picture to focus the mind
Devotional images were often used as an aid to yoga meditation. This painting dates from the 17th or 18th century and shows the sacred lotus flower surrounding a figure seated in the 'lotus position' with legs crossed and feet drawn up onto the thighs. The painting comes from Rajasthan in north-west India and belongs to the Jain religious tradition which acquired yogic teachings from Hinduism. Adherents of Jainism practise reverence for all forms of life, and believe that the soul is reincarnated many times before achieving perfection and being liberated from earthly existence.

ARTHRITIS, MULTIPLE SCLEROSIS and DIABETES, for cerebral palsy, for learning difficulties, for OSTEOPOROSIS, for postnatal depression, and to prepare pregnant women for childbirth (see NATURAL CHILDBIRTH).

Finding a therapist or teacher For difficult health problems make sure to consult a skilled yoga therapist. There is still a shortage of experienced therapists since therapeutic yoga remains in its infancy. Your GP or physiotherapist may be able to recommend a suitable person.

For minor problems you will receive adequate help from an ordinary yoga teacher. A teacher is also essential if you wish to take up yoga for general physical and mental health. In the more difficult early stages a regular class with an experienced teacher will prove invaluable, not only for physical guidance but to help you strengthen your mental control and concentration.

Information about classes can be obtained from sports centres, health clubs and some health shops, as well as from the advertising columns of health and fitness magazines.

There are several schools of yoga, so be sure to choose one to suit your interest; for example, those who want to explore the spiritual side of yoga would not be content with what is principally an exercise class.

Postural alignment, with the focus on correct breathing, is emphasised in the system made famous by B K S Iyengar. For information about this method, and for addresses of teachers, write (enclosing a stamped, self-addressed envelope) to the B K S Iyengar Yoga Institute of Southern Africa, 309 Lawley Street, Waterkloof 0181. At the Young Yoga Institute – Duplex 4, Bellevue Heights, 47 Bellevue Road, Durban 4001 – the Iyengar method is taught with a difference, for the teaching has a Christian background.

Those who follow the teachings of the late Swami Sivananda adhere to an integral, classical system of yoga in which all its aspects are practised. Information about this school can be obtained by writing (enclosing a stamped, self-addressed envelope) to the Ananda Kutir Yoga Centre, 24 Sprigg Road, Rondebosch East 7780; or to the Sivananda School of Yoga, 4 Tyson Road, Parkview 2122. Yoga of the classical kind is taught, too, at the Mandana Yoga Institute, 136 Prince Edward Street, Durban 4001.

Addresses of teachers can also be obtained from the Yoga Teachers Fellowship of Southern Africa, P O Box 6929, Brackendowns 1454; or from the International Yoga Teachers Association, 501 Herschel Oaks, Herschel Road, Claremont 7700.

Seeing a therapist or teacher A yoga therapist will tailor routines to suit each individual case. No set pattern exists. The growing awareness and control of the patient and the insight of the therapist, as well as the condition itself, will determine the exact form of the therapy.

When you attend a yoga class, you will be expected to perform the exercises along with all the other class members, led by the teacher. Classes generally last about 1 – 1½ hours. Some classes are designed specifically for beginners, others for more advanced students. There is a spirit of friendly working together, rather than competition.

Self help Progress in yoga is said to come gradually through persistent development of flexibility, strength and mental poise. To aid this development, regular practice at home is recommended, as well as attending classes. Using the class work as the basis, you can plan a routine to follow at home. The following exercises, just three of the hundreds of yoga exercises, could form part of this home routine. Wear loose or stretchy clothing and do the exercises on a thick mat or folded blanket on the floor of a warm, well-ventilated room.

The cobra This exercise aims to develop flexibility and muscle tone in the back.

Lie face down with toes pointed, elbows bent and close to the body, and palms down on the floor beside your shoulders. As you breathe in, raise your head slowly, looking upwards. Hold the position while you breathe out. Then, breathing in again, slowly raise your chest as far as you can, using your back and abdominal muscles to do so, not your arms. Breathe out.

Then, breathing in once more, slowly arch further upwards, using your arms to help. Arch up as far as you can without lifting your navel from the floor and hold the position for two or three normal breaths. Then lower yourself, uncoiling vertebra by vertebra until your face is back on the floor. Rest for a time with your head turned to the side.

Half shoulderstand This inverted posture benefits the abdominal organs and refreshes you when you are tired. But avoid it if you have high blood pressure, are overweight, or are pregnant or menstruating.

Lie on your back with legs together and arms by your sides. As you breathe in, raise your legs until they are vertical; bend your knees if necessary and keep your lower back close to the floor. Pause for a short time in this position.

Then, as you breathe out, continue the leg movement, taking your legs right back over your head and raising your lower back off the floor. Put your hands on your lower back, keeping your elbows on the floor, to give you support. Adjust the angle of your legs to give an easy, relaxed balance. Rest there for one to three minutes, breathing normally. Then lower your arms, breathe in, and gently roll out of the posture.

Tense and relax This exercise makes you aware of your muscles and helps you to relax them at will. The whole sequence should take about two minutes.

Lie on your back with your legs together and arms by your sides. Tighten all your muscles, working slowly from toes to head. As you start to breathe in deeply, tighten first your toes, then your feet, then ankles, calves, kneecaps, thigh muscles. As you breathe out, tighten your abdomen, clench your fists, then tighten your lower arms, upper arms and your shoulders. Breathe in deeply and tighten your chest, throat and face. Make yourself tighter all over.

Hold this position for as long as your breath lasts, then release all the muscles. Move your legs apart and your arms out with the palms upwards. Relax your whole body completely so that you feel as if you are sinking into the floor.

An orthodox view

Yoga, like other forms of meditation and relaxation, helps to relieve many conditions. Provided the exercises are carried out properly, they will improve mobility and circulation; being non-competitive, they should pose no danger of injury.

If yoga is to be used to treat a specific condition, it is essential that the condition should first be properly diagnosed by a qualified doctor. A few doctors do refer patients to yoga therapists and some doctors are taking part in controlled trials to measure the results produced by yoga. Most doctors, however, still see yoga only as a beneficial form of gentle exercise.

YOGHURT

The benefits of yoghurt come from 'acidophilus' bacteria in it. These convert milk into yoghurt by forming lactic acid, which partially curdles the milk and suppresses the growth of harmful bacteria. Eating live yoghurt strengthens the natural bacteria population of the gut, helping to fight off infections.

Most yoghurts are sold with these bacteria still alive but kept dormant by refrigeration, and develop a sharp, acid taste if the bacteria in them are allowed to be active. In heat-treated yoghurt the bacteria have all been killed off, but the lactic acid has by then already been produced and the growth of harmful bacteria inhibited. However, once the carton has been opened, the yoghurt is then still subject to bacterial contamination.

Yoghurt is a source of protein, natural sugars, fat, calcium and other minerals, as well as of B vitamins. The amount of fat it contains

Making your own yoghurt

Bring 600 ml of milk slowly to the boil in a thick-bottomed saucepan. Let it cool to blood heat – test by sprinkling a few drops on the inside of your wrist; it should feel neither hot nor cold.

Stir in a tablespoon of live yoghurt (from your last bought carton), then pour the mixture into a clean vacuum flask, screw on the top and leave for six to eight hours. Alternatively, pour the mixture into a clean shallow dish, wrap it in a linen cloth and then in a thick towel, and put it in a warm airing cupboard for six to eight hours.

The yoghurt will keep for up to six days in the refrigerator. Use the last tablespoonful for the next batch.

depends on the milk used. Yoghurts sold as low-fat are less than 2 per cent fat, compared with about 3,5 per cent fat in whole-milk yoghurt.

ZEN

A Buddhist path to self-discovery

The Japanese form of Buddhism known as Zen is a system of MEDITATION and sustained self-discipline aimed at transforming completely the everyday experience of its adherents through teachings of insight and self-awareness.

Buddhism began in India in the 6th century BC, from where it was taken to China in AD 520 by a monk named Bodhidharma. The type of meditation he taught became known in China as ch'an. In the 12th century it was introduced into Japan, where it has flourished ever since as Zen.

Zen meditation is aimed at achieving direct insight into yourself at a level too deep to be expressed in words. When attained, this is known as enlightenment. Like other forms of Buddhism, Zen also teaches that unhappiness comes from longing for things to be other than they really are, and that learning to accept the real world is an important step on the road to enlightenment.

In Buddhism, the sense of a fixed personal identity is seen as the strongest illusion standing in the way of enlightenment. Everyone wants to believe that the 'self' or personality with which they identify is a permanent one, but Buddhism holds that everything has to change – including this. Teaching centres on helping you to see yourself as part of a never-ending process of change, and of loosening your attachment to a particular self-image.

Who it can help Zen meditation and training aims to help anyone who feels the need for a deeper level of insight and self-awareness in his daily life, or is dissatisfied with the materialistic 'I-centred' way of life that dominates Western society. The new perspective taught by Zen and the effects of practising techniques such as meditation may also help with problems such as STRESS, ANXIETY and DEPRESSION that are aspects of daily life for many Westerners.

Finding a teacher Zen is taught as a form of apprenticeship – each student gets personal tuition from a particular teacher. The teacher's role is to guide, encourage and, if necessary, challenge the pupil's progress. To find a teacher, or for further information, you should write to the Dharma Centre, Heldervue Homestead, 16 Prunus Street, Heldervue, Somerset West 7130.

Seeing a teacher Zen aims at developing a kind of direct understanding based on intuition and going beyond normal thought and reason. Three main techniques are used: daily life practice, meditation, and special anecdotes, riddles and puzzles which are designed to carry thought beyond the limits of the intellect.

Daily life practice The aim is to apply the Buddhist principle of 'mindfulness' in every waking moment. This means being continually aware of your own responses to outside stimuli, and devoting yourself fully to each activity as you perform it, rather than wishing you were doing something else or saying, 'I want ...' or, 'If only ...'

The difficulty here lies in overcoming the common desire to hang onto your illusions and desires – even though they can cause anger, frustration and disappointment.

Zen teaches that by seeing these negative feelings for what they really are, by accepting and 'suffering through' them, the wilful, demanding side of the personality can be tamed. In this state happiness and good fortune are gratefully accepted when they come, but the student does not become attached to them, since he knows that, like everything else, they will pass.

Meditation Known as za-zen (literally, 'sitting meditation'), this is really a special kind of daily life practice. Meditators sit crosslegged on cushions, with weight balanced equally on buttocks and knees, the spine erect and the head balanced upright.

At first, they learn to meditate by silently counting their breaths from one to ten. When other thoughts arise, the meditator must set them aside without dwelling on them, and start the count again.

Za-zen is often both physically and mentally uncomfortable. Maintaining the same posture for long periods can be painful, and meditation forces students to confront the turmoil of their own restless thoughts.

With practice, however, meditators learn to let thoughts come and go without making judgments about them. Eventually, a state is reached where the sitter is aware without there being a personal 'I' who is aware.

Za-zen is practised daily, either privately or in a group. Occasionally, there are longer periods of meditation known as sesshin, which can go on for hours or even days.

Anecdotes, riddles and puzzles Zen abounds with stories, conundrums, parables and paradoxes intended to 'trap' or jolt the rational mind, freeing the student for new ways of thinking. For example, one story tells of two monks looking at a flag flapping in the breeze and arguing. One says: 'The flag is moving.' The other insists: 'No, the wind is moving.' A passing master rebukes them, saying: 'It is your minds that are moving.' Even this, teachers say, is not the last word.

More advanced Zen students are sometimes given a koan to meditate on by their teacher. These are puzzles that cannot be understood or solved by reason. Two examples are: 'What is the sound of one hand clapping?' and 'Show me your original face before you were born.'

The effect is to confront the intellect with a barrier which no amount of logical thinking can penetrate. Instead, insight may burst in with a response born of the immediate moment – a smile, a shout, the sight of raindrops trickling down a windowpane, for example. The answer is to 'un-ask' the question; the problem lies in calling it a problem.

Zen teaches that with each moment of insight, the stranglehold of the personal 'I' on the student's way of thinking is loosened and a new, deeper understanding grows. With this understanding comes an ability to live comfortably in the present – whatever the circumstances – and a feeling of 'travelling light', without strong attachments, in the everyday world.

An orthodox view

There is a theoretical danger that the very unfamiliarity of Zen could make it attractive to some people who happen to be damaged by or out of touch with everyday life. However, Zen is not a form of psychotherapy and cannot provide easy relief from various mental or emotional troubles. The amount of self-confrontation involved may even make it unsuitable for some people with weak psychological defences.

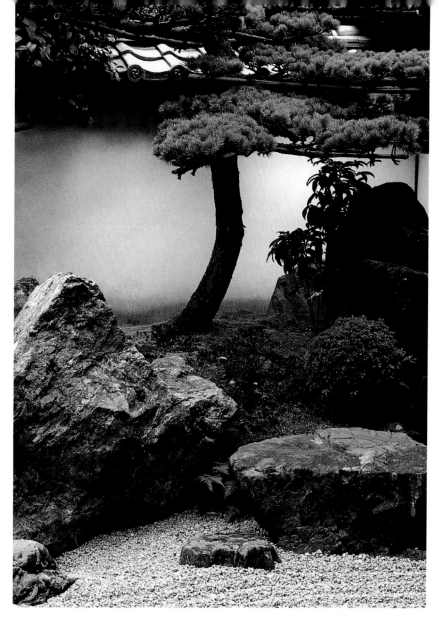

The Zen garden at the working temple of Daitoku-ji, in Kyoto, is among the most celebrated of those found in Japan. Simplicity is the keynote, and the 'shrine' of grey rocks is fronted by well-raked gravel and backed by shrubs and conifers. The garden is revered by the temple monks and admired by visitors.

ZEN GARDEN

The main purpose of a Zen garden is to provide an ideal outdoor setting for MEDITATION – which Zen Buddhists regard as the basis of their religion and their chief way of reaching spiritual enlightenment. To this end the garden's traditional focal point is a rock, or small group of rocks, which are meant to take those who view them out of the immediate, everyday world and into a state of mind in which thought can flourish freely.

The rocks are framed in a setting – such as a small backyard, or a corner of a back garden – which separates and distinguishes them from their wider surroundings. The size and nature of the setting, however, is immaterial. The important thing is that the spectator's eye is led up towards the 'shrine' by the layout of the area.

At its simplest, a Zen garden can consist of three or four strategically placed stones, with a foreground of smoothly raked gravel or closely cropped grass. If you already have a garden which is well-planted and secluded, all you need to do is put your 'shrine' in place and possibly put down some gravel or a short stretch of grass.

If you have the space, however, you can create a more elaborate garden, with converging lines of flowerbeds rising to form a mound behind the rocks. A backdrop of plants can be chosen to match and enhance the shape and size of the rocks. The picture can be 'framed' by an overhanging tree. Finally, the setting should be enclosed by a wall, fence, or dense, evergreen bushes which will cut it off from the outside world. This sense of privacy is essential for the setting to be free of everyday associations.

But no two Zen gardens are exactly alike, and a well-designed garden should reflect its creator's artistic and aesthetic tastes. To achieve this, careful thought should be given to the proportions of the various elements which make up the garden.

The size of the 'shrine' must fit in with the total size of the garden. It must not be so large that it dominates the scene, or so small that it may be overlooked at first sight. Consideration must also be given to the amount of earth used for the mound and flanking flowerbeds; to the right amount of open space needed in the foreground; and to the height

and bulk of the plants used. The exact balance between these elements is up to you. If you wish, the arrangement can be a mixture of interwoven shapes and colours – simple overall but rich in complex and stimulating detail. On the other hand, it can be uncontrived.

However, two important aspects must be borne in mind. Firstly, the rocks should be set off-centre so that they do not merely blend in with the symmetry of the walls behind and on either side of them. Secondly, to achieve the maximum, concentrated effect, the rocks should be arranged as simply and naturally as possible – their different shapes and sizes creating a pleasing but uneven pattern.

The power of such simplicity is graphically shown in the gardens of the Zen Buddhist temples of Daitoku-ji and Ryoan-ji, on the outskirts of the former imperial capital of Japan, Kyoto. Laid out in the late 15th century, the Ryoan-ji garden consists of 15 large stones set in an expanse of grey-white gravel,

which is raked daily. Apart from a few mosses, there are no plants. Even so, the bare beauty of the rocks and their surroundings inspire people throughout the world.

But whichever form of garden is chosen, it should provide the perfect setting to nurture deep and contemplative thought.

ZONE THERAPY

Dr William H Fitzgerald, who introduced RE-FLEXOLOGY to the West around 1913, originally called it zone therapy. Fitzgerald, an American ear, nose and throat specialist, divided the body into ten zones, or energy channels, and applied healing pressure to points on them, using his hands or special instruments. The zones ran from the toes up through the body to the head, then down to the fingers.

377

Alternative and orthodox action in emergencies

Knowing how to give first aid in emergencies can, and does, save many lives. Common emergencies and the techniques used to deal with them are listed alphabetically in this section of the book.

Whenever possible, alternative treatments accompany conventional ones; but where there are no appropriate alternatives, orthodox methods are used.

Remember, however, that it is essential to call a doctor – or an ambulance – for any serious injury or illness. If you are taking herbal or homoeopathic preparations, always tell your GP, as some orthodox treatments may not combine well with these particular medicines.

Using the list as a guide, conventional home or travel first-aid kits of plasters, bandages, antiseptics and so on can be supplemented by various commonly used alternative medicines – including calendula ointment, lavender oil, marjoram and Bach Rescue Remedy.

Artificial respiration: the ABC

When dealing with seriously ill or unconscious patients, there are three main priorities, which can be remembered as A, B and C (Airway, Breathing and Circulation).

● **A. Airway** Check that nothing is blocking the patient's airway to the lungs, and remove anything (such as false teeth) that may be obstructing breathing.

● **B. Breathing** Check that the victim is breathing by watching the chest or holding your cheek close to the mouth or nose. If the victim is not breathing, start ARTIFICIAL RESPIRATION (opposite).

● **C. Circulation** Check if the victim's heart is beating. If not, start CHEST COMPRESSION (p. 382).

Artificial respiration: applying it

● Clear casualty's mouth of blood or vomit.

● Tilt head up so that back is resting on ground with chin well up.

● Pinch casualty's nose shut with your fingers (above).
● Seal your lips around casualty's open mouth.
● Breathe into casualty's mouth until chest rises.
● Remove your mouth (below).
● Keep nose pinched shut with one hand.
● Turn your head to watch casualty's chest fall.

● Replace your mouth and start to breathe into casualty's mouth again. Continue at normal breathing rate of 12-16 a minute (15-30 breaths a minute for children).
● If the casualty starts to vomit during resuscitation turn the head to one side and clear mouth with your finger.
● When mouth is clear, tilt the casualty's head again and resume resuscitation.

Babies and children

Head should not be tilted back too far. In infants, cover nose and mouth with mouth. Perform resuscitation just enough to make chest rise. Give faster breaths – 15-30 a minute – depending on size of child. (The smaller the child the faster the breaths.)

Asphyxiation

Orthodox treatment
● Check casualty is breathing.
● Drag casualty from any danger.
● Untie or cut any cord or other material around neck.
● Clear casualty's airway by lying him on his back, supporting chin, and removing any debris from mouth with finger.

● If airway is blocked by food, treat for CHOKING.
● Check breathing and pulse, see PULSE AND RESPIRATION.
● If you can't see, hear, or feel any breathing, give mouth-to-mouth resuscitation.
● Once breathing is normal, turn casualty on side in recovery position, see UNCONSCIOUSNESS.
● Again make sure casualty's airway is clear.
● Monitor breathing; give artificial respiration again if it falters.
● Get immediate medical aid, if you can do so without leaving casualty unattended.

Bandages

Using a triangular bandage

● Lay out bandage on clean, flat surface ready for use.

● Make broader bandage for emergencies by folding top point of triangle to middle of base.
● Fold bandage once more in same direction.
● To turn broad bandage into narrow one, fold it a third time in same direction.
● Use to bind hands, arms and legs.

Bandages: *making raised pads*

- Put clean cloth over wound.

- Make at least two curved pads by rolling cotton wool or any other material in clean cloth.
- If possible, make pads higher than foreign body in wound.

- Place pads around foreign body and bandage on with diagonal strips of material.
- If foreign body is higher than pads, don't cross bandage over it.
- You then have raised pads to prevent pressure on a wound that has a foreign object in it, such as a piece of glass.

Bites and stings

Alternative treatment (*bites*)

Homoeopathy   Be sure to clean all animal bites with pure tincture of *Hypericum*, or a dilution in cold, boiled water.
- For pain and swelling, try *Apis* 6X.

Orthodox treatment (*bites*)

- Wash the affected area with warm water and soap, or a mild antiseptic preparation.

- Dry gently, wiping down and away from wound.
- Cover with clean dressing. Fix dressing with sterile bandage or plaster.
- If wound is extensive or dirty, take casualty to hospital. Injections against tetanus may be needed, or a course of antibiotics.

Alternative treatment (*stings*)

Traditional Medicine   For insect stings in general, rub affected area with crushed dock leaves, found near nettle-beds.
- For bee stings – in which both sting and poison bag are left in casualty – apply crumbled leaves of plantain to area.
- Alternatively, heat crumbled leaves over flame until they wilt without becoming burnt, squeeze them and rub on juice.
- For wasp stings – in which only poison is left in casualty – dab sting with vinegar.
- Chewed or moist tobacco placed on sting may help to ease pain.
Homoeopathy   For bee stings *Ledum* may help to relieve redness, swelling and pain. Take one dose every hour or two until discomfort stops.
Naturopathy   Immerse affected area in bowl of cold water containing ice cubes and teaspoon of baking soda. This slows circulation and helps prevent poison spreading.
- Alternatively, hold fresh slice of raw onion over area, or cover with wheat-germ oil. Put ice bag on top and apply calendula cream to soothe.
Herbal Medicine   For bee stings apply ice-cold water containing a little bicarbonate of soda on sting.
- For wasp stings put some drops of lemon juice in water and apply.
- Alternatively, apply plain ice cube.
- Marigold ointment may help to reduce swelling.

Orthodox treatment (*stings*)

- Scrape out bee sting and poison bag with fingernail, or any blunt edge.
- Avoid squeezing bag as this spreads poison.
- Apply antihistamine cream or calamine lotion to relieve itching.

- If casualty reacts strongly to bee or wasp sting, or if sting seems infected, get medical help.
- In rare cases, casualty may be allergic to stings. This can be fatal – get specialist help as soon as possible.
- If you know you are allergic to stings, ask your doctor for pre-filled syringe of adrenaline to inject in an emergency.

Bleeding

Orthodox treatment

Treat deep cuts to chest with casualty sitting up and inclined towards injured side.
You should treat deep cuts to the stomach, leg or back with the casualty lying down as comfortably as possible.

- Gently remove clothing from around wound (above).
- Press down firmly on the wound with clean, absorbent material or bare hands.
- If possible, raise injured leg, arm or head to slow bleeding (below).
- Maintain pressure on the wound for 5-15 minutes.
- When bleeding stops, put absorbent pad – such as sterile gauze or clean, folded handkerchief – over wound.

- Bandage firmly with scarf or clean piece of linen.
- If blood seeps through dressing, put another on top.
- Get medical attention, if you can do so without leaving casualty for more than a minute or two.
- Don't give anything to eat or drink.
- Regularly check casualty's pulse and breathing.
- Be ready to give first aid for other injuries if necessary.

Warning Don't touch any foreign object firmly embedded in wound. Never pull out object that has made puncture – such as knife – as it may be plugging wound.
- Put raised pad of clean material around wound – preferably higher than object – to prevent pressure on it, see BANDAGES.
- Bandage pad with diagonally applied strips of material that don't go over foreign object.
- Get medical attention as soon as possible.
- If casualty bleeds from ear, mouth or nose, this can indicate serious injury to head or chest.
- In this case, put casualty in half-sitting position.
- If nose is bleeding, pinch bridge just below bone with your fingers and apply firm pressure for at least 5 minutes.
- Cover other bleeding points with clean cloth. Don't apply pressure.
- Get medical aid immediately.
- If casualty becomes unconscious, place in recovery position, see UNCONSCIOUSNESS.

Alternative treatment (*cuts*)

Herbal Medicine Apply calendula ointment after washing cut in running water, or warm, soapy water to remove any surrounding dirt. Alternatively, soak cut with calendula tincture.

Orthodox treatment (*cuts*)

- Take clean piece of cloth and press it on cut, or around edges if foreign body is in it.
- When bleeding stops, take pad away and remove any dirt or gravel that comes out easily.
- Gently wipe wound outwards with swab soaked in warm, soapy water. Use fresh swab for each wipe.
- Gently dry around wound with clean swab and apply plaster or bandage.

Warning Never apply tourniquet as this reduces supply of oxygen in blood and can permanently damage tissues, leading to gangrene and possible amputation.

Blisters

Alternative treatment

Biochemic Tissue Salts Adults should take four tablets of Nat. *mur.* half-hourly; children should take two tablets half-hourly.
Aromatherapy Dab lavender oil on blister.
Traditional Medicine Applying the leaves of the spekboom, the water lily or traveller's joy are among traditional South African means of relieving blisters. Blisters can also be soothed by the fruit and leaf of the bitter apple.

Orthodox treatment

- Gently wipe blister with cotton wool soaked in methylated spirit.
- Alternatively, wash it with soap and water, or antiseptic wipe.
- A blister should not be burst because the underlying damaged tissue could become infected. You should see your doctor about large, troublesome blisters, sometimes called bullae.

Burns and scalds

Alternative treatment (*burns*)

Homoeopathy For superficial burns apply *Hypericum* lotion to burnt area.

Orthodox treatment (*burns*)

- Bathe burnt area in cold water for 10-15 minutes.

- Remove any jewellery or rings and cover area with clean bandages or clean handkerchief.
- Do *not* apply butter or fat.

Warning Don't try to treat deep burns or those that blister. Seek expert medical help without delay.

Alternative treatment (*scalds*)

Homoeopathy Apply *Hypericum* lotion to scalded area. Dosage is about 10 drops of lotion in cup of water.
- Take some drops of Bach Rescue Remedy in glass of cold water.

Orthodox treatment (*scalds*)

- Cool scalded area with cold water.
- Cover scald with clean, non-fluffy material such as linen handkerchief.
- If scald is serious, get medical aid.

Chest compression

Providing artificial pump for blood if heart has stopped beating

● Give 2 inflations of casualty's lungs and then feel for carotid pulse for at least 5 seconds.
,● If pulse can't be detected, and if casualty's complexion is blue-grey, place on firm surface and start chest compression.

● Feel for breastbone.

● Place heel of one hand on casualty's chest, two fingers up from bottom of breastbone.
● Keep thumb and fingers raised and off chest.

● Keep heel of hand in place and put other hand over it, fingers locked, thumb and finger raised.
● Press down 40-50 mm. Let chest rise.
● Give 15 presses, then inflate lungs twice by ARTIFICIAL RESPIRATION.

● Check carotid pulse after 1 minute.
● Continue chest compression until pulse returns, and give artificial respiration until casualty breathes.
Adults   Repeat pressure at normal pulse rate: 80 times a minute.

Children   Lightly repeat pressure 80-100 times a minute, according to size of child. (The smaller the child the faster the rate.)
● Press lightly with heel of one hand on lower part of breastbone to depth of 25-40 mm.
● After pressing breastbone down, let it rise.
● Give 5 presses followed by 1 lung inflation.
● Repeat until pulse beats unaided.
● Continue if necessary.

Babies   Very lightly repeat pressure with two fingers 120 times a minute.
● Support baby along one arm, with your hand cradling its head, which should be tilted slightly down. (Artificial respiration can also be given in this position.)
● Press middle of breastbone down about 13 mm, using two fingers, and let it rise.
● Give 5 presses followed by 1 small lung inflation.
● Repeat until pulse beats unaided.
Warning   Chest compression should only be used if casualty's

heart has stopped beating altogether and he seems likely to die. Ideally, it should be learned from a qualified instructor, and should be applied only by someone who has been trained. If applied wrongly or unnecessarily it could be fatal.

Choking

Orthodox treatment

Tell casualty to cough vigorously. If obstruction isn't cleared, apply following:
Back slaps   Give 3 or 4 sharp, flat slaps between casualty's shoulder blades with palm of hand.

● If casualty is young child, turn upside down while giving slaps.
● Rest older child face down across your thigh while giving slaps.

The Heimlich Manoeuvre or abdominal thrust (conscious adult) Stand behind casualty and put arms around waist, making fist with one hand.

● Place thumb side slightly above casualty's navel and below rib cage.
● Hold fist with other hand and give 3 or 4 strong pulls diagonally upwards and towards you.
● Use hands to exert pressure; don't just squeeze with arms.
● Once obstruction has been cleared, reassure casualty and give frequent sips of water. Adults should sip cup of water over 10 minutes to help recovery.
Abdominal thrust (unconscious adult) Turn victim face up, kneel astride hips, put hand above navel.

● Push on it with your other hand, thrusting at an angle downwards and towards casualty's head.
● Clear mouth with finger. If necessary, give ARTIFICIAL RESPIRATION and CHEST COMPRESSION if the heart has stopped.

● Once casualty's breathing is normal, put in recovery position.
● Give casualty something to drink when fully conscious.
Abdominal thrust (self help)
Below left: clench the fist and place it, thumb side against abdomen, above the navel.

● With other hand, jerk fist inwards and upwards repeatedly. Alternatively use back of chair or table edge.
● Lean over edge, supported by hands on either side. Thrust inwards and upwards 3 or 4 times.

Abdominal thrust (conscious child) Sit child on your lap, facing away from you.
● Put tips of two fingers of each hand side by side, just above navel.
● Press gently but firmly upwards.
Abdominal thrust (unconscious child) Lie child face up.
● Put tips of two fingers of each hand side by side, just above navel.
● Press gently but firmly upwards.
● Clear mouth of any object.
● Give child water to sip when consciousness returns.

Concussion

A sharp blow to the head can shake and disturb the brain, causing concussion. Symptoms may include confusion, slurred speech, vomiting, unsteadiness, inability to follow commands, or loss of consciousness.

Orthodox treatment

● Get expert medical help urgently.
● On recovery, casualty may suffer nausea and vomiting.
● Following head injury, any pressure on brain – from blood, fluid or fracture of skull – can cause compression, affecting casualty's alertness and level of consciousness.
● Compression may develop immediately after injury, or more slowly after casualty has apparently recovered from concussion.
● Again, get urgent medical help.

Drowning

Orthodox treatment

● Keep casualty's head and upper chest clear of water.
● Remove any debris from mouth.
● If casualty's breathing has stopped, start mouth-to-mouth ARTIFICIAL RESPIRATION.
● Move carefully towards dry land.
● Once in shallow water continue artificial respiration. Don't waste time bringing up water from lungs.
● Take casualty's pulse, see PULSE AND RESPIRATION. If there's no pulse, start CHEST COMPRESSION.
● Once breathing has re-started, turn casualty into recovery position, see UNCONSCIOUSNESS.
● Cover casualty with blankets or towels and treat any injuries.
● Get medical help immediately.
Note Don't stop artificial respiration, even if situation looks hopeless. Recovery can be achieved even after apparent death for a long period. Nobody should be regarded as dead if the body is cold from immersion or exposure.

Electric shock

Orthodox treatment

● Turn off power. If casualty is holding frayed wire from electric lead, and power can't be switched off, rescuer may receive shock.

● With such accidents, lever casualty away from source of electricity with long, thick, dry piece of wood – such as broom handle.
● If possible, stand on dry, insulating material such as rubber mat or pile of newspapers.
● Once casualty is safely removed from contact with electric source, smother any burning clothes with blanket or towel.
● If impact of shock has thrown casualty to ground, check to see if breathing and heartbeat have stopped, see Pulse and Respiration.
● If necessary, apply Artificial Respiration and Chest Compression.
● Once casualty is breathing naturally, place in recovery position, see Unconsciousness.
● Check for broken bones and give appropriate treatment, see Fractures.
● Treat minor burns by cooling with cold water, then cover with dressings or suitable material.
● Call ambulance as soon as possible.

Exposure

Orthodox treatment

● Wrap casualty in spare, dry clothes or blankets, or put sleeping-bags over clothes.
● Get casualty to tent or other spot sheltered from wind and rain.
● Lie casualty on blanket or groundsheet to prevent further heat loss.
● Remove wet clothes and put casualty into sleeping-bag, or cover with blankets or spare clothes.
● Wrap any windproof material – such as polythene or aluminium foil – on top of clothes for extra protection.
● Use a space blanket if one is available.
● Check casualty's breathing and pulse, see Pulse and Respiration.
● Be ready to give Artificial Respiration and Chest Compression if necessary.
● Give warm, sweet, non-alcoholic drink and chocolate or biscuits if possible.
● Give warm (not hot) bath and get casualty into warm bed.
● Do not give up resuscitation until a doctor has declared that death has occurred.

Eye injuries

Orthodox treatment

Chemical burns Tilt casualty's head with injured eye pointing down.
● Flood eye with gently running cold or lukewarm water.
● Alternatively, wash chemical away by splashing water from basin.
● Lightly put the pad over the eye and get the casualty to hospital without delay.
Impaled objects Don't try to remove an impaled object from eye.
● Cut hole in piece of gauze and put over injured eye.
● Place soft pad, paper cup or similar object over gauze. This keeps gauze in place and should be secured by bandage.

● Cover uninjured eye as well to reduce eye movement.
● Get immediate medical aid.
Cut eyebrows Make casualty sit down with head erect. This will reduce bleeding by lowering the blood pressure to the head.
● Firmly put gauze pad over cut.
● Once bleeding is controlled, leave pad in place and put retaining bandage over it. Be careful not to put pressure on eye itself.
● Get immediate medical aid.

Fainting

Alternative treatment

Bach Remedies As casualty comes round, place few drops of Rescue Remedy on tongue, or offer in water or tea.
Homoeopathy Give *Aconite* after faint from fright, *Arsenicum album* after faint from exhaustion or cold, and *Carbo vegetalis* after faint from lack of air.
Acupressure Use fingernail to stimulate firmly point on midline two-thirds of way up, between casualty's top lip and nose.

Orthodox treatment

● If casualty has passed out, but is breathing normally, lay on back with legs raised above level of head.
● Make sure casualty can still breathe, if necessary by supporting chin.
● Hold legs up, or prop them on chair or anything else suitable.
● Loosen clothing at neck, chest and waist and ensure casualty gets plenty of fresh air. If casualty is indoors, open windows.
● If casualty is out of doors, do the same and protect from sun.
● Casualty should stay lying down for a few minutes after recovering, before attempting to rise.
● If casualty has difficulty in breathing, ensure that airway is clear and, if necessary, apply Artificial Respiration.

Fractures

Alternative treatment

Homoeopathy To help relieve pain offer casualty *Asafoetida* 6 or 6X.
● Get expert medical help.

Orthodox treatment

● Gently remove clothing from any open wound over break, making sure to move affected area as little as possible.
● Cover wound with clean piece of lint. If bone protrudes, place gauze raised pad over area, see BANDAGES.
● Support injured part, ensuring circulation is not restricted.
● If break is in leg, use uninjured leg as splint by tying it to other leg with bandages at knees and ankles and around feet. Pad between legs.
● Broken arm can be supported in sling, see SLINGS.
● Broken finger can be taped to adjacent finger.

Frostbite

Alternative treatment

Traditional Medicine For early stage of minor frostbite put slices of peeled cucumber dipped in warm water on affected area. Alternatively, use slices of raw onion.

Orthodox treatment

● Do *not* apply any form of direct heat – such as from fire – to frostbitten skin, and do *not* rub skin.
● Instead, warm area slowly between your hands until circulation returns.
● With frostbitten foot, remove casualty's shoe and sock and cover foot with linen pad.
● Cover foot with warm sock, blanket or sleeping-bag.
● Bandage frostbitten hands and cover in similar manner.
● Make sure casualty is wrapped warmly with coats or blankets and give plenty of hot, sweet drinks and painkillers as needed.

Head and facial injuries

Orthodox treatment

Scalp injuries Place clean pad or your hands on wound to stop the bleeding.
● Cover wound with clean dressing. If foreign object is present, or if fracture is suspected, put dressing on lightly with pad on top of it to avoid causing further injury.
● Fix dressing or pad with bandage around head or chin, depending on position of wound.
● Keep casualty's head as steady as possible.
Broken jaw If jaw is broken or dislocated, make sure mouth is clear of blood or debris and that casualty can breathe.
● Put makeshift pad under point of chin.
● Put narrow bandage or scarf under chin.
● Tie ends of bandage on top of head in double knot.
● Make sure bandage is tight enough to support jaw, but not so tight casualty's teeth are clenched.
Bleeding face Press sterile pad or clean handkerchief against wound to stem bleeding.
● Seek medical aid.

Heart attack and stroke

Orthodox treatment (heart attack)

Symptoms are sudden crushing pain in chest, often spreading to the arms, neck and jaw. Possibly also breathlessness.
● Check victim's breathing and pulse, see PULSE AND RESPIRATION.
● If necessary, give ARTIFICIAL RESPIRATION and, if there's no pulse, CHEST COMPRESSION.
● If victim is conscious, put in half-sitting position, with head and shoulders supported with pillows or cushions, and cushion under knees.
● If there's loss of consciousness, lie victim flat.
● Loosen clothing at neck, chest and waist.

● Send for medical aid immediately.
● Comfort victim and stop any onlookers from crowding around.
● Give two soluble aspirin tablets in water to reduce blood clotting.

Orthodox treatment (stroke)

Symptoms may include paralysis down one side of body, difficulty in swallowing and speaking. Possibly confusion and loss of consciousness.
● If victim is conscious, lay down with head and shoulders slightly raised and supported with pillow.
● If victim is not conscious, place on side in recovery position, see UNCONSCIOUSNESS.
● Send for medical aid immediately.
● Comfort victim and stop any onlookers from crowding around.

Heat stroke

Orthodox treatment (heat stroke)

● Remove victim from source of heat, preferably to cool room.
● Undress victim and wrap in sheet or towels soaked in tepid water.
● Fan regularly.
● Take victim's temperature every 5 minutes.
● When temperature is down to 38°C (101°F), remove wet sheet, but continue fanning.
● If temperature rises again, restart cooling treatment.
● If victim is unconscious, place on side in recovery position, see UNCONSCIOUSNESS.
● If victim is conscious, you can give a cup of weakly salted water every 10 minutes.
● Use level teaspoon of salt to each litre of water. Add fruit juice to improve taste.

Motion sickness

Alternative treatment

Acupressure Press point three fingers' width above wrist crease on inner wrist, centrally, in line with middle finger. Apply pressure towards centre of wrist.
● Alternatively, wristbands applying similar pressure can be worn. Get them from chemists, airports or seaports and main travel stations.
Homoeopathy Try *Petroleum* for nausea and vomiting; *Tabacum* for nausea, sweating and giddiness; and *Borax* for turbulence during air travel.

Orthodox treatment

● Travel-sickness and seasickness tablets are available from chemists. Take one about ½-1 hour before setting out on a journey.
● If driving, do *not* take tablets containing antihistamine, which can cause drowsiness.
● Fresh air and regular breaks should help ward off sickness.

Overdose

Orthodox treatment

● If breathing stops, start ARTIFICIAL RESPIRATION immediately, with CHEST COMPRESSION if there's no pulse.
● If casualty is breathing but unconscious, place on side in recovery position and treat for UNCONSCIOUSNESS.
● If casualty is conscious, treat for POISONING.
● Get medical aid immediately, even if casualty seems to have recovered.
● Keep any vomit, tablets, bottles or containers which will help identify overdose drug.
Warning Try to keep casualty awake, but do not give coffee or help him to walk about. Wait until stomach has been pumped out.

Poisoning

Orthodox treatment

● If casualty isn't breathing give ARTIFICIAL RESPIRATION with CHEST COMPRESSION if necessary.
● If casualty is unconscious, but breathing, turn on side in recovery position, see UNCONSCIOUSNESS.
● Check that airway is clear.
● If necessary, hold chin forwards so that tongue doesn't fall back into casualty's throat.
● If casualty is conscious and has swallowed something caustic, give half a litre of milk to be sipped slowly to dilute poison in stomach.
● Don't deliberately make casualty vomit without medical advice.
● Get medical help immediately.

Pulse and respiration

Two places to take pulse

On inside of wrist (above) About 25 mm below base of casualty's thumb and 13 mm in from edge of arm.
● Place three fingers on pulse and press slightly.
● Time the beats.
On carotid area (below) On outer side of neck, by windpipe and just over halfway to jawline.
● Place three fingers on pulse and press slightly.
● Time the beats.

● Take casualty's pulse and respiration rates as you are treating him – except in cases of minor injuries.
● Bend casualty's arm at elbow so that it rests across chest near opposite shoulder, if that won't worsen injuries.
● Raise wrist slightly and feel for pulse with your fingertips – not your thumb.
● Count beats for 30 seconds and remember figure.
● Keep holding wrist and count number of times casualty's chest rises in next 30 seconds.
● Double pulse and respiration figures to express them per minute.
● Write them down, or have them noted by helper.

Normal pulse rate

Adults 60-80 beats a minute; average 72.
Children 90-100 beats a minute.
Babies Up to 140 beats a minute.

Normal respiration rate

Adults 12 times a minute when at rest.
Children and babies 20-40 times a minute.

Shock

Symptoms may include grey or pallid skin, cold and moist to touch; fast, shallow breathing and rapid, weak and thin pulse; dizziness or faintness; blurred vision; nausea or vomiting; thirst; anxiety and restlessness, sometimes leading to loss of consciousness.

Orthodox treatment

● Lay casualty down and treat any obvious injury or underlying condition which has caused shock.
● Reassure casualty.
● Loosen casualty's clothing at neck, chest and waist. Lightly cover with coat or single blanket.
● If possible, raise casualty's legs to return blood supply to brain.

- If casualty complains of thirst, moisten lips but don't give anything to drink.
- Try to comfort and calmly reassure casualty.
- Don't move casualty unnecessarily.
- If casualty is unconscious, put on side in recovery position, see UNCONSCIOUSNESS.
- Try to get immediate medical aid, but don't leave casualty unattended.

Slings

Making a triangular sling

- If the casualty's hand or forearm is injured, first raise the arm so that the hand rests on the opposite shoulder. Get the casualty to hold it in place if possible.

- Put one point of base of sling over casualty's shoulder on uninjured side, with point extended well beyond elbow. Sling should hang over injured arm (above).
- Gently push base of sling under hand, forearm and elbow of injured limb. Bring lower end of base up and around casualty's back on injured side (below).

- Bring two ends of sling together round back of casualty on injured side. Tie at uninjured shoulder.

- Fold top of sling at elbow and fasten with pin or tape, or tuck it in.
- Check nail beds to make sure they haven't turned blue, indicating constricted blood supply. If they have, ease sling or bandage.

Improvising sling

- Use belt, tie, narrow scarf, or roller bandage.
- For injured upper arm, wrap improvised sling round casualty's wrist on injured side.

- Bring other end of sling across casualty's chest and around back of neck.

- Tie ends in hollow above collar-bone on uninjured side.

Splinters

Orthodox treatment

- Sterilise pair of tweezers by passing them through flame. Be sure not to wipe any soot from them.
- Alternatively, boil tweezers in water for 10 minutes.
- Wash the skin around injury carefully with warm, soapy water. Make sure that you wipe outwards from wound.
- Dry skin carefully. ·
- Using tweezers, pull splinter out.
- When splinter has been removed, wash wound with mild antiseptic and dry gently.

- Cover wound with plaster or sterile dressing.
- If splinter can't be removed, or becomes painful, get medical aid.

Warning Unskilled person should *not* put splint on broken limb. Fractures should only be splinted by skilled person if casualty has to undergo long or rough journey to receive medical aid.

- If casualty faces long or rough journey to receive medical aid, use five bandages.

- Tie feet and ankles together with bandage.

Splints

Improvising bandage splint

- If one leg is injured, prepare to bandage to other leg.
- Carefully and gently move uninjured leg to it.
- Place plenty of padding between legs – especially knees and ankles.
- Carefully and gently move uninjured leg to injured.

Improvising blanket splint
- Roll blanket lengthways as tightly as possible.

- Tie casualty's feet and ankles together (above).
- Tie knees together with bandage knotted on uninjured side (below).
- Tie extra bandages above and below fracture site.

- Tie broad fold bandage around knees.

- Place one end between casualty's legs, starting at crotch.
- Bring blanket around foot of injured leg and take other end alongside leg up to thighs.
- Tie legs together with two bandages.

- Tie knot on uninjured leg.
- Tie third and fourth bandages above and below fracture site.
- Tie fifth bandage around casualty's thigh or calf, depending on where fracture is.

Sprains and strains

Alternative treatment (*sprains*)

Homoeopathy Take A*rnica* 30 as soon as possible after accident, hourly for 6 doses.
Aromatherapy Apply hyssop and marjoram as soon as possible after accident and massage area gently.
● Use 2 drops of each oil in teaspoon of vegetable carrier oil.
● Apply compress made with 5 drops of each oil and enough water to soak through compress.
● Hold compress in place with clingfilm and leave for several hours.

Orthodox treatment (*sprains*)

● For indoor ankle sprains remove casualty's shoe.
● For outdoor ankle sprains leave shoe on.
● In either case, apply cold compress to injury and elevate foot.
● Place bandage over compress.
● Make one turn around ankle, then go over instep, under foot, back across instep, around ankle again and pin.
● Bandage over shoe.
● For wrist sprains, apply cold compress and bandage in place.
● Consult doctor to exclude fracture.

Orthodox treatment (*strains*)

● Steady and support casualty's injured part.
● Gently apply cold compress.
● Keep injured part steady and well supported.
● Bandage firmly but not too tightly as muscles may swell, causing further discomfort.
● Get medical aid.

Sunburn

Alternative treatment

Herbal Medicine Apply cold water then add 1 or 2 drops of lavender oil.
● Alternatively, apply cold compress of marigold infusion.

Marigold or comfrey cream may ease large, mild burns.
● Apply fresh leaves of houseleeks or plaintain to small burns.
Naturopathy Immerse small burns in cold water for 2 or 3 minutes, then dab dry. Immerse large burns in cold bath, then apply vitamin E moisturising cream.
Traditional Medicine Try lotion made from dock roots or mixture of water and vinegar.

Orthodox treatment

● Rest casualty in shade and give plenty of liquids to drink.
● Don't let casualty out in sun again without covering affected areas with light, loose clothing.
● Soothe mild cases of sunburn by bathing in cool water, or applying calamine lotion, witch hazel or proprietary after-sun lotion or cream to affected areas.
● If sunburn is severe, get medical help.
Warning Never deliberately burst blisters caused by sunburn.

Unconsciousness

Orthodox treatment

● Check to see if casualty is still breathing.
● Put your ear to casualty's nose or mouth and listen.
● Watch chest to see if it rises and falls, or rest your hand lightly on it to feel for movement.
● If there's no breathing, give ARTIFICIAL RESPIRATION.
● Check casualty's pulse, see PULSE AND RESPIRATION.
● If there's no pulse, start CHEST COMPRESSION.
● If and when casualty is breathing, loosen his clothing at neck, chest and waist.
● Turn casualty to recovery position (see illustration).
● Open doors and windows for fresh air.
● Check for injuries or bruises and stem any bleeding.
● Get medical assistance as soon as possible.

Recovery position

● Turn casualty on side by kneeling and tucking near arm under body, palm upwards.

● Cross ankle farthest away from you over one nearest to you.
● Put other arm over chest.

● Turn casualty towards you, supporting head with your hand.
● Place your other hand on his hip and roll him gently towards you.
● Hold casualty's chin forwards.
● Bend casualty's knee to stop him rolling over too far.

● Pull the other arm out behind the body so that casualty is prevented from rolling back.

● Pull up casualty's arm nearest to you so that point of elbow is in line with shoulder.
● Don't leave casualty unattended.

Index

Acknowledgments

The publishers wish to thank the following individuals, companies and organisations for their assistance in the preparation of this book.

Chris Albertyn; Ericka Allison; Atomic Energy Corporation of South Africa; Meloma Balaskas; Dr Cyril Beardwood; Dr Ruth Bloch; Charlene Bluett; Bric A Brac Lane; Esme Butler; Kevin Campbell; Sarah Campbell; The Camphill Farm Community; Barbara Cohen; Peter Collis; Wendy Cullinan; Dr Jean-Claude Degueldre; Miss Rose De La Hunt; Earthlife Africa; Denise Findley; Mannie Finger; Anne Fiske; J A Folliott; Dr Peter Frazer; Garon Foods; Dr Raoul Goldberg; Dr A Grazioli; Dr Christa Hall-Sandford; George Heye; Professor Justus Hofmeyr; Jackie Holzen; Shirley Horwitz; Marius Hulsman; Lilian Jones; Dr Mark Jury; Dr M R Khan; Dr Frans Kromhout; Polly Lansdown; Priscilla Lazarus; Dr Vaughan Leader; Dr Barbara Lewis; Charles Liggins; Heiner Lotzer; Robyn MacLean; Martha's Vineyard; Dr K R Matthews; Arthur Miller; Dr Geraldine Mitten; Miss Linda Muller; Natural Remedies Centre; Naturama; Dalene Newbould; Lindsey Nicholls; Dr Michael O'Brien; Swami Parvathi; Jill Persson; Pick 'n Pay Stores; David Plank; Dr Bernie Radomsky; Helen Ranger; Leslie Reed; Peter Roux; Imam Achmat Salie; Betty Salmon; Dr Y Saloojee; Dr A E Saon; Professor Diana Schmukler; Dr Peter Smith; Imam Hassan Solomon; Michele Stalling; Adam Struben; A Swanepoel; Pat Swilling; Sheila To; David Townsend; Joan van Alphen; Marguerite van der Merwe; Dr W C van der Veen; Dr Gert van der Walt; Peggy Walford; Carol Watkins; The Wellstead.

The photographs and drawings in *The Family Guide to Natural Medicine* were supplied by the following sources. Names printed in *italics* refer to illustrations that are Reader's Digest copyright. Where ambiguous, the position of an illustration on the page is indicated by letters in brackets, as follows: T = top; C = centre; B = bottom; L = left; R = right.

11 Sheila Brandt; 13 Biz Hull; 14 Rosalyn Kennedy; 15 Biz Hull; 16 (T) Michael Holford, (B) ET Archive/National Palace Museum, Taiwan; 21 Diana Miller; 22 Biz Hull; 23 (L) Rosalyn Kennedy, (TR) Glynn Macdonald; 24 Rosalyn Kennedy; 31 Biz Hull; 32 (L) Mansell Collection, (R) P Blundell-Jones/The Architectural Association; 35 The Ancient Art & Architecture Collection; 36 Biz Hull; 39 Richard Bonson; 40 Rosalyn Kennedy; 44 CNRI/Science Photo Library; 47-48 Biz Hull; 50 The Hulton Picture Company; 52 Biz Hull; 54 Tim Pearce; 55 Rosalyn Kennedy; 56-57 Biz Hull; 58-59 Rosalyn Kennedy; 60-62 Biz Hull; 65 Archiv fur Kunst und Geschichte, Berlin; 68 Biz Hull; 69 Baird Harris Ltd; 73 Rosalyn Kennedy; 78-79 CNRI/Science Photo Library; 83 Rosalyn Kennedy; 86 (T) The Scofield Chiropractic Clinic, (BL) Dr Brian Hammond, (BR) Biz Hull; 96 Baird Harris Ltd; 99 J Paisley/Photo Access Library; 100 Biz Hull; 102 John Walmsley/Impact Photos; 104-5 Biz Hull (from photos by Bronwen Burford); 110 (L) Biz Hull, (R) Rosalyn Kennedy; 111 Rosalyn Kennedy; 112 Mary Evans Picture Library; 119-25 Diana Miller; 129 Biz Hull; 130 Tim Pearce; 133 Baird Harris Ltd; 134-5 Rosalyn Kennedy; 137 Biz Hull; 138 Rosalyn Kennedy; 140 The Floatarium, Brighton; 142-3 The Image Bank; 144 Reader's Digest;

145 Diana Miller; 147 Reader's Digest; 151 Biz Hull; 153 ET Archive; 155 Diana Miller; 156 Mary Evans Picture Library; 162-3 Biz Hull; 166 Mansell Collection; 168 Diana Miller; 170 (L) High Rustenberg, (R) Reader's Digest; 171 Andra Nelki; 172-3 Richard Bonson; 175 Photo Source/Photo Access Library; 176-7 Richard Bonson; 180 Biz Hull; 181 David Thorpe; 182 Michael Holford; 184 Rosalyn Kennedy; 185 (T) Garden Picture Library, (BL) Richard Bonson, (BR) Elizabeth Whiting & Associates; 186-7 Vernon Morgan; 192 (L) Ted Lau/Time magazine, (R) The Bettmann Archive; 194 Biz Hull; 202 Julie Busby; 204 Tim Pearce; 205 (TL) CNRI/Science Photo Library, (TC) Oxford Molecular Biophysics Laboratory/Science Photo Library, (TR) Biology Media/Science Photo Library, (B) Richard Bonson; 206 (T) Dr Steve Patterson/Science Photo Library, (B) Richard Bonson; 207 Baird Harris Ltd; 208 (T) Gordon Garradd/Science Photo Library, (C) Julian Nieman/Susan Griggs Agency, (B) Biz Hull; 210 (T) Baird Harris Ltd, (BL) Biz Hull, (BR) Peter Enkel; 213 Rosalyn Kennedy; 214 (L) CNRI/Science Photo Library, (R) Tim Pearce; 215-17 Biz Hull; 218 Dr Leonard W Konikiewicz; 220 ET Archive; 223 Françoise Sauze/Science Photo Library; 225 Biz Hull; 226-7 Rosalyn Kennedy; 230 Joanna Walker; 232-3 Diana Miller; 239-40 Biz Hull; 244 Mary Evans Picture Library; 247 Biz Hull; 248 Gamma/Frank Spooner; 253 National Medical Slide Library; 254 Reader's Digest 255 (T & BL) Rosalyn Kennedy, (R) Andra Nelki; 258 Mary Evans Picture Library; 259 Rosalyn Kennedy; 260 Petit Format; 261 (T) Mary Evans Picture Library, (B) Sally & Richard Greenhill; 262 (T) Rosalyn Kennedy, (B) Biz Hull; 265 Biz Hull; 269 Popperfoto; 270 Biz Hull; 277 Shirley Harris; Chapman/Collins & Partners; 280-4 Rosalyn Kennedy; 290 (R) Freud Museum, (L) Mary Evans Picture Library/Sigmund Freud Collection; 293 Zefa; 295 Baird Harris; 296-8 Biz Hull; 299 Tim Pearce.; 300 Rosalyn Kennedy; 303 (TR & BR) Biz Hull, (BL) Karsh of Ottawa; 304 Biz Hull; 305 Ann Ronan Picture Library; 309-10 Biz Hull; 316 (L) Biz Hull, (R) Rosalyn Kennedy; 320 Richard Bonson; 323 Malcolm Porter; 333 Joanna Walker; 334-5 Sally & Richard Greenhill, (B) Biz Hull; 336 Biz Hull; 337 Richard Bonson; 338 (T) Lorraine Rorke, (B) Dave Stock; 345 Rosalyn Kennedy; 346 Roger de la Harpe; 347 (T) Jean Morris, (B) Shaen Adey; 348 South African Library; 351 Richard Bonson; 356-7 Diana Miller; 359 Narodni Galerie, Prague/Bridgeman Art Library; 369 Rex Features; 370-3 Rosalyn Kennedy; 374 Werner Forman Library; 377 Marijke Heuff/The Garden Picture Library; 378-89 Andrew Aloof.

The publishers acknowledge their indebtedness to the following books and journals, which were consulted for reference.
The Alternative Dictionary of Symptoms and Cures by Dr Caroline M Shreeve (Century); *The Alternative Health Guide* by Brian Inglis and Ruth West (Michael Joseph); *A-Z of the Human Body* (Reader's Digest); *Beating Back Pain* by Dr John Tanner (Dorling Kindersley); *Bibliography: Guide to Natural Medicine* The American Medical Association Encyclopedia of Medicine (Randon House, New York); *Biochemic Tissue Salts* by Andrew Stanway (Thorsons); *Bloomsbury Good Health Guide* (Bloomsbury); *Boiling Energy* by Richard Katz (Harvard University Press); *Chiropractice* by Arthur G Scofield (Thorsons); *Clinical Medicine: A Textbook for Medical Students and Doctors* edited by Parveen J Kumar & Michael L Clark (ELBS); *The Complete Manual of Fitness and Well-Being* (Reader's Digest); *The Complete Natural Health Consultant* by Michael van Straten (Ebury Press); *Concise Medical Dictionary* (Oxford University Press); *Coping with Old Age* by Pat Blair (Optima); *Cures that Work* by Janet Pleshette (Century Arrow); *The Dictionary of Medical Folklore* by Carol Ann Rinzler (Magnum); *The Encyclopedia of Herbs and Herbalism* edited by Malcolm Stuart (Orbis); *The Face and Body Book* edited by Miriam Stoppard (Windward); *The Family Guide to Homeopathy* by Dr Andrew Lockie (Elm Tree Books); *Family Medical Adviser* (Reader's Digest); *First Aid with Herbs* by Yvette van Wijk (Blackwoods Herbs); *Good Things Come in Small Packages: The Why's & How's of Turner Syndrome* by Diana Plumridge (Oregon Health Sciences University); *Grandmother's Secrets* by Jean Palaiseul (Penguin); *Gray's Anatomy* edited by Roger Warwick and Peter L Williams (Longman); *Guide to Alternative Medicine* by Dr Vernon Coleman (Corgi); *A Guide to Chiropractic* by Susan Moore (Hamlyn); *The Handbook of Complementary Medicine* by Stephen Fulder (Coronet); *The Health and Fitness Handbook* edited by Miriam Polunin (Windward); *The Herb User's Guide* by David L Hoffmann (Thorsons); *Here's Health* (Argus Health Publications; monthly); *Holistic First Aid* by Dr Michael Nightingale (Optima); *Holistic Living: A Guide to Self Care* by Patrick Pietroni (Dent); *Indigenous Healing Plants* by Margaret Roberts (Southern Book Publishers); *Iridology* by Farida Sharan (Thorsons); *Journal of Alternative and Complementary Medicine* (Green Library Ltd; monthly); *Living in Two Worlds* by M Vera Buhrmann (Human & Rousseau); *Living with Fear* by Isaac M Marks (McGraw-Hill); *McCance and Widdowson's The Composition of Foods* by A Paul and D A T Southgate (HMSO); *Medical Philosophy in Islam* by Syed Habibul Haq Nadvi (Academia); *The Metamorphic Technique* by Gaston Saint-Pierre and Debbie Shapiro (Element Books); *Mitchell Beazley Atlas of the Body and Mind* (Mitchell Beazley); *Natural Choice* (Orbis; partwork); *The Natural Family Doctor* edited by Dr Andrew Stanway (Century); *The Natural House Book* by David Pearson (Conran Octopus); *The Polarity Process* by Franklyn Sills (Element Books); *Potter's New Cyclopedia of Botanical Drugs and Preparations* by R C Wren (C W Daniel Co); *Reader's Digest Atlas of Southern Africa* (Reader's Digest Association, Cape Town); *Reflexology – A Way to Better Health* by Nicola M Hall (Pan); *South African Family Medical Adviser* (Reader's Digest Association, Cape Town); *Standard Encyclopedia of South Africa* (Nasionale Boekhandel); *Stay Younger Longer* by Bronwen Meredith (Michael Joseph); *Thorsons Complete Guide to Alternative Living* by David Harvey (Thorsons); *Traditional Healers* by Dr M V Gumede (Skotaville Publishers); *Treat Your Own Back* by Robin McKenzie (Spinal Publications, New Zealand); *Turner Syndrome: A Guide for Physicians* by Dr R G Rosenfeld; *A Visual Encyclopaedia of Unconventional Medicine* edited by Ann Hall (New English Library); *Vogue Beauty and Health Encyclopedia* by Christina Probert (Octopus); *Vogue Complete Diet and Exercise* by Deborah Hutton (Octopus); *What To Do In An Emergency* (Reader's Digest Association, Cape Town); *Which? Way to Health* (Consumers' Association; bi-monthly); *Yoga for Common Ailments* by R Nagarathna, H R Nagendra and Robin Monro (Gaia Books).